Introduction to Audiology

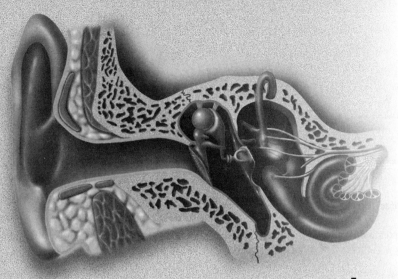

Introduction to Audiology

TWELFTH EDITION

Frederick N. Martin

The University of Texas at Austin

John Greer Clark

University of Cincinnati

Clark Audiology, LLC

PEARSON

Boston   Columbus   Indianapolis   New York   San Francisco   Upper Saddle River
Amsterdam   Cape Town   Dubai   London   Madrid   Milan   Munich   Paris   Montreal   Toronto
Delhi   Mexico City   São Paulo   Sydney   Hong Kong   Seoul   Singapore   Taipei   Tokyo

Vice President and Editor in Chief: Jeffery W. Johnston
Executive Editor: Ann Davis
Media Development: Christina Robb
Executive Field Marketing Manager: Krista Clark
Senior Product Marketing Manager: Christopher Barry
Project Manager: Annette Joseph
Full-Service Project Management: Jouve North America
Composition: Jouve India
Cover Designer: Suzanne Duda
Cover Image: Victor Habbick Visions/Science Photo Library/Corbis

Credits and acknowledgments borrowed from other sources and reproduced, with permission, in this textbook appear on the appropriate page within text.

ADDITIONAL CREDITS

Design: Chapter opener image (internal ear), BSIP/Universal Images Group/Getty Images; ear against digital background, Magictorch/Photographer's Choice RF/Getty Images; "Check Your Understanding" icon, Frender/iStock/360/Getty Images; "Activities" icon, Pagadesign/E+/Getty Images; sound wave, Hong Li/iStock Vectors/Getty Images.

Part Opener Images: Part 1 (page 2), John Greer Clark; Part II (page 68), Natus Medical Incorporated; Part III (page 216), John Greer Clark; Part IV (page 362), John Greer Clark.

All photos not credited on their respective page are courtesy of the authors.

10 9 8 7 6 5 4 3 2 1

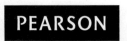

ISBN-10: 0-13-349146-3
ISBN-13: 978-0-13-349146-3

To Cathy, my wife and best friend for almost six decades, for her support, encouragement, and love. To my son David, an anesthesiologist, who, with his generosity of spirit, does great good both within and outside the practice of medicine. To my daughter, Leslie Anne, a professional in human resources whose talents include a large measure of humanity, and who is a wonderful and sweet friend. To my daughter-in-law, April, an attorney and managed-care professional who leads a large network of hospitals. To my dear friend and colleague of nearly 60 years, Dr. Mark Ross, for his many contributions to audiology. To my many students and teaching assistants, especially Dr. John Greer Clark, who made mine a marvelous career. Finally, to my magnificent rescue dogs, Fearless-Bluedog and Gaia, who fill my life with joy, and to the memories of Decibelle and Compass Rose, whose presence on this earth blessed every day.

FNM

To my wife and partner, Suzanne, and our children and petite-fille, who make everything worthwhile; to Kitty, my first and favorite editor, good friend and mother; and to my students, who continue to challenge and teach me.

JGC

Brief Contents

PART I   **Elements of Audiology**   **2**

1   **The Profession of Audiology**   *4*
2   **The Human Ear and Simple Tests of Hearing**   *16*
3   **Sound and Its Measurement**   *30*

PART II   **Hearing Assessment**   **68**

4   **Pure-Tone Audiometry**   *70*
5   **Speech Audiometry**   *98*
6   **Masking**   *126*
7   **Physiological Tests of the Auditory System**   *150*
8   **Pediatric Audiology**   *186*

PART III   **Hearing Disorders**   **216**

9   **The Outer Ear**   *218*
10   **The Middle Ear**   *238*
11   **The Inner Ear**   *273*
12   **The Auditory Nerve and Central Auditory Pathways**   *315*
13   **Nonorganic Hearing Loss**   *343*

PART IV   **Management of Hearing Loss**   **362**

14   **Amplification/Sensory Systems**   *364*
15   **Audiological Treatment**   *398*

About the Authors

Following a four-year enlistment in the U.S. Air Force, Frederick Martin returned to college to complete his bachelor's and master's degrees and embarked on a career as a clinical audiologist. After eight years of practice, he returned to graduate school and earned his Ph.D., then he joined the faculty at The University of Texas at Austin, where he taught and did research for 38 years. He is now the Lillie Hage Jamail Centennial Professor Emeritus in Communication Sciences and Disorders.

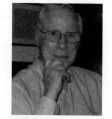

Frederick N. Martin

In addition to the twelve editions of *Introduction to Audiology*, six of which were co-authored by Dr. John Greer Clark, Martin has authored seven books, co-authored another seven, edited thirteen, and co-edited three. He has written 24 chapters for edited texts, 122 journal articles, 104 convention or conference papers, and 5 CD-ROMs. He served as a reviewer for the most prominent audiology journals and for years co-edited *Audiology: A Journal for Continuing Education*.

During his tenure at The University of Texas, Martin won the Teaching Excellence Award of the College of Communication, the Graduate Teaching Award, and the Advisor's Award from the Texas Alumni Association. The National Student Speech-Language-Hearing Association named him Professor of the Year in Communication Sciences and Disorders at The University of Texas for 2002–2003. He was the 1997 recipient of the Career Award in Hearing from the American Academy of Audiology, and in 2006, he was the first to receive the Lifetime Achievement Award from the Texas Academy of Audiology. In 2009, Martin was honored by the Arkansas Hearing Society with the Thomas A. LeBlanc Award. His book, *Introduction to Audiology*, was a finalist for the prestigious Hamilton Book Award of The University of Texas in 2006. He is a Fellow of the American Academy of Audiology and the American Speech-Language-Hearing Association and is an Honorary Lifetime Member of the American Speech-Language-Hearing Association and the Texas Speech-Language Hearing Association, and was the first and remains the only recipient of Honorary Lifetime Membership in the Austin Audiology Society.

The College of Communication of The University of Texas at Austin established the Frederick N. Martin Endowed Scholarship in 2011. Funds from this scholarship are awarded annually to an outstanding graduate student at The University who plans to pursue a career in audiology. The scholarship is designed to continue in perpetuity.

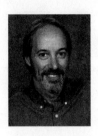

John Greer Clark

Dr. Clark received his bachelor of science from Purdue University and his master's degree from The University of Texas at Austin. Following post-graduate studies at Louisiana State University, he completed his doctoral degree at the University of Cincinnati.

A recipient of both the Prominent Alumni and Distinguished Alumnus Awards from the University of Cincinnati and the Honors of the Ohio Speech and Hearing Association, Dr. Clark was elected a Fellow of the American Speech-Language-Hearing Association in 1996. He is a Past President of the Academy of Rehabilitative Audiology, Past Chair of the American Board of Audiology, and a Fellow of the American Academy of Audiology. He served four years on the Board of Directors of the American Academy of Audiology and the Ohio Academy of Audiology, and, with his wife, was co-founder of the Midwest Audiology Conference, which subsequently evolved into separate conferences for the states of Indiana, Ohio, and Kentucky.

A presenter at local, national, and international association meetings and conventions, Dr. Clark has served as faculty for the Ida Institute, and as associate editor, editorial consultant, and reviewer for a number of professional journals. His more than 100 publications include three edited textbooks, a variety of co-authored texts, two single-authored books, 15 book chapters, and a range of journal articles on various aspects of communication disorders. His current research interests are within the areas of adult audiologic rehabilitation, audiologic counseling, and animal audiology.

Dr. Clark's professional career started with the Louisiana Department of Health and Human Resources, where he served as audiologist for the Handicapped Children's Program and coordinator for the Geriatric Pilot Project in Communicative Disorders. He was an Assistant Clinical Professor within the Department of Otolaryngology and Maxillofacial Surgery at the University of Cincinnati Medical Center before embarking on a successful private practice, which he left after 15 years to serve as the Director of Clinical Services of Helix Hearing Care of America. Currently, he is an Associate Professor in Communication Sciences and Disorders at the University of Cincinnati; a Faculty Fellow of the Ida Institute in Naerum, Denmark; a visiting professor at the University of Louisville; and president of Clark Audiology, LLC.

Preface

The founders of audiology could not have envisioned the many ways in which this profession would evolve to meet the needs of children and adults with hearing and balance disorders. Breakthroughs continue to come in all areas of audiological diagnosis and treatment, resulting in a profession that is more exciting and rewarding today than ever before.

Treatment is the goal of audiology, and treatment is impossible without diagnosis. Some people have developed the erroneous opinion that audiology is all about doing hearing tests. Surely, testing the hearing function is essential; however, it might appear that many tests could be performed by technical personnel who lack the education required to be total hearing healthcare managers. Historically, the profession has rejected this approach and has developed a model wherein one highly trained, self-supervised audiologist carries the patient and family from taking a personal history through diagnosis and into management. Toward this end, the development of a humanistic, relationship-centered, patient–professional approach to hearing care has evolved, one in which the audiologist guides patients and families to the highest success levels possible.

The profession has moved away from requiring a master's degree to requiring the Doctor of Audiology (AuD) as the entry-level degree for those wishing to enter the profession of audiology. This is due in part to recognition of the fact that additional education and training are necessary for those practicing audiology so that they can meet the demands of an expanding scope of practice and continuing technological growth.

New to This Edition

With each new edition of this book, we strive not only to update the material to keep content current with recent research, but also to make it more user-friendly for students. Although a great deal of advanced material has been added, the primary target of this book continues to be the new student in audiology. While providing an abundance of how-to information, every effort is made to reveal to the novice that audiology can be a rewarding and fascinating career. In this edition, a number of features have been added or enhanced, including:

- Expansion of the Evolving Case Studies to include more cases.
- A new list of frequently asked questions (FAQs) in each chapter. These lists are derived from students' actual queries in class and during instructor office hours.
- Updated references to reflect the most recent research.

In addition, for the first time, *Introduction to Audiology* is available in a whole new format as an eText. The advantages provided in this electronic version are numerous.

The eText Advantage

Publication of *Introduction to Audiology* in an eText format allows for several advantages over a traditional print format. In addition to greater affordability, this format provides a search function that allows the reader to locate coverage of concepts efficiently. **Bold** key terms are clickable and take the reader directly to the glossary definition. Index entries are also hyperlinked and take the reader directly to the relevant page of the text. Navigation to particular sections of the book is also possible by clicking on desired sections within the expanded table of contents. Sections of text may be highlighted and reader notes can be typed onto the page for enhanced review at a later date.

All websites provided are now active eText links to aid interested readers in additional research on a topic. It should be noted that neither the authors nor Pearson Education endorse or approve, nor are they responsible for, the content of any third-party website linked to this text. The authors and Pearson Education make no representations as to the content or accuracy of any linked websites.

To further enhance assimilation of new information, links to 20 video clips are interspersed throughout the text and are available through the eText. These video clips demonstrate different aspects of audiological practice. They include illustration of otoscopic technique and basic hearing test procedures, as well as more advanced electroacoustic and electrophysiologic tests, earmold impression technique, hearing aid assessment measures, and more.

At the end of each chapter, readers can access interactive eText multiple-choice Check Your Understanding questions to assess comprehension of text concepts as well as a variety of Activities designed to facilitate learning. Immediate feedback is provided on the appropriateness of responses. We believe use of this material can increase confidence in preparation for examinations and other challenges. In their diagnostic form, these questions and activities can help identify points of knowledge and areas of weakness or knowledge gaps to direct students in their review of materials.

It is our hope that this new eText format will enrich the student's learning experience and further enhance the learning process. To learn more about the enhanced Pearson eText, go to www.pearsonhighered.com/etextbooks.

How to Use This Book

Throughout this book's history of nearly four decades, its editions have been used by individuals in classes ranging from introductory to advanced levels. Students who plan to enter the professions of audiology, speech-language pathology, and education of children with hearing impairment have used it. All of these individuals are charged with knowing all they can learn about hearing disorders and their ramifications. To know less is to do a disservice to those children and adults who rely on professionals for assistance.

The chapter arrangement in this book differs somewhat from most audiology texts in several ways. The usual approach is to present the anatomy and physiology of the ear first, and then to introduce auditory tests and remediation techniques. After an introduction to the profession of audiology, this book first presents a superficial look at how the ear works. With this conceptual beginning, details of auditory tests can be understood as they relate to the basic mechanisms of hearing. Thus, with a grasp of the test principles, the reader is better prepared to benefit from the many examples of theoretical test results that illustrate different disorders in the auditory system. Presentations of anatomy and physiology, designed for greater detail and application, follow the descriptions of auditory disorders.

The organization of this book has proved useful because it facilitates early comprehension of what is often perceived as difficult material. Readers who wish a more traditional approach may simply rearrange the sequence in which they read the chapters. Chapters 9 through 12, on the anatomy, physiology, disorders, and treatments of different parts of the auditory apparatus, can simply be read before Chapters 4 through 8 on auditory tests. At the completion of the book, the same information will have been covered.

The teacher of an introductory audiology course may feel that the depth of coverage of some subjects in this book is greater than desired. If this is the case, the primary and secondary headings allow for easy identification of sections that may be deleted. If greater detail is desired, the suggested reading lists at the end of each chapter can provide more depth. The book may be read in modules so that only specified materials are covered.

Each chapter in this book begins with an introduction to the subject matter and a statement of instructional objectives. Liberal use is made of headings, subheadings, illustrations, and figures. A summary at the end of each chapter repeats the important portions. Terms that may be new or unusual appear in **bold** print and are defined in the book's comprehensive glossary. Review tables summarize the high points within many chapters. Readers wishing to test their understanding of different materials may find the questions at the end of each chapter useful. For those who wish to test their ability to synthesize what they learn and solve some practical clinical problems, the Evolving Case Studies in selected chapters provide this opportunity. The indexes at the back of this book are intended to help readers to find desired materials rapidly.

Acknowledgments

The authors would like to express their appreciation to Christina Robb for guiding us through the process of updating and converting *Introduction to Audiology* from print to digital format. The authors would also like to express their appreciation to the reviewers of this edition: Frank Brister, Stephen F. Austin State University; Nancy Datino, Mercy College; John Ribera, Utah State University; and Renee Shellum, Minnesota State University–Mankato. We also want to thank John Shannon at Jouve North America, who oversaw the many details involved getting from manuscript to finished product. Finally, we want to thank Steve Dragin who served as executive editor for well over a dozen of our books. We will miss his guidance and wish him great success in all future endeavors.

Contents

PART I Elements of Audiology 2

1 The Profession of Audiology 4

The Evolution of Audiology 5
Licensing and Certification 6
Prevalence and Impact of Hearing Loss 7
A Blending of Art and Science 8
Audiology Specialties 9
Employment Settings 13
Professional Societies 14
Summary 14
Websites 15
Frequently Asked Questions 15
Suggested Reading 15
Endnote 15

2 The Human Ear and Simple Tests of Hearing 16

Anatomy and Physiology of the Ear 17
Pathways of Sound 17
Types of Hearing Loss 18
Hearing Tests 20
Tuning Fork Tests 20
Summary 27
Frequently Asked Questions 28
Endnotes 29

3 Sound and Its Measurement 30

Sound 31
Waves 31
Vibrations 34
Frequency 35
Resonance 36

Sound Velocity   36
Wavelength   37
Phase   38
Complex Sounds   39
Intensity   41
The Decibel   44
Environmental Sounds   49
Psychoacoustics   49
Impedance   53
Sound Measurement   54
Summary   65
Frequently Asked Questions   66
Suggested Reading   67
Endnotes   67

PART II   Hearing Assessment   68

4   Pure-Tone Audiometry   70

The Pure-Tone Audiometer   71
Test Environment   72
The Patient's Role in Manual Pure-Tone Audiometry   74
The Clinician's Role in Manual Pure-Tone Audiometry   76
Air-Conduction Audiometry   77
Bone-Conduction Audiometry   85
The Audiometric Weber Test   88
Audiogram Interpretation   88
Automatic Audiometry   93
Computerized Audiometry   93
Summary   95
Frequently Asked Questions   96
Suggested Reading   97
Endnotes   97

5   Speech Audiometry   98

The Diagnostic Audiometer   99
Test Environment   99
The Patient's Role in Speech Audiometry   99
The Clinician's Role in Speech Audiometry   100
Speech-Threshold Testing   100
Bone-Conduction SRT   104

Most Comfortable Loudness Level   *106*

Uncomfortable Loudness Level   *106*

Range of Comfortable Loudness   *107*

Speech-Recognition Testing   *107*

Computerized Speech Audiometry   *118*

Summary   *120*

Frequently Asked Questions   *124*

Suggested Reading   *125*

Endnote   *125*

6   Masking   *126*

Cross Hearing in Air- and Bone-Conduction Audiometry   *127*

Masking   *128*

Masking for the Speech-Recognition Threshold   *142*

*Cross Hearing and Masking in Speech-Recognition
Score Testing*   *145*

Summary   *148*

Frequently Asked Questions   *149*

Suggested Reading   *149*

Endnote   *149*

7   Physiological Tests of the Auditory System   *150*

*Combined Speech and Pure-Tone Audiometry with
Immittance Measures*   *151*

Acoustic Immittance   *151*

Acoustic Reflexes   *159*

Otoacoustic Emissions (OAEs)   *165*

Laser-Doppler Vibrometer Measurement   *168*

Auditory-Evoked Potentials   *169*

A Historical Note   *180*

Summary   *183*

Frequently Asked Questions   *184*

Suggested Reading   *185*

8   Pediatric Audiology   *186*

Auditory Responses   *187*

Identifying Hearing Loss in Infants under 3 Months of Age   *188*

Objective Testing in Routine Pediatric Hearing Evaluation   *193*

*Behavioral Testing of Children from Birth to Approximately
2 Years of Age*   *196*

Behavioral Testing of Children Approximately 2 to 5 Years of Age   199

Language Disorders   205

Auditory Processing Disorders   206

Auditory Neuropathy in Children   207

Psychological Disorders   207

Developmental Disabilities   207

Identifying Hearing Loss in the Schools   207

Nonorganic Hearing Loss in Children   211

Summary   213

Frequently Asked Questions   214

Suggested Reading   215

Endnotes   215

PART III   Hearing Disorders   216

9   The Outer Ear   218

Anatomy and Physiology of the Outer Ear   219

Development of the Outer Ear   223

Hearing Loss and the Outer Ear   224

Disorders of the Outer Ear and Their Treatments   224

Summary   234

Frequently Asked Questions   235

Suggested Reading   237

Endnotes   237

10   The Middle Ear   238

Anatomy and Physiology of the Middle Ear   239

Development of the Middle Ear   244

Hearing Loss and the Middle Ear   245

Disorders of the Middle Ear and Their Treatments   245

Other Causes of Middle-Ear Hearing Loss   269

Summary   270

Frequently Asked Questions   271

Suggested Reading   272

Endnotes   272

11   **The Inner Ear**   *273*

Anatomy and Physiology of the Inner Ear   *274*
Development of the Inner Ear   *285*
Hearing Loss and Disorders of the Inner Ear   *286*
Causes of Inner-Ear Disorders   *286*
Summary   *311*
Frequently Asked Questions   *312*
Suggested Reading   *314*
Endnotes   *314*

12   **The Auditory Nerve and Central Auditory Pathways**   *315*

From Cochlea to Auditory Cortex and Back Again   *316*
Hearing Loss and the Auditory Nerve and Central Auditory Pathways   *319*
Disorders of the Auditory Nerve   *319*
Disorders of the Cochlear Nuclei   *327*
Disorders of the Higher Auditory Pathways   *329*
Tests for Auditory Processing Disorders   *331*
Summary   *340*
Frequently Asked Questions   *341*
Suggested Reading   *342*
Endnotes   *342*

13   **Nonorganic Hearing Loss**   *343*

Terminology   *344*
Patients with Nonorganic Hearing Loss   *346*
Indications of Nonorganic Hearing Loss   *347*
Performance on Routine Hearing Tests   *348*
Tests for Nonorganic Hearing Loss   *350*
Tinnitus   *356*
Management of Patients with Nonorganic Hearing Loss   *357*
Summary   *359*
Frequently Asked Questions   *360*
Suggested Reading   *361*

PART IV **Management of Hearing Loss** **362**

14 **Amplification/Sensory Systems** *364*

Hearing Aid Development *365*
Hearing Aid Circuit Overview *366*
Electroacoustic Characteristics of Hearing Aids *367*
Bilateral/Binaural Amplification *371*
Types of Hearing Aids *371*
Selecting Hearing Aids for Adults *382*
Selecting Hearing Aids for Children *386*
Hearing Aid Acceptance and Orientation *387*
Dispensing Hearing Aids *388*
Hearing Assistance Technologies *389*
Summary *396*
Frequently Asked Questions *396*
Suggested Reading *397*

15 **Audiological Treatment** *398*

Patient Histories *399*
Referral to Other Specialists *402*
Audiological Counseling *406*
Management of Adult Hearing Impairment *413*
Management of Childhood Hearing Impairment *418*
The Deaf Community *423*
Management of Auditory Processing Disorders *424*
Management of Tinnitus *426*
Hyperacusis *428*
Vestibular Rehabilitation *429*
Multicultural Considerations *431*
Evidenced-Based Practice *432*
Outcome Measures *433*
Summary *436*
Frequently Asked Questions *437*
Suggested Reading *438*
Endnote *438*

Glossary **439**

References **453**

Author Index **473**

Subject Index **477**

Introduction to Audiology

ELEMENTS OF AUDIOLOGY

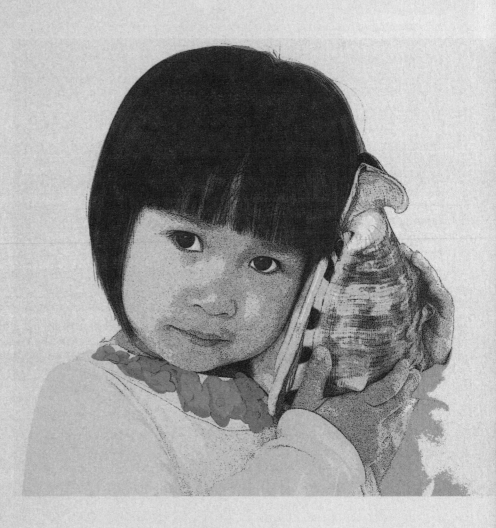

The first part of this book requires no foreknowledge of audiology. Chapter 1 presents an overview of the profession of audiology, its history, and directions for the future. Chapter 2 is an elementary look at the anatomy of the auditory system to the extent that basic types of hearing loss and simple hearing tests can be understood. Oversimplifications are clarified in later chapters. Tuning-fork tests are described here for three purposes: first, because they are practiced today by many physicians; second, because they are an important part of the history of the art and science of audiology; and third, because they illustrate some fundamental concepts that are essential to understanding contemporary hearing tests. Chapter 3 discusses the physics of sound and introduces the units of measurement that are important in performing modern audiologic assessments. Readers who have had a course in hearing science may find little new information in Chapter 3 and may wish to use it merely as a review. For those readers for whom this material is new, its comprehension is essential for understanding what follows in this text.

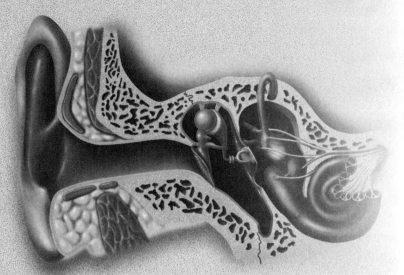

CHAPTER 1

The Profession of Audiology

LEARNING OBJECTIVES

The purpose of this opening chapter is to introduce the profession of audiology, from its origins through its course of development to its present position in the hearing-healthcare delivery system. At the completion of this chapter, the reader should be able to

- Describe the evolution of audiology as a profession.
- Discuss the impact of hearing impairment on individuals and society.
- List specialty areas within audiology and the employment settings within which audiologists may find themselves.
- Describe the reasons that speech-language pathologists may interact closely with audiologists as they provide services within their chosen professions.

THE PROFESSION OF AUDIOLOGY has grown remarkably since its inception only a little more than 70 years ago. What began as a concentrated effort to assist hearing-injured veterans of World War II in their attempts to reenter civilian life has evolved into a profession serving all population groups and all ages through increasingly sophisticated diagnostic and rehabilitative instrumentation. The current student of audiology can look forward to a future within a dynamic profession, meeting the hearing needs of an expanding patient base.

The Evolution of Audiology

Prior to World War II, hearing-care services were provided by physicians and commercial hearing aid dealers. Because the use of hearing protection was not common until the latter part of the war, many service personnel suffered the effects of high-level noise exposure from modern weaponry. The influx of these service personnel reentering civilian life created the impetus for the professions of **otology** (the medical specialty concerned with diseases of the ear) and speech pathology (now referred to as **speech-language pathology**) to work together to form military-based **aural rehabilitation** centers.

These centers met with such success that, following the war, many of the professionals involved in the programs' development believed that their services should be made available within the civilian sector. It was primarily through the efforts of the otologists that the first rehabilitative programs for those with hearing loss were established in communities around the country, but it was mainly those from speech-language pathology, those who had developed the audiometric techniques and rehabilitative procedures of the military clinics, who staffed the emerging community centers (Henoch, 1979).

[handwritten margin note: OTOLOGY & speech lang & path worked together to make aural rehab centers]

Audiology developed rapidly as a profession distinct from medicine in the United States. While audiology continues to evolve outside the United States, most professionals practicing audiology in other countries are physicians, usually otologists. Audiometric technicians in many of these countries attain competency in the administration of hearing tests; however, it is the physician who dictates the tests to be performed and solely the physician who decides on the management of each patient. Some countries have developed strong academic audiology programs and independent audiologists, like those in the United States, but, with the exception of geographically isolated areas, most audiologists around the globe look to American audiologists for the model of autonomous practice that they wish to emulate.

The derivation of the word *audiology* is itself unclear. No doubt purists are disturbed that a Latin root, *audire* (to hear), was fused with a Greek suffix, *logos* (the study of), to form the word *audiology*. It is often reported that *audiology* was coined as a new word in 1945 simultaneously, yet independently, by Captain Raymond Carhart[1] and Dr. Norton Canfield, both active in the establishment of military aural rehabilitation programs. However, a course established in 1939 by the Auricular Foundation Institute of Audiology entitled "Audiological Problems in Education" and a 1935 instructional film developed under the direction of Mayer Shier titled simply *Audiology* clearly predate these claims (Skafte, 1990). Regardless of the origin of the word, an audiologist today is defined as an individual who, "by virtue of academic degree, clinical training, and license to practice and/or professional credential, is uniquely qualified to provide a comprehensive array of professional services related to the audiologic identification, assessment, diagnosis, and treatment of persons with impairment of auditory and vestibular function, and to the prevention of impairments associated with them" (American Academy of Audiology, 2004).

[handwritten margin note: audiology has expanded b/c technology is advancing]

Academic Preparation in Audiology

In the United States, educational preparation for audiologists evolved as technology expanded, leading to an increasing variety of diagnostic procedures and an expanded professional scope of practice (American Academy of Audiology, 2004; American Speech-Language-Hearing Association, 2004b). Audiology practices have grown to encompass the identification of hearing loss, the differential diagnosis of hearing impairment, and the nonmedical treatment of hearing impairment and balance disorders. What began as a profession with a bachelor's level preparation quickly transformed into a profession with a required minimum of a master's degree to attain a state license, now held forth as the mandatory prerequisite for clinical practice in most states. More than a quarter of a century ago, Raymond Carhart, one of audiology's founders, recognized the limitations imposed by defining the profession at the master's degree level (Carhart, 1975). Yet it was another 13 years before a conference, sponsored by the Academy of Dispensing Audiologists, set goals for the profession's transformation to a doctoral level (Academy of Dispensing Audiologists, 1988).

In recent years academic programs have transitioned to the professional doctorate for student preparation in audiology, designated as the doctor of audiology (Au.D.). At most universities, the Au.D. comprises four years of professional preparation beyond the bachelor's degree, with heavy emphasis on didactic instruction in the early years gradually giving way to increasing amounts of clinical practice as students progress through their programs. The final (fourth) year consists of a full-time clinical placement usually in a paid position.

Although the required course of study to become an audiologist remains somewhat heterogeneous, course work generally includes hearing and speech science, anatomy and physiology, fundamentals of communication and its disorders, counseling techniques, electronics, computer science, and a range of course work in diagnostic and rehabilitative services for those with hearing and balance disorders. Through this extensive background, university programs continue to produce clinicians capable of making independent decisions for the betterment of those they serve.

 ## Licensing and Certification

The practice of audiology is regulated in the United States through license or registration in every state of the union and the District of Columbia. Such regulation ensures that audiology practitioners have met a minimum level of educational preparation and, in many states, that a minimum of continuing study is maintained to help ensure competencies remain current. A license to practice audiology or professional registration as an audiologist is a legal requirement to practice the profession of audiology. Licensure and registration are important forms of consumer protection, and loss or revocation of this documentation prohibits an individual from practicing audiology. To obtain an audiology license, one must complete a prescribed course of study, acquire approximately 2,000 hours of clinical practicum, and attain a passing score on a national examination in audiology.

In contrast to state licensure and registration, certification is not a legal requirement for the practice of audiology. Audiologists who choose to hold membership in the American Speech-Language-Hearing Association (ASHA) are required by ASHA to hold the Certificate of Clinical Competence in Audiology, attesting that a designated level of preparation as an audiologist has been met and that documented levels of continuing education are maintained throughout one's career. Many audiologists select certification from the American Board of Audiology as a fully voluntary commitment to the principles of lifelong continuing education. ABA certification is an attestation that one holds him- or herself to a higher standard than may be set forth by professional associations or in the legal documents of licensure or registration.

The use of support personnel within a variety of practice settings is growing. The responsibilities of these "audiologist assistants" have been delineated by the American Academy of Audiology (1997). Licensing laws in nearly half of the states define permitted patient care assignments for audiology assistants. Assistants can be quite valuable in increasing practice efficiency and meeting the needs of a growing population with hearing loss. It is audiologists' responsibility to ensure that their assistants have the proper preparation and training to perform assigned duties adequately.

Prevalence and Impact of Hearing Loss

Although the profession of audiology was formed under the aegis of the military, its growth was rapid within the civilian sector because of the general prevalence of hearing loss and the devastating impact that hearing loss has on the lives of those affected. The reported prevalence of hearing loss varies somewhat depending on the method of estimation (actual evaluation of a population segment or individual response to a survey questionnaire), the criteria used to define hearing loss, and the age of the population sampled. However, following the world health organization's definition for hearing loss, prevalence in the United States may be as high as 30 million Americans with hearing loss in both ears or as many as 48 million with hearing loss in at least one ear (see Table 1.1).

The **prevalence** of hearing loss increases with age, and it has been estimated that the number of persons with hearing loss in the United States over the age of 65 years will reach nearly 13 million by 2015. The number of children with permanent hearing loss is far lower than the number of adults. However, the prevalence of hearing loss in children is almost staggering if we consider those children whose speech and language development and academic performances may be affected by mild transient ear infections so common among children. While not all children have problems secondary to ear pathologies, 75 percent of children in the United States will have at least one ear infection before 3 years of age (National Institute on Deafness and Other Communication Disorders, 2010a).

For children with recurrent or persistent problems with ear infections, the developmental impact may be significant. Studies have shown that children prone to ear pathologies may lag behind their peers in articulatory and phonological development, the ability to receive and express thoughts through spoken language, the use of grammar and syntax, the acquisition of vocabulary, the development of auditory memory and auditory perception skills, and social maturation (Clark & Jaindl, 1996). There is indication, however, that children with early history of ear infections, while initially delayed in speech and language, may catch up with their peers by the second year of elementary school (Roberts, Burchinal, & Zeisel, 2002; Zumach, Gerrits, Chenault, & Anteunis, 2010). Even so, a study reporting no significant differences in speech understanding in noise between groups of third- and fourth-grade students with and without histories of early ear infections did, however, find a much greater range in abilities for those with a positive history of ear infections (Keogh et al., 2005). This study demonstrated that some of these children experience considerable difficulty in speech understanding.

TABLE 1.1 Prevalence of Hearing Loss and Related Disorders

50 million people have tinnitus (ear or head noises).
30 million are exposed to hazardous noise levels or ototoxic chemicals at work.
48 million people are hard of hearing in one or both ears.
10 million people have some degree of permanent, noise-induced hearing loss.
2 million people are classified as deaf.
6 of every 1,000 children may be born with hearing impairment.
1 in 6 baby boomers (ages 41 to 59) have a hearing problem.
1 in 14 Generation Xers (ages 29 to 40), or 7.4%, already have hearing loss.
15% of school-age children may fail a school hearing screening mostly due to a transient ear infection.
90% of children in the United States will have had at least one ear infection before the age of 6 years.

Sources: Johns Hopkins Medical Center (www.ata.org); Tinnitus Association (www.ata.org); Centers for Disease Control and Prevention (www.cdc.gov); National Institute for Occupational Safety and Health (www.cdc.gov/niosh/topics/noise); Better Hearing Institute (www.betterhearing.org).

The fact that many children with positive histories of ear infection develop no speech, language, or educational delays suggests that factors additional to fluctuating hearing abilities may also be involved in the learning process (Davis, 1986; Williams & Jacobs, 2009), but this in no way reduces the need for intervention. The impact of more severe and permanent hearing loss has an even greater effect on a child's developing speech and language and educational performance (Diefendorf, 1996) and also on the psychosocial dynamics within the family and among peer groups (Altman, 1996; Clark & English, 2014).

Often, the adult patient's reaction to the diagnosis of permanent hearing loss is to feel nearly as devastated as that of the caregivers of young children with newly diagnosed hearing impairment (Martin, Krall, & O'Neal, 1989). Yet the effects of hearing loss cannot be addressed until the reason for the hearing loss is diagnosed. Left untreated, hearing loss among adults can seriously erode relationships both within and outside the family unit. Research has demonstrated that, among older adults, hearing loss is related to overall poor health, decreased physical activity, and depression. Indeed, Bess, Lichtenstein, Logan, Burger, and Nelson (1989) demonstrated that progressive hearing loss among older adults is associated with progressive physical and psychosocial dysfunction.

In addition to the personal effects of hearing loss on the individual, the financial burden of hearing loss placed upon the individual, and society at large, is remarkable. The National Institute on Deafness and other Communication Disorders (2010b) reports that the total annual costs for the treatment of childhood ear infections may be as high as $5 billion in the United States. When one adds to this figure the costs of educational programs and (re)habilitation services for those with permanent hearing loss and the lost income when hearing impairment truncates one's earning potential, the costs become staggering. Northern and Downs (1991) estimate that for a child of 1 year of age with severe hearing impairment and an average life expectancy of 71 years, the economic burden of deafness can exceed $1 million.

A survey conducted by the Better Hearing Institute of over 44,000 American families reported that those who are failing to treat their hearing problems are collectively losing at least $100 billion in annual income (National American Precis Syndicated, 2007). While many people think of hearing loss as affecting mainly older individuals, most people with hearing loss are in the prime of their lives, including one out of six baby boomers ages 41 to 59 years. While the Better Hearing Institute study reported that the use of hearing aids can reduce the effects of lost income by nearly 50 percent, only one in four with hearing problems seeks treatment.

A Blending of Art and Science

Audiology is a scientific discipline based upon an ever-growing body of research on the fundamentals of hearing, the physiologic and psychosocial impacts of lost hearing, and the technological aspects of both hearing diagnostics and pediatric and adult hearing-loss treatments. Over the years, some have cautioned that audiology should avoid becoming mired in the technological aspects of service delivery. Indeed, as Hawkins (1990) points out, the importance of the many technological advances seen in audiology may be of only minor importance to the final success with patients when compared to the counseling and rehabilitative aspects of audiological care.

The blending of the science of audiology with the art of patient treatment makes audiology a highly rewarding profession. The humanistic side of professional endeavors in audiology is what brings audiologists close to the patients and families they serve and makes the outcomes of provided services rewarding for both the practitioner and the recipient of care. All patients bring to audiology clinics their own life stories, personal achievements, and recognized (and unrecognized) limitations. Audiologists must learn to listen supportively, thus allowing patients to tell their own stories, so that both diagnostics and rehabilitation may be tailored to individual needs effectively (Clark & English, 2014).

Clinical COMMENTARY

Speech-language pathologists often find that they work in close concert with audiologists. This may be true with children, whose hearing loss can have a direct impact on speech and language development, as well as with older adults, who have a higher incidence of age-related communication disorders. The frequent coexistence of hearing disorders and speech and language problems has led the American Speech-Language-Hearing Association to include hearing-screening procedures, therapeutic aspects of audiological rehabilitation, and basic checks of hearing aid performance within the speech-language pathologist's scope of practice (ASHA, 2001, 2004a).

Audiology Specialties

Most audiology training programs prepare audiologists as generalists, with exposure and preparation in a wide variety of areas. Following graduation, however, many audiologists discover their chosen practice setting leads to a concentration of their time and efforts within one or more specialty areas of audiology. In addition, many practice settings and specialty areas provide audiologists with opportunities to participate in research activities to broaden clinical understanding and application of diagnostic and treatment procedures. When those seeking audiological care are young or have concomitant speech or language difficulties, a close working relationship of audiologists with professionals in speech-language pathology or in the education of those with hearing loss often develops.

The varied nature of the practice of audiology can make an audiology career stimulating and rewarding. Indeed, the fact that audiologists view their careers as both interesting and challenging has been found to result in a high level of job satisfaction within the profession (Martin, Champlin, & Streetman, 1997). In 2013, audiology was ranked as the fourth most desirable profession in the United Sates out of 200 rated occupations, based on five criteria including hiring outlook, income potential, work environment, stress levels, and physical demand (CareerCast, 2013). The appeal of audiology as a career choice is hightened by the variety of specialty areas and employment settings available to audiologists.

Medical Audiology

The largest number of audiologists are currently employed within a medical environment, including community and regional hospitals, physicians' offices, and health maintenance organizations. Audiologists within military-based programs, Department of Veterans Affairs medical centers, and departments of public health often work primarily within the specialty of medical audiology. Many of the audiology services provided within this specialty focus on the provision of diagnostic assessments to help establish the underlying cause of hearing or balance disorders (see Figure 1.1). The full range of diagnostic procedures detailed in this

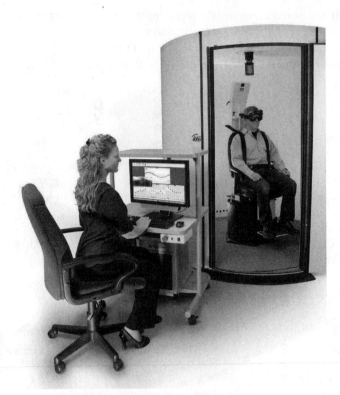

FIGURE 1.1 A computerized rotational chair allows the audiologist to attain a comprehensive evaluation of patients suffering with balance disorders. (*Source:* Micromedical Technologies, 10 Kemp Drive, Chatham, IL 62629.)

text may be employed by the medical audiologist with patients of all ages. Results of the final audiological assessment are combined with the diagnostic findings of other medical and non-medical professionals to yield a final diagnosis. Medical audiologists may also work within newborn-hearing-loss-identification programs and monitor the hearing levels of patients being treated with medications that can harm hearing. Additional responsibilities frequently include nonmedical endeavors such as hearing aid dispensing.

Educational Audiology

Following the federal mandates dictated by Public Law 94-142, the Education for All Handicapped Children Act, in 1975 and Public Law 99-457, the Education for the Handicapped Amendments, in 1986, the need for audiologists within the schools has increased. Yet fewer than half the audiologists required to meet the needs of children in the public schools are serving in that capacity. Educational audiologists bear a wide range of responsibilities in minimizing the devastating impact that hearing loss has on the education of young children, and in the educational setting they may work closely with professionals in the education of deaf and hearing-impaired children and speech-language pathology. Audiologists in this specialty are responsible for the identification of children with hearing loss and referral to medical and other professional services as needed; the provision of rehabilitative activities, including auditory training, speechreading, and speech conservation; the creation of hearing-loss-prevention programs; counseling and guidance about hearing loss for parents, pupils, and teachers; and the selection and evaluation of individual and group amplification (Johnson & Seaton, 2011).

Pediatric Audiology

Work with children and their families has perhaps more far-reaching effects than any other challenge audiologists undertake. In addition to developing a honed proficiency in the special considerations involved with the diagnostic evaluation of young children, pediatric audiologists must be prepared to bring to their clinical endeavors an empathy that will help guide parents and families through what is an exceptionally difficult time in their lives. One of the pediatric audiologist's primary roles is facilitating parents' efforts to meet the many (re)habilitative challenges the child and family will face.

Nonaudiology professionals who work in the areas of communication and education for children with hearing loss frequently work closely with pediatric audiologists. Audiologists within a variety of employment settings may work with children and their families. However, those within pediatric hospitals, large rehabilitation centers, and community-based hearing and speech centers often see a higher percentage of the pediatric population.

Dispensing/Rehabilitative Audiology

Nearly 40 years ago, ASHA rescinded its previous ban on the dispensing of hearing aids by audiologists. Since that time, audiologists have become increasingly active in the total hearing rehabilitation of their patients. (See Chapter 14.) While many audiologists establish their dispensing/rehabilitative practices within hospitals or physicians' offices, a growing number are attracted to the greater autonomy afforded by an independent practice within their communities. Regardless of employment setting, hearing aid dispensing is part of the audiologist's responsibilities.

Industrial Audiology

As discussed in Chapter 11, exposure to high levels of noise is one of the primary contributors to insidious hearing loss. Many of today's industries produce noise levels of sufficient intensity to damage employees' hearing permanently. According to the National Institute for Occupational Safety and Health (2001), more than 30 million U.S. workers are exposed to hazardous noise levels, resulting in noise-induced occupational hearing loss being one of the the most common occupational diseases and the second most commonnly reported occupational injury. Allowable levels and duration of employee noise exposure have been set by the U.S. Department of Health. To ensure that adequate hearing protection is provided by the employer *and* used effectively by the employee, audiologists who work in industry design hearing-conservation programs to identify and measure excessive noise areas, consult in the reduction of noise levels produced by industrial equipment, monitor employee hearing levels, educate employees on the permanent consequences of excessive noise exposure, and fit hearing protection for those employees with excessive exposure. While some audiologists practice full-time exclusively within industrial settings, most who work with industry provide these services as part-time contracted consultants, or as an adjunct to their work within other practice settings. As consultants to industry, audiologists may work in conjunction with attorneys, industrial physicians and nurses, industrial hygienists, safety engineers, and industrial relations and personnel officers within management and unions.

Tele-Audiology

The practice of tele-medicine is finding ways to reach out to remote areas of the world to serve patients whose inaccessible locations preclude inclusion for medical diagnosis and treatment in traditional ways. This branch of audiology has proven to be especially valuable for those living in remote and developing areas of the world. Further discussion of **tele-audiology** can be found in Chapter 15. The World Health Organization (WHO) reports that hearing loss is now the number one disability, so it was inevitable that tele-audiology would become more important. As a matter of fact, the vast majority of individuals, perhaps as many as 90 percent of those in need (Nemes, 2010), live away from centers that deliver traditional audiological diagnosis and treatment and can benefit from this novel approach.

Using tele-audiology, an entire battery of hearing-care services can be delivered to persons in need who do not have the means or opportunity to travel sometimes great distances to receive services traditionally located in urban areas. These regions literally encompass the entire world, but they can also include low-income areas in the United States. This is what has led to the development and implementation of the tele-audiology network.

Special models need to be developed with application to different geographic, cultural, and financial situations. There is little doubt that the desire of the profession of audiology to reach all those in need of hearing healthcare will lead to many changes and improvements in this unique specialty.

Recreational and Animal Audiology

While some audiologists will find themselves working largely or wholly within other specialty areas of audiology, most who work within either recreational or animal audiology do so as a smaller part of their employment responsibilities. Chapter 11 details the deleterious effects of intense sounds on human hearing. One must only wonder at the human proclivity to place one's sense of hearing willingly in harm's way. Yet it is true that many activities, ranging from the enjoyment of music and the use of firearms to the growing recreational use of motorboats, snowmobiles, motorbikes, and racecars, can have a negative impact on human hearing. Recreational audiologists continue to find opportunities to provide hearing-conservation services to those who enjoy excessively loud forms of recreation.

An even more recent, and smaller, specialty area in audiology lies in the audiological assistance given to nonhuman animals, particularly the canine, "man's best friend" (see Figure 1.2). There are more than 80 breeds of dogs with documented congenital hearing loss, and many dogs experience the same age-related declines in hearing seen in humans. Counseling about dog safety and communication issues is an important service provided by

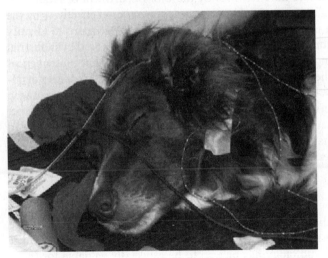

FIGURE 1.2 The identification, diagnosis, and management of canine hearing loss should be carried out through a systematic protocol by qualified practitioners. Objective hearing assessments designed for humans as described in Chapter 7 can be completed successfully on dogs with mild sedation. (*Source:* The Facility for the Education and Testing of Canine Hearing and the Laboratory for Animal Bioacoustics [FETCH~LAB], University of Cincinnati.)

animal audiologists (Scheifele, Clark, & Scheifle, 2012). Hearing conservation for service animals, especially military working dogs, is also a concern of animal audiologists and these dogs' handlers, especially considering the substantial time and money that is invested in the training of these animals. Ongoing research continues on effective hearing-loss prevention and management for canines.

Employment Settings

While some audiologists list their primary employment function as a researcher, administrator, or university teacher, more than 82 percent consider themselves to be direct clinical service providers (American Academy of Audiology, 2010). As noted in Figure 1.3, more audiologists deliver services within a medical environment than within any other single employment setting. Private practice constitutes the second largest employment affiliation for audiologists.

The trend of most students in master's degree programs to state a preference for employment within a medical setting may be giving way to Au.D. students' aspirations of future employment within private practice (Freeman & Doyle, 2001). By far the most rapidly growing employment setting for audiologists is that of private practice. Today, private-practice audiology concentrates on the dispensing/rehabilitative efforts of the audiologist; however, a number of practices offer a wide array of diagnostic services as well.

FIGURE 1.3 An American Academy of Audiology membership survey reports that the majority of audiologists are employed within a medical setting (hospital, clinic, or physician's office). More than 82 percent of surveyed audiologists report that they are direct providers of clinical services. Unlike just a few years ago, the single primary employment setting for audiologists is private practice.

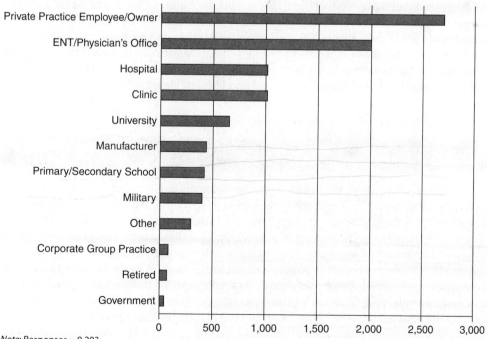

Note: Responses = 9,203.

(*Source:* American Academy of Audiology, Membership Demographics, 2010.)

Professional Societies

A number of professional societies for the advancement of the interests of audiologists and those they serve has evolved as the profession itself has grown. The American Speech Correction Association (originally founded in 1927 as the American Society for the Study of Disorders of Speech) adopted the new profession of audiology in 1947 when its name was changed to the American Speech and Hearing Association (ASHA). Renamed the American Speech-Language-Hearing Association in 1978 (while retaining its recognized acronym), ASHA was instrumental in setting standards for the practice of audiology and for the accreditation of academic programs for audiologists and speech-language pathologists. ASHA provides continuing education and professional and scientific journals for these two professions, which share a common heritage.

Because of the need for a strong national association that could represent the unique needs and interests of the audiology profession, the American Academy of Audiology (AAA) was founded in 1988. Rapidly embraced by the profession, AAA became the home of more than 6,000 audiologists before it was 10 years old and well over 10,000 by the time the academy was 20 years old. The academy is committed to the advancement of audiological services through increased public awareness of hearing and balance disorders among the U.S. population as well as national governmental agencies and congressional representatives. The academy's journals and continuing education programs are instrumental for audiologists' maintaining a high level of expertise in their chosen profession. AAA, along with ASHA, continues to set and revise practice standards, protocols, and guidelines for the practice of audiology to ensure quality patient care.

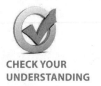

CHECK YOUR UNDERSTANDING

ACTIVITIES

In addition to belonging to one or both of the national associations for audiology as well as their state academy of audiology, many practitioners belong to organizations that promote their chosen area of expertise. Audiologists may affiliate with other audiologists with similar interests through the Academy of Rehabilitative Audiology, the Academy of Doctors of Audiology, or the Educational Audiology Association. The American Auditory Society presents a unique opportunity for audiologists to interact with a variety of medical and nonmedical professionals whose endeavors are largely directed toward work with those who have hearing impairment. Some audiologists find professional growth through affiliation with one or more of the primarily consumer-oriented associations such as the Hearing Loss Association of America and the Alexander Graham Bell Association for the Deaf and Hard of Hearing.

Summary

Relative to other professions in the health arena, audiology is a newcomer, emerging from the combined efforts of otology and speech pathology during World War II. Following the war, this new area of study and practice grew rapidly within the civilian sector because of the high prevalence of hearing loss in the general population and the devastating effects on individuals and families when hearing loss remains untreated. To support the needs of those served most fully, especially within the pediatric population, audiologists often maintain a close working relationship with speech-language pathologists and educators of those with hearing impairment. A mutual respect for what each profession brings to the (re)habilitation of those with hearing impairments leads to the highest level of remediation for those served.

Today the profession of audiology supports a variety of specialty areas. Given projected population demographics, students choosing to enter this profession will find themselves well placed for professional growth and security.

Websites

The following websites will help you connect to professional and consumer organizations related to audiological concerns, professional issues, legislative initiatives, service providers, and consumer education.

- Academy of Doctors of Audiology, *www.audiologist.org*
- Academy of Rehabilitative Audiology, *www.audrehab.org*
- Alexander Graham Bell Association for the Deaf and Hard of Hearing, *www.agbell.org*
- American Academy of Audiology, *www.audiology.org*
- American Auditory Society, *www.amauditorysoc.org*
- American Board of Audiology, *www.americanboardofaudiology.org*
- American Speech-Language-Hearing Association, *www.asha.org*
- American Tinnitus Association, *www.ata.org*
- Better Hearing Institute, *www.betterhearing.org*
- Educational Audiology Association, *www.edaud.org*
- Facility for the Education and Testing of Canine Hearing/Laboratory for Animal Bioacoustics, *www.fetchlab.org*
- Hearing Health Fundation, *www.hearinghealthfoundation.org*
- Hearing Loss Association of America, *www.hlaa.org*
- Military Audiology Association, *www.militaryaudiology.org*

 ## Frequently Asked Questions

Q How do you know when to go to a physician and when to go to an audiologist?

A *Generally audiologists see patients whose primary concern is hearing loss, and physicians see those with a history of pain or disease.*

Q Is it possible to lose one's hearing completely?

A *Yes, this is possible, but total loss of hearing is extremely rare.*

Q What is an otologist? Does it relate to an otolaryngologist (ENT)?

A *Otologists are otolaryngologists who limit their practices to diseases of the ear. Other ENT specialists may concentrate only on diseases of the nose (rhinologists) or throat (laryngologists).*

Q Does the field of audiology exist in other countries?

A *Yes, but the requirements for practice vary. In Australia, New Zealand, and Canada, requirements for certification are similar to the United States. Most other countries require audiologists to be physicians, usually otolaryngologists, who supervise the more technical aspects of the field (like testing), which is carried out by technicians.*

Q What is the difference between a license in audiology and certification in audiology?

A *A license, or registration with the state, is required by all 50 states and the District of Columbia to practice audiology, while certification is not. Certification in audiology is available through both the American Board of Audiology and the American Speech-Language-Hearing Association. Certification is not legally required to practice audiology.*

Q What is the difference between the two certifying agencies for audiology?

A *Certification through the American Board of Audiology (ABA) is a voluntary certification designed to demonstrate a practitioner's dedication to a high level of continuing education. ABA certification is independent of membership in any of the national audiology associations. Those holding certification through the American Speech-Language-Hearing Association (ASHA) must maintain membership in ASHA.*

Q Do many audiologists conduct research outside a university setting?

A *The majority of research publications are associated with universities, but many come from other places, such as private practice, community speech and hearing centers, and Veterans Administration hospitals. The exact numbers are not known.*

 ## Suggested Reading

American Academy of Audiology. (2004). Audiology: Scope of practice. *Audiology Today, 16*(30), 44–45.

American Speech-Language-Hearing Association. (2004). Scope of practice in audiology. *Asha, 24* (Suppl.), 35–37.

 ## Endnote

1. Dr. Raymond Carhart (1912–1975), largely regarded as the father of audiology.

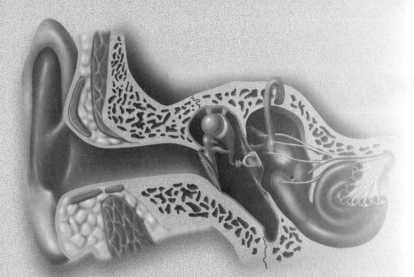

CHAPTER 2

The Human Ear and Simple Tests of Hearing

LEARNING OBJECTIVES

The purpose of this chapter is to present a simplified explanation of the mechanism of human hearing and to describe tuning-fork tests that provide information about hearing disorders. Because of the structure of this chapter, some of the statements have been simplified. These basic concepts are expanded in later chapters in this book. At the completion of this chapter, the reader should be able to

- Define basic vocabulary relative to the ear.
- Understand the core background for study of more sophisticated hearing tests.
- Describe the general anatomy of the hearing mechanism and its pathways of sound.
- List and describe the three types of hearing loss presented.
- Outline the expected tuning-fork test results for different types of hearing loss.

ANATOMY IS CONCERNED with how the body is structured, and physiology is concerned with how it functions. To facilitate understanding, the anatomist neatly divides the mechanisms of hearing into separate compartments, at the same time realizing that these units actually function as one. Sound impulses pass through the **auditory** tract, where they are converted from acoustical to mechanical to hydraulic to chemical and electrical energy, until finally they are received by the brain, which makes the signal discernible.

We test human hearing by two sound pathways: **air conduction (AC)** and **bone conduction (BC)**. Tests of hearing utilizing **tuning forks** are by no means modern, but they illustrate hearing via these two pathways. Tuning-fork tests may compare the hearing of the patient to that of a presumably normal-hearing examiner, the relative sensitivity by air conduction and bone conduction, the effects on bone conduction of closing the opening into the ear, and the lateralization of sound to one ear or the other by bone conduction.

Anatomy and Physiology of the Ear

A simplified look at a coronal section through the ear (see Figure 2.1) illustrates the division of the hearing mechanism into three parts. The **outer ear** comprises a shell-like protrusion from each side of the head, a canal through which sounds travel, and the **eardrum membrane** (more correctly called the tympanic membrane) at the end of the canal. The **middle ear** consists of an air-filled space with a chain of tiny bones, the third of which, the stapes, is the smallest in the human body. The portion of the **inner ear** that is responsible for hearing is called the **cochlea**; it is filled with fluids and many microscopic components, all of which serve to convert waves into a message that travels to the stem (base) of the brain via the **auditory nerve**. The brain stem is not coupled to the highest auditory center in the cortex by a simple neural connection. Rather, there is a series of waystations that receive, analyze, and transmit impulses along the auditory pathway. Stimuli reaching the inner ear directly by bone conduction bypass the conductive mechanisms of the outer ear and the middle ear.

Pathways of Sound

Those persons whose primary interest is in the measurement of hearing sometimes divide the hearing mechanism differently than do anatomists. Audiologists and physicians separate the ear into the conductive portion—consisting of the outer and middle ears—and the sensory/neural portion—consisting of the inner ear and the auditory nerve. This type of breakdown is illustrated in the block diagram in Figure 2.2.

Any sound that courses through the outer ear, middle ear, inner ear, and beyond is heard by air conduction. It is possible to bypass the outer and middle ears by vibrating the skull mechanically and stimulating the inner ear directly. In this way, the sound is heard by bone

FIGURE 2.1 Cross-section of the ear showing the air-conduction pathway and the bone-conduction pathway.

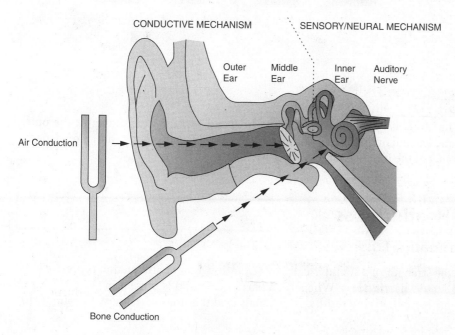

FIGURE 2.2 Block diagram of the ear. A conductive hearing loss is illustrated by damage to the middle ear. Damage to the outer ear would produce the same effect. Similarly, a sensory/neural hearing loss could be demonstrated by damage to the hearing nerve as well as to the inner ear.

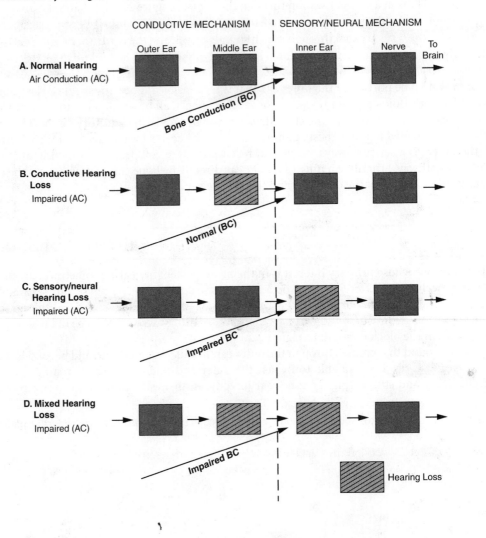

conduction. Therefore, hearing by air conduction depends on the functioning of the outer, middle, and inner ear and of the neural pathways beyond; hearing by bone conduction depends on the functioning of the inner ear and beyond.

Types of Hearing Loss

Conductive Hearing Loss

A decrease in the strength of a sound is called **attenuation**. Sound attenuation is precisely the result of a conductive hearing loss. Whenever a barrier to sound is present in the outer ear or middle ear, some loss of hearing results. Individuals find that their sensitivity to sounds that are introduced by air conduction is impaired by such a blockage. If the sound is introduced by bone conduction, it bypasses the obstacle and goes directly to the sensory/neural mechanism. Because the inner ear and the other sensory/neural structures are unimpaired, the hearing by bone conduction is normal. This impaired air conduction with normal bone conduction is called a **conductive hearing loss** and is diagrammed in Figure 2.2B. In this illustration, the **hearing loss** is caused by damage to the middle ear. Outer ear abnormalities produce the same relationship between air and bone conduction.

Sensory/Neural Hearing Loss

If the disturbance producing the hearing loss is situated in some portion of the sensory/neural mechanism, such as the inner ear or the auditory nerve, a hearing loss by air conduction results. Because the attenuation of the sound occurs along the bone-conduction pathway, the hearing loss by bone conduction is as great as the hearing loss by air conduction. When a hearing loss exists in which there is the same amount of attenuation for both air conduction and bone conduction, the conductive mechanism is eliminated as a possible cause of the difficulty. A diagnosis of **sensory/neural hearing loss** can then be made. In Figure 2.2C, the inner ear was selected to illustrate a sensory/neural disorder, although the same principle would hold if the auditory nerve were damaged.

Hearing loss resulting from damage to the inner ear or to the auditory nerve was once called either a "perceptive loss" or a "nerve loss." Both these terms are inaccurate (although the latter is, regrettably, still used today by some individuals). The term *perceptive loss* is misleading as perception is achieved by centers in the brain and thereby removed from either the inner ear or the auditory nerve. The term *nerve loss* is equally misleading given that the auditory nerve is far less common than the inner ear as the site of these hearing losses.

Several decades ago the term *sensori-neural* was introduced to suggest that the problem involved the inner ear and/or the auditory nerve. This was a considerable advance toward accuracy in scientific terminology, although technically a hyphenated word must contain two accepted words and *sensori* does not appear in the dictionary. The term *sensori-neural* also suffers from the fact that a hyphen implies a connection between two words, but not one and/or the other. Over time the hyphen was dropped and the compound word *sensorineural* was coined, a term that fails to acknowledge that such losses are rarely both sensory and neural. The term adopted for this book uses the slash with a slight spelling change, namely, *sensory/ neural,* because this more strongly indicates that the damage may be to the inner ear, to the auditory nerve, or possibly both. Diagnostic audiology is well on its way toward differentiating sensory from neural hearing losses, and when that eventuality is fully realized, the use of hyphens, slashes, or compound words will no longer be necessary.

Mixed Hearing Loss

Problems can occur simultaneously in both the conductive and sensory/neural mechanisms, as illustrated in Figure 2.2D. This results in a loss of hearing sensitivity by bone conduction because of the sensory/neural abnormality, but an even greater loss of sensitivity by air conduction. This is true because the loss of hearing by air conduction must include the loss (by bone conduction) in the sensory/neural portion plus the attenuation in the conductive portion. In other words, sound traveling on the bone-conduction pathway is attenuated only by the defect in the inner ear, but sound traveling on the air-conduction pathway is attenuated by both middle-ear and inner-ear problems. This type of impairment is called a **mixed hearing loss**.

Nonorganic Hearing Loss

Individuals are sometimes seen whose test results show some degree of hearing loss, usually sensory/neural, but who either have normal hearing or insufficient auditory pathology to explain the extent of the loss. The mechanisms for this phenomenon are explained more fully in Chapter 13, but the underlying psychodynamics may be quite complex. In the past, a simple, popular dichotomy said that patients with **nonorganic hearing loss** were either consciously faking the problem for some financial or other gain, or there was some psychological disorder that manifested in the symptom of a hearing loss. The former condition is called **malingering** and the latter one **psychogenic hearing loss**. Some explanation of this oversimplification will be found later in this text.

Hearing Tests

Some of the earliest tests of hearing probably consisted merely of producing sounds of some kind, such as clapping the hands or making vocal sounds, to see if an individual could hear them. Asking people if they could hear the ticking of a watch or the clicking of two coins together may have suggested that the examiner was attempting to sample the upper pitch range. Obviously, these tests provided little information of either a quantitative or a qualitative nature.

Tuning Fork Tests

The tuning fork (see Figure 2.3) is a device, usually made of steel, magnesium, or aluminum, that is used to tune musical instruments or by singers to obtain certain pitches. A tuning fork emits a tone at a particular pitch and has a clear musical quality. When the tuning fork is vibrating

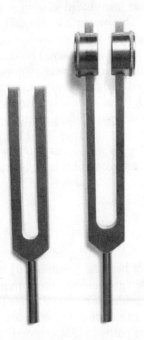

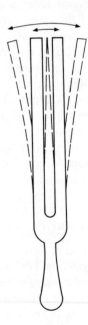

FIGURE 2.3 Several tuning forks. The larger forks vibrate at lower frequencies (produce lower-pitched tones) than the smaller forks. (*Source:* Fosterdesigns/iStock/360/Getty Images.)

FIGURE 2.4 Vibration pattern of tuning forks.

properly, the tines move alternately away from and toward one another (see Figure 2.4), and the stem moves with a piston action. The air-conduction tone emitted is relatively pure, meaning that it is free of overtones (more on this subject in Chapter 3).

The tuning-fork tests described in this chapter are named for the four German otologists (ear specialists) who described them in the middle 19th to early 20th centuries. They are rarely used by audiologists, who prefer more sophisticated electronic devices. However, tuning-fork tests serve to illustrate the principles involved in certain modern tests.

The tuning fork is set into vibration by holding the stem in the hand and striking one of the tines against a firm but resilient surface. The rubber heel of a shoe does nicely for this purpose, although many physicians prefer the knuckle, knee, or elbow. If the fork is struck against too solid an object, dropped, or otherwise abused, its vibrations may be considerably altered. To see how a tuning fork is activated, see the **video** titled Tuning Fork Tests.

The tuning fork was adopted as an instrument for testing hearing over a century ago. It held promise then because it could be quantified, at least in terms of the pitch emitted. Several forks are available that usually correspond to notes on the musical scale of C. By using tuning forks with various known properties, hearing sensitivity through several pitch ranges may be sampled. However, any diagnostic statement made on the basis of a tuning-fork test is absolutely limited to the pitch of the fork used because hearing sensitivity is often different for different pitches.

The Schwabach Test

The **Schwabach test**,[1] introduced in 1890, is a bone-conduction test. It compares the hearing sensitivity of a patient with that of an examiner. The tuning fork is set into vibration, and the stem is placed alternately against the **mastoid process** (the bony protrusion behind the ear) of the patient and of the examiner (see Figure 2.5A). Each time the fork is pressed against the patient's head, the patient indicates whether the tone is heard. The vibratory energy of the tines of the fork decreases over time, making the tone softer. When the patient no longer hears the tone, the examiner immediately places the stem of the tuning fork behind his or her own ear and, using a watch, notes the number of seconds that the tone is audible after the patient stops hearing it.

This test assumes that examiners have normal hearing, and it is less than worthless unless this is true. If both examiners and patients have normal hearing, both stop hearing the tone emitted by the fork at approximately the same time. This is called a *normal Schwabach*. If patients have sensory/neural hearing loss, hearing by bone conduction is impaired, and they stop hearing the sound much sooner than the examiner. This is called a *diminished Schwabach*. The test can be quantified to some degree by recording the number of seconds an examiner continues to hear the tone after a patient has stopped hearing it. If an examiner hears the tone for 10 seconds longer than a patient, the patient's hearing is "diminished 10 seconds." If patients have a conductive hearing loss, bone conduction is normal, and they hear the tone for at least as long as the examiner, sometimes longer. In some conductive hearing losses, the patient's hearing in the low-pitch range may appear to be better than normal. When this occurs, the result is called a *prolonged Schwabach*.

Difficulties arise in the administration and interpretation of the Schwabach test. Interpretation of test results in cases of mixed hearing losses is especially difficult. Because both inner ears are very close together and are embedded in the bones of the skull, it is almost impossible to stimulate one without simultaneously stimulating the other. Therefore, if there is a difference in sensitivity between the two inner ears, a patient will probably respond to sound heard through the better ear, which can cause a *false normal Schwabach*. Thus, the examiner may have difficulty determining which ear is actually being tested. To see a demonstration of the Schwabach test, see the **video** titled Tuning Fork Tests.

FIGURE 2.5 Positions of tuning fork during tuning-fork tests.

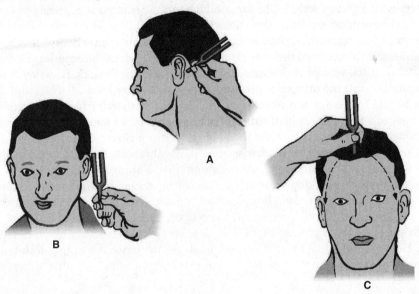

The Rinne Test

The **Rinne test**[2] compares patients' hearing sensitivity by bone conduction to their sensitivity by air conduction. This is done by asking them to state whether the tone is louder when the tuning-fork stem is held against the bone behind the ear, as in the Schwabach test (see Figure 2.5A), or when the tines of the fork that are generating an air-conducted sound are held next to the opening of the ear (see Figure 2.5B). Because air conduction is a more efficient means of sound transmission to the inner ear than bone conduction, people with normal hearing hear a louder tone when the fork is next to the ear than when it is behind the ear. This is called a *positive Rinne*. A positive Rinne also occurs in patients with sensory/neural hearing loss. The attenuation produced by a problem in the sensory/neural mechanism produces the same degree of loss by air conduction as by bone conduction (see Figure 2.2C).

If patients have more than a mild conductive hearing loss, their bone-conduction hearing is normal (see Figure 2.2B), and they hear a louder tone with the stem of the fork behind the ear (bone conduction) than with the tines at the ear (air conduction). This is called a *negative Rinne*. Sometimes patients manifest what has been called the *false negative Rinne,* which occurs when the inner ear not deliberately being tested responds to the tone. As mentioned in the discussion of the Schwabach test, this may happen readily during bone-conduction tests. For example, if the right ear is the one being tested, the loudness of the air-conducted tone in the right ear may inadvertently be compared to the loudness of the bone-conducted tone in the left ear. If the left-ear bone conduction is more sensitive than the right-ear bone conduction, a false negative Rinne may result, giving rise to an improper diagnosis of conductive hearing loss. To see a demonstration of the Rinne test, see the video titled Tuning Fork Tests.

The Bing Test

It has been known for some time that when persons with normal hearing close off the opening into the ear canal, the loudness of a tone presented by bone conduction increases. This phenomenon has been called the **occlusion effect (OE)**, and it is observed primarily for low-pitched sounds. This effect is also evident in patients with sensory/neural hearing loss, but it is absent in patients with conductive hearing loss. This is the premise of the **Bing test**.[3]

When performing the Bing test, the tuning fork handle is held to the mastoid process behind the ear (see Figure 2.5A) while the examiner alternately closes and opens the ear canal with a finger. For normal hearers and those with sensory/neural hearing loss, the result is a pulsating sound, or a sound that seems to get louder and softer (called a *positive Bing*). For patients with conductive hearing losses, no change in the loudness of the sound is noticed (*negative Bing*). The examiner must not suggest to patients what their responses should be. As in the Schwabach and Rinne tests, the danger of a response to the tone by the nontest ear is ever present.

The Weber Test

Since its introduction, the **Weber test**[4] has been so popular that it has been modified by many audiologists for use with modern electronic testing equipment. It is a test of **lateralization**; that is, patients must state where they hear the tone (left ear, right ear, both ears, or midline).

When performing the Weber test, the tuning fork is set into vibration, and the stem is placed on the midline of the patient's skull. Figure 2.5C shows placement on the forehead, which is probably the most popular location. Other sites are also used, such as the top or the back of the head, the chin, or the upper teeth. In most cases the upper teeth produce the loudest bone-conducted sound. Patients are simply asked in which ear they hear a louder sound. Often the reply is that they hear it in only one ear.

People with normal hearing or with equal amounts of the same type of hearing loss in both ears (conductive, sensory/neural, or mixed) report a midline sensation. They may say that the tone is equally loud in both ears, that they cannot tell any difference, or that they hear the tone as if it originated somewhere in the middle of the head. Patients with sensory/neural hearing loss in one ear hear the tone in their better ear. Patients with conductive hearing loss in one ear hear the tone in their poorer ear.

The midline sensation is easy to understand. If the ears are equally sensitive and equally stimulated, equal loudness should logically result. One explanation of the Weber effect in sensory/neural cases is based on the Stenger principle. The **Stenger principle** states that if two tones that are identical in all ways except loudness are introduced simultaneously into both ears, only the louder tone will be perceived. When the bone-conduction sensitivity is poorer in one ear than in the other, the tone being introduced to both ears with equal energy will be perceived as softer or will not be perceived at all in the poorer ear.

Results on the Weber test are most poorly understood in unilateral conductive hearing losses. The explanation for the tone being louder in the ear with a conductive loss than in the normal ear is probably based on the same phenomenon as prolonged bone conduction, described briefly in the discussion of the Schwabach test.

The Weber test has been known to avert misdiagnosis of unilateral sensory/neural hearing loss as conductive when false normal Schwabach or false negative Rinne results are seen, but the tone is heard in the poorer-hearing ear rather than the expected better-hearing ear. The Weber test is quick, easy, and often helpful, although like most auditory tests, it has some drawbacks. Clinical experience has shown that many patients with a conductive hearing loss in one ear report hearing the tone in their better ear because what they are actually experiencing seems incorrect or even foolish to them. Again, care must be taken not to lead patients into giving the kind of response they think is "correct." Interpretation of the Weber test is also difficult in mixed hearing losses.

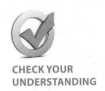

CHECK YOUR UNDERSTANDING

ACTIVITIES

Clinical COMMENTARY

Electronic tests for testing hearing by bone conduction have largely supplanted tuning-fork tests in audiological testing; however, tuning-fork tests continue to be used by many otologists. The Bing and Weber tests can be performed easily with today's electronic test equipment and can prove useful in separating conductive from sensory/neural hearing loss if other testing proves somewhat ambiguous.

EVOLVING CASE STUDIES

As you read the following case histories, try to see why they have been placed in their different diagnostic categories. For each of the cases, predict what the results would be on the Rinne, Schwabach, and Weber tuning-fork tests when these are possible. Make your predictions before you read the Test Results and Conclusions. In later chapters, you will be asked to conjecture about a variety of other, more sophisticated test and management procedures for these six cases as diagnostic and treatment information about these cases unfolds in the ensuing chapters.

Case Study 1: Conductive Hearing Loss—Outer Ear Disorder

The parents of a 9-year-old boy bring him to the audiology clinic. The most noticeable details about this child are that he has downward slanting eyes, a small lower jaw, underdeveloped cheekbones, drooping lower eyelids, and absent external ears and ear canals. He appears bright and friendly and communicates fairly well using a bone-conduction hearing aid. The parents and the child have been seen by several ear, nose, and throat specialists and told that nothing medically or surgically can be done to correct his problems. He has been referred to you by a speech-language pathologist to see whether the child may be helped further.

Case Study 2: Conductive Hearing Loss—Middle Ear Disorder

This 23-year-old woman has a history of middle-ear infections and drainage in both ears since early childhood. She says that while she is always aware of a hearing loss, it appears to vary in degree. She says she can understand speech well if people are close to her or speak loudly. The otologist who referred her for testing says that, while there is evidence of past infection, her eardrum membranes are both intact.

Case Study 3: Sensory/Neural Hearing Loss—Inner Ear Disorder

This 79-year-old male denies any history of ear infection or exposure to loud noise. He first noticed some difficulty in hearing in both ears about 10 years earlier and says that it has progressed. He notes that he does much better in quiet surroundings than in noisy places or when several people are speaking at the same time. His difficulty in correctly identifying words is more bothersome than the loss of the loudness of speech and he does not like people shouting at him. His wife volunteers that in recent years the patient has significantly reduced his interactions with others and avoids movies, the theater, and religious services because he has so much trouble understanding words. The cause of the hearing loss appears to be aging but that is a conclusion that should await further testing.

Case Study 4: Sensory/Neural Hearing Loss—Auditory Nerve Disorder

This 36-year-old woman presents with a main complaint that the hearing in her left ear has diminished gradually over the previous several years. Because her hearing is normal in the right ear, she communicates pretty well except when there is a lot of background noise or when several people speak at once. She has recently seen a neurologist because of dizziness and headaches, and he has ordered several tests, which have not yet been performed. Because of the gradual and unilateral nature of the hearing loss, it is precautionary to suspect a possible lesion on the left auditory nerve.

Case Study 5: Nonorganic Hearing Loss

This patient, a 45-year-old male who works in a factory, has recently brought a legal suit against his employer because of a claimed hearing loss. He states that one day at work there was a very loud explosion about 10 yards to his left, and since that time he can hear nothing in his left ear and has a very loud ringing in that ear. He states that he has no trouble hearing in his right ear. When you stand several feet away on his right side, he is able to answer all your questions. He claims that he cannot hear people if they speak to him on his left side. He speaks adamantly about his belief that his work setting is responsible for his difficulty and also claims to have very loud ringing in his left ear.

Case Study 6: Pediatric Patient

Interview with the parents indicates that your patient is a 3-year-old-female who uses no spoken language. The parents have sought a diagnosis of her delayed language from a variety of specialists, including her pediatrician and a psychologist. Several tentative diagnoses have been made, including mental handicap and autism. Her older brother was speaking in complete sentences when he was much younger than this little girl. The parents are desperate for a diagnosis so they can begin to try to help their child. Recently the patient was seen by a speech-language pathologist who suggested the possibility of hearing loss as an etiological factor and referred her to you. The child has no history of ear infections and there is no known family history of childhood hearing loss. She is reported to respond inconsistently to sound, although her mother has always believed that some hearing loss exists. This child passed a neonatal hearing screening before she was released from the hospital, but the possibility, however small, of a false negative test result or a later onset hearing loss must be borne in mind given the history.

Tuning-Fork Test Results and Conclusions

Case Study 1: Conductive Hearing Loss—Outer Ear Disorder

Most audiologists do not do tuning-fork tests. However, given this child's age of 9 years, he would undoubtedly respond very well to tuning-fork tests if they were completed. The results would be as follows: Schwabach—normal in both ears, Rinne—negative in both ears, Weber—not lateralized. These are all consistent with a conductive hearing loss, but even with these results, it cannot be determined at this point whether the loss is caused entirely by the absent ear canals or whether the middle ear is also involved.

Case Study 2: Conductive Hearing Loss—Middle Ear Disorder

The patient would show a negative Rinne in both ears and a normal Schwabach, and the tone would not lateralize on the Weber test, but rather would be heard equally loud in both ears or in the middle of her head. These results are consistent with a conductive hearing loss and her history of ear infections, but more sophisticated testing must be done to determine the extent of the loss and related factors.

Case Study 3: Sensory/Neural Hearing Loss—Inner Ear Disorder

This patient would show a positive Rinne and a prolonged (lengthened) Schwabach in both ears. The Weber would be unlateralized. The case history, especially the difficulty in speech understanding even when the signal is sufficiently loud, is consistent with a sensory/neural hearing loss, which would be borne out by these tuning-fork test results. Given the age of onset of the hearing loss, it can be supposed that his hearing loss was produced by aging and suggests that the primary problem exists in the cochlea of the inner ear. Further testing is obviously needed.

Case Study 4: Sensory/Neural Hearing Loss—Auditory Nerve Disorder

The Rinne would be positive and the Schwabach would be normal on the right side. When using a high-frequency tuning fork on the left side, the patient would respond that the tones are heard in her right ear. On the Weber test, the patient would reports hearing the tone in both ears using a lower-pitched tuning fork and in the right ear using a higher-pitched one. These results would bear out the patient's report of a hearing loss only in the left ear in the higher frequencies but possibly normal hearing in the right.

Case Study 5: Nonorganic Hearing Loss

Results would show a positive Rinne for the right ear and the patient, as is reported in such cases, would claim that the tone in the left ear cannot be heard by either air conduction or bone conduction. The Schwabach would be normal on the right side, and the patient would claim that he does not hear any of the bone-conducted tones at all on the left side. The Weber would be reported as lateralizing to the right ear.

Suspicion of a feigned or exaggerated (nonorganic) hearing loss is first raised by the legal action, with promise of financial gain, and by the fact that a noise loud enough to cause a hearing loss in his left ear would probably have caused some hearing loss in his right ear as well. It is also true that he should have heard speech in his right ear that was directed to his left side because the shadow of sound (the amount of energy lost as a signal travels from one side of the head to the other) is only about 13 dB. If he truly had a sensory/neural hearing loss in his left ear, he would have been able to hear the bone-conducted signals on the Rinne and the Schwabach in his right ear (with the tuning fork placed on his left mastoid) because practically no sound intensity is lost as the signal travels through the skull from one side of the head to the other.

Case Study 6: Pediatric Patient

Tuning-fork tests are inappropriate for children at this age. Your casual observation of the child suggests that she does not appear to respond to environmental sounds. Your first session consisted of observation and the introduction of earphones without an insistence to place the inserts in the child's ears. A technique presenting sounds through loud speakers was briefly attempted but abandoned, as the child grew restless. The little girl was allowed to play with some toys and was observed to relax. After taking a complete history, the parents were encouraged to observe the child's reactions to environmental sounds, follow up with the speech-language pathologist, and return in several days for further audiometric testing. The parents appeared relieved and made a new appointment. Before departure, several foam insert earphone plugs were given to the parents to acclimate the child to plug insertion at home to help ensure greater success in the clinic on the family's return.

Summary

The mechanisms of hearing may be roughly broken down into conductive and sensory/neural portions. Tests by air conduction measure sensitivity through the entire hearing pathway. Tests by bone conduction sample the sensitivity of the structures from the inner ear and beyond, up to the brain. The Schwabach test compares the bone-conduction sensitivity of the patient to that of a presumed normal-hearing person (the examiner). The Rinne tuning-fork test compares patients' own hearing by bone conduction to their hearing by air conduction in order to sample for conductive versus sensory/neural loss. The Bing test samples for conductive hearing loss by testing the effect of occluding the ear. The Weber test checks for lateralization of a bone-conducted tone presented to the midline of the skull to determine if a loss in only one ear is conductive or sensory/neural.

REVIEW TABLE 2.1 Types of Hearing Loss

Anatomical Area	Purpose	Type of Loss
Outer ear	Conduct sound energy	Conductive
Middle ear	Conduct sound energy Increase sound intensity	Conductive
Inner ear	Convert mechanical to hydraulic to electrochemical energy	Sensory/neural
Auditory nerve	Transmit electrochemical (nerve) impulses to brain	Sensory/neural

REVIEW TABLE 2.2 Tuning-Fork Tests

Test	Purpose	Fork Placement	Normal Hearing	Conductive Loss	Sensory/Neural Loss
Schwabach	Compare patient's BC to normal	Mastoid process	Normal Schwabach—Patient hears tone as long as examiner	Normal or Prolonged Schwabach—Patient hears tone as long as or longer than examiner	Diminished Schwabach—Patient hears tone for shorter time than examiner
Rinne	Compare patient's AC to BC	Alternate between mastoid process and opening to ear canal	Positive Rinne—Louder at the ear	Negative Rinne—Louder behind the ear	Positive Rinne—Louder at the ear
Bing	Determine presence or absence of occlusion effect	Mastoid process	Positive Bing—Tone is louder with ear occluded	Negative Bing—Loudness does not change with ear occluded	Positive Bing—Tone is louder with ear occluded
Weber	Check lateralization of tone in unilateral losses	Midline of head	Tone equally loud in both ears	Tone louder in poorer ear	Tone louder in better ear

REVIEW TABLE 2.3 Relationship Between Air Conduction and Bone Conduction for Different Hearing Conditions

Finding	Condition
Normal air conduction	Normal hearing
Normal bone conduction	Normal hearing or conductive hearing loss
Poorer hearing for air conduction than for bone conduction	Conductive or mixed hearing loss
Hearing for air conduction the same as hearing for bone conduction	Normal hearing or sensory/neural hearing loss

Frequently Asked Questions

Q What portion of the inner ear is responsible for hearing?

A *The cochlea is the end organ for hearing and the utricle, sacccule, and semicircular canals are the end organs for balance.*

Q What is attenuation? How does it relate to a conductive hearing loss?

A *The dictionary defines attenuation as "weakening in force, amount, or value; reduction." The attenuation of a sound is the reduction of intensity. It is commonly believed that this is the only symptom experienced by people with conductive hearing losses; that is, sounds are merely weaker for them than they are for those with normal hearing. Patients with sensory/neural hearing losses report that, even when sounds are made louder, they are not always entirely clear, suggesting that some distortion exists.*

Q Why would a mixed hearing loss not simply be the sum of the hearing loss produced by the abnormalities of the conductive and sensory/neural mechanisms?

A *It is generally accepted that the air-conduction threshold represents the entire hearing loss, the bone-conduction threshold the sensory/neural component, and the air-bone gap represents the conductive component of a hearing loss.*

As the sensory/neural component of a mixed loss increases over time, the air-bone gap is sometimes seen to decrease. This is probably due to the fact that the decibel is a logarithmic, rather than a linear, unit of measurement.

Q Is a hearing loss from the auditory nerve (VIIIth nerve) considered a sensory/neural hearing loss?

A *Yes. Losses produced by lesions in either the cochlea or on the VIIIth nerve are traditionally grouped together as sensory/neural. Newer audiological tests are capable of separating these loses as either sensory (cochlear) or neural (auditory nerve and beyond).*

Q Why do we study tuning forks when audiometric equipment is so much more advanced?

A *We study tuning forks for several reasons. They illustrate some principles about the relationships between air conduction and bone conduction, which makes the understanding of pure-tone audiometry easier. They have an important place in the history of the development of hearing tests. And many physicians conduct tuning-fork tests and audiologists must be prepared to interpret those results.*

Q Why does a unilateral sensory/neural hearing loss produce a false negative on the Rinne test?

A *Unless the better ear is masked, it will hear the tone when the stem of the tuning fork is placed on the mastoid at the poorer ear. The result is that sound is louder than the air-conducted sound when the tines of the fork are held next to the poorer ear. When asked if the tone is louder in the front of the ear or behind, patients indicate that it is louder behind the ear, which can falsely be interpreted as a negative Rinne and a misdiagnosis of conductive hearing loss.*

Q Why do audiologists prefer not to use tuning forks if their audiometric findings are sometimes found to be incorrect by physicians who use them?

A *There is no reason for an audiometric test to produce inaccurate results that may be discovered by a physician doing a tuning-fork test. Rather than performing tuning-fork tests themselves, audiologists should concentrate on using careful, scientific audiometric practices as a cross-check.*

Q During the Rinne test, what is the stem of the tuning fork held against?

A *Traditionally it is held against the mastoid, which is appropriate because a bone-conducted tone is loudest from that position.*

Q Does the Schwabach test compare the patient's BC or AC to the examiner's BC or AC, respectively?

A *The Schwabach is a bone-conduction test.*

Endnotes

1. Named for Dr. Dabobert Schwabach (1846–1920).
2. Named for Dr. Heinrich Rinne (1819–1868).
3. Named for Dr. Albert Bing (1844–1922).
4. Named for Dr. Friedrich Weber (1832–1891).

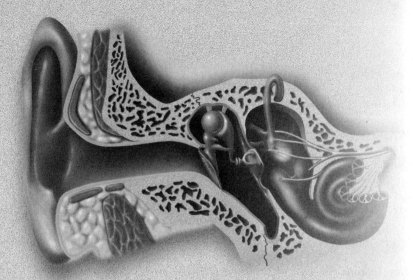

CHAPTER 3

Sound and Its Measurement

LEARNING OBJECTIVES

Understanding this chapter requires no special knowledge of mathematics or physics, although a background in either or both of these disciplines is surely helpful. At the completion of this chapter, the reader should be able to

- Describe sound waves and their common attributes, and express the way these characteristics are measured.

- Discuss the basic interrelationships among the measurements of sound and be able to do some simple calculations (although at this point it is more important to grasp the physical concepts of sound than to gain skill in working equations).

- Understand the different references for the decibel and when they are used.

- State the difference between physical acoustics and psychoacoustics.

- Discuss the reasons for audiometer calibration and what this may entail in general terms.

IT IS IMPOSSIBLE to study abnormalities of human hearing without a basic understanding of the physics of sound and some of the properties of its measurement and perception. Sound is generated by vibrations and is carried through the air around us in the form of pressure waves. It is only when a sound pressure wave reaches the ear that hearing may take place.

Many factors may affect sound waves during their creation and propagation through the air, and most are specified physically in terms of the frequency and intensity of vibrations.

Human reactions to sound are psychological and reflect subjective experiences such as pitch, loudness, sound **quality,** and the ability to tell the direction of a sound source.

Sound

Sound may be defined in terms of either psychological or physical phenomena. In the psychological sense, a sound is an auditory experience—the act of hearing something. In the physical sense, sound is a series of disturbances of molecules within, and propagated through, an elastic medium such as air.

Sound may travel through any elastic medium, although our immediate concern is the propagation of sound through air. Every cubic inch of the air that surrounds us is filled with billions and billions of tiny molecules. These particles move about randomly, constantly bouncing off one another. The **elasticity,** or springiness, of any medium is increased as the distance between the molecules is decreased. If a springy object is distorted, it returns to its original shape. The rate at which this occurs is determined by the elasticity of the object. Molecules are packed more closely together in a solid than in a liquid and more closely in a liquid than in a gas. Therefore, a solid is more elastic than a liquid, and a liquid is more elastic than a gas.

When water is heated in a kettle, the molecules begin to bounce around, which in turn causes them to move farther apart from one another. The energy increases until steam is created, resulting in the familiar teakettle whistle as the molecules are forced through a small opening. As long as there is any heat in the air, there is particle vibration. The rapid and random movement of air particles is called **Brownian motion**[1] and is affected by the heat in the environment. As the heat is increased, the particle velocity is increased.

Waves

Whenever air molecules are disturbed by a body that is set into **vibration,** they move from the point of disturbance, striking and bouncing off adjacent molecules. Because of their elasticity, the original molecules bounce back after having forced their neighbors from their previous positions. When the molecules are pushed close together, they are said to be condensed or compressed. When a space exists between areas of compression, this area is said to be rarefied.

The succession of molecules being shoved together and then pulled apart sets up a motion called **waves.** Waves through the air, therefore, are made up of successive **compressions** and **rarefactions.** Figure 3.1A illustrates such wave motion and shows the different degrees of particle density. Figure 3.1B illustrates the same wave motion as a function of time.

Transverse Waves

The molecular motion in **transverse waves** is perpendicular to the direction of wave motion. The example of water is often useful in understanding transverse wave motion. If a pebble is dropped into a water tank, a hole is made in the area of water through which the pebble falls (see Figure 3.2A). Water from the surrounding area flows into the hole to fill it, leaving a circular trough around the original hole (see Figure 3.2B). Water from the area surrounding the trough then flows in to fill the first trough (see Figure 3.2C). As the circles widen, each trough becomes shallower, until the troughs are barely perceptible. As the water flows in to fill the hole, the waves move out in larger and larger circles. In water, then, a float would illustrate a

FIGURE 3.1 Simple wave motion in air showing (A) particle displacement (movement of pressure waves through space) and (B) sinusoidal waveform (the pressure wave displayed as a function of time). Note the compressions (C) and rarefactions (R).

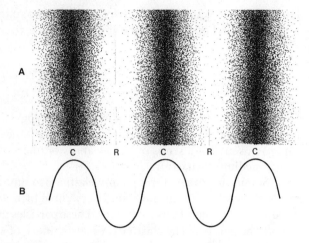

fixed point on the surface, which could be seen to bob only up and down. In fact, the movement of the float would describe a circle or ellipse on a vertical axis, while the waves moving outwardly would describe movement on the horizontal axis. This horizontal movement creates what are called transverse waves.

Longitudinal Waves

Another kind of wave, which is more important to the understanding of sound, is the **longitudinal wave.** This wave is illustrated by the motion of wheat blowing in a field, with the tips of the stalks representing the air particles. The air molecules, like the grains of wheat, move along the same axis as the wave itself when a force, such as that provided by the wind, is applied.

Sine Waves

Sound waves pass through the air without being seen. Indeed, they are real, even if there is no one there to hear them. It is useful to depict sound waves in a graphic way to help explain them. Figure 3.3 assists with a pictorial representation if the reader concedes a bird's-eye

FIGURE 3.2 Wave motion in water as an example of transverse waves. A hole in the water is produced by a pebble (A); the first trough is produced when water flows in to fill the hole (B); the second trough is produced when water flows in to fill the first trough (C). A cork on the surface bobs up and down in a circular fashion.

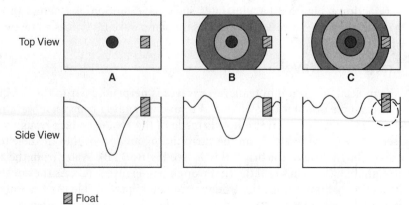

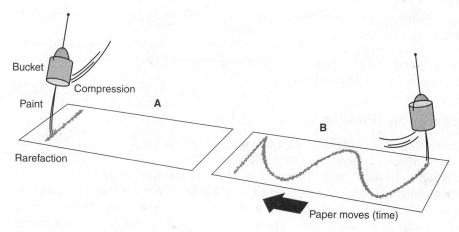

FIGURE 3.3 Sinusoidal motion. Bird's-eye view of a stream of paint from a bucket tracing a line forward (compression) and backward (rarefaction) on a sheet of paper (A). When the paper is moved to the left to represent the passage of time (B), the paint traces a sinusoidal wave.

view of a bucket of paint suspended by a string above a sheet of paper. If the bucket is pushed forward and backward, a small hole in its bottom allows a thin stream of paint to trace a line on the paper. We assume that forward motions of the bucket stand for compressions of molecules and backward motions for rarefactions. If the bucket continues to swing at the same rate, and if the paper is moved in a leftward direction to represent the passage of time, a smooth wave is painted on the paper; this represents each **cycle,** consisting of its compression and rarefaction, as a function of time. If the movement of the paper takes one second, during which two complete cycles take place, the **frequency** is two cycles per second (cps), and so forth.

A body moving back and forth is said to oscillate. One cycle of vibration, or **oscillation,** begins at any point on the wave and ends at the identical point on the next wave. This definition of an oscillation allows for a number of mathematical analyses that are important in the study of acoustics. Such waves are called **sine waves** or **sinusoidal waves.** When a body oscillates sinusoidally, showing only one frequency of vibration with no tones superimposed, it is said to be a **pure tone.** The number of complete sine waves that occur in one second constitutes the frequency of that wave. The compression of a sine wave is usually shown by the extension of the curve upward, and rarefaction is usually shown by the extension of the curve downward. One cycle may be broken down into 360 degrees (see Figure 3.4). Looking at a sine wave in terms of degrees is useful, which we will see later in this chapter. When a wave begins at 90 degrees rather than at 0 degrees, it is called a **cosine wave.**

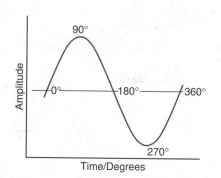

FIGURE 3.4 Denotation of a sine wave into 360 degrees.

Vibrations

Given the proper amount of energy, a mass can be set into vibration. The properties of its vibration may be influenced by a number of factors.

Effects of Energy on Vibration

Figure 3.5 illustrates the effects of energy on a sine wave. When the oscillating body has swung from point A to point B, it must come to a stop before the onset of the return swing because the paint bucket in Figure 3.3 must cease its forward swing before it can swing back. At this point, there is no **kinetic energy** (moving energy), but rather all the energy is **potential energy.** As the vibrating body picks up speed going from B to D, it passes through point C, where there is maximum kinetic energy and no potential energy. As point D is approached, kinetic energy decreases and potential energy increases, as at point B.

Free Vibrations

An object that is allowed to vibrate—for example, a weight suspended at the end of a string (see Figure 3.6A)— encounters a certain amount of opposition to its movement by the molecules in the air. This small amount of friction converts some of the energy involved in the initial movement of the object into heat. Friction has the effect of slowing down the distance of the swing until eventually all swinging stops. If no outside force is added to perpetuate the swinging, the movement is called a **free vibration.** When the vibrations of a mass decay gradually over time, the system is said to be lightly damped. Heavy **damping** causes the oscillations to cease rapidly. When the oscillations cease before a single cycle is completed, the system is said to be critically damped.

Forced Vibrations

If an outside force is added to a swinging motion that controls the vibration (see Figure 3.6B), swinging continues unaltered until the outside force is removed. Such movement is called a **forced vibration.** When the external force is removed, the object simply reverts to a condition of free vibration, decreasing the distance of its swing until it becomes motionless. In both free and forced vibrations, the number of times the weight moves back and forth (the frequency) is unaltered by the distance of the swing (the amplitude). As the amplitude of particle movement decreases, the velocity of movement also decreases.

FIGURE 3.5 The effects of energy on a vibrating object. The object is at rest at point A. At point B, maximum excursion from the resting position has occurred, and all motion stops prior to the return swing. At point B, all energy is potential with zero kinetic energy. At point C, maximum velocity is reached, so all energy is kinetic and none is potential. Swinging slows down as point D is approached (the same as at point B), and when point D is reached, all energy is potential again.

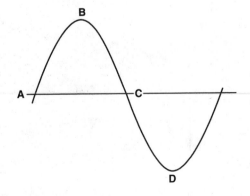

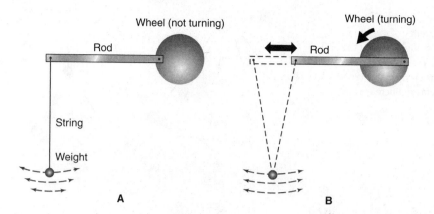

FIGURE 3.6 Free and forced vibrations. If the weight at the end of the string in A is pushed, the swinging back and forth decreases until it stops. If the rod is caused to move back and forth because of the motion of the wheel (B), the distance of the swing of the weight remains uniform until the wheel ceases to turn. A illustrates free vibration; B, forced vibration.

Frequency

You may ask how often, or how frequently, an event occurs during some period of time. Occurrences may be rated by using units such as the day or minute; in acoustics, however, when referring to events per unit of time, the duration usually used is the second. Consider the familiar metronome, whose pendulum swings back and forth. Any time the pendulum has moved from any still position to the far right, then past the original position to the far left, and then back to the point of origin, one cycle has occurred. Other motions, such as from far left to far right and back again, would also constitute one cycle. If the time required to complete a cycle is one second, it could be said that the frequency is 1 cycle per second (cps). For some time the term **hertz (Hz),** [2] instead of cps, has been adopted as the unit of frequency. The metronome may be adjusted so that the swings of the pendulum occur twice as often. In this way each journey of the pendulum must be made in half the time. This would mean that the time required for each cycle (the **period**) is cut to one-half second. Consequently, the frequency is doubled to 2 Hz. This reciprocal relationship between frequency and period always exists and may be expressed as:

$$Period = 1/frequency$$

Effects of Length on Frequency

With a little imagination, the swinging of an object suspended at the end of a string can be seen to move slowly back and forth (see Figure 3.7A). If the length of the string were suddenly shortened by holding it closer to the weight (see Figure 3.7B), the number of swings per second would increase, causing the weight to swing back and forth more frequently. Thus, as length decreases, frequency increases. Conversely, as length increases, the number of hertz decreases. The musical harp exemplifies the effects of length on frequency: As the strings get shorter, they are easily seen (and heard) to vibrate at a higher frequency. For a demonstration of frequency, see the video entitled Sound Waveforms.

Effects of Mass on Frequency

A greater **mass** of an oscillating system results in a decrease in velocity to keep the kinetic energy constant. Simply stated, as the mass is increased, the frequency of vibration is decreased. For example, consider that the increased thickness of the larger strings of a harp produces lower notes.

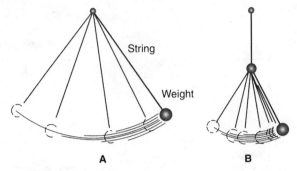

FIGURE 3.7 Effects of the length of a pendulum on the frequency of the vibration. Given a length of string, the weight at the end swings back and forth a specific number of times per second. If the string is shortened (B), the weight swings faster (increase in frequency).

Effects of Stiffness on Frequency

As a body vibrates, it exhibits a certain amount of compliance (the reciprocal of **stiffness**). As the compliance increases, the frequency at which the body is most easily made to vibrate (the resonant frequency) decreases. Systems that have more elasticity vibrate better at higher frequencies than at lower frequencies.

Resonance

Almost any mass, regardless of size, may be set into vibration. Because of its inherent properties, each mass has a frequency at which it vibrates most naturally—that is, the frequency at which it is most easily set into vibration and at which the magnitude of vibration is greatest and decays most slowly. The natural rate of vibration of a mass is called its **resonant frequency.** Although a mass may be set into vibration by a frequency other than its resonant frequency, when the external force is removed, the oscillation reverts to the resonant frequency until it is damped.

Musical notes have been said to shatter a drinking glass. This is accomplished when the resonant frequency of the glass is produced, and the **amplitude** of the sound (the pressure wave) is increased until the glass is set into vibration that is sympathetic to (the same as) the sound source. If the glass is made to vibrate with sufficient amplitude, its shape becomes so distorted that it shatters.

Sound Velocity

The **velocity** of a sound wave is the speed with which it travels from the source to another point. Sound velocity is determined by a number of factors, one of the most important of which is the density of the medium. As stated earlier, molecules are packed closer together in a solid than in a liquid or gas, and more closely in some solids (or liquids or gases) than in others. The closer together the molecules, the shorter the journey each particle makes before striking its neighbor, and the more quickly the adjacent molecules can be set into motion. Therefore, sounds travel faster through a solid than through a liquid and faster through a liquid than through a gas. In audiology, our concern is with the movement of sound through air. The velocity of sound in air is approximately 344 meters (1,130 feet) per second at standard temperature-pressure conditions (20° Celsius at sea level). When temperature and humidity are increased, the speed of sound increases. At higher altitudes the speed of sound is reduced because the distance between molecules is greater.

The velocity of sound may be determined at a specific moment; this is called the instantaneous velocity. In many cases, sound velocity fluctuates as the wave moves through a medium. In such cases, the average velocity of the wave may be determined by dividing the distance traveled by the time interval required for passage. Although we often think of velocity in miles per hour (mph), we can shift our thinking to meters per second (m/s) or centimeters per second (cm/s). When velocity is increased, acceleration takes place. When velocity is decreased, deceleration occurs.

As a solid object moves through air, it pushes the air molecules it strikes out of the way, setting up a wave motion. If the object itself exceeds the speed of sound, it causes a great compression ahead of itself, leaving a partial vacuum behind. The compressed molecules rushing in to fill the vacuum result in a sudden overpressure, called the sonic boom. An aircraft flying faster than the speed of sound is first seen to pass by; followed by the boom; followed by the sound of the aircraft approaching, flying overhead, and departing. The loud sound of a gun discharging is made not so much by the explosion of gunpowder as by the breaking of the sound barrier (exceeding the speed of sound) as the bullet leaves the barrel.

Wavelength

A characteristic of sound proportionately related to frequency is **wavelength.** The length of a wave is measured from any point on a sinusoid (any degree from 0 to 360) to the same point on the next cycle of the wave (see Figure 3.8). The formula for determining wavelength is $w = v/f$, where w = wavelength, v = the velocity of sound, and f = frequency. To solve for velocity, the formula $v = fw$ is used; to solve for frequency, $f = v/w$ is used. As frequency goes up, wavelength decreases. For example, the wavelength of a 250 Hz tone is 4.5 feet ($w = 1,130/250$), whereas the wavelength of an 8000 Hz tone is 0.14 feet ($w = 1,130/8,000$). Expressed in the metric system, the wavelength for a 250 Hz tone is 1.4 meters ($w = 344/250$) and for an 8000 Hz tone, 0.04 meters ($w = 344/8,000$).

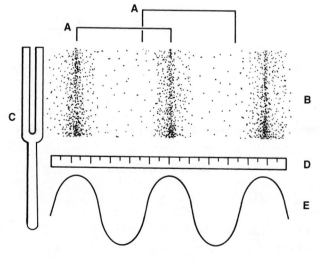

FIGURE 3.8 Wavelength (A) is measured from any point on the pressure wave to the same point (in degrees) on the next wave. Pressure waves (B) are set up in the air by the vibrating tines of the tuning fork (C). These waves move a given distance, as measured by the meter stick (D), and also may be displayed as a function of time (E).

Clinical **COMMENTARY**

A common complaint among those with hearing loss is difficulty hearing someone speaking from another room. The reason for this difficulty is more easily understood when one is familiar with the wavelength of sounds. The longer wavelengths of the lower-frequency sounds of vowels move around corners and obstructions more easily than do the shorter wavelengths of the higher frequencies contained in many of the consonants of speech. For a demonstration of the effects of frequency on wavelength, see the video entitled Sound Waveforms.

Phase

It is convenient to discuss the relationships among corresponding points on different waves in terms of the angular measurements used to describe circular motion. Any point on a sine wave (expressed in degrees) may be compared to a standard. This standard is considered to be 0 degrees. If an oscillation has a beginning at 0 (or 360) degrees, it is said to be in **phase** with the standard (see Figure 3.9A). Tones presented out of phase (see Figure 3.9B, C, and D) are discussed in terms of differences in degrees from the standard function of time.

Interference

Whenever more than one tone is introduced, there are interactions among sound waves. Such interactions are determined by the frequency, intensity, and phase relationships of the different waves. At any given moment, the instantaneous amplitudes of concurrent sound waves

FIGURE 3.9 Relationship of phase on four waves of identical frequency.

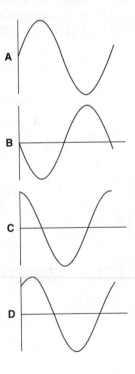

are summed. Two tones of the same frequency and phase relationship reinforce each other, increasing the amplitude. Two tones of identical frequency, but 180 degrees out of phase, cancel each other, resulting in 0 amplitude at any given moment. Away from laboratory conditions, there are usually more than two concomitant signals, so complete **cancellation** and complete reinforcement rarely occur in the real world.

Beats

When two tones of almost identical frequency are presented (e.g., 1000 and 1003 Hz), there is a noticeable increase and decrease in the resulting sound intensity, which is determined by the separation of the tones in frequency (in this illustration, 3 Hz). These changes in amplitude are perceived as **beats.** When one hears two tones of different frequencies, and the difference between the two frequencies is increased, the number of beats per second increases, changing to a pulsing, then to a roughness, and finally to a series of complex sounds. Depending on the starting frequency, when the difference in frequency between two tones becomes large enough, the ear recognizes a number of tones, including the higher one, the lower one, the **difference tone,** and the summation tone, all of which may be expressed in hertz as multiples of the original two tones.

Complex Sounds

Pure tones, as described in this chapter, seldom appear in nature. When they are created, it is usually by devices such as tuning forks or electronic sine-wave generators. Most sounds, therefore, are characterized as containing energy at a number of different frequencies, amplitudes, and phase relationships. Fourier[3] first showed that any **complex wave** can be analyzed in terms of its sinusoidal **components.**

Fundamental Frequency

When a number of pure tones are presented, one of them will naturally have a frequency lower than the others. The lowest rate of a sound's vibration is called the **fundamental frequency,** which is determined by the physical properties of the vibrating body. Some complex sounds repeat over time, as do many of the sounds of speech and music. Such sounds are called **periodic sounds. Aperiodic sounds** vary randomly over time, do not have fundamental frequencies, and are usually perceived as noise.

Harmonics

In a periodic complex sound, all frequencies are whole-number multiples of the fundamental. These tones, which occur over the fundamental, are called **harmonics** or **overtones.** The **spectrum** of a sound with a 100 Hz fundamental would therefore contain only higher frequencies of 200 Hz, 300 Hz, 400 Hz, and so on. With respect to periodic signals, the only difference between overtones and harmonics is the way in which they are numbered: The first harmonic is the fundamental frequency, the second harmonic is twice the fundamental, and so on. The first overtone is equal to the second harmonic, and further overtones are numbered consecutively.

Spectrum of a Complex Sound

When two or more pure tones of different frequencies are generated simultaneously, their combined amplitudes must be summed at each instant in time. This is illustrated in Figure 3.10, which shows that a new and slightly different waveform appears. Adding a fourth and fifth tone would further alter the waveform. Complex waves of this nature can be synthesized in the laboratory and constitute, in essence, the opposite of a **Fourier analysis.**

Although the fundamental frequency determines all the harmonic frequencies, the harmonics do not all have equal amplitude (see Figure 3.11A). In any wind instrument, the fundamental frequency is determined by a vibrating body: in a clarinet, the reed; in a trombone, the lips within the mouthpiece; and in that peculiar wind instrument called the human vocal tract, the vocal folds in the larynx. The length and cross-sectional areas of any of these wind instruments may be varied: in the trombone, by moving the slide; in the clarinet, by depressing keys; and in the vocal tract, by raising or lowering the tongue and moving it forward or back. In this way, even though the fundamental and harmonic frequencies may be the same, the amplitudes of different harmonics vary from instrument to instrument, resulting in the different harmonic spectrum (see Figure 3.11B and C) and characteristic qualities of each.

FIGURE 3.10 Synthesis of a complex waveform (D) from three sine waves (A, B, C) of different frequency and/or amplitude. Note that the amplitudes are summed at each moment in time, resulting in a new waveform.

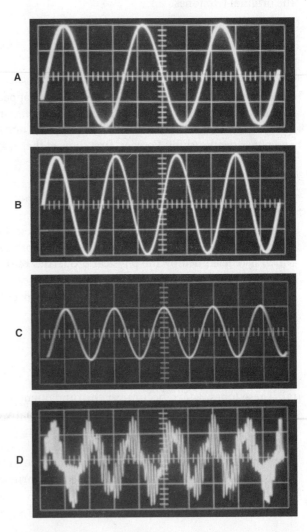

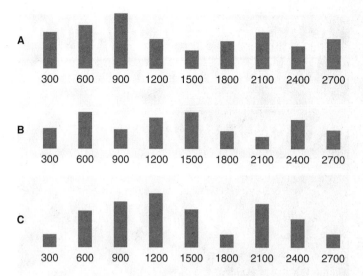

FIGURE 3.11 Histograms showing the spectra of three wind instruments. The fundamental frequency is the same in each (300 Hz), but the amplitudes of the harmonics differ.

During speech, altering the size and shape of the vocal tract, mostly by moving the tongue, results in frequency and intensity changes that emphasize some harmonics and suppress others. The resulting waveform has a series of peaks and valleys. Each of the peaks is called a **formant,** and it is manipulation of formant frequencies that facilitates the recognition of different vowel sounds. The peaks are numbered consecutively and are expressed as the lowest, or first, formant (F1), the second formant (F2), and so on. The spectrum of a musical wind instrument may be similar to that of a vowel and is also determined by the resonances of the acoustic systems.

Once the harmonic structure of a wave has been determined by the fundamental, the fundamental is no longer critical for the clear perception of a sound for persons with normal hearing. This is exemplified by the telephone, which does not allow frequencies below about 300 Hz to pass through. Although a man's fundamental vocal frequency averages about 85 to 150 Hz and a woman's about 175 to 250 Hz (both the consequences of laryngeal size, shape, and subglottal pressure), the sex of the speakers, as well as their identities, is often evident over a telephone even though the fundamental frequency is filtered out.

Intensity

Up to this point, we have concerned ourselves with the frequency of vibration and its related functions. It is important that we know not only how fast but also how far a body vibrates—its **intensity.** Figure 3.12A shows two tones of identical frequency; however, there is a difference in the maximum excursions of the two waves. Obviously, a greater **force** has been applied to the wave on the top than to the wave on the bottom to cause this difference to occur. The distance the mass moves from the point of rest is called its amplitude. Because our concern is with particle motion in air, it is assumed that if a greater force is applied to air molecules, they will move further from their points of rest, causing greater compressions and greater rarefactions, increasing the particle displacement and therefore the amplitude. Figure 3.12B shows two tones of identical amplitude and starting phase but of different frequency. Figure 3.12C shows two tones with the same amplitude and frequency but different phase.

FIGURE 3.12 (A) Two tones of different amplitude (frequency and phase constant), (B) two tones of different frequency (amplitude and phase constant), and (C) two tones differing in phase (amplitude and frequency constant).

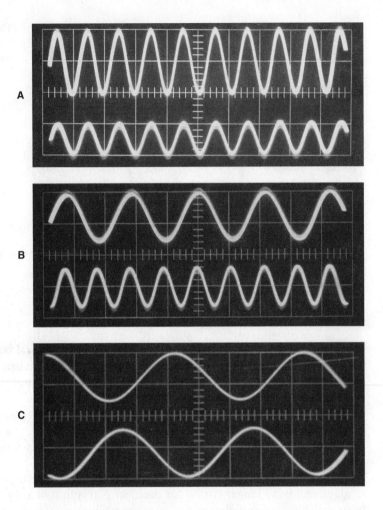

Force

When vibrating bodies, such as the tines of a tuning fork, move to and fro, they exert a certain amount of force on adjacent air molecules. The greater the force, the greater the displacement of the tines, and therefore the greater the amplitude of the sound wave. Because of the human ear's extreme sensitivity to sound, only very small amounts of force are required to stimulate hearing. The **dyne (d)** is a convenient unit of measurement for quantifying small changes in force.

One dyne is a force sufficient to accelerate a mass of 1 gram at 1 centimeter per second squared. If a mass of 1 gram (1/30 ounce) is held at sea level, the force of gravity on this mass is about 1,000 dynes. The **Newton (N)**[4] has been used more recently as a force measurement in the United States. One Newton is a force that accelerates a 1 kg mass at $1 \, m/s^2$.

Pressure

Pressure is generated whenever force is distributed over a surface area. An example is the number of pounds per square inch used in tire-pressure measurements. Normal atmospheric pressure is $14.7 \, lb/in^2$, 1 million dynes/cm^2, or 105 **Pascals (Pa)**.[5] If a given area remains constant, the pressure increases as the force is increased.

A word might be said here regarding units of measurement. The metric centimeter-gram-second (CGS) system has been popular among scientists in the United States for many years, but is being replaced by the meter-kilogram-second (MKS) system. What might eventually be used exclusively is the International System of Units, abbreviated SI, taken from the French Le Système International d'Unites. In the CGS system, pressure is expressed in dynes/cm^2, and in the SI system, it is expressed as Pascals.

Because of the sensitivity of human hearing, micropascals—millionths of a Pascal (μPa)—are used to express sound pressure in the audible range of intensities for humans and most animals. The smallest pressure variation required to produce a just-audible sound to healthy young ears is approximately 0.0002 dyne/cm^2, or 20 μPa. Sound waves that may be damaging to the ear have a pressure of about $2 \times 10^8 \mu$Pa.

Work

When any mass, such as a group of air particles, is moved, a certain amount of **work** is done as energy is expended. The amount of work done may be expressed as the force exerted times the distance the mass is moved. One **erg (e)** is the amount of work done when a 1 dyne force displaces an object by 1 cm; one **joule (J)**[6] is 10 million ergs.

Power

Power is the capacity to exert physical force or energy and is expressed as the rate at which energy is expended. Familiar units of power are horsepower and watts.[7] Because human hearing is extremely sensitive, small units of power, such as the erg per second, are used in acoustics. One watt is equal to 1 million ergs/second or 10^{21} joule per second, and 1 horsepower is equal to 746 watts. Power is a common measure of the magnitude of a sound. As the distance from the source is increased, the sound energy that reaches a given point decreases because the sound's power is spread out over a larger area.

Intensity of a Sound Wave

In any vibration, more air particles are displaced as the distance from the source increases. However, when the intensity of sound is measured, interest is usually centered on a small area at the point of measurement. The intensity of a sound wave is the amount of force per unit of area. It decreases proportionately to the square of the distance from the sound source (the **inverse square law**), so an intensity of 10^{-12} watt/m^2 (or 10^{-16} watt/cm^2) at 1000 Hz will produce a just-audible sound if that intensity reaches the ear.

Assuming that sound radiates in a spherical pattern from a source, this relationship can be expressed by the following formula:

$$\text{Intensity} \left(\text{watts/cm}^2 \text{ or watts/m}^2 \right) = \frac{\text{power (watts)}}{4\pi \times \text{radius}^2 \text{ (cm or m)}}$$

Common units of measurement, such as the pound or the mile, are additive in nature. As an example, ten 1-pound weights equal exactly 10 pounds. However, because the range of human hearing is so great, using such units results in very large, cumbersome numbers. It is convenient to discuss one intensity in terms of the number of times it is multiplied by another intensity—that is, in terms of a ratio between the two. The **decibel (dB)** is commonly used for this purpose.

The Decibel

A convenient way of expressing a ratio between two lengthy numbers is to use the **logarithm.** One unit established in such a way is the **Bel,** named for Alexander Graham Bell.[8] Because a Bel may have a rather large value, the decibel, which is one-tenth of a Bel, is the unit of measurement of intensity used in acoustics and in audiometrics.

Five important aspects of the decibel must be remembered: (1) It involves a ratio; (2) it utilizes a logarithm; (3) it is therefore nonlinear; (4) it may be expressed in terms of various reference levels, which must be specified; and (5) it is a relative unit of measure.

Logarithms

A logarithm (log) is simply a number expressed as an **exponent** (or power) that tells how often a number (the base) is multiplied by itself. In the expression 10^2 (ten squared), the log (2) tells us that the base (10) is multiplied by itself one time ($10 \times 10 = 100$). The exponent is the power, which tells us how many times the base is used in multiplication (e.g., $10^3 = 10 \times 10 \times 10 = 1,000$).

Although any base may be used, the base 10 is most common in acoustics. This is convenient because the log simply tells how many zeros appear after the 1. Table 3.1A and B shows a natural progression of logarithms with the base 10. It is important to note that the log of 1 is zero.

The logarithm is useful in expressing a **ratio** between two numbers. Remember that a ratio is shown when any number is divided by another number. If a number is divided by itself (e.g., $25 \div 25$), the ratio is always one to one (1:1), a fact regardless of the magnitude of the numbers. When numbers with identical bases are used in division, the log of the denominator is subtracted from the log of the numerator (e.g., $10^3 \div 10^2 = 10^1$). These mathematics do not change, regardless of whether the numerator or the denominator is the larger (e.g., $10^2 \div 10^3 = 10^{-1}$). When a ratio is expressed as a fraction, the denominator becomes the reference to which the numerator is compared. Ratios expressed without a specific reference are totally meaningless, as in those commercial ads that claim a product is twice as good, three times as bright, or 100 percent faster, and so on, without saying what it is better, brighter, or faster than.

Intensity Level

Under some circumstances, it is useful to express the decibel with an intensity reference. A practical unit in such cases is the watt per meter squared (watt/m^2). The intensity reference in a given system may be expressed as I_R (the number of **watts** of the reference intensity). The output (e.g., a loudspeaker) of the system may be expressed as I_O, so that a ratio may be set up between the intensity reference and the intensity output. In solving for the number of decibels using an intensity reference, the formula is

$$dB = 10 \times \log (I_O/I_R)$$

The usual intensity reference (I_R) is 10^{-12} watt/m^2 (or sometimes 10^{-16} watt/cm^2), although this may be changed if desired. The exponent tells the number of places the decimal points must be moved to the right or left of the number 1. If the exponent is positive (or unsigned), the number of zeros is added following the 1. If the exponent is negative, the number of zeros placed before the 1 is equal to the exponent minus 1, with a decimal point before the zeros. If the exponent is positive, it suggests a large number; if it is negative, it

TABLE 3.1 Ratios, Logarithms, and Outputs for Determining Number of Decibels with Intensity and Pressure References

A Ratio	B Log	C Intensity Outputs (I_O) CGS (watt/cm²)	C Intensity Outputs (I_O) SI (watt/m²)	D dB IL*	E Equal Amplitudes	F dB SPL†	G Pressure Outputs (P_O) CGS (dyne/cm²)	G Pressure Outputs (P_O) SI (μPa)
1:1	0	10^{-16}	10^{-12}	0	Threshold of Audibility	0	.0002	$20.0 \ (2 \times 10^1)$
10:1	1	10^{-15}	10^{-11}	10		20	.002	$200.0 \ (2 \times 10^2)$
100:1	2	10^{-14}	10^{-10}	20		40	.02	$2,000.0 \ (2 \times 10^3)$
1,000:1	3	10^{-13}	10^{-9}	30		60	.2	$20,000.0 \ (2 \times 10^4)$
10,000:1	4	10^{-12}	10^{-8}	40		80	2.0	$200,000.0 \ (2 \times 10^5)$
100,000:1	5	10^{-11}	10^{-7}	50		100	20.0	$2,000,000.0 \ (2 \times 10^6)$
1,000,000:1	6	10^{-10}	10^{-6}	60		120	200.0	$20,000,000.0 \ (2 \times 10^7)$
10,000,000:1	7	10^{-9}	10^{-5}	70		140	2000.0	$200,000,000.0 \ (2 \times 10^8)$
100,000,000:1	8	10^{-8}	10^{-4}	80				
1,000,000,000:1	9	10^{-7}	10^{-3}	90				
10,000,000,000:1	10	10^{-6}	10^{-2}	100				
100,000,000,000:1	11	10^{-5}	10^{-1}	110				
1,000,000,000,000:1	12	10^{-4}	10^{0}	120				
10,000,000,000,000:1	13	10^{-3}	10^{1}	130				
100,000,000,000,000:1	14	10^{-2}	10^{2}	140	Threshold of Pain			

*The number of dB with an intensity reference ($I_R = 10^{-12} watt/m^2$) uses the formula: $dB \ (IL) = 10 \times \log (I_O/I_R)$.

†The number of dB with a pressure reference ($P^R = 20 \ \mu Pa$) uses the formula: $dB \ (SPL) = 20 \times \log (P_O/P_R)$.

suggests a small number, less than 1. Therefore, 10^{-12} watt/m^2 is an extremely small quantity (0.000000000001 watt/m^2).

If the intensity reference of a sound system (I_R) is known, the preceding equation may be used to determine the number of decibels of the output above (or below) the reference. As mentioned earlier, it is essential that the reference always be stated. When the reference is 10^{-12} watt/m^2, the term **intensity level (IL)** may be used as shorthand to imply this reference.

If the intensity output and the intensity reference are exactly the same ($I_O = I_R$), the ratio is 1:1. Because the log of 1 is 0, use of the formula shows the number of decibels to be 0. Therefore, 0 dB does not mean that sound is absent, but rather that the intensity output is the same as the intensity reference. If I_O were changed to 10^1 watt/m^2, the number of decibels (IL) would be 130. Table 3.1 shows that as the intensity output (C) increases, the ratio (A) increases, raising the power of the log (B) and increasing the number of decibels (D).

Remember that the decibel is a logarithmic expression. When the intensity of a wave is doubled—for example, by adding a second loudspeaker with a sound of identical intensity to the first—the number of decibels is not doubled but is increased by three. This occurs because the intensity outputs of the two signals, and not the number of decibels, are added algebraically according to the principles of wave interference and the rules for working with logs. For example, if loudspeaker A creates a sound of 60 dB IL (10^{-6} watt/m^2) and loudspeaker B also creates a sound of 60 dB IL (10^{-6} watt/m^2) to the same point in space, the result is 63 dB IL (2×10^{-6} watt/m^2).

Sound-Pressure Level

Audiologists and acousticians are more accustomed to making measurements of sound in pressure than in intensity terms. Such measurements are usually expressed as **sound-pressure level (SPL)**. Because intensity is known to be proportional to the square of pressure, the conversion from intensity to pressure may be made as follows:

$$\text{Intensity reference: dB (IL)} = 10 \times \log (I_O/I_R)$$

$$\text{Pressure reference: dB (SPL)} = 10 \times \log (P_O{}^2/P_R{}^2)$$

Intensity is proportional to pressure squared, so to determine the number of decibels from a pressure reference, I_R may be written as $P_R{}^2$ (pressure reference) and I_O may be written as $P_O{}^2$ (pressure output). It is a mathematical rule that when a number is squared, its log is multiplied by 2; therefore, the formula for dB SPL may be written as:

$$\text{dB (SPL)} = 10 \times \log (P_O{}^2/P_R{}^2)$$

$$\text{or}$$

$$\text{dB (SPL)} = 10 \times 2 \times \log (P_O/P_R)$$

$$\text{or}$$

$$\text{dB (SPL)} = 20 \times \log (P_O/P_R)$$

As in the case of decibels with an intensity reference, when P_O is the same as P_R, the ratio between the two is 1:1 and the number of decibels (SPL) is zero. Just as in the case of intensity, 0 dB SPL does not mean silence; it means only that the output pressure is 0 dB above the reference pressure.

One dyne/cm^2 is equal to 1 **microbar** (μ**bar**) (one-millionth of normal barometric pressure at sea level), so the two terms are frequently used interchangeably. The pressure of 0.0002 dyne/cm^2 has been the sound-pressure reference in physics and acoustics for some time. It is being replaced, however, by its SI equivalent, 20 micropascals (μPa). This is the reference used for most **sound-level meters** (see Figure 3.13), devices designed to measure the sound-pressure levels in various acoustical environments. Therefore, 20 μPa is 0 dB SPL. The threshold of pain at the ear is reached at 140 dB SPL. The term *dB SPL* implies a pressure reference of 20 μPa. Table 3.1 shows that increases in the number of μPa (or dyne/cm^2) (G) is reflected in the ratio (A), the log (B), and the number of dB SPL (F).

Because the decibel expresses a ratio between two sound intensities or two sound pressures, decibel values cannot be simply added and subtracted. Therefore, 60 dB plus 60 dB does not equal 120 dB. When sound-pressure values are doubled, the number of decibels is increased by six. Therefore, 60 dB (20,000 μPa) plus 60 dB (20,000 μPa) equals 66 dB (40,000 μPa). In actual fact, the SPL increases by a factor of 3 dB unless the two waves are in perfect correspondence. Also, because of the special relationship between intensity and sound pressure, a 6 dB increase will be shown if the number of loudspeakers is quadrupled, unless they are all in phase.

Note that the amplitude of a wave, whether expressed in decibels with an intensity reference or a pressure reference (see columns C and G in Table 3.1), is the same as long as the number of decibels is the same. Intensity and pressure are simply different ways of looking at the same wave. Column E of Table 3.1 is designed to illustrate this point.

Hearing Level

The modern audiometer was designed as an instrument to test hearing sensitivity at a number of different frequencies. Originally, each audiometer manufacturer determined the SPL required to barely stimulate the hearing of an average normal-hearing individual. Needless to

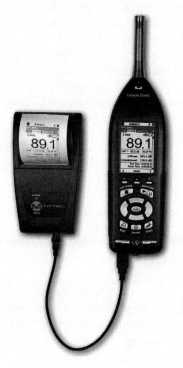

FIGURE 3.13 A commercial sound-level meter designed to measure the sound-pressure levels in various acoustical environments. (*Source:* Soundtrack LXT photo courtesy of Larson-Davis Laboratory, a Division of PCB Piezotronics, Inc. [www.larsondavis.com])

say, there were some differences from manufacturer to manufacturer. Studies were then conducted (e.g., Beasley, 1938) in which the hearing of many young adults was carefully measured. The resulting data culminated in the standard adopted in 1951 by the American Standards Association (ASA). This organization has been renamed the **American National Standards Institute (ANSI).**

The lowest sound intensity that stimulates normal hearing is called zero **hearing level (HL).** Because the ear shows different amounts of sensitivity to different frequencies (being most sensitive in the 1000 to 4000 Hz range), different amounts of pressure are required for 0 dB HL at different frequencies. Even early audiometers were calibrated so that hearing could be tested over a wide range of intensities, up to 110 dB HL (above normal hearing thresholds) at some frequencies. The pressure reference for decibels on an audiometer calibrated to ASA-1951 specifications was therefore different at each frequency, but the hearing-level dial was calibrated with reference to normal hearing (audiometric zero).

An international organization covering 148 countries (with one member per country) was created to establish a wide variety of standards in various practices. This organization is called the International Organization for Standardization and has a Central Secretariat in Geneva, Switzerland, where the organization is based. It was recognized that a single international abbreviation was needed for the organization to be recognized around the world, but due to differences in languages this presented a problem. For example, the abbreviation would be "IOS" in English, "OIN" in French (for Organisation Internationale de Normalisation), and so on. The decision was to use a word derived from the Greek *isos,* meaning, "equal." Therefore, the organization's name is ISO in all countries regardless of language.

Audiometers manufactured in different countries had slightly different SPL values for audiometric zero until a standard close to what had been used in Great Britain was adopted by the **International Organization for Standardization (ISO).** This revised standard, which was called ISO-1964, showed normal hearing to be more sensitive than the 1951 ASA values, resulting in a lowering of the SPL values averaging approximately 10 dB across frequencies. Differences between the two standards probably occurred because of differences in the studies during which normative data were compiled, in terms of test environment, equipment, and procedure.

Audiologists who had experience testing normal-hearing persons on the ASA standard had noted that many such subjects had hearing better than the zero reference, often in the −10 dB HL range, and welcomed the conversion to the ISO standard. More recently, a new American standard has been published by the American National Standards Institute (American National Standards Institute, 2004) showing SPL values for normal hearing using supra-aural audiometer earphones close to the ISO levels (see Table 3.2). These values are termed the reference equivalent threshold sound-pressure levels (RETSPLs).

Sensation Level

Another reference for the decibel may be the auditory **threshold** of a given individual. The threshold of a pure tone is usually defined as the level at which the tone is so soft that it can be perceived only 50 percent of the time it is presented; however, the 50 percent response criterion is purely arbitrary. The number of decibels of a sound above the threshold of a given individual is the sound's **sensation level (SL)** in decibels.

If a person can barely hear a tone at 5 dB HL at a given frequency, a tone presented at 50 dB HL is 45 dB above his or her threshold, or, stated another way, 45 dB SL. The same 50 dB HL tone presented to a person with a 20 dB threshold has a sensation level of 30 dB. It is important to recognize that a tone presented at threshold has a sensation level of 0 dB. To state the number of dB SL, the threshold of the individual (the reference) must be known.

TABLE 3.2 Reference Equivalent Threshold Sound Pressure Levels (RETSPLs) (dB re 20 μPa) for Supra-Aural Earphones (ANSI, 2004)

Frequency Hz	TDH Type JE318C IEC318	TDH 39 NBS9A	TDH 49/50 BS9A
125	45.0	45.0	47.5
160	38.5		
200	32.5		
250	27.0	25.5	26.5
315	22.0		
400	17.0		
500	13.5	11.5	13.5
630	10.5		
750	9.0	8.0	8.5
800	8.5		
1000	7.5	7.0	7.5
1250	7.5		
1500	7.5	6.5	7.5
1600	8.0		
2000	9.0	9.0	11.0
2500	10.5		
3000	11.5	10.0	9.5
3150	11.5		
4000	12.0	9.5	10.5
5000	11.0		
6000	16.0	15.5	13.5
6300	21.0		
8000	15.5	13.0	13.0
Speech	20.0	19.5	20.0

Environmental Sounds

Earlier we saw that the range of sound intensities, from threshold of audibility to pain in the ear, is extremely wide. All of the sounds that normal-hearing persons may hear without discomfort must be found within this range. Table 3.3 gives examples of some ordinary environmental sounds and their approximate intensities. This table may help the reader to develop a framework from which to approximate the intensities of other sounds.

Psychoacoustics

Thus far in this chapter, attention has been focused on physical acoustics. These factors are the same with or without human perception. It is also important that consideration be allocated to psychoacoustics, the study of the relationship between physical stimuli and the psychological responses to which they give rise.

Pitch

Pitch is a term used to describe the subjective impressions of the "highness" or "lowness" of a sound. Pitch relates to frequency; in general, pitch rises as the frequency of vibration increases, at least within the range of human hearing (20 to 20,000 Hz). The Western world uses the

TABLE 3.3 Scale of Intensities for Ordinary Environmental Sounds

Decibels*	Sound
0	Just audible sound
10	Soft rustle of leaves
20	A whisper at 4 feet
30	A quiet street in the evening with no traffic
40	Night noises in the city
50	A quiet automobile 10 feet away
60	Department store
70	Busy traffic
60–70	Normal conversation at 3 feet
80	Heavy traffic
80–90	Niagara Falls
90	Truck traffic
100	Snowmobile, Motorcycle
110	iPod at full volume (average)
115	Loud rock concert
120	Amplified rock music at 4 to 6 feet
125	Pain begins
140	Even short-term exposure can cause permanent hearing loss
165	12 gauge shotgun blast
194	Highest level sound possible

*The reference is 10^{-16} watt/cm^2.
Sources: Van Bergeijk, Pierce, & David, 1960; http://www.gcaudio.com/resources/howtos/loudness.html.

octave scale in its music. When frequency is doubled, it is raised one octave, but raising (or lowering) a sound one octave does not double (or halve) its pitch. Intensity also contributes to the perception of pitch, although to a lesser extent than does frequency. For a demonstration of the effects of frequency on pitch perception, see the video entitled Sound Waveforms.

The subjective aspect of pitch can be measured by using a unit called the mel. One thousand mels is the pitch of a 1000 Hz tone at 40 dB SL. Frequencies can be adjusted so that they sound twice as high (2000 mels), half as high (500 mels), and so on. Except for the fact that the number of mels increases and decreases with frequency, apart from 1,000 Hz, the numbers do not correspond. Although the task sounds formidable, pitch scaling can be accomplished on cooperative, normal-hearing subjects with great accuracy after a period of training. The mel scale is illustrated in Figure 3.14.

Loudness

Loudness is a subjective experience, as contrasted with the purely physical force of intensity. The thinking reader has realized, to be sure, that a relationship exists between increased intensity and increased loudness. The decibel, however, is not a unit of loudness measurement, and thus such statements as "The noise in this room is 60 dB loud" are erroneous. The duration and frequency of sounds contribute to the sensation of loudness.

As stated earlier, the ear is not equally sensitive at all frequencies. It is also true that the subjective experience of loudness changes at different frequencies. Comparing the loudness of different frequencies to the loudness of a 1000 Hz tone at a number of intensity levels determines the **loudness level** of the different frequencies. Figure 3.15 shows that loudness grows faster for low-frequency tones and certain high-frequency tones than for mid-frequencies. The unit of loudness level is the **phon.**

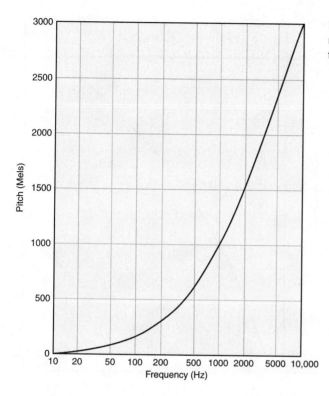

FIGURE 3.14 The mel scale, showing the relationship between pitch (in mels) and frequency (in hertz).

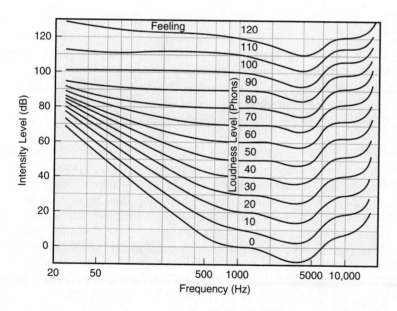

FIGURE 3.15 Equal loudness contours showing the relationship between loudness level (in phons) and intensity (in dB) as a function of frequency.

The term *sone* refers to the comparison of the loudness of a 1000 Hz tone at different intensities. One sone is the loudness of 1000 Hz at 40 dB SL. The intensity required for subjects to perceive half the loudness of 1 sone is 0.5 sone; the intensity for twice the loudness is 2 sones, and so forth. Loudness level (in phons) can be related to loudness (in sones) but, as Figure 3.16 shows, the measurements do not correspond precisely.

FIGURE 3.16 Loudness function showing the relationship between loudness (in sones) and loudness level (in phons).

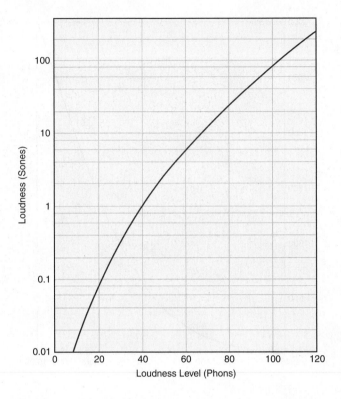

Localization

Hearing is a distance sense, unaffected by many barriers that interfere with sight, touch, and smell. Sound can bend around corners with little distortion, although as frequencies get higher, they become more unidirectional. Under many conditions it is possible, even without seeing the source of a sound, to tell the direction from which it comes. This ability, called **localization,** is a complex phenomenon resulting from the interaction of both ears. The localization of sound, which warned our ancestors of possible danger, was probably a major contributor to the early survival of our species.

Localization is possible because of the relative intensities of sounds and their times of arrival at the two ears (i.e., phase). The greatest single contributors to our ability to localize are interaural phase differences in the low frequencies (below 1500 Hz) and intensity differences in the higher frequencies. Naturally, in an acoustical environment with hard surfaces, reverberation may occur, and the sound may be perceived to come from a direction other than its source. An area in which there are no hard surfaces to cause reverberation is called a free field. Free fields actually exist only in exotic areas such as mountaintops and specially built anechoic chambers (see Figure 3.17).

Masking

When two sounds are heard simultaneously, the intensity of one sound may be sufficient to cause the other to be inaudible. This change in the threshold of a sound caused by a second sound with which it coexists is called **masking.** There is surely no one who has not experienced masking in noisy situations in the form of speech interference. The noise that causes the interference is called the masker. Because masking plays an important role in some aspects of clinical audiology, it is discussed in detail in Chapter 6.

FIGURE 3.17 The inside of an anechoic chamber designed to eliminate sound reverberation. (*Source:* Orfield Laboratories.)

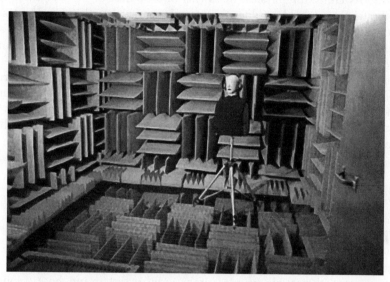

Impedance

Any moving object must overcome a certain amount of resistance to its movement. A sound wave moving through air strikes surfaces that impede or retard its progress. The impedance of a medium is the opposition it offers to the transmission of acoustic energy.

As a general rule, as a surface that is placed in the path of a sound wave is made more dense, it offers greater impedance to the wave. For example, when a sound strikes a closed door, some of the energy is reflected because the door is so much denser than the air on either side of it. If the sound is to be carried to the adjacent room, the door itself must be set into vibration, whereupon the opposite side of the door, moving against the air molecules in the next room, generates new sound waves. The amount of impedance of the door determines the amplitude of the waves in the next room. The greater the impedance of the door, the smaller the amplitude of the waves transmitted to the adjacent room.

Given sufficient energy to overcome its inertia, a mass may be set into vibration. The resonant characteristics of a body or medium determine its frequencies of most efficient and least efficient vibration. **Resonance** is determined by the mass, elasticity, and frictional characteristics of an object (or medium). Therefore, resonance characteristics are defined by impedance. In the case of sound moving past an object, like a door, there is more impedance to some frequencies than to others. As a rule, the mass of the door attenuates high-frequency sounds more than low-frequency sounds, which is what makes the sound on the opposite side of the door appear muffled.

Total impedance (Z) is determined by two factors. The first is simple resistance (R)—that is, resistance that is not influenced by frequency of vibration. This simple resistance is analogous to electrical resistance in a direct-current system, such as a battery, in which electrons move in a single direction from a negative to a positive pole. The second factor is complex resistance, or **reactance.** Reactance is influenced by frequency, so that the opposition to energy transfer varies with frequency. Reactance is seen in alternating-current electrical systems, such as household current, in which the flow of electrons is periodically reversed (60 Hz in the United States).

Total reactance is determined by two subsidiary factors called **mass reactance** and **stiffness reactance.** As either the physical mass (M) of an object or the frequency (f) at which the object vibrates is increased, so does the mass reactance. In other words, mass reactance is directly related to both mass and frequency. Stiffness (S) reactance behaves in an opposite manner. As the physical stiffness of an object increases, so does stiffness reactance. As frequency increases, however, stiffness reactance decreases (an inverse relationship).

Together, simple resistance, mass reactance, and stiffness reactance all contribute to the determination of total impedance. All four terms are given the same unit of measurement, the **ohm** (Ω).[9] In the formula for computing impedance, Z is the total impedance, R is the simple resistance, $2\pi fM$ is the mass reactance, and $S/2\pi f$ is the stiffness reactance. This equation shows that mass reactance and stiffness reactance combine algebraically:

$$Z = \sqrt{R^2 + \left(2\pi fM - \frac{S}{2\pi f}\right)^2}$$

Sound Measurement

Audiologists are generally interested in making two kinds of measurements: those of the hearing ability of patients with possible disorders of the auditory system and those of sound-pressure levels in the environment. The first modern step toward quantifying the amount of a patient's hearing loss came with the development of the pure-tone audiometer. This device allows for a comparison of any person's hearing threshold to that of an established norm. Hearing threshold is usually defined as the intensity at which a tone is barely audible. Hearing sensitivity is expressed as the number of decibels above (or below) the average normal-hearing person's thresholds for different pure tones (0 dB HL). Speech audiometers were designed, in part, to measure thresholds for the spoken word.

The Pure-Tone Audiometer

A pure-tone audiometer is diagrammed in Figure 3.18. It consists of an audio oscillator, which generates pure tones of different frequencies, usually at discrete steps of 125, 250, 500, 750, 1000, 1500, 2000, 3000, 4000, 6000, and 8000 Hz. Each tone is amplified to a maximum of about 110 dB HL in the frequency range of 500 to 4,000 Hz, with less output above and below those frequencies.

The tones are attenuated with the use of a manual dial or electronic attenuator, which is numbered (contrary to attenuation) in decibels above the normal threshold for each frequency. As the number of decibels is increased, the attenuation is decreased. The audiometer is provided with a silent switch that can introduce or interrupt a tone. The signal is routed, via an

FIGURE 3.18 Block diagram of a pure-tone audiometer.

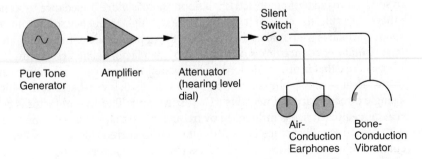

output selection control, to a right or left earphone or to a bone-conduction vibrator. A photograph of a pure-tone audiometer is shown in Figure 3.19.

Air Conduction

Earphones are held in place by a steel headband that fits over the top of the head. The phones themselves are connected to the headband by two small metal yokes. The earphone consists of a magnetic device that transduces the electrical translations supplied by the audiometer to a small diaphragm that vibrates according to the acoustic equivalents of frequency and intensity. Around the earphone is a rubber cushion that may fit around the ear (circumaural) or, more usually, over the ear (supra-aural). Circumaural earphones are rarely used with audiometers because they are difficult to calibrate. The movement of the earphone diaphragm generates the sound, which enters the ear directly, resulting in an air-conduction signal. Supra-aural audiometric earphones are shown in Figure 3.20.

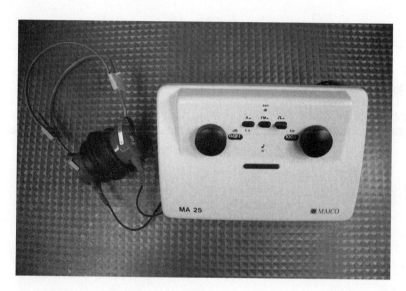

FIGURE 3.19 A pure-tone audiometer designed to deliver preselected frequencies at examiner-selected intensities to determine an individual's hearing sensitivity. (*Source:* MAICO.)

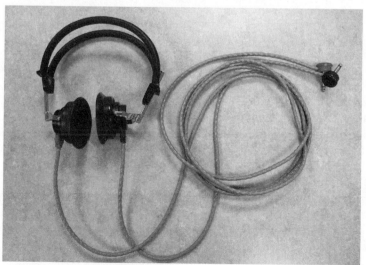

FIGURE 3.20 A set of supra-aural air-conduction receivers.

FIGURE 3.21 A pair of insert receivers.
(*Source:* Etymotic Research.)

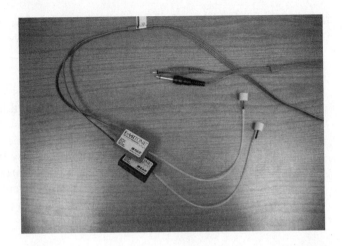

For some time it has been recognized that there are distinct advantages to using earphones that are inserted into the external ear canal for air-conduction testing. These advantages will be discussed in some detail later in this text, but one of them includes a significant increase in comfort for the patient. Insert earphones that are appropriate for audiometry are shown in Figure 3.21.

Clinical COMMENTARY

The sound pressure level to reach audiometric zero is different for supra-aural air conduction receivers (earphones) than it is for insert receivers (See Tables 3.2 and 3.5.) Accurate hearing test results cannot be attained when one earphone type is exchanged for another without recalibration.

Bone Conduction

Selection of the bone-conduction output of the audiometer causes the signal to terminate in a small plastic device with a slight concavity on one side for comfortable fit against the skull. The principle of the bone-conduction vibrator is the same as that of the air-conduction receiver except that, instead of moving a waferlike diaphragm, the plastic shell of the vibrator must be set into motion. Because they must vibrate a greater mass (the skull), bone-conduction vibrators require greater energy than air-conduction receivers to generate a vibration level high enough to stimulate normal hearing. For this reason, the maximum power outputs are considerably lower for bone conduction, usually not exceeding 50 to 80 dB HL, depending on frequency. Frequencies of 250 through 4000 Hz are usually available for bone-conduction testing.

The bone-conduction vibrator is held against the skull at either the forehead or the mastoid process. When the forehead is the placement site, a plastic strap is used that circles the head to hold the vibrator in place. When the bone behind the ear is the desired place for testing, a spring-steel headband that goes over the top of the skull is employed. A bone-conduction vibrator is shown in Figure 3.22.

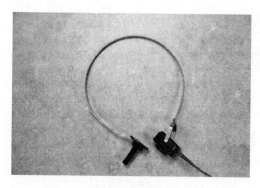

FIGURE 3.22 A bone-conduction vibrator through which pure tones may be routed using a pure-tone audiometer to measure bone-conduction sensitivity. (*Source:* Clark Audiology.)

The Speech Audiometer

As will be discussed later in this text, measurements made with speech stimuli are very helpful in the diagnosis of auditory disorders. A speech audiometer is required for such measurements. The speech audiometer is usually part of a clinical audiometer (see Figure 3.23) that can also perform pure-tone tests.

The diagram in Figure 3.24 shows that the speech circuit of an audiometer can have an input signal provided by a microphone, a compact disc (CD) player, or other audio imput. The input level of the speech signal is monitored by an averaging voltmeter called a volume units (VU) meter. Such a meter reads in dB VU, implying an electrical reference in watts. The signal is amplified and attenuated as in a pure-tone audiometer, with the hearing-level dial calibrated in decibels with reference to audiometric 0 for speech (20 dB SPL on the ANSI-2004 standard for a TDH-49 earphone). Some audiometers use light-emitting diodes in lieu of a VU meter.

Air Conduction

Most of the measurements made on speech audiometers are accomplished through air-conduction receivers. Testing may be carried out by selecting the right ear, the left ear, or both ears. The usual range is from −10 to 110 dB HL.

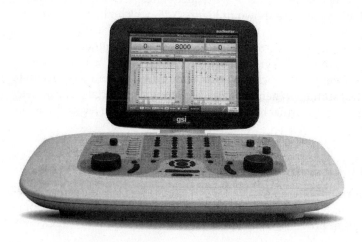

FIGURE 3.23 A diagnostic audiometer measures hearing sensitivity for speech and for tones via either air or bone conduction. (*Source:* Grason-Stadler Co.)

FIGURE 3.24 Block diagram of the speech circuit of a diagnostic audiometer.

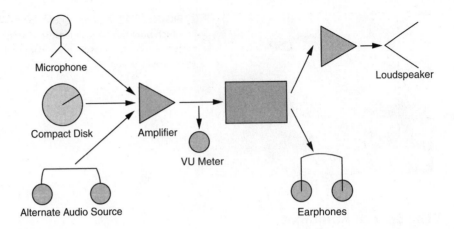

Sound Field

It is often desirable to test with speech in the sound field—that is, to feed the speech signal into the room rather than directly into the ears by using one or more loudspeakers. The signal generated by the audiometer is designed for air-conduction earphones and does not have sufficient power to drive a larger loudspeaker. When the speaker output of the audiometer is selected, the speech signal is fed to an auxiliary amplifier that augments the intensity of the signal, creating the additional power necessary to drive the loudspeaker.

Sound-Level Meters

As mentioned earlier, airborne sounds are measured by devices called sound-level meters. These consist of a microphone, amplifier, attenuator, and meter that pick up and transduce pressure waves in the air, measure them electrically, and read out the sound-pressure levels in decibels. The usual reference for sound-level meters is $20\,\mu\text{Pa}$.

Because the human ear responds differently to different frequencies, many sound-level meters contain systems called weighting networks, which are filters to alter the response of the instrument, much as the ear does at different levels. The phon lines (see Figure 3.15) show that the ear is not very sensitive to low frequencies at low SPLs and that, as the sound increases in intensity, the ear is capable of better and better low-frequency response. The three usual weighting networks of sound-level meters are shown in Figure 3.25, which illustrates how the meters respond.

Sound-level meters are useful in the study of acoustics and are common tools in industry as concern over noise pollution grows. Background noise levels can play a major role in the testing of hearing because, if they are sufficiently high, they may interfere with accurate measurement by masking the test stimuli. Whenever hearing testing is undertaken, especially with persons who have normal or near-normal hearing, the background noise levels should be known.

Acceptable Noise Levels for Audiometry

Table 3.4 shows the maximum room noise allowable for air-conduction testing using supra-aural and insert earphones on the ANSI-1999 scale. To determine the allowable levels for bone-conduction testing, the attenuation provided by the usual audiometer earphone and cushion

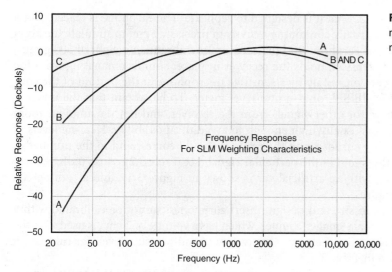

FIGURE 3.25 Weighting networks for sound-level meters.

TABLE 3.4 Maximum Permissible Ambient Noise Sound Pressure Levels in Octave Bands for Audiometric Testing with Ears Covered Using Supra-Aural or Insert Earphones and Test Frequency Ranges 125 to 8,000, 250 to 8,000, and 500 to 8,000 Hz*

Octave Band Intervals	Supra-Aural Earphones			Insert Earphones		
	125 to 8,000 Hz	250 to 8,000 Hz	500 to 8,000 Hz	125 to 8,000 Hz	250 to 8,000 Hz	500 to 8,000 Hz
125	35.0	39.0	49.0	59.0	67.0	78.0
250	25.0	25.0	35.0	53.0	53.0	64.0
500	21.0	21.0	21.0	50.0	50.0	50.0
1000	26.0	26.0	26.0	47.0	47.0	47.0
2000	34.0	34.0	34.0	49.0	49.0	49.0
4000	37.0	37.0	37.0	50.0	50.0	50.0
8000	37.0	37.0	37.0	56.0	56.0	56.0

*Table values are in dB re: 20 μPa rounded to the nearest 0.5 dB.
Source: American National Standards Institute, 1999.

must be subtracted from the maximum allowable levels for air conduction because the ear remains uncovered during bone-conduction audiometry.

Calibration of Audiometers

Although periodic factory checks on audiometer calibration are desirable, many audiologists also perform frequent checks on the operation of their equipment on-site in the clinic. In the early days of audiometers, checks on the reliability of the hearing level were conducted by testing a group of subjects with known normal hearing—the "psychoacoustic method." This is done by taking the median of the threshold findings and posting a correction chart on the audiometer to remind the audiologist to correct any readings obtained on a patient by the number of decibels the audiometer had drifted out of calibration.

Many audiology clinics today are equipped with meters and also couplers so that the task of level checking may be accomplished electroacoustically. The coupler is often called an **artificial ear** because that is what it is designed to replicate. The earphone is placed over a carefully machined coupler, usually containing a cavity of precisely 6 cm³ to simulate the average volume of air between the earphone and the eardrum membrane. A weight of 500 grams, or a spring with equivalent tension, holds the receiver in place. Sounds emanating from the diaphragm of the receiver are picked up by a sensitive microphone at the bottom of the coupler, amplified, and read in dB SPL on a sound-level meter. To be certain that the meter is reading the level of the tone (or other signal) from the receiver, and not the ambient room noise, the level of the signal is usually high enough to avoid this possibility. Hearing levels of 70 dB are convenient for this purpose, and the readout should correspond to the number of decibels required for the threshold of the particular signal (see Table 3.2), plus 70 dB. A form designed for level checking with an artificial ear is shown in Figure 3.26, and a commercial testing unit is shown in Figure 3.27.

Because of differences in size and design, insert earphones cannot be calibrated with a standard 6 cm³ coupler. Rather, a smaller coupler, which has a volume of 2 cm³, is used with the calibration device described earlier. Reference equivalent sound-pressure levels for calibrating insert earphones are shown in Table 3.5.

When calibrating the speech circuit of an audiometer, a signal must be fed through one of the inputs. A pure tone, a noise containing approximately equal intensity at all frequencies, or a sustained vowel sound, may be used. The signal is adjusted so that the VU or equivalent meter reads 0. With the hearing-level dial set at 70 dB, and with the earphone on the coupler, the signal should read 90 dB SPL on the meter (70 dB HL plus 20 dB SPL required for audiometric 0 for speech) for the most commonly used earphone.

Calibration of the bone-conduction systems of audiometers may be accomplished in several ways. One method of field calibration involves the use of several patients with known sensory/neural losses. Their air- and bone-conduction thresholds are compared, and median values for the differences are taken at each frequency. The amounts by which the bone-conduction thresholds differ from the (calibrated) air-conduction thresholds are averaged, and corrections are posted on the audiometer. Persons with normal hearing cannot be used because of the danger of masking their uncovered ears by ambient room noise.

The **artificial mastoid** (see Figure 3.28) is a device that allows for electronic calibration of the bone-conduction system of an audiometer. The procedure is similar to that for testing air-conduction calibration. The bone-conduction vibrator is placed on the artificial mastoid, which has properties similar to the human skull, scalp, and skin. Vibrations are transduced into electrical currents, which are then converted to decibels for direct readout. The form shown in Figure 3.26 allows for calibration to the ANSI standard for bone-conduction testing on either the forehead or the mastoid. The reference equivalent threshold force levels (RETFLs) are shown in Table 3.6.

Calibration of a loudspeaker system with an audiometer requires either the testing of a number of normal-hearing subjects or the use of a sound-level meter. A heavy chair that is difficult to move should be placed before the speaker at a distance of about three times the diameter of the loudspeaker, plus one foot, or often just at one meter. This allows the subject to be placed in the "far field." The sound-level meter should be placed in the same position as the head of a patient seated in that same chair.

The loudspeaker output for 0 dB HL in the sound field, when listening with both ears, should be 14.5 dB SPL for speech. If the hearing-level dial is set to 70 dB, the sound-level meter should read 70 dB, plus 20 dB for audiometric 0 for speech, minus 5.5 dB (84.5 dB SPL). Five and one-half decibels are subtracted because thresholds for pure tones determined under earphones, called the minimum audible pressure (MAP) (Sivian & White, 1933), are slightly higher (require greater intensity) than thresholds determined in a free sound field, the minimum audible field (MAF) (Fletcher & Munson, 1933). When an external auxiliary amplifier is

FIGURE 3.26 Sample of form for field check of audiometer level and frequency.

University of Texas Speech and Hearing Center
AUDIOMETER CALIBRATION

For TDH-49 Earphone

Calibrated By _____   Audiometer _____   Serial No. _____   Date _____

Attn. HL		Frequency					Right Air Output*			Left Air Output*				Mastoid Output #			Forehead Output #		
Obs.	HL	Obs.	Err.	Dial	Count	HL	Obs.	Cor.	Err.	Obs.	Cor.	Err.	HL	Obs.	Cor.	Err.	Obs.	Cor.	Err.
	110			125		70		117.5	—		117.5			—						
	105																			
	100			250		70		96.5			96.5		25		66.4			79.9		
	95																			
	90			500		70		83.5			83.5		40		70.7			85.7		
	85																			
	80			750		70		78.5			78.5		40		59.3			71.8		
	75																			
	70			1000		70		77.5			77.5		40		56.9			66.9		
	65																			
	60			1500		70		77.5			77.5		40		55.4			66.4		
	55																			
	50			2000		70		81.0			81.0		40		48.1			56.6		
	45																			
	40			3000		70		79.5			79.5		40		46.6			54.1		
	35																			
	30			4000		70		80.5			80.5		40		51.2			57.7		
	25																			
	20			6000		70		83.5			83.5		—								
	15																				
	10			8000		70		83.0			83.0		—								
	5																				
	0			Speech		70		90.0			90.0		40		( )			( )		
	Ttl Err.																			

FUNCTIONAL CHECKS WITH TOLERANCES:

Rise Time (20 — 100 milliseconds) _____ .

Fall Time (5 — 100 milliseconds) _____ .

Overshoot and ringing (± 1dB) _____ .

Total Harmonic Distortion (max. —30dB) _____ .

Comments:

*Figures in this column are dB re 20 μPa for proposed ANSI standards for use with TDH-49 receivers mounted in MX-41/AR cushions.

#These figures include corrections for the B&K Model 4930 artificial mastoid for a B—70A bone-conduction vibrator.

FNM/80

FIGURE 3.27 A commercial audiometer calibration device. A supra-aural earphone is placed on an artificial ear for calibration. A separate, smaller, artificial ear is used for calibration of insert receivers.
(*Source:* AUDit™ with System 824 photo courtesy of Larson-Davis Laboratory, a Division of PCB Piezotronics, Inc. [www.larsondavis.com])

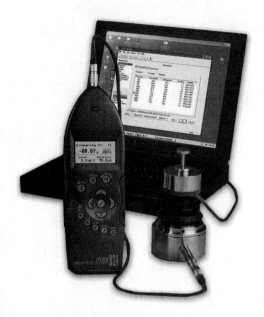

TABLE 3.5 Reference Equivalent Threshold Sound Pressure Levels (RETSPLs) (dB re 20 μPa) for Calibration of Insert Earphones to the ANSI (2004) Standard

Frequency (Hz)	Occluded Ear Simulator	HA-2 with Rigid Tube	HA-1
125	28.0	26.0	26.5
160	24.5	22.0	22.0
200	21.5	18.0	19.5
250	17.5	14.0	14.5
315	15.5	12.0	15.0
400	13.0	9.0	10.5
500	9.5	5.5	6.0
630	7.5	4.0	4.5
750	6.0	2.0	2.0
800	5.5	1.5	1.5
1000	5.5	0.0	0.0
1250	8.5	2.0	1.0
1500	9.5	2.0	0.0
1600	9.5	2.0	1.5
2000	11.5	3.0	2.5
2500	13.5	5.0	4.5
3000	13.0	3.5	2.5
3150	13.0	4.0	2.5
4000	15.0	5.5	0.0
5000	18.5	5.0	1.5
6000	16.0	2.0	−2.5
6300	16.0	2.0	−2.0
8000	15.5	0.0	−3.5
Speech	18.0	12.5	12.5

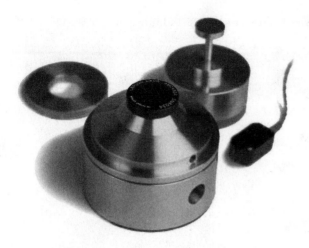

FIGURE 3.28 An artificial mastoid assembly for calibration of the bone-conduction system of an audiometer. The artificial mastoid has properties similar to the human skull, scalp, and skin. Here the bone-conduction vibrator of an audiometer is placed on the artificial mastoid, which is then attached to the audiometer calibration device.

(*Source:* AMC493B photo courtesy of Larson-Davis Laboratory, a Division of PCB Piezotronics, Inc. [www.larsondavis.com])

TABLE 3.6 Reference Equivalent Threshold Force Levels (RETFLs) for Bone Vibrators

Frequency Hz	Mastoid (dB re 1μN)	Forehead (dB re 1μN)	Forehead Minus Mastoid
250	67.0	79.0	12.0
315	64.0	76.5	12.5
400	61.0	74.5	13.5
500	58.0	72.0	14.0
630	52.5	66.0	3.5
750	48.5	61.5	13.0
800	47.0	59.0	12.0
1000	42.5	51.0	8.5
1250	39.0	49.0	10.0
1500	36.5	47.5	11.0
1600	35.5	46.5	11.0
2000	31.0	42.5	11.5
2500	29.5	41.5	12.0
3000	30.0	42.0	12.0
3150	31.0	42.5	11.5
4000	35.5	43.5	8.0
5000	40.0	51.0	11.0
6000	40.0	51.0	11.0
6300	40.0	50.0	10.0
8000	40.0	50.0	10.0
Speech	55.0	63.5	8.5

Source: American National Standards Institute, 2004.

used to power the loudspeaker, its volume control may often be adjusted to produce the proper level. Many modern diagnostic audiometers contain their own "booster" amplifiers and cannot be easily adjusted in the field. Reference equivalent sound-pressure levels for sound-field testing are shown in Table 3.7.

Whenever the audiometer differs from the required level at any frequency by more than 2.5 dB, a correction should be added to the hearing-level dial setting during audiometric testing. Corrections are rounded to the nearest multiple of 5 dB. Although this may seem superficially illogical, if the calibration procedure reveals that the system is putting out too low a level,

TABLE 3.7 Reference Equivalent Threshold Sound Pressure Levels (RETSPLs) (dB re 20 μPa) for Sound-Field Testing

Frequency (Hz)	Binaural Listening* in a Free Field	Monaural Listening in a Free Field		
	0 Degree Incidence	0 Degree Incidence	45 Degree Incidence	90 Degree Incidence
125	22.0	24.0	23.5	23.0
160	18.0	20.0	19.0	18.5
200	14.5	16.5	15.5	15.0
250	11.0	13.0	12.0	11.0
315	8.5	10.5	9.0	8.0
400	6.0	8.0	5.5	4.5
500	4.0	6.0	3.0	1.5
630	2.5	4.5	1.0	−0.5
750	2.0	4.0	0.5	−1.0
800	2.0	4.0	0.5	−1.0
1000	2.0	4.0	0.0	−1.5
1250	1.5	3.5	−0.5	−2.5
1500	0.5	2.5	−1.0	−2.5
1600	0.0	2.0	−1.5	−2.5
2000	−1.5	0.5	−2.5	−1.5
2500	−4.0	−2.0	−5.5	−4.0
3000	−6.0	−4.0	−9.0	−6.5
3150	−6.5	−4.5	−9.5	−6.5
4000	−6.5	−4.5	−8.5	−4.0
5000	−3.0	−1.0	−7.0	−5.0
6000	2.5	4.5	−3.0	−5.0
6300	4.0	6.0	−1.5	−4.0
8000	11.5	13.5	8.0	5.5
9000	13.5	15.5	10.5	8.5
10,000	13.5	15.5	11.0	9.5
11,200	12.0	14.0	10.0	7.0
12,500	11.0	13.0	11.5	5.0
14,000	16.0	18.0		
16,000	43.5	44.5		
Speech	14.5	16.5	12.5	11.0

ISO 389–7 Reference Threshold of Hearing Under Free Field and Diffuse Field Conditions.
Source: American National Standards Institute, 2004.

the number of decibels of deviation must be subtracted from the hearing-level dial setting during any given test. If the intensity is too high, the correction is added during testing. Whenever level calibration reveals marked differences from specification, the audiometer should be sent for recalibration. Audiologists should never assume that their audiometers, even when new, are in proper calibration unless they have verified this for themselves.

In addition to level checking, on pure-tone audiometers it is important to check for changes in frequency to be sure that the ANSI frequency limitations have not been exceeded. This may be done with a frequency counter.

The linearity of the attenuator dial is most easily tested electronically with a voltmeter. Checks should be made through the entire intensity range to be certain that when the hearing-level dial is moved a given number of decibels, the level actually changes by this precise amount, plus or minus the stated tolerance per 5 dB step. In addition, the total error in the hearing-level dial linearity cannot exceed a set degree of error, depending on frequency. The form shown in Figure 3.26 provides space for checking attenuator linearity.

CHECK YOUR UNDERSTANDING

ACTIVITIES

Even though the audiometer generates a pure tone, it is likely that distortion in the system (often the earphone) results in the emission of the second harmonic of the tone; that is, if a 1000 Hz tone is generated, some energy at 2000 Hz is present. ANSI standards state how much lower the second harmonic must be relative to the fundamental (the test frequency) to meet tolerance. This can be checked with special equipment, such as frequency counters.

Summary

Sound may be regarded objectively if we consider its waves in terms of their frequency, intensity, phase, and spectrum. Sounds may also be studied subjectively, in terms of pitch, loudness, or the interactions of signals producing masking or localization. In discussing sound energy, it is always important to specify precisely the various aspects and appropriate measurement references, such as hertz, decibels (IL, SPL, HL, or SL), mels, sones, or phons.

Hearing tests measure responses to pure tones as well as speech and other complex signals. These tests cannot be performed accurately unless all signals are calibrated in accordance with specifications set by the American National Standards Institute. Accurate testing is further ensured when test environments are determined not to exceed acceptable noise levels for audiometry. These noise levels as well as environmental and employment noise levels can be determined through the use of a sound-level meter.

REVIEW TABLE 3.1 Common Units of Measurement in Acoustics

Unit (Abbreviation in Parentheses)			Abbreviation		
Measurement	*CGS*	*SI*	*CGS*	*SI*	*Equivalents*
Length	Centimeter (cm)	Meter (m)	cm	m	1 cm = 0.01 m 1 m = 100 cm
Mass	Gram	Kilogram	g	kg	1 g = 0.001 kg 1 kg = 1000 g
Area	Square centimeter	Square meter	cm^2	m^2	1 cm^2 = 0.0001 m^2 1 m^2 = 10,000 cm^2
Work	Erg	Joule	e	J	1 e = 0.0000001 J 1 J = 10,000,000 e
Power	Ergs per second	Joules per second	e/sec	J/sec	1 e/sec = 0.0000001 J/sec 1 J/sec = 10,000,000 e/sec
	Watts	Watts	w	w	1 w = 1 J/sec 1 w = 10,000,000 e/sec
Force	Dyne	Newton	d	N	1 d = 0.00001 N 1 N = 100,000 d
Intensity	Watts per centimeter squared	Watts per meter squared	w/cm^2	w/m^2	1 w/cm^2 = 10,000 w/m^2 1 w/m^2 = 0.0001 w/cm^2
Pressure	Dynes per centimeter squared	Newtons* per meter squared	d/cm^2	N/m^2	1d/cm^2 = 0.1Pa
		Pascal		Pa	1 Pa = 10 d/cm^2 1 Pa = 1 N/m^2
Speed (velocity)	Centimeters per second	Meters per second	cm/sec	m/sec	1 cm/sec = 0.01 m/sec 1 m/sec = 100 cm/sec
Acceleration	Centimeters per second squared	Meters per second squared	cm/sec^2	m/sec^2	1 cm/sec^2 = 0.01 m/sec^2 1 m/sec^2 = 100 cm/sec^2

*Related to but not strictly on the SI scale.

REVIEW TABLE 3.2 Determinants Contributing to Psychological Perceptions of Sound

Perception	Prime Determinant	Other Determinants
Pitch	Frequency	Intensity
Loudness	Intensity	Frequency, duration
Quality	Spectrum	

REVIEW TABLE 3.3 Psychological Measurements of Sound

Measurement	Unit	Reference	Physical Correlate
Pitch	Mel	1,000 mels (1000 Hz at 40 dB SL)	Frequency
Loudness	Sone	1 sone (1000 Hz at 40 dB SL)	Intensity
Loudness level	Phon	0 phons (corresponding to threshold at 1,000 Hz)	Intensity
Quality			Spectrum

REVIEW TABLE 3.4 Physical Measurements of Sound

Measurement	Unit	Reference	Formula	Psychological Correlate
Frequency	cps/Hz			Pitch
Intensity level	dB IL	10^{-16} watt/cm (CGS) 10^{-12} watt/m^2 (SI)	$NdB = 10 \log I_O/I_R$	Loudness
Sound-pressure level	dB SPL	0.0002 dyne/cm^2 (CGS) 20 μPa(SI)	$NdB = 20 \log P_O/P_R$	Loudness
Hearing level	dB HL	ANSI (2004)	$NdB = 20 \log P_O/P_R$	Loudness
Sensation level	dB SL	Hearing threshold of subject	$NdB = 20 \log P_O/P_R$	Loudness
Impedance	ohm		$Z = \sqrt{R^2 + (2\pi fM - S/2\pi f)^2}$	

Frequently Asked Questions

Q Why is there an increase or decrease in the resulting sound intensity when two tones of almost identical frequency are presented?

A *The interaction of two tones that are out of phase results in their amplitudes varying, depending on the interactions at various places on the sound wave. The difference in frequency between the two tones becomes the number of beats per second.*

Q What is a Fourier analysis?

A *This is a process by which a complex sound is broken down into its pure-tone components.*

Q Why does raising a sound one octave not result in a doubling of pitch?

A *Although pitch and frequency are directly related, this relationship is not on a one-to-one basis. Pitch measurements use the mel scale.*

Q When do we use HL to reference a dB level, and when do we use SPL?

A *The HL (hearing level) reference is used only for audiometric purposes and has as its reference the average normal-hearing person's thresholds at each frequency. SPL (sound-pressure level) is used for most other measurements and has as its reference 20 micropascals or 0.0002 dyne/cm^2.*

Q How are air-conduction receivers calibrated?

A *A coupler (sometimes called an artificial ear) is used to connect (or couple) the air-conduction receiver (earphone) to a sound-level meter. The level of measured sound coming from the earphone is compared to the audiometric dial reading. Of course, the audiometric dial is in dB HL and the meter reads the output in dB SPL, so conversion corrections must be added.*

Q What does ANSI stand for?

A *ANSI is the abbreviation for the American National Standards Institute. It sets the standards for a wide variety of instruments, including audiometers.*

Q How is loudness measured electronically?

A *Loudness is a purely subjective (psychological) experience, so it cannot be measured using instruments. Its cognate, intensity, can be measured using a sound-level meter.*

Q Why can't loudness be measured in decibels?

A *The decibel is a unit of sound pressure or sound power and is an objective, mathematical unit. Loudness is a psychological phenomenon and is measured in phons or sones.*

Q What is a mel?

A *A mel is a unit of pitch measurement. One thousand mels are said to be equal to the pitch of a 1,000 Hz tone at 40 dB SL. A sound twice the pitch is called 2,000 mels, and so forth.*

Q Can individuals taking hearing tests be made more comfortable by using those large donut-shaped earphones that fit around the ears?

A *You refer to circumaural receivers that cannot be calibrated to an audiometer using conventional instrumentation. The acceptable audiometric earphones fit over the ear (supra-aural) or within the ear (insert).*

Q What does the term *sensation level* mean?

A *The term is often misunderstood as have something to do with the way the human ear senses sound. It simply means the number of decibels above the listener's hearing threshold.*

Q How does one hear by bone conduction?

A *A tuning fork, or the bone-conduction oscillator of an audiometer, is pressed against the skull and when it is set into vibration (as with a pure tone), it causes the skull to vibrate sympathetically. The acceleration of the skull distorts the bones that house the cochlea of the inner ear, thereby disturbing the fluids and cells within it. This disturbance generates patterns that the brain interprets as sound.*

Suggested Reading

Frank, T. (2007). Basic instrumentation and calibration. In R. J. Roeser, M. Valente, & H. Hosford-Dunn (Eds.), *Audiology diagnosis* (pp. 195–237). New York: Thieme.

Hamill, T. A., & Price, L. L. (2007). *The hearing sciences.* San Diego: Plural Publishing.

Endnotes

1. For Robert Brown, British botanist, 1773–1858.
2. For Dr. Heinrich Hertz, German physicist, 1857–1894.
3. For Jean Baptiste Joseph Fourier, French mathematician and physicist, 1768–1830.
4. For Sir Isaac Newton, British mathematician, astronomer, and physicist, 1643–1727.
5. For Blaise Pascal, French mathematician and philosopher, 1623–1662.
6. For James Prescott Joule, British physicist, 1818–1889.
7. For James Watt, Scottish inventor, 1736–1819.
8. American of Scottish descent. Renowned educator of children with hearing loss and inventor of the telephone, 1847–1922.
9. For Georg Simon Ohm, German mathematician and physicist, 1787–1854.

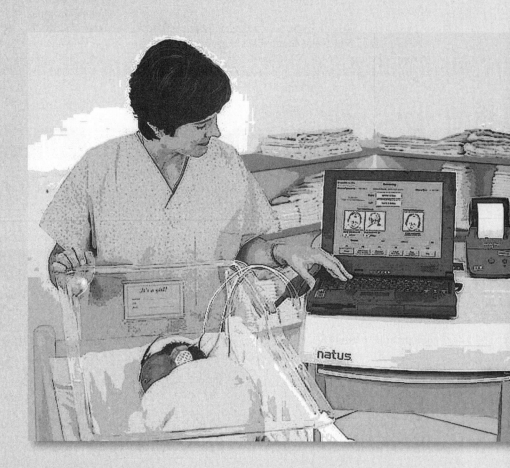

There is evidence that even seasoned clinicians do not carry out some hearing tests in precise and scientific ways. Often it is the basic tests that do not get the care and attention they deserve. Part II of this text covers the tests that are performed as part of a complete audiological evaluation. Chapter 4 is concerned with pure-tone tests, which are in some ways quantifications of the results found on the tuning-fork tests described in Chapter 2. Chapter 5 presents different forms of speech audiometry and describes ways in which tests carried out with speech stimuli assist in diagnosis and treatment. Determination of the need for and appropriate use of masking are described in Chapter 6. Tests for determining the sites in the auditory system that produce different kinds of auditory disorders are described in Chapter 7. These tests include both electrophysiological and electroacoustical procedures, wherein relatively objective determinations can be made of a lesion site, and behavioral measures, in which the patient plays an active role. In many cases, step-by-step procedures are outlined, along with test interpretations. Special diagnostic procedures for testing children are described in Chapter 8. The importance of using an entire battery of tests in making a diagnosis is stressed.

Any test must be subjected to scrutiny to determine its specific usefulness in a particular situation. Questions arise about two factors—reliability and validity. *Reliability* has to do with how well a test result is repeatable. Poor reliability can make a test useless, but good reliability does not necessarily make it valuable unless it is also valid. Questions of *validity* ask whether a test measures what it is supposed to measure. Any single test can turn out in one of four ways:

1. *True positive:* The test indicates a disorder correctly.
2. *True negative:* The test correctly eliminates an incorrect diagnosis.
3. *False positive:* The test suggests a diagnosis incorrectly.
4. *False negative:* The test incorrectly eliminates a correct diagnosis.

Audiological tests can be subjected to a set of mathematical models by **clinical decision analysis (CDA)**. The CDA asks questions about each test's **sensitivity** (how well it correctly diagnoses disorder—true positive), its **specificity** (the inverse of sensitivity—how well it rejects an incorrect diagnosis—true negative), its **efficiency** (the percentage of false positive and false negative results), and its **predictive value** (the percentage of true positive and true negative results).

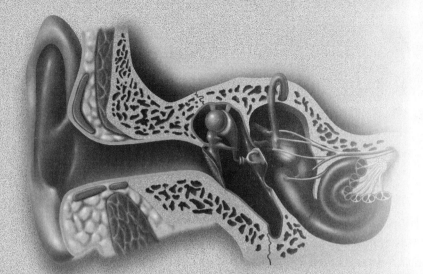

CHAPTER 4

Pure-Tone Audiometry

LEARNING OBJECTIVES

It is assumed that the reader has access to an audiometer in good working condition and the opportunity for supervised experience. At the completion of this chapter, the reader should be able to

■ Describe the fundamentals underlying pure-tone audiometry and the components of a reliable **audiogram**.

■ Demonstrate how different pure-tone tests are performed.

■ Interpret several pure-tone tests.

P URE-TONE TESTS OF HEARING, performed with an **audiometer,**[1] are electronic tests developed along the same conceptual line as tuning-fork tests such as the Schwabach and Rinne. When such tests are carried out, the procedure is called audiometry. The main disadvantage of the tuning-fork tests is that they are difficult to quantify. That is, although the Schwabach might suggest sensory/neural sensitivity that is poorer than normal, it does not tell how much poorer; although the Rinne might suggest the presence of a conductive component, it does not tell how large that component is.

The purpose of testing hearing is to aid in the process of making decisions regarding the type and extent of a patient's hearing loss and developing a habilitative/rehabilitative plan to address the impact of the loss. Because some of these decisions may have profound effects on the patient's medical, social, educational, and psychological status, accurate performance and careful interpretation of hearing tests are mandatory. The reliability of any test is based on interrelationships among factors such as calibration of equipment, test environment, patient performance, and examiner sophistication. In the final analysis, it is not hearing that we measure; rather, we measure responses to a set of acoustic signals that we interpret as representing hearing. The vocabularies in Chapters 2 and 3 are relied upon extensively within this chapter as the reader is exposed to new concepts and problems. Some of these problems can be solved; others can only be compensated for and understood.

The Pure-Tone Audiometer

Pure-tone audiometers have been in use for over a hundred years as devices for determining hearing **thresholds,** which are then compared to established norms at various frequencies. The original audiometers were electrically driven tuning forks that generated a number of pure tones of different frequencies. In later designs the tones were generated electrically. With the advent of the electronic era, audiometers incorporated vacuum tubes, then transistors, and then the integrated circuits of today. Like other electronic items, audiometers vary considerably in cost. Specifications of the American National Standards Institute (American National Standards Institute, 2004) are imposed on all audiometers so that price differences should not reflect differences in quality of manufacture or in performance.

A common type of audiometer, which is sometimes portable, tests hearing sensitivity by air conduction and bone conduction. A switch allows for easy selection of pure tones. The testable frequencies for air conduction with these audiometers usually include 125, 250, 500, 750, 1000, 1500, 2000, 3000, 4000, 6000, and 8000 Hz. The range of intensities begins at –10 dB HL and goes to 110 dB HL at frequencies between 500 and 6000 Hz, with slightly lower maximum values at 125, 250, and 8,000 Hz. Some special devices, called extended high-frequency audiometers, test from 8,000 to 20,000 Hz and have specific diagnostic value. A matched pair of earphones is provided and an output switch directs the tone to either earphone.

Usually only the range from 250 through 4000 Hz may be tested by bone conduction. The maximum testable hearing level for bone conduction is considerably lower than for air conduction, not exceeding 50 dB at 250 Hz and 70 or 80 dB at 500 Hz and above. Maximum outputs for bone conduction are lower than for air conduction for several reasons. The power required to drive a bone-conduction vibrator is greater than for an air-conduction earphone. When the bone-conduction vibrator is driven at high intensities, harmonic distortion occurs, especially in the low frequencies. High-intensity sounds delivered by a bone-conduction oscillator may result in the patient's feeling rather than hearing the stimulus. In addition to air- and bone-conduction capability, a *masking* control is usually provided that allows for introduction of a noise to the nontest ear when needed during audiometry. For some audiometers, the **masking** noise is not of a specific spectrum and is not well calibrated for practical clinical purposes. Persons who rely solely on portable air- and bone-conduction audiometers are often unsophisticated about the need for and proper use of masking. Most pure-tone audiometers, however, contain excellent masking-noise generators and can be used for a variety of pure-tone audiometric procedures (see Figure 4.1). The reasons for masking and how to accomplish effective masking are discussed in Chapter 6.

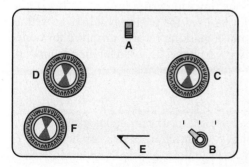

FIGURE 4.1 Typical face of a pure-tone audiometer. (A) On-off power switch. (B) Output selector switch. Selects right ear, left ear, or bone conduction. Masking delivered to nontest earphone for air conduction and to left earphone for bone conduction. (C) Frequency selector dial. Air conduction selects 125, 250, 500, 750, 1000, 1500, 2000, 3000, 4000, 6000, or 8000 Hz. Bone conduction selects 250, 500, 750, 1000, 1500, 2000, 3000, or 4000 Hz. (D) Hearing-level dial. Air-conduction range: –10 to 110 dB HL (500 to 6000 Hz), –10 to 90 dB HL (250 and 8000 Hz), and –10 to 80 dB HL (125 Hz). Bone-conduction range: –10 to 50 dB HL (250 Hz), –10 to 70 dB HL (500 Hz), and –10 to 80 dB HL (750 to 4000 Hz). (E) Tone-presentation bar. Introduces tone with prescribed rise and fall time and no audible sound from the switch. (F) Masking-level dial. Controls intensity of masking noise in the nontest ear. Spectrum and intensity range vary with manufacturer.

Test Environment

Table 3.4 showed the maximum ambient sound-pressure levels allowable for air-conduction and bone-conduction testing. Rooms in which such standards can be met are not always utilized. This is true in the case of hearing test sites in industry or in the public schools. Regardless of the practical limitations imposed by a given situation, the person responsible for audiometric results must realize that background noise may affect audiometric results by elevating auditory thresholds or causing unnecessary screening failures. Ambient room noise may be attenuated in three major ways: by using specially designed earphone enclosures, by testing through receivers that insert into the ear, and by using sound-treated chambers.

Earphone Attenuation Devices

Audiometer earphone and cushion combinations do not provide sufficient attenuation of most background noises to allow determination of threshold down to 0 dB HL for people with normal hearing. Several devices are available that allow the supra-aural audiometer earphone and cushion to be mounted within a larger cup, which assists in the attenuation of background noise (see Figure 4.2). Most use a fluid-filled cushion to achieve a tight seal against the head. Such enclosures may be effective, but differences exist in the efficiency of different models (Franks, Engel, & Themann, 1992).

Problems with regard to **calibration** are encountered in the use of some earphone enclosures. The phones cannot be placed on the usual 6 cm^3 coupler of an artificial ear. Even if the earphone is checked and found to be in proper calibration before it is placed into the enclosure, mounting may alter the calibration slightly, especially in the low frequencies. Because bone-conduction testing is done with the ears uncovered, the masking effects of room noise may affect these test results without affecting the air-conduction results, possibly causing a misdiagnosis. Children often find these earphone devices heavy and uncomfortable.

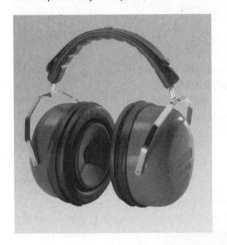
FIGURE 4.2 Commercial earphone enclosure device used to attenuate room noise during threshold audiometry. (*Source:* Audiocups courtesy of Amplivox, Ltd.)

Insert Earphones

Testing hearing with receivers that insert directly into the ear has a number of advantages audiometrically, including further reduction of background noise compared to supra-aural earphones and better infection control because the inserts are disposed of following testing. If the foam is inserted deep into the ear, just short of causing discomfort, even more attenuation is obtained. It is desirable to have patients open and close their mouths three or four times to ensure proper seating of the cushion. Insert earphones can be used for testing children as well as adults. Problems with room-noise masking remain unsolved for bone-conduction testing, even if insert earphones are used for air conduction.

Clinical COMMENTARY

During all patient contact for hearing testing and subsequent treatment, audiologists should be conscious of effective infection-control procedures. Harmful organisms can be passed from person to person through direct patient contact or indirect contact when test instruments are used without proper cleaning. The importance of this area of clinical care cannot be overemphasized.

Sound-Isolated Chambers

The term *soundproof room* is often used erroneously. Totally soundproofing a room—that is, removing all sound—is impossible. All that is necessary in clinical audiometry is to keep the noise in the room below the level of masking that would cause a threshold shift in persons with normal hearing. Sound-isolated rooms may be custom-built or purchased commercially in a prefabricated form.

The primary objective in sound-treating a room is to isolate it acoustically from the rest of the building in which it is housed. This usually involves the use of mass (such as cinder blocks), insulating materials (such as fiberglass), and dead air spaces. The door must be solid and must close with a tight acoustic seal. Sometimes two doors are used, one opening into the room and the other opening out. The inside walls are covered with soft materials, such as acoustic tile, to help minimize reverberation. Some such chambers contain large wedge-shaped pieces of soft material such as fiberglass on all walls, ceilings, and floors, with a catwalk provided for the subject. Rooms in which reverberation is markedly diminished are called anechoic chambers. An example of such a room was shown in Figure 3.17.

Audiometric suites may be designed for either one-room or two-room use. In the one-room arrangement, examiners, their equipment, and the patient are all together in the same room, or the patient is within the room and the clinician just outside. In the two-room arrangement, the examiner and audiometer are in the equipment room and the patient is in the examining room. Windows provide visual communication between the rooms. As a rule, several panes of glass attenuate the sounds that emanate from the equipment room. Moisture-absorbing materials must be placed between the panes of glass to keep the windows from fogging. Electrical connections between the rooms are necessary so that signals can be directed from the audiometer to the earphones. In addition, a talkback device, consisting of a microphone, amplifier, and speaker and/or earphone, enables the examiner to hear patients when they speak.

In customizing sound-isolated rooms, a great deal of attention is often paid to attenuating sound from adjoining spaces outside the walls of the room, but insufficient care is given to building-borne vibrations that may enter the room from the floor or ceiling. It does little good to have four-foot walls of solid concrete when footsteps can be heard from the floor above.

When sufficient space, money, and architectural know-how are available, custom sound rooms may be the proper choice. Contemporary audiology centers, however, lean more toward the commercially prefabricated sound room, which is made of steel panels and can be installed with wiring included for a two-room operation (see Figure 4.3). The manufacturer does not guarantee the noise level within the sound room after installation, but only the amount of attenuation the room can provide under specific laboratory conditions, a fact often not fully understood by many purchasers. Therefore, it is necessary to prepare the room that will enclose the prefabricated booth by making this area as quiet and nonreverberant as possible.

Prefabricated sound booths are available in one- and two-room suites. Windows with several panes of glass are installed to enable the examiner to observe the patient. The inside walls of the booth are constructed of perforated steel and filled with sound-absorbing materials. Some booths are double-walled; that is, there is one booth inside another, larger one. Prefabricated booths are freestanding, touching none of the walls of the room in which they stand, and are isolated from the ceiling by air and from the floor by specially constructed sound rails.

One of the great weaknesses of audiometric rooms, whether custom or commercial, is their ventilation systems. Rooms that are to be tightly closed must have adequate air circulation, requiring the use of fans and motors. Sometimes the air-intake system is coupled directly with the heating and air-conditioning ducts of the building. In such cases, care must be taken to minimize the introduction of noise through the ventilation system.

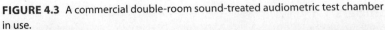

FIGURE 4.3 A commercial double-room sound-treated audiometric test chamber in use.

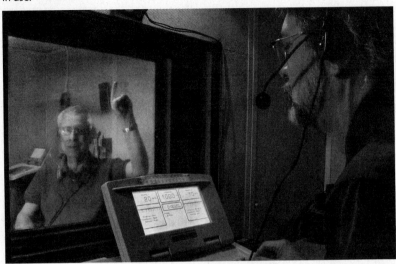

Lighting for both kinds of rooms should be incandescent, but if the use of fluorescent lighting is desired, the starters must be remotely mounted. Starters for fluorescent tubes often put out an annoying 60 Hz hum that can be heard by the patient or picked up by the audiometer.

The Patient's Role in Manual Pure-Tone Audiometry

Patients seeking hearing tests vary a great deal in age, intelligence, education, motivation, and willingness to cooperate. The approach to testing is very different for an adult compared to a child, or for an interested person compared to one who is frightened, shy, or even hostile. Procedures also vary depending on the degree of the patient's spoken language skills and if the patient and examiner share a common language. Test results are most easily obtained when a set of instructions can be given orally to a patient, who then complies. As any experienced audiologist can testify, things do not go equally well with all patients.

In pure-tone audiometry, regardless of how the message is conveyed, patients must learn to accept their responsibility in the test if results are to be valid. Spoken instructions, written instructions, gestures, and/or demonstrations may be required. In any case, patients must become aware that they are to indicate when they hear a tone, even when that tone is very soft. The level at which tones are perceived as barely audible is the threshold of hearing sensitivity. Auditory thresholds at different frequencies form the basis for pure-tone audiometry.

Patient Response

After patients understand the instructions and know what they are listening for, they must be given some way of indicating that they have heard. Some audiologists request that patients raise one hand when a tone is heard. They then lower the hand when they no longer hear the tone. Sometimes patients are asked to raise their right hands when they hear the tone in the right ear and their left hands when they hear the tone in the left ear. The hand signal is probably the most popular response system used in pure-tone audiometry. Many audiologists like this method because they can observe both *how* the patient responds and the hearing level that produces the response. Often, when the tones are close to threshold, patients raise their hands more hesitatingly than when they are clearly audible. Problems occur with this response system when patients either forget to lower their hands or keep them partially elevated.

As with the hand signal, patients may simply raise one index finger when the tone is heard and lower it when it is not heard. This system has the same advantages and disadvantages as the hand-signal system. It is sometimes difficult, however, to see from an adjacent control room when the patient raises only a finger.

The patient may be given a signal button with instructions to press it when the tone is heard and release it when the tone goes off. Pressing the button illuminates a light on the control panel of the audiometer and/or makes a sound. The use of signal buttons limits the kind of subjective information the audiologist may glean from observing hand or finger signals because the pushbutton is an all-or-nothing type of response. Reaction time is sometimes another important drawback to pushbutton signaling because some people may be slow in pushing and releasing the button. Often, if the button is tapped very lightly, the panel light may only flicker, and the response may be missed. Pushbuttons are usually not a good idea for children or the physically disabled, although they are standard equipment on many audiometers. For young adults, however, research does suggest a slight decrease in the length of testing and a patient preference for the use of pushbuttons (DiGiovanni & Repka, 2007).

Some audiologists prefer vocal responses like "now," "yes," or "I hear it" whenever the tone is heard. This procedure is often useful with children, although some patients have complained that their own voices "ring" in the earphones after each utterance, making tones close to threshold difficult to hear. Play and other motivational techniques are often necessary when testing children or other difficult-to-test persons. Some of these methods are discussed in the chapter on pediatric audiology (Chapter 8). As you watch this video of pure-tone Air-Conduction Testing, you will see the standard threshold search method of decreasing sound intensity by 10 dB when a response is given until the tone is inaudible and then raising the tone in 5 dB steps until the next response is obtained.

False Responses

False responses are common during behavioral audiometry, and the alert clinician is always on guard for them because they can be misleading and can cause serious errors in the interpretation of test results. A common kind of false response occurs when patients fail to indicate that they have heard a tone. Some patients may have misunderstood or forgotten their roles in the test. Such **false negative responses,** which tend to suggest that hearing is worse than it actually is, are also seen in patients who deliberately feign or exaggerate a hearing loss (see Chapter 13).

False positive responses, where the patient responds when no tone has been presented, are often more irritating to the clinician than are false negatives. Most patients respond with some false positives if long silent periods occur during the test, especially if they are highly motivated to respond. When false positive responses obscure accurate test results, the clinician must slow down the test to watch for them, which encourages even more false positives. Sometimes even reinstructing the patient fails to alleviate this vexing situation. Some patients who suffer from ringing sounds in their ears complain that this is often confused with the test tone.

The Clinician's Role in Manual Pure-Tone Audiometry

As stated earlier, the first step in manual pure-tone testing is to make patients aware of their task in the procedure. If verbal instructions are given, they may be something like this:

> You are going to hear a series of tones, first in one ear and then in the other. When you hear a tone, no matter how high or low in pitch, and no matter how loud or soft, please signal that you have heard it. Raise your hand when you first hear the tone, and keep it up as long as you hear it. Put your hand down quickly when the tone goes away. Remember to signal every time you hear a tone. Are there any questions?

If a different response system is preferred, it may be substituted. There is an advantage to asking the patient to signal quickly to both the onset and the offset of the tone. This permits two responses to each presentation of the tone to be observed. If the patient responds to both the introduction and the discontinuation of the tone, the acceptance of false responses may be avoided.

There are some distinct advantages to providing written instructions to patients before they undergo a hearing evaluation. These instructions can be mailed so that they can be read at home before patients arrive at the audiology clinic, or they can be provided when the patients check in with the receptionist, to be read while waiting to be seen by the audiologist. In addition to augmenting verbal instructions, printed instructions can be retained by the patient after the appointment to help clarify what the different tests were intended to measure. Printed instructions should never be used to replace verbal instructions.

Patient's Position During Testing

It is of paramount importance that the patient is never in a position to observe the clinician during pure-tone testing. Even small eye, hand, or arm movements by the clinician may cause patients to signal that they have heard a tone when they have not. In one-room situations, patients should be seated so that they are at right angles to the audiometer (see Figure 4.4). Some audiologists prefer to have the patient's back to the audiometer to eliminate any possibility of visual cues; however, this is disconcerting to some patients and eliminates observation of the patient's facial expression, which is often helpful to the audiologist in interpreting responses.

Even if the audiologist and patient are in different rooms, care must be taken to ensure that the patient cannot observe the clinician's movements. Figure 4.5 illustrates one satisfactory arrangement. Of course, the patient must always be clearly observable by the audiologist.

FIGURE 4.4 Proper positioning during pure-tone audiometry carried out with a single sound-treated room for (A) examiner, (B) audiometer, and (C) patient.

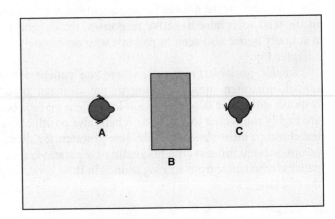

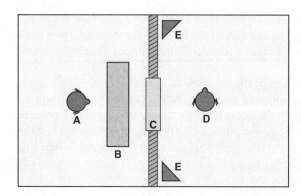

FIGURE 4.5 Proper positioning during pure-tone audiometry conducted in a two-room suite for (A) examiner, (B) audiometer, (C) window separating rooms, (D) patient, and (E) loudspeakers. For sound field testing the patient would be turned to face the window placing loudspeakers (E) at 45 degree azimuth to each ear.

Air-Conduction Audiometry

The purpose of air-conduction audiometry is to specify the amount of a patient's hearing sensitivity at various frequencies. If there is a loss of hearing, air-conduction test results can specify the degree of loss but not whether the deficit is produced by abnormality in the conductive mechanism, the sensory/neural mechanism, or both.

Proper placement of supra-aural earphones is shown in Figure 4.6A. The headband should be placed directly over the top of the head. All interfering hair should be pushed out of the way and earrings should be removed, when possible. Eyeglasses should also be removed as they sometimes lift the cushion of the earphone away from the ear and may become uncomfortable as the earphone cushion presses on the temple bar of the eyeglasses. Some patients are reluctant to remove their eyeglasses because they feel more relaxed when they can see clearly. This is another advantage to insert receivers, which do not interfere at all with the wearing of eyeglasses during testing.

When insert earphones are not used, earphone cushions are usually the hard rubber, supra-aural type that fit tightly against the external ear. The phones should be positioned so that their diaphragms are aimed directly at the opening into the ear canal. The yokes that hold

FIGURE 4.6 Properly placed supra-aural (A) and insert (B) air-conduction earphones.

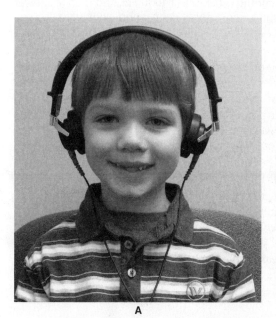

A

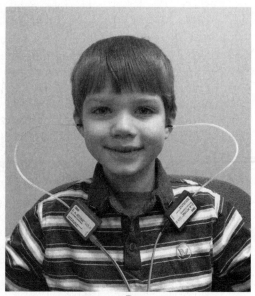

B

the phones may be pulled down so that the headset is in its most extended position. While the clinician is holding the phones against the ears, the size of the headset can be readjusted for a tight fit. Because this may pull the ear up and cause discomfort, the phones should be gently lifted away from the head and then replaced.

Some patients' outer ears collapse because of the pressure of the earphones. This creates an artificial conductive hearing loss, usually showing poorer sensitivity in the higher frequencies, which can be misleading in diagnosis. It is advisable to check for ear canal collapse prior to beginning air-conduction testing. This may be accomplished by pressing the **pinna** against the head during ear canal inspection and observing any potential canal-wall collapse. When this occurs, or when the clinician suspects that it may take place because the ear seems particularly supple, certain steps can be taken to overcome the difficulty. One easy solution is to place a small piece of foam rubber (cut in the shape of a behind-the-ear hearing aid) under the pinna (the protrusion of the ear at the side of the head). It is useful to have a number of these small pieces on hand, precut in different sizes for use when they are needed.

The use of insert receivers for air-conduction testing is becoming routine in most clinics and provides an immediate solution when collapsing ear canals are a potential problem. The foam insert must be compressed with the fingers and can be slipped into a small plastic sleeve to maintain this compression until insertion is made into the external ear canal. After the insert is in place, the foam quickly expands. The transducer itself is built within a plastic housing to which the foam tip is attached or is mounted at the end of a 250 mm plastic tube that may be clipped to a blouse or shirt. As with supra-aural phones, insert receivers are colored red and blue for testing the right and left ears, respectively. Properly placed insert earphones are shown in Figure 4.6B. For a demonstration of the proper placement of supra-aural audiometer earphones and the preferred insert audiometer earphones, see the video titled Air-Conduction Receiver Placement.

Procedure for Air-Conduction Audiometry

The selection of which ear to test first is purely arbitrary unless a difference in hearing sensitivity between the ears is known or suspected, in which case the better ear should be tested first. Frequency order probably does not affect results, although most audiologists prefer to test at 1,000 Hz initially, test higher frequencies in ascending order, retest 1000 Hz, and then test lower frequencies in descending order (1000, 2000, 3000, 4000, 6000, 8000, 1000, 500, 250 Hz, etc.). Some audiologists feel that useful information is gained from the 125 Hz threshold, while others believe that thresholds at this frequency can most often be predicted from the 250 Hz results.

Many audiologists sample hearing only at octave points, whereas others prefer the detail resulting from testing the mid-octave frequencies (750, 1500, 3000, and 6000 Hz). In its guidelines for manual pure-tone audiometry, the American Speech-Language-Hearing Association (2005) prudently recommends that mid-octave points be tested when a difference of 20 dB or more is seen in the thresholds of adjacent octaves between 500 and 2000 Hz. ASHA also recommends routine testing of the inter-octave frequencies 3000 and 6000 Hz, which frequently turns up notches in the audiogram that would otherwise be missed. To hear samples of audiometric pure-tone stimuli, go to the **audiograms** illustrations.

Over the years, a number of different procedures have been devised for determining pure-tone thresholds. Some audiologists have used automatically pulsing tones and some have used manually pulsed tones. Some have used a descending technique, whereby the tone is presented above threshold and lowered in intensity until patients signal that they can no longer hear it. Others have used an ascending approach, increasing the level of the tone from below threshold until a response is given. Still others have used a bracketing procedure to find threshold.

When the profession of audiology was still quite new, Carhart and Jerger (1959) investigated several pure-tone test procedures and found that there were no real differences in results obtained with different methods. Nevertheless, they recommended that a particular procedure be followed, and this procedure appears to have been widely accepted. The procedure recommended here, based on Carhart and Jerger's suggestion, is to begin testing at 1,000 Hz because this frequency is easily heard by most people and has been said to have high test-retest reliability. In practice, it may be advisable in some cases to begin testing at other frequencies, perhaps lower ones, in cases of severe hearing loss in which no measurable hearing may be found at 1,000 Hz and above.

Following the American Speech-Language-Hearing Association (2005) guidelines, a pure tone is presented initially at 30 dB HL. If a response is obtained from the patient, it suggests that the 30 dB tone is above the patient's threshold. If no response is seen, the level is raised to 50 dB HL, introduced, and then raised in 10 dB steps until a response is obtained or the limit of the audiometer is reached for the test frequency.

After a response is obtained, the level is lowered in 10 dB steps. Each time a tone is introduced, it is maintained for one or two seconds. The hearing-level dial is never moved while the tone is in the "on" position because a scratching sound may occur in the earphone, causing the patient to respond as if to a tone. All ascending movements of the hearing-level dial from this point are made in steps of 5 dB. When the tone is lowered below the patient's response level, it is then raised in 5 dB steps until it is audible again, then lowered in 10 dB steps and raised in 5 dB steps until the 50 percent threshold response criterion has been met. The threshold is the lowest level at which the patient can correctly identify at least two out of three tone presentations. This usually, but not always, implies that a point 5 dB above this level evokes more than a 50 percent response. Levels accepted as threshold are often in the 75 percent to 100 percent response range.

Although the majority of audiologists use continuous tones during pure-tone testing, Burk and Wiley (2004) find that automatically pulsed tones have several advantages. The results of tests done using both measures are similar in terms of false responses, test reliability, and test time. However, test subjects reported increased awareness of the pulsed tones. This study was done on subjects with normal hearing, but it would appear to have some advantages for those with hearing loss, especially those complaining of interfering ear or head noises. For these patients, there is also a benefit in using frequency-modulated signals called **warble tones.** Franklin, Johnson, Smith-Olinde, and Nicholson (2009) report findings consistent with past research that there is no significant difference in thresholds obtained with normal hearing listeners regardless of whether the stimulus is a pulsed pure tone or a steady or pulsed warble tone. Caution should be exercised, however, when using warble tones with patients who exhibit steeply sloping audiometric curves.

Some audiologists prefer to record their results numerically on a specially prepared score sheet. The form shown in Figure 4.7A has proven to be very useful, especially in the training of new clinicians. This form allows recording the audiometric data numerically before plotting the graph, for a retest of 1000 Hz, and, if necessary, for retest of all frequencies with masking as discussed in Chapter 6. Determination of the need for masking can be made using this form and the appropriate effective-masking levels recorded. Accuracy criteria must be satisfied before the graph is drawn. Some clinics use a form that contains only numerical data and does not employ a graph at all (see Figure 4.8). These forms contain space for a number of tests and are useful where serial audiometric data are required. Many audiologists prefer to record the results directly onto a graph called an audiogram, using symbols to depict the threshold of each ear as a function of frequency and intensity, with reference to normal thresholds (see Figure 4.7B).

FIGURE 4.7 (A) Example of a form used to show pure-tone and speech test results in numerical format. The need to mask and appropriate opposite-ear effective masking levels are shown. (B) Example of an audiogram. The information listed below is included on the form:

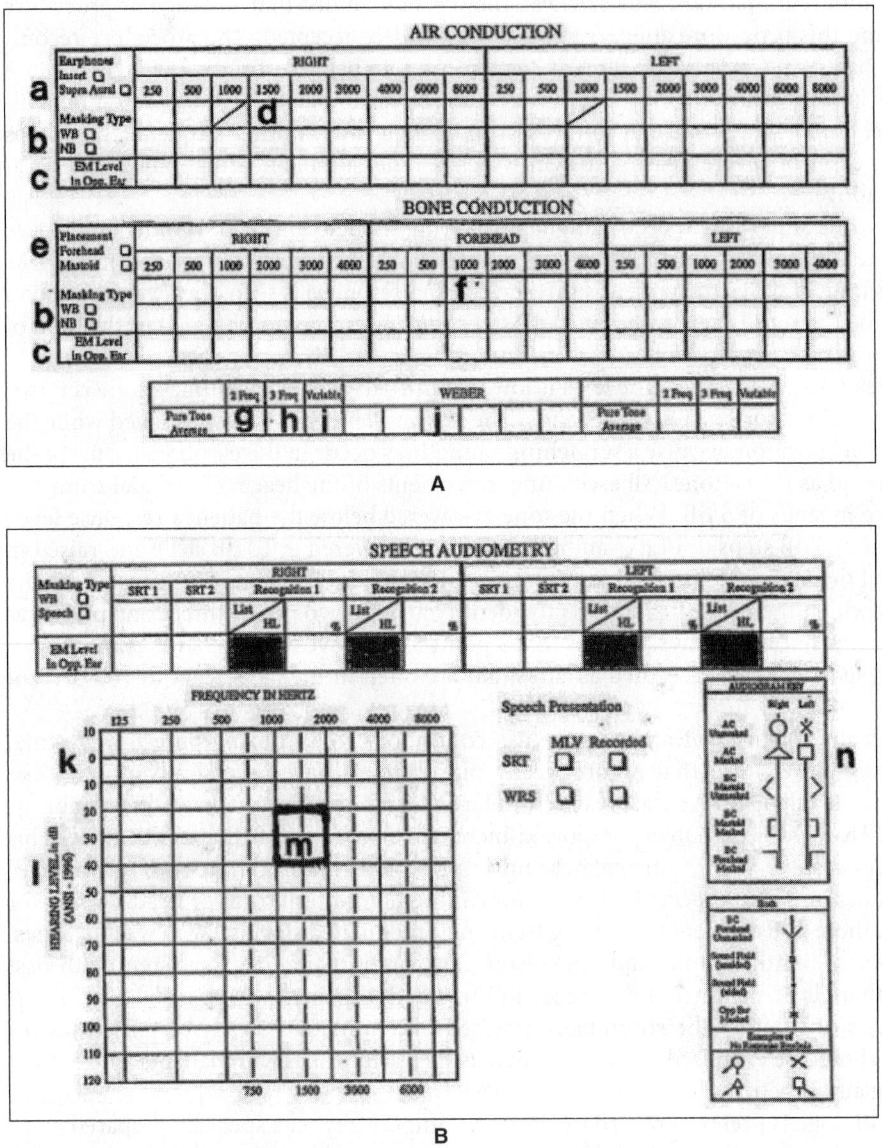

A

B

a. Type of earphone used for air-conduction tests
b. Masking type used in the nontest ear, as discussed in Chapter 6
c. Effective masking levels in the nontest ear, as discussed in Chapter 6
d. Air-conduction thresholds—a second set of cells is provided for repeated measurements of air-conduction tests, sometimes with opposite-ear masking, as discussed in Chapter 6.
e. Bone-conduction oscillator placement
f. Bone-conduction thresholds for either the forehead or the right and left mastoid—a second set of cells is provided for repeated measurements of bone-conduction tests, sometimes with opposite-ear masking.
g. Two-frequency pure-tone average (lowest two thresholds at 500, 1000, and 2000 Hz)
h. Three-frequency pure-tone average (500, 1000, and 2000 Hz)
i. Variable pure-tone average (average of the three poorest [highest] thresholds at 500, 1000, 2000, and 4000 Hz
j. Audiometric Weber results
k. The audiogram
l. Indication that hearing levels refer to ANSI values
m. A square to illustrate that the distance of 1 octave (across) is the same as 20 dB (down) at any place on the audiogram
n. Symbols used for plotting the audiogram

FIGURE 4.8 A form used to collect serial audiometric data. This form allows for recording of ten hearing evaluations so that comparisons may be made to check for progression or improvement of a hearing loss.

SERIAL AUDIOMETRIC DATA

Patient's Name _____

		RIGHT EAR									LEFT EAR							
		250	500	1000	2000	3000	4000	8000		250	500	1000	2000	3000	4000	8000	
Date	Air								Air								Air
	Bone							XXXX	Bone							XXXX	Bone
Date	Air								Air								Air
	Bone							XXXX	Bone							XXXX	Bone
Date	Air								Air								Air
	Bone							XXXX	Bone							XXXX	Bone
Date	Air								Air								Air
	Bone							XXXX	Bone							XXXX	Bone
Date	Air								Air								Air
	Bone							XXXX	Bone							XXXX	Bone
Date	Air								Air								Air
	Bone							XXXX	Bone							XXXX	Bone
Date	Air								Air								Air
	Bone							XXXX	Bone							XXXX	Bone
Date	Air								Air								Air
	Bone							XXXX	Bone							XXXX	Bone
Date	Air								Air								Air
	Bone							XXXX	Bone							XXXX	Bone
Date	Air								Air								Air
	Bone							XXXX	Bone							XXXX	Bone

Any audiometric worksheet should have some minimal identifying information—the patient's name, age, and sex as well as the date of the examination, the equipment used, and the examiner's name. Some estimate of the test reliability should also be noted. After the air-conduction thresholds have been recorded, the average threshold levels for each ear at 500, 1,000, and 2,000 Hz should be recorded. This is called the **pure-tone average (PTA),** and it is useful for predicting the threshold for speech as well as for gaining a gross impression of the degree of communication impact imposed by a hearing loss. Table 4.1 shows the degree of communication impact created by various degrees of sensitivity loss. Even though this table is based in part on the recommendations made by Stewart and Downs (1984) for children, it has applications for adults as well. The two-frequency pure-tone average (lowest two thresholds at 500, 1000, and 2000 Hz) may be recorded as well and is often a better predictor of hearing for speech than the three-frequency average. A **variable pure-tone average (VPTA)** (Clark, 1981) consisting of the poorest of three thresholds obtained at 500, 1000, 2000, and 4000 Hz may be more effective than the traditional pure-tone average in estimating the degree of communication impact of a given hearing loss.

Many laypersons are accustomed to expressing the degree of hearing impairment as a percentage because they are unfamiliar with concepts such as frequency and intensity. Many physicians also calculate the percentage of hearing impairment, probably because they believe it is easier for their patients to understand. Although percentage of hearing impairment is an outmoded concept, its continued use mandates mention here; keep in mind, however, that for practical application in the counseling of patients, it is considered inappropriate and even misleading in many cases (Clark, 1981, 1982).

One weakness in the concept of percentage of hearing impairment is that it ignores audiometric configuration and looks only at the average hearing loss. The addition of 3000 Hz to the formula by the American Academy of Ophthalmology and Otolaryngology (AAOO) (1979) improves the situation somewhat. The formula, as modified slightly by Sataloff, Sataloff, and Vassallo (1980), works as follows:

1. Compute the average hearing loss (in decibels) from the threshold responses at 500, 1000, 2000, and 3000 Hz for each ear.

2. Subtract 25 dB—considered to be the lower limit of normal hearing by the AAOO.

3. Multiply the remaining number by 1.5 percent for each ear. This gives the percentage of hearing impairment for each ear.

4. Multiply the percentage of hearing impairment in the better ear by 5, add this figure to the percentage of hearing impairment in the poorer ear, and divide this total by 6. This gives the binaural (both ears) hearing impairment in percentage form.

Obviously, in addition to being somewhat misleading, the computation of percentage of hearing impairment is time-consuming. It is likely that patients are frequently confused by what they have been told about their hearing losses. For example, Table 4.1 indicates that a 25 dB pure-tone average constitutes a slight hearing impairment, but such a loss would prove to be 0 percent by using the AAOO method. This latter figure suggests to patients that their hearing is normal. Likewise, it can be seen that a 92 dB pure-tone average would be shown as 100 percent impairment, which would suggest total deafness to many laypersons. Patients with a 92 dB hearing level often prove to have considerable residual hearing.

When an audiogram is used, the graph should conform to specific dimensions. As Figure 4.7B illustrates, frequency (in hertz) is shown on the abscissa and intensity (in dB HL) on the ordinate. The space horizontally for one octave should be the same as the space vertically for 20 dB, forming a perfect square (20 dB by 1 octave). Unlike most graphs, the audiogram is drawn with 0 at the top rather than the bottom. This often leads to confusion for individuals new to the study of audiology because *lower* thresholds (better hearing) are shown by symbols *higher* on the audiogram, and *higher* thresholds (poorer hearing) are shown by symbols *lower* on the audiogram.

TABLE 4.1 Scale of Hearing Impairment Based on the Variable Pure-Tone Average of the Poorest Three Thresholds at 500, 1,000, 2,000, and 4,000 Hz*

VPTA (dB)	Degree of Communication Impact	Consider Hearing Aid	Consider Communication Training
–10 to 15	None	No	No
16 to 25	Slight	Possibly, especially for children	Possibly
26 to 40	Mild	Probably for adults, definitely for children	Probably
41 to 55	Moderate	Definitely	Definitely
56 to 70	Moderately severe	Definitely	Definitely
71 to 90	Severe	Definitely	Definitely
>91	Profound	Consider cochlear implant	Definitely

Hearing levels refer to the ANSI-2004 scale.

After a hearing threshold is obtained, a symbol is placed under the test frequency at a number corresponding to the hearing-level dial setting (in decibels) that represents threshold. The usual symbols for air conduction are a ○ representing the right ear and an X representing the left ear. After all the results are plotted on the audiogram, the symbols are usually connected with a solid red line for the right ear and a solid blue line for the left ear. When masking is used in the nontest ear, the symbol Δ (in red) is used for the right ear and the symbol □ (in blue) is used for the left ear.

When no response (NR) is obtained at the highest output for the frequency being tested, the appropriate symbol is placed at the point on the intersection of the maximum testable level for the test frequency; an arrow pointing down indicates no response. Because a significant number of individuals (usually children) have hearing that is more sensitive than the lower limit of intensities shown on standard audiograms (–10 dB HL), Halpin (2007) recommends that an arrow pointing up be placed next to symbols when threshold readings of –10 dB HL are found. This is a logical recommendation.

The American Speech-Language-Hearing Association (1990) has recommended a set of symbols that has been widely adopted. The currently used symbols are shown in Figure 4.9.

FIGURE 4.9 Symbols for unmasked and masked thresholds (top) and no response (bottom) recommended by the American Speech-Language-Hearing Association (1990) for use in pure-tone audiometry.

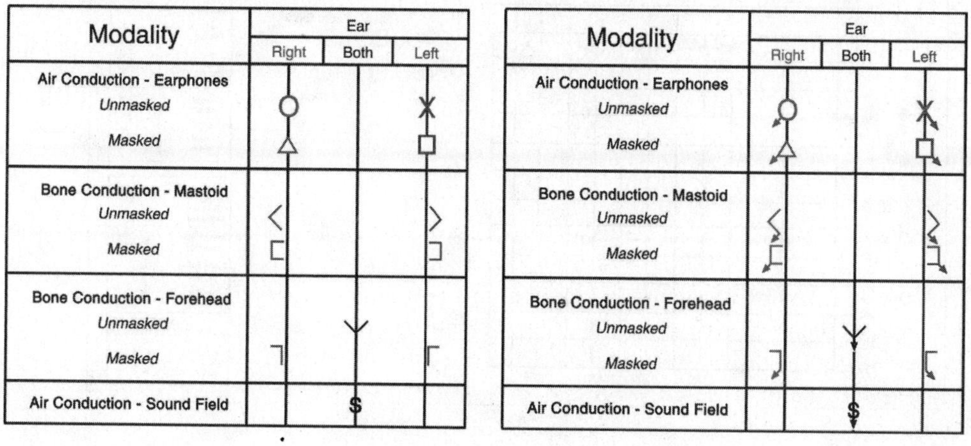

The obvious reason for using standardized symbols is to improve communication and minimize confusion when audiograms are exchanged among different clinics. Because audiograms are often faxed or photocopied to other clinics, many clinicians record their data in black ink. For this reason careful use of the proper symbols is mandated.

Figure 4.10 shows an audiogram that illustrates normal hearing for both ears. Note that the normal audiometric contour is flat because the normal threshold curve, with a sound-pressure-level reference, has been compensated for in calibration of the audiometer, which uses a hearing-level reference.

FIGURE 4.10 (A) Worksheet showing normal hearing in both ears. Note that no hearing level by either air conduction or bone conduction exceeds 15 dB HL. (B) Audiogram using the tabulated results in 4.10A. The three-frequency pure-tone averages are 7 dB HL in each ear. Naturally the two-frequency averages are slightly lower and the variable average is slightly higher.

AIR CONDUCTION

Earphones: Insert ☒ / Supra Aural ☐	RIGHT 250	500	1000	1500	2000	3000	4000	6000	8000	LEFT 250	500	1000	1500	2000	3000	4000	6000	8000
Masking Type	5	10	5/5	5	5	0	10	10	15	10	5	5/5	10	10	5	15	10	10
WB ☐ NB ☐																		
EM Level in Opp. Ear																		

BONE CONDUCTION

Placement: Forehead ☒ / Mastoid ☐	RIGHT 250	500	1000	2000	3000	4000	FOREHEAD 250	500	1000	2000	3000	4000	LEFT 250	500	1000	2000	3000	4000
Masking Type							5	5	5	10	10	10						
WB ☐ NB ☐																		
EM Level in Opp. Ear																		

	2 Freq	3 Freq	Variable	WEBER							2 Freq	3 Freq	Variable
Pure Tone Average	5	7	8	M	M	M	M	M	M	Pure Tone Average	5	7	10

A

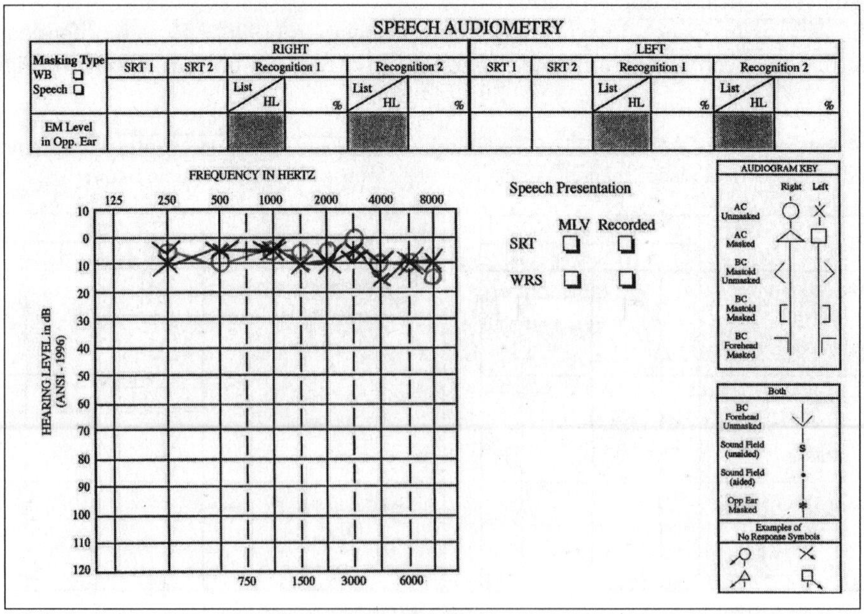

B

Bone-Conduction Audiometry

The purpose of measuring hearing by bone conduction is to determine the patient's sensory/neural sensitivity. The descriptions offered in Chapter 2 were very much oversimplified because bone conduction is an extremely complex phenomenon. Actually, hearing by bone conduction arises from the interactions of at least three different phenomena.

When the skull is set into vibration, as by a bone-conduction vibrator or a tuning fork, the bones of the skull become distorted, resulting in distortion of the structures of hearing within the cochlea of the inner ear. This distortion activates certain cells and gives rise to electrochemical activity that is identical to the activity created by an air-conduction signal. This is called **distortional bone conduction**.

bones become distorted from how tight the vibrator is. still need hair cells to be excited

While the skull is moving, the chain of tiny bones in the middle ear, owing to its inertia, lags behind so that the third bone, the stapes, moves in and out of an oval-shaped window into the cochlea. Thus, activity is generated within the cochlea as in air-conduction stimulation. This mode of inner-ear stimulation is appropriately called **inertial bone conduction**.

activates ossicular chain bc of bone distortion; inertia causes stapes to go into the oval window

Simultaneously, oscillation of the skull causes vibration of the column of air in the outer-ear canal. Some of these sound waves pass out of the ear, whereas others go further down the canal, vibrating the tympanic membrane and following the same sound route as air conduction. This third mode is called **osseotympanic bone conduction**. Hearing by bone conduction results from an interaction of these three ways of stimulating the cochlea.

hearing a combination of BC & AC; primarily by BC

For many years, the prominent bone behind the ear (the mastoid process) has been the place on the head from which bone-conduction measurements have been made. The mastood process was probably chosen because (1) bone-conducted tones are loudest from the mastoid in normal-hearing persons and (2) each mastoid process is close to the ear being tested. Probably the bone-conducted tone is loudest from behind the ear because the chain of middle ear bones is driven on a direct axis, taking maximum advantage of its hinged action. The notion that placing a vibrator behind the right ear results in stimulation of only the right cochlea is false because vibration of the skull from any location results in approximately equal stimulation of both cochleas (see Figure 4.11).

FIGURE 4.11 Vibrations of the skull result in bone-conducted stimulation of both inner ears, whether the vibrator is placed on (A) the mastoid or (B) the forehead.

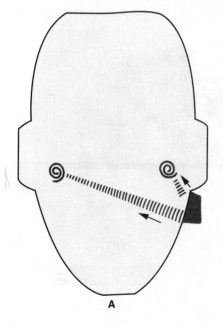

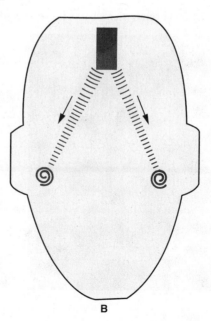

A

B

Years ago, Studebaker (1962) demonstrated that the forehead is in many ways superior to the mastoid process for measurement of clinical bone-conduction thresholds. Variations produced by vibrator-to-skull pressure, artifacts created by abnormalities of the sound-conducting mechanism of the middle ear, test-retest differences, and so on, are all of smaller consequence when testing from the forehead than from the mastoid. The greater amount of acoustic energy generated in the outer ear canal when the mastoid is the test site, as compared to the forehead, is further evidence of the advantage of forehead testing (Fagleson & Martin, 1994).

In addition to the theoretical advantages of forehead bone-conduction testing, there are numbers of practical conveniences. The headband used to hold the bone-conduction vibrator is much easier to affix to the head than the mastoid headband. Also, eyeglasses need not be removed when the vibrator is placed on the forehead, which is the case for mastoid placement.

The main disadvantage of testing from the forehead is that about 10 dB greater intensity is required to stimulate normal thresholds, resulting in a decrease of the maximum level at which testing can be carried out. Although bone-conduction testing should sometimes be done from both the forehead and the mastoid, the forehead is recommended here for routine audiometry. Despite negative reports on mastoid test accuracy and other problems that go back many years (e.g., Barany, 1938), a national survey (Martin, Champlin, & Chambers, 1998) shows that the mastoid process continues to be the preferred bone-conduction vibrator site among audiologists. Clinical observations suggest that this has not changed in spite of evidence supporting forehead placement.

When the mastoid is the place of measurement, a steel headband that crosses over the top of the head is used (see Figure 4.12A). If testing is to be done from the forehead, the bone-conduction vibrator should be affixed to the centerline of the skull, just above the eyebrow line. A plastic strap encircles the head, holding the vibrator in place (see Figure 4.12B). All interfering hair must be pushed out of the way, and the concave side of the vibrator should be placed against the skull. When you watch the video on Bone Conduction Receiver Placement, you will see demonstration of both forehead and mastoid placements as well as placement of air-conduction receivers when masking is used. Note that the preferred insert air-conduction receiver can be used for masking with either bone-conduction receiver placement site.

FIGURE 4.12 Bone-conduction vibrator placement on (A) the mastoid process and (B) the forehead.

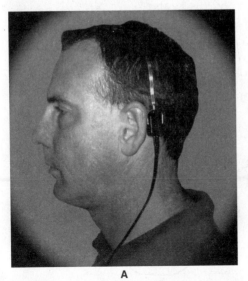

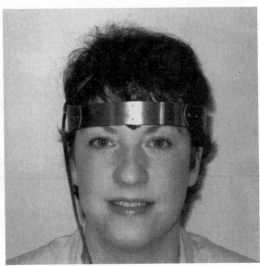

A   B

Both ears must be uncovered during routine bone-conduction audiometry. When normal ears and those with sensory/neural impairments are covered by earphones or occluded by other devices, there is an increase in the intensity of sound delivered by a bone-conduction vibrator to the cochlea. This intensity occurs partly because of changes in osseotympanic bone conduction. This phenomenon, called the occlusion effect (OE), occurs at frequencies of 1000 Hz and below. The occlusion effect is rare in patients with conductive hearing losses (e.g., problems in the middle ear) because the increase in sound pressure created by the occlusion is attenuated by the hearing loss. The occlusion effect (see Table 4.2) explains the results on the Bing tuning-fork test described in Chapter 2. Research findings confirm previous notions that the occlusion effect is the result of the increase in sound-pressure level in the external ear canal when the outer ear is covered (Fagelson & Martin, 1994; Martin & Fagelson, 1995). Dean and Martin (2000) compared supra-aural earphones to insert earphones with slight and deep insertion and found the occlusion effect to be markedly decreased when the insert phone was deeply inserted, nearly eliminating it at 1000 Hz. This has profound effects when masking for bone conduction, as will be discussed in Chapter 6.

Procedure for Bone-Conduction Audiometry

The decision about which ear to test first in mastoid bone-conduction audiometry is unimportant. As is illustrated in Figure 4.11, clinicians really cannot be certain which cochlea they are testing. The procedure for actual testing is identical to that for air conduction, although the range of frequencies to be tested and the maximum intensities emitted are more limited for bone conduction than for air conduction.

Bone-conduction thresholds may be recorded in identical fashion to those for air conduction, using the appropriate spaces on the audiometric worksheet. All audiograms should contain a key that tells the reader the symbols used and what they represent. The symbol for forehead (or ear unspecified) bone conduction is a black V when no masking is used. When the nontest ear is masked for forehead bone-conduction testing, a red ⌐ is used as a symbol for the right ear and a blue ⌐ for the left ear. If the mastoid is the test site, a red arrowhead pointing to the reader's left (<) is used for the right ear and a blue arrowhead pointing to the reader's right (>) is used for the left ear. If the printed page is viewed as the patient's face looking at the reader, the symbols for right and left are logical. When masking is used in the nontest ear, the symbols are changed to square brackets, [in red for the right ear and] in blue for the left ear. Some audiologists prefer to connect the bone-conduction symbols on the audiogram with a dashed red line for the right ear and a dashed blue line for the left ear. Others prefer not to connect the symbols at all. The latter is the preference in this text. At times, a patient may give no response at the maximum bone-conduction limits of the audiometer. When this occurs, the appropriate symbol should be placed under the test frequency where that line intersects the maximum testable level. An arrow pointing down indicates no response at that level. Figure 4.10 shows the recording of results and plotting of an audiogram for a hypothetical normal-hearing individual.

TABLE 4.2 Occlusion Effect for Bone Conduction Produced When a Supra-Aural Earphone-Cushion Is Placed over the Ear During Bone-Conduction Tests*

Frequency (Hz)	250	500	1000	2000	4000
Occlusion Effect (dB)					
Elpern & Naunton (1963)	30	20	10	0	0
Hodgson & Tillman (1966)	22	19	7	0	0
Martin et al (1974)	20	15	5	0	0

*The amounts shown indicate central tendencies and the range of occlusion effects may be considerable.

The Audiometric Weber Test

The Weber test, described in Chapter 2, can be performed by using the bone-conduction vibrator of an audiometer. The vibrator is placed on the midline of the skull, just as for forehead bone-conduction testing, and the level of the tone is raised until it is above the patient's hearing threshold. Tones of different frequencies are then presented, and patients are asked to state whether they hear them in the left ear, in the right ear, or in the midline. Midline sensations are sometimes described as being heard in both ears or as unlateralized.

It is expected that, during the Weber test, tones will be referred to the poorer-hearing ear in a conductive loss, to the better ear in a sensory/neural loss, and to the midline in symmetrical losses or normal hearing. It has been suggested that the **audiometric Weber test** be used to determine which ear to mask during bone-conduction testing. This notion is not encouraged here because there are several reasons why the Weber may be misleading. Weber results help in the confirmation or denial of results obtained from standard pure-tone audiometry, and the probable results on this test are illustrated in all of the audiograms in this text.

Audiogram Interpretation

Whether the audiometric results have been recorded as numbers or plotted on a graph, they are interpreted in the same way. Results must be looked at for each frequency in terms of (1) the amount of hearing loss by air conduction (the hearing level), (2) the amount of hearing loss by bone conduction, and (3) the relationship between air-conduction and bone-conduction thresholds.

A wide variety of pure-tone configurations may be seen among patients and within various pathologies. While some configurations may be suggestive of a given pathology, it is not always possible to identify pathology by audiometric configuration alone. Some distinct gender effects have been noted in audiometric configuration with a wider variation in configuration and a greater preponderance of more steeply sloping audiograms reported for men (Ciletti & Flamme, 2009).

The audiometric results depicted in Figure 4.13A and B illustrate a **conductive hearing loss** in both ears. There is approximately equal loss of sensitivity at each frequency by air conduction. Measurements obtained by bone conduction show normal hearing at all frequencies. Therefore, the air-conduction results show the loss of sensitivity (about 35 dB); the bone-conduction results show the amount of sensory/neural impairment (none); and the difference between the air- and bone-conduction thresholds, which is called the **air-bone gap (ABG)**, shows the amount of conductive involvement (35 dB).

Figure 4.14 shows an audiogram similar to that in Figure 4.13; however, Figure 4.14 illustrates a bilateral **sensory/neural hearing loss.** Again, the air-conduction results show the total amount of loss (35 dB), the bone-conduction results show the amount of sensory/neural impairment (35 dB), and the air-bone gap (0 dB) shows no conductive involvement at all.

The results shown in Figure 4.15A and B suggest a typical **mixed hearing loss** in both ears. In this case, the total loss of sensitivity is much greater than in the previous two illustrations, as shown by the air-conduction thresholds (60 dB). Bone-conduction results show that there is some sensory/neural involvement (35 dB). The air-bone gap shows a 25 dB conductive component.

Sometimes high-frequency tones radiate from the bone-conduction vibrator when near-maximum hearing levels are presented by bone conduction. If the patient hears these signals

FIGURE 4.13 (A) Worksheet illustrating a bilateral conductive hearing loss. Bone-conduction thresholds were obtained from the forehead, first without masking and then with masking, and the appropriate masking is recorded on the form. The determination of need for and correct amounts of masking are covered in detail in Chapter 6. (B) Audiogram using the tabulated results in Figure 14.3A illustrating a conductive hearing loss in both ears. The three-frequency pure-tone averages are 35 dB HL in each ear. There are air-bone gaps of about 35 dB (conductive component) in both ears. An asterisk is used to denote that nontest-ear masking was used. Bone-conduction results obtained from the forehead with the left ear masked are assumed to come from the right cochlea, and bone-conduction results obtained from the forehead with the right ear masked are assumed to come from the left cochlea. No lateralization is seen on the Weber test at any frequency.

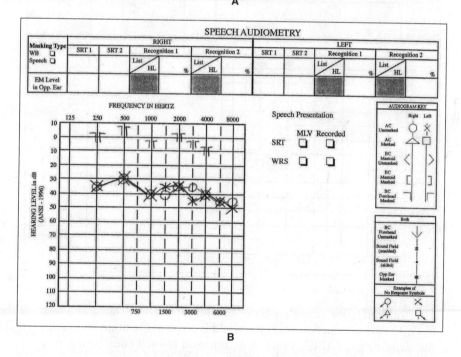

by air conduction, the false impression of an air-bone gap may be made. Because this occurs only at 3000 and 4000 Hz, it is unlikely that a misdiagnosis of conductive hearing loss would be made. This small inaccuracy can be ameliorated by testing bone conduction from the forehead. Harkrider and Martin (1998) found less acoustic radiation in the high frequencies from the forehead than from the ipsilateral mastoid.

FIGURE 4.14 (A) Worksheet illustrating a relatively symetrical sensory/neural hearing loss in both ears. (B) Audiogram using the tabulated results in Figure 14.4A illustrating sensory/neural hearing loss in both ears. The air-conduction thresholds average 35 dB HL, and the bone-conduction thresholds (obtained from the forehead) are about the same (33 dB HL). Tones are heard in the midline at all frequencies on the Weber test.

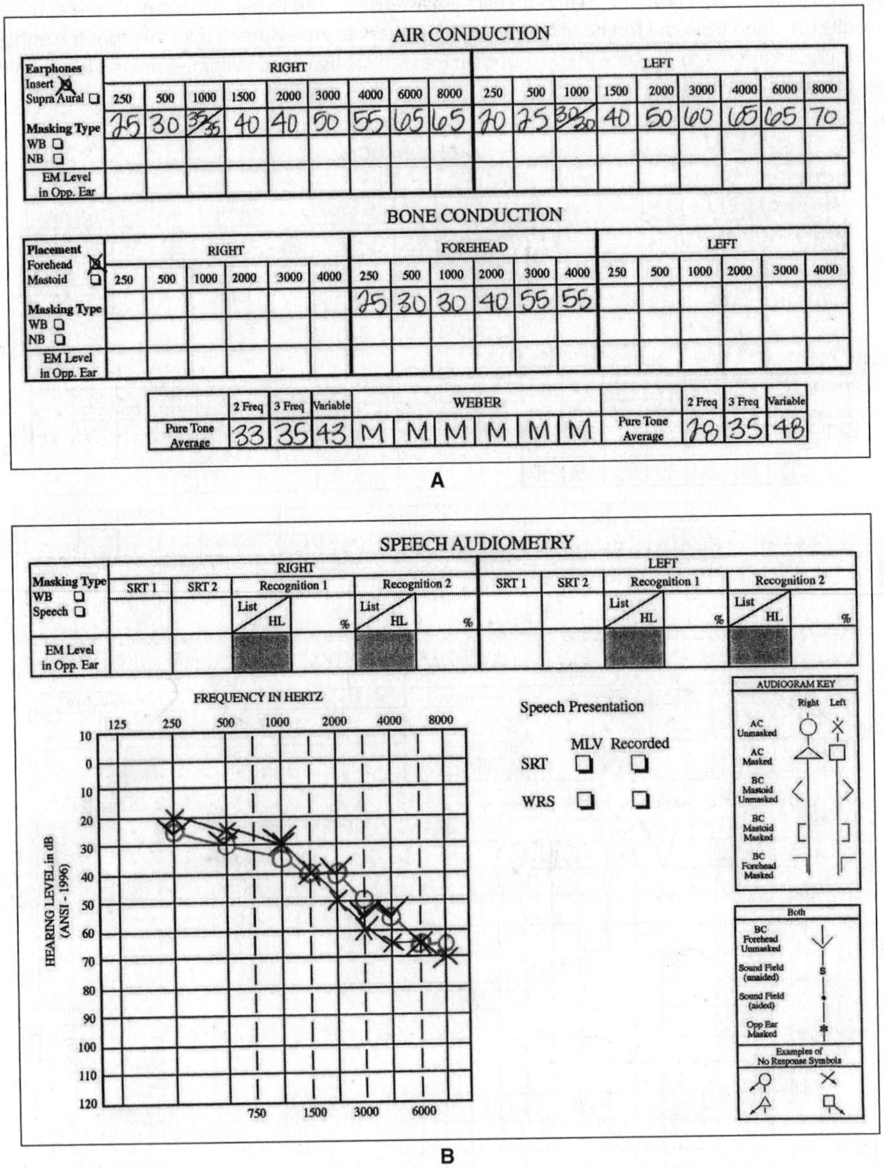

A

B

Interpretation of the air-bone relationships can be stated as a formula that reads as follows: The air-conduction (AC) threshold is equal to the bone-conduction (BC) threshold plus the air-bone gap (ABG), which is determined at each audiometric frequency. With this formula, the four audiometric examples just cited would read

Formula: **AC = BC + ABG**
Figure 4.10: $5 = 5 + 0$ (normal)
Figure 4.13: $35 = 0 + 35$ (conductive loss)
Figure 4.14: $35 = 35 + 0$ (sensory/neural loss)
Figure 4.15: $60 = 35 + 25$ (mixed loss)

FIGURE 4.15 (A) A form showing a mixed hearing loss, Masking (explained in Chapter 6) was required for all frequencies for bone conduction. (B) Audiogram using the tabulated results in Figure 14.15A that illustrates a mixed hearing loss in both ears. The air-conduction thresholds average about 60 dB HL (total hearing loss), whereas the bone-conduction thresholds average 35 dB HL (sensory/neural component). There is an air-bone gap of about 25 dB (conductive component). Tones on the Weber test do not lateralize.

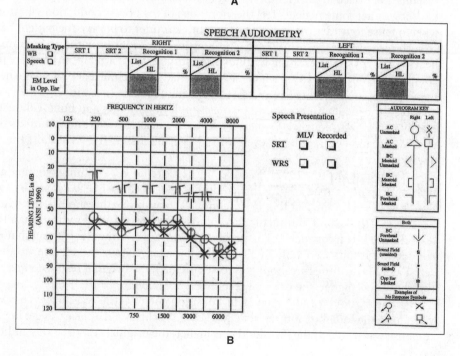

A

B

Air-Bone Relationships

Figure 2.2 suggested that (1) hearing by bone conduction is the same as by air conduction in individuals with normal hearing and in patients with sensory/neural impairment (no air-bone gap) and (2) hearing by air conduction is poorer than by bone conduction in patients with conductive or mixed hearing losses (some degree of air-bone gap), but (3) hearing by bone conduction that is poorer than by air conduction should not occur because both routes ultimately measure the integrity of the sensory/neural structures. It has been shown that, although assumptions 1 and 2 are correct, 3 may be false. There are several reasons why bone-conduction thresholds may be slightly poorer than air-conduction thresholds, even when properly calibrated audiometers are used. Some of these reasons arise from changes in the inertial and osseotympanic bone-conduction modes produced by abnormal conditions of the outer or middle ears. Many decades ago, Studebaker (1967) demonstrated that slight variations between air-conduction and bone-conduction thresholds are bound to occur based purely on normal statistical variability. Slight differences between air- and bone-conduction thresholds are to be anticipated (Barry, 1994) and are built into the American National Standards Institute (1992) standard for bone conduction. Because no diagnostic significance can be attached to air-conduction results being better than those obtained by bone conduction, the insecure clinician may be tempted to alter the bone-conduction results to conform to the usual expectations. Such temptations should be resisted because (in addition to any ethical considerations) they simply propagate the myth that air-conduction thresholds can never be lower than bone-conduction thresholds.

Tactile Responses to Pure-Tone Stimuli

At times, when severe losses of hearing occur, it is not possible to be certain about whether responses obtained at the highest limits of the audiometer are auditory or tactile. Nober (1970) has shown that some patients feel the vibrations of the bone-conduction vibrator and respond when intense tones are presented, causing the examiner to believe the patient has heard them. In such cases, a severe sensory/neural hearing loss may appear on the audiogram to be a mixed hearing loss, possibly resulting in unjustified surgery in an attempt to alleviate the conductive component. Martin and Wittich (1966) found that some children with severe hearing impairments often could not differentiate tactile from auditory sensations. Nober found that it is possible for patients to respond to tactile stimuli to both air- and bone-conducted tones, primarily in the low frequencies, when the levels are near the maximum outputs of the audiometer. When audiograms show severe mixed hearing losses, the validity of the test should be questioned.

Dean and Martin (1997) describe a procedure for ascertaining whether a severe mixed hearing loss has a true conductive component or if the ABG is caused by tactile stimulation. It is based on the fact that bone-conduction auditory thresholds are higher on the forehead than the mastoid, but tactile thresholds are lower on the forehead than the mastoid, at least for the low frequencies. The procedure works as follows (assuming that original bone-conduction results were obtained from the forehead): Move the vibrator to the mastoid and retest at 500 Hz. If the threshold gets lower (better), the original response was auditory. If the threshold gets higher, the original response was tactile.

If the mastoid was the original test position and a **tactile response** is suspected, move the vibrator to the forehead and retest at 500 Hz. If the threshold appears to get lower, the original response was tactile. If the threshold gets higher, the original response was auditory.

Cross Hearing

When there are differences in hearing sensitivity between the two ears, there may be a risk that sounds that are presented to one ear (the test ear) may actually be heard in the opposite (nontest) ear. It is important for clinicians to be alert to these possibilities and to deal with them effectively. These matters are addressed in detail in the chapter on masking (Chapter 6).

Automatic Audiometry

Some audiometers allow patients to track their own auditory thresholds while they are automatically recorded in the form of a graph on a special form. Automatic audiometers can test discrete frequencies or may use a variable oscillator with a range from 100 to 10,000 Hz. The tones may be either automatically pulsed (200 msec on/200 msec off), or presented continuously. The tone gradually increases in intensity and begins at an inaudible level. When patients hear the tone, they press a hand switch, which reverses the attenuator, causing the signal to get weaker. When the tone becomes inaudible, the hand switch is released and the tone is allowed to increase in intensity again. Frequency can be either set or can continue to increase whether the intensity is increasing or decreasing. This procedure is called **Békésy audiometry.**[2] Upon completion of the test, an audiogram has been drawn that represents the patients' thresholds for discrete frequencies or over a continuous frequency range (Békésy, 1947).

Although popular for a time as a test for auditory site of lesion, the clinical use of automatic audiometry has faded from prominence. While there is value in testing between the normal discrete audiometric frequencies, the limited use of automatic audiometry is largely found in industrial settings.

Computerized Audiometry

Computers may be programmed to control all aspects of administering pure-tone air- and bone-conduction stimuli, recognize the need for masking, determine the appropriate level of masking, regulate the presentation of the masker to the nontest ear, analyze the subject's responses in terms of threshold-determination criteria, and present the obtained threshold values in an audiogram format at the conclusion of the test. **Computerized audiometry** is performed on a device that is microprocessor-controlled, and the audiometric data may be "dumped" into a computer file for later retrieval.

Possibly due to economic considerations, several companies have been formed that specialize in hearing testing performed by nonaudiologists, sometimes called para-audiologists or oto-techs. These individuals, many of whom have no academic training in hearing and its disorders, are trained to use automated devices that are programmed to complete pure-tone audiometry, and speech audiometry (Chapter 5), as well as immittance measures (Chapter 7), in a matter of 20 minutes. The claims by these firms are that the results are reliable, but this has not been empirically verified. Certainly automated audiometry cannot be used reliably with noncooperative patients (Chapter 13) or with young children or the very elderly, who may need more personalized modifications in test procedure and speed to accommodate the test situation.

CHECK YOUR UNDERSTANDING

Presumably, in these computerized hearing settings physicians carry out the counseling and follow-up. This leaves the patients without the special training of clinical audiologists in the areas of counseling, therapy, and amplification systems. Despite its sophistication, the computer has not replaced, nor is it likely to replace, the clinical audiologist in the performance of auditory tests, except for its possible use with test-cooperative patients. The fact that computers can make step-by-step decisions in testing helps to prove that many hearing tests can be carried out logically and scientifically.

ACTIVITIES

EVOLVING CASE STUDIES

You were introduced to six theoretical case studies in Chapter 2. The next step is to predict, based on your reading of Chapter 4, what the pure-tone audiometric results would be for each of these cases. Review the case study descriptions at the end of Chapter 2 before reading the discussion below. Then sketch an audiogram for each case and compare your results to the given information, bearing in mind that there will naturally be some differences.

Case Study 1: Conductive Hearing Loss—Outer Ear Disorder

Because this child has no external auditory canals, insert receivers could not be used. Supra-aural earphones were placed on this child's head with the receivers positioned where his ears would normally be. He took a reliable hearing test and results showed large air-bone gaps in both ears, with air-conduction thresholds about 50 to 60 dB HL, similar to Figure 9.10. Bone-conduction thresholds were normal with the bone oscillator applied to the forehead. Masking cannot be successfully accomplished given that the masking signal via supra-aural headphones, to be audible, would be of sufficient intensity to create a confounding dilemma known as cross-masking (see Chapter 6). It is possible that further electrophysiologic testing can shed light on this.

Case Study 2: Conductive Hearing Loss—Middle Ear Disorder

Audiometric findings for this patient should be similar to what is observed in Figure 4.13. Note that there is a moderate hearing loss by air conduction for both ears but that the bone-conduction thresholds are normal, indicating normal sensory/neural sensitivity. The resultant air-bone gaps show the degree of conductive involvement. A great deal of masking was required in this case (see Chapter 6). These results do not indicate the cause of the hearing loss, but the tests described in later chapters will assist in this regard. The history of ear infections suggests the infections may be the cause of the hearing loss but may be misleading.

Case Study 3: Sensory/Neural Hearing Loss—Inner Ear Disorder

Compare the audiogram you have drawn to Figure 4.14. Results should be similar but surely will not be identical. You should have shown a moderate loss, in this case approximately 45 dB HL based, on the variable pure-tone average, but the air-conduction and bone-conduction thresholds should be about the same. The lack of an air-bone gap indicates that the loss is entirely sensory/neural and probably cochlear. The case history points to aging as the cause, but further tests, as described in later chapters, can help to determine the site of the pathology.

Case Study 4: Sensory/Neural Hearing Loss—Auditory Nerve Disorder

Audiometric findings are consistent with the patient's report of a unilateral (left) hearing loss (see Figure 12.2). Masking (to be explained in Chapter 6) was required for several tests. It appears that the hearing loss in the left ear is sensory/neural because there are no air-bone gaps in that ear. Speech audiometry (discussed in Chapter 5) will be an essential part of the diagnosis for this patient. The history and nature of the audiogram suggest a possible lesion on the auditory nerve, but more testing is required before this diagnosis is confirmed. This is potentially a serious medical matter.

Case Study 5: Nonorganic Hearing Loss

What you have drawn should closely resemble Figure 13.2A. The patient is reporting normal hearing in his right ear and gives no response by either air conduction or bone conduction at the highest intensities in his left ear. This is actually impossible because at some intensity (possibly as low as 40 dB HL for supra-aural earphones and 70 dB HL for insert earphones) the sound would have lateralized (crossed the skull) and been heard in the right ear. This total lack of response is a clear indication that the hearing loss in the left ear cannot be of the degree claimed, but based on the present information, it cannot be learned just how much loss exists in the left ear, if any. Chapter 5 will allow for more insights about this case, and Chapter 13 will describe tests that are specific to nonorganic hearing loss.

Case Study 6: Pediatric Patient

The test procedures described in Chapter 4 are designed for adults and older children, or young children who are particularly cooperative. Some youngsters can take adult-level tests that have been modified by an audiologist who provides significant social reward for accurate responses. Using a variety of pediatric techniques (to be described in Chapter 8), an audiogram has been obtained, as will be discussed later.

Summary

For pure-tone hearing tests to be performed satisfactorily, control is needed over factors such as background noise levels, equipment calibration, patient comprehension, and clinician expertise. The audiologist must be able to judge when responses are accurate and to predict when a sound may have actually been heard in the ear not being tested. When this cross hearing occurs, proper masking procedures must be instituted to overcome this problem, as discussed in Chapter 6. Although at times the performance of pure-tone hearing tests is carried out as an art, it should, in most cases, be approached in a scientific manner using rigid controls.

REVIEW TABLE 4.1 Summary of Pure-Tone Hearing Tests*

Test	*Air Conduction (AC)*	*Bone Conduction (BC)*
Purpose	Hearing sensitivity for pure tones	Sensory/neural sensitivity for pure tones
Interpretation	AC audiogram shows amount of hearing loss at each frequency	BC audiogram shows degree of sensory/neural loss at each frequency
		Air-bone gap shows amount of conductive impairment at each frequency

*Minimal interaural attenuation is considered to be 40 dB for supra-aural earphones and 70 dB for insert earphones.

REVIEW TABLE 4.2 Possible Findings for Air Conduction (AC) and Bone Conduction (BC)

Finding	Possibilities	Eliminate
Normal AC	Normal hearing	Conductive loss Sensory/neural loss Mixed loss
Normal BC	Normal hearing Sensory/neural loss	Conductive loss Mixed loss
Impaired AC	Conductive loss Sensory/neural loss Mixed loss	Normal hearing
Impaired BC	Sensory/neural loss Mixed loss	Normal hearing Conductive loss

Frequently Asked Questions

Q What term is used when a patient fails to respond to a stimulus that has been heard?

A *When a patient fails to respond to a stimulus, we use the term* negative response. *If the signal has actually not been heard, this is a true negative. If the patient hears the signal but does not respond, this is a false negative and can be caused by a variety of factors.*

Q Under what circumstances will an audiologist see a mixed hearing loss?

A *A mixed hearing loss is a combination of a conductive and sensory/neural loss. This occurs regardless of the causes of the different disorders.*

Q Why does it matter which way a patient faces during a test?

A *The most important thing is for the patient not to be able to watch the clinician during the test because this can result in false positive responses. The patient seated at right angles to the clinician is probably the best arrangement.*

Q How do you tell from the audiogram to which ear the tone lateralizes in the Weber test?

A *The Weber principle states that a bone-conducted tone originating from an oscillator placed in the midline of the head (the forehead is usually used) will refer to the better ear in a unilateral sensory/neural hearing loss and to the poorer ear in a unilateral conductive loss. If audiometric thresholds are about the same in both ears, the tone is usually heard in the middle of the head or in both ears. Several factors can alter these results.*

Q When is 1500 Hz tested?

A *ASHA's older guideline recommended that clinicians test any mid-octave point when there is a difference in threshold at adjacent octaves of 20 dB or more. This is still the recommendation for 750 Hz and 1500 Hz. The newer guidelines recommend routine testing of the mid-octave points at 3000 Hz and 6000 Hz.*

Q Why does a profound bilateral sensory/neural hearing loss sometimes look like a mixed hearing loss?

A *This happens because patients respond to bone-conducted tones when they feel them rather than when they hear them. This usually occurs near the bone-conduction limits of the audiometer below 1000 Hz.*

Q How do you know if the earphones or audiometer are calibrated correctly?

A *The only way to know is to test the audiometer using electroacoustic instruments. Audiologists should be trained to do this to be certain that their equipment is functioning correctly. Usually technicians correct the errors if they are present, but some audiologists do this themselves.*

Q What does the air-bone gap tell us?

A *The air-conduction threshold shows the total amount of hearing loss, the bone-conduction threshold shows the sensory/neural component of a hearing loss, and the air-bone gap (the difference between the AC and BC thresholds) shows the conductive portion of a hearing loss.*

Q According to the Rinne tuning fork test, air conduction is better than bone conduction in normal-hearing individuals. On an audiogram, however, patients with normal hearing hear bone-conducted tones at the same intensities as those for air conduction. Which is better, air conduction or bone conduction?

A *In the real world, hearing by air conduction for those with normal hearing is more efficient than for bone conduction. That is why people with normal hearing and those with sensory/neural hearing losses hear a tuning fork louder at the ear than behind the ear. Audiometers electronically increase the intensity of bone-conducted signals over that required for air conduction because it takes more energy to drive a plastic bone-conduction oscillator, which then must drive the skull, than it does to drive the thin diaphragm of* *an air-conduction receiver, which must move the very thin eardrum membrane.*

Q How much does each of the three types of bone conduction (distortional, inertial, and osseotympanic) factor into the total measurement of the auditory threshold for bone conduction?

A *Distortional bone conduction, the actual distortion of the cochlear shell, is the primary means by which we hear by bone conduction. The other modes augment distortional bone conduction and vary depending on the integrity of the conductive system.*

Q When explaining to a patient his or her degree of hearing loss, should an audiologist refer to pure-tone averages (PTAs)? If so, how does one determine which type of PTA (two-frequency, three-frequency, variable) should be used?

A *Counseling may well be the most important thing the audiologist does. Experience dictates how much detail of test findings should be related to the patient or caregiver. In any event, any question asked should be answered in what is determined to be the correct amount of detail. If you are reporting pure-tone averages, you may want to use the two-frequency PTA for steeply sloping audiometric configurations. If you are trying to demonstrate agreement between the PTA and SRT, you may want to use the three-frequency PTA for flatter configurations. You may want to use the variable PTA for high-frequency hearing loss if you want the reported PTA to reflect the impact of the hearing loss on speech communication.*

Suggested Reading

Bankaitis, A. U., & Kemp, R. J. (2003). *Infection control in the audiology clinic.* Boulder, CO: Auban.

Schlauck, R. S., & Nelson, P. (2009). Puretone evaluation. In J. Katz, L. Medwetsky, R. Burkhard, & L. Hood (Eds.), *Handbook of clinical audiology* (pp. 30–49). Baltimore: Lippincott Williams & Wilkins.

Endnotes

1. The term *audiometer* was first coined by an English physician, Benjamin Richardson, in 1879. It was not until 1919 that the first clinically useful audiometer, the pitch range audiometer, was developed by Lee Dean and Cordia Bunch.

2. This test was suggested by Dr. Georg von Békésy, the Hungarian-born physicist (1899–1976) who won the Nobel Prize in 1961 for his contributions to the understanding of the human cochlea.

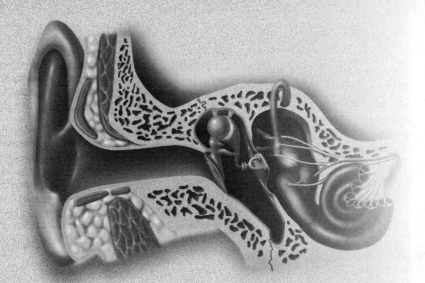

CHAPTER 5

Speech Audiometry

LEARNING OBJECTIVES

Chapter 4 introduced the concept of pure-tone audiometry and described its administration and interpretation. This chapter acquaints the reader with speech audiometry and some of its ramifications. The new vocabulary in this chapter, which is included in the glossary, is indispensable for understanding the concepts that follow in this text. At the completion of this chapter, the reader should be able to

- Understand the measures obtained with speech audiometry such as threshold for speech, most comfortable and uncomfortable loudness levels, and word-recognition ability.

- Interpret speech audiometric results; relate them to pure-tone threshold tests; and, after some supervised practice with an audiometer, actually perform the tests described in this chapter.

- Understand the implications of speech audiometric tests to speech-language therapy planning and goal setting.

THE HEARING IMPAIRMENT INFERRED from a pure-tone audiogram cannot depict, beyond the grossest generalizations, the degree of disability in speech communication caused by a hearing loss. Because difficulties in hearing and understanding speech evoke the greatest complaints from patients with hearing impairments, it is logical that tests of hearing function should be performed with speech stimuli. Modern diagnostic audiometers include circuitry for measuring various aspects of receptive speech communication (Figures 3.23 and 3.24, pages 57 and 58). Using speech audiometry, audiologists set out to answer questions regarding patients' degree of hearing loss for speech; the levels required for their most comfortable and uncomfortable loudness levels; their range of comfortable loudness; and, perhaps most important, their ability to recognize and discriminate the sounds of speech. Speech-language pathologists use reported findings of speech audiometric results in both therapy planning and client and family counseling.

The Diagnostic Audiometer

In the early days of speech audiometry, separate speech audiometers were used to perform the measurements to be described in this chapter. Modern devices have these circuits incorporated, along with circuitry for pure tones, into a single unit. Diagnostic audiometers are either accompanied by or have auxiliary inputs for testing with microphones, compact disks, or other audio files. A volume units (VU) meter is used to monitor the intensity of the input source visually.

Diagnostic audiometers contain a circuit for masking the nontest ear or for mixing a noise with a speech signal in the same ear. Tests can usually be carried out in either ear (**monaural**) or in both ears simultaneously (**binaural**), or speech can be channeled to one or more loudspeakers for testing in the sound field. Hearing level controls that usually have a range of 120 dB (from −10 to 110 dB HL, according to ANSI-2004 values) are provided. A talkback system is available for communication between separate rooms that hold the clinician and the patient.

Test Environment

Most speech audiometry is carried out with the patient isolated from the examiner in either one- or two-room sound-treated suites (see Figure 4.3 on page 74 for an example). This is mandatory when **monitored live-voice (MLV)** testing is used because, if examiners and patients are in the same room, there is no way to ensure that the patients are responding to sounds channeled to them through the audiometer rather than directly through the air in the room. If prerecorded materials are used, as should be standard practice, same-room operation is possible. Problems of ambient noise levels are very much the same for speech audiometry as for pure-tone tests, as discussed in Chapter 4.

Using recorded materials has significant advantages. Primarily, they provide a consistency of presentation that is independent of the expertise of the clinician. Most audiologists appear to prefer monitored live-voice testing because they feel it provides more flexibility in delivering the stimuli and that it takes less time. With the advent of the CD, some of these objections have been overcome, and, for the most part, the CD or audio files should be used instead of live-voice testing.

The Patient's Role in Speech Audiometry

To use speech audiometry, patients must know and understand reasonably well the words with which they are to be tested. Depending on the type of test, a response must be obtainable in the form of an oral reply, a written reply, or the identification of a picture or object.

Although spoken responses are more necessary in some speech tests than in others, they have certain advantages and disadvantages. One advantage is in the speed with which answers can be scored. Also, a certain amount of rapport is maintained through the verbal interplay between the patient and the audiologist. One serious drawback is the possible misinterpretation of the patient's response. Many people seen for hearing evaluation have speech and/or language difficulties that make their responses difficult to understand. For example, Nelson, Henion, and Martin (2000) found that non-native speakers of Spanish were less accurate at scoring recorded Spanish word-recognition tests than were native speakers. Also, discrepancies occur in the scoring of some speech tests when verbal responses are obtained because audiologists tend to score some incorrectly spoken responses as correct.

In addition, for reasons that have never become completely clear, the talkback systems on many audiometers are often of poor quality, sounding very little better than inexpensive intercom systems. This creates an additional problem in interpreting responses.

Written responses lend themselves only to tests that can be scored upon completion. When responses require an instantaneous value judgment by the audiologist, written responses are undesirable. When used, however, written responses do eliminate errors caused by difficulties in discriminating the patient's speech; they also provide a permanent record of the kinds of errors made. Having patients write down or otherwise mark responses may slow down some test procedures and necessitate time at the end of the test for scoring. Difficulties with handwriting and spelling provide additional, although not insurmountable, problems.

The use of pictures or objects is generally reserved for small children, who otherwise cannot or will not participate in a test. Adults with special problems are sometimes tested by this method, in which the patient is instructed to point to a picture or object that matches a stimulus word.

False responses may occur in speech audiometry as well as in pure-tone audiometry. False positive responses are theoretically impossible because patients cannot correctly repeat words or sentences that have been presented to them below their thresholds, unless, through the carelessness of the examiner, they have been allowed some visual cues and have actually lipread the stimulus words. False negative responses, however, do occur. The audiologist must try to make certain that the patient completely understands the task and responds in the appropriate manner whenever possible.

No matter how thorough the attempt to instruct patients, it is impossible to gain total control over the internal response criteria each individual brings to the test. It has been suspected, for example, that aging might affect the relative strictness of these criteria. Jerger, Johnson, and Jerger (1988) demonstrated, however, that aging alone does not appear to affect the criteria that listeners use in giving responses to speech stimuli. All the alert clinician can do is to instruct patients carefully and be aware of overt signs of deviation from expected behaviors.

The Clinician's Role in Speech Audiometry

First and foremost in speech audiometry, through whatever means necessary, the audiologist must convey to patients what is expected of them during the session. A combination of written and verbal instructions is usually successful with adults and older children, whereas gestures and pantomime may be required for small children and certain adults. At times, the instructions are given to patients through their hearing aids or, if this is not feasible, through a portable amplifier or the microphone circuit of the audiometer.

It is just as important that the patient not observe the examiner's face during speech audiometry as it is during pure-tone audiometry, and even more so if monitored live-voice testing is used. The diagram in Figure 4.5 (page 77) shows a desirable testing arrangement.

Speech-Threshold Testing

The logic of pure-tone threshold testing carries over to speech audiometry. If a patient's thresholds for speech can be obtained, they can be compared to an average normal-hearing individual's thresholds to determine the patient's degree of hearing loss for speech. Speech thresholds may be of two kinds: the **speech-detection threshold (SDT)** and the **speech-recognition threshold (SRT)**.

The terminology used in speech audiometry has been inconsistent. Konkle and Rintelmann (1983) feel that the word *speech* itself may be too general and that the specific speech stimuli in any test should always be specified. Likewise, they are concerned with the conventional term *speech-reception threshold* because the listener is asked to recognize, rather than receive, the words used in the test. In the "Guidelines for Determining Threshold Level for Speech," the American Speech-Language-Hearing Association (1988) also recommends the term *speech-recognition threshold* as preferable to the earlier term *speech-reception threshold*.

Speech-Detection Threshold

The speech-detection threshold (SDT) may be defined as the lowest level, in decibels, at which a subject can barely detect the presence of speech and identify it as speech. The SDT is sometimes called the speech-awareness threshold (SAT). This does not imply that the speech is in any way understood—rather, merely that its presence is detected. One way of measuring the SDT is to present to the patient, through the desired output transducer, some continuous discourse. The level of the speech is raised and lowered in intensity until the patient indicates that he or she can barely detect the speech and recognize it as speech.

Sentences are preferable to isolated words or phrases for finding the SDT. The sentences should be presented rapidly and monotonously so that there are few peaks above and below zero on the VU meter, or series of light-emitting diodes designed to control the input level of the speech signal. The materials should be relatively uninteresting, hence the term **cold running speech**.

Whether the right ear or the left ear is tested first is an arbitrary decision. Sometimes tests of SDT are run binaurally, or through the sound-field speakers, either with or without hearing aids. Patients may respond verbally, with hand or finger signals, or with a pushbutton to indicate the lowest level, in dB HL, at which they can barely detect speech.

Speech-Recognition Threshold

The speech-recognition threshold (SRT) may be defined as the lowest hearing level at which speech can barely be understood. Most audiologists agree that the speech should be so soft that about half of it can be recognized. For a number of reasons, the SRT has become more popular with audiologists than the SDT and is thus the preferred speech-threshold test. In this text, very little attention is paid to the SDT, although it has some clinical usefulness. SRTs have been measured with a variety of speech materials using both continuous discourse, as in measurement of the SDT, and isolated words.

Today most SRTs are obtained with the use of **spondaic words**, often called *spondees*. A spondee is a word with two syllables, both pronounced with equal stress and effort. Although spondees do not occur naturally in spoken English, it is possible, by altering stress slightly, to force such common words as *baseball, hot dog,* and *toothbrush* to conform to the spondaic configuration. Whether the spondees are spoken into the microphone or introduced by disk or preset audiofiles within the audiometer's software, both syllables of the word should peak at zero VU. Although it takes practice for the student to accomplish this equal peaking on the VU meter when using monitored live voice, most people can acquire the knack relatively quickly. There is no advantage to using recorded material for SRT testing unless the examiner has an accent different from the clinical population being served.

When a prerecorded list of spondaic words is to be used, it is common to find a calibration tone recorded on a special band. The calibration signal is played long enough so that the gain control for the VU meter can be adjusted with the needle at zero VU. On some prerecorded spondee lists, a **carrier phrase** precedes each word, for example, "Say the word . . . ," followed by the stimulus word. Although some clinicians prefer the use of a carrier phrase, many do not. No real advantage of using a carrier phrase with spondaic words has been proved.

SRT Testing with Cold Running Speech

When connected speech is used to measure the SRT, patients are instructed to indicate the level at which the speech is so soft that they can barely follow about half of what is being said. Sometimes this involves using a verbal or hand signal. The level of the speech may be raised and lowered, usually in steps of 5 dB. Several measurements should be taken to ensure accuracy.

SRT Testing with Spondaic Words

The SRT is usually defined as the lowest hearing level at which 50 percent of a list of spondaic words is correctly identified. This definition appears incomplete, however, because it does not specify how many words are presented at threshold before the 50 percent criterion is invoked. Also, many methods used for SRT measurement in the past were rather vague, suggesting that the level should be raised and lowered but not giving a precise methodology.

Martin and Stauffer (1975) recommended testing for the SRT in 5 dB steps, rather than the previous traditional 2 dB steps, which greatly increased test speed without sacrificing test accuracy. Additionally, if the SRT is to serve as an independent measurement of hearing and a check of the reliability of pure-tone thresholds, it should be accomplished without knowledge of the pure-tone thresholds with which it is compared. To attain this goal, Martin and Dowdy (1986) recommend a procedure based on previously recommended outlined steps (Tillman and Olsen, 1973), which is summarized as follows:

1. Set the start level at 30 dB HL. Present one spondee. If a correct response is obtained, this suggests that the word is above the patient's SRT.

2. If no correct response is obtained, raise the presentation level to 50 dB HL. Present one spondee. If there is no correct response, raise the intensity in 10 dB steps, presenting one spondee at each increment. Stop at the level at which either a correct response is obtained or the limit of the equipment is reached.

3. After a correct response is obtained, lower the intensity 10 dB and present one spondee.

4. When an incorrect response is given, raise the level 5 dB and present one spondee. If a correct response is given, lower the intensity 10 dB. If an incorrect response is given, continue raising the intensity in 5 dB steps until a correct response is obtained.

5. From this point on, the intensity is increased in 5 dB steps and decreased in 10 dB steps, with one spondee presented at each level until three correct responses have been obtained at a given level.

6. Threshold is defined as the lowest level at which *at least* 50 percent of the responses are correct, with a minimum of at least three correct responses at that intensity.

The American Speech-Language-Hearing Association (1988) method for determining SRT provides recommendations to ensure patient familiarity with the test vocabulary prior to testing. This goal can be accomplished by allowing the patient to listen to the words as presented through the audiometer and is important regardless of the method employed to measure SRT. Words that present any difficulty should be eliminated from the list. While the American Speech-Language-Hearing Association (ASHA) recommendation to familiarize patients with test stimuli is important, the actual ASHA recommended test methods (American Speech-Language-Hearing Association, 1978, 1988) never enjoyed full acceptance (Martin, Champlin, & Chambers, 1998), possibly due to several procedural limitations.

To ensure familiarity with the test, it is advisable, whenever possible, to give the patient a list of the words before the test begins, together with printed instructions for the entire test procedure. Although written instructions may serve as an adjunct, they should not routinely replace spoken directions for taking a test. Proper instructions are of great importance in test results. One usable set of instructions follows:

> The purpose of this test is to determine the faintest level at which you can hear and repeat some words. Each word you hear will have two syllables, like *hot dog* or *baseball,* and will be selected from the list of words that you have been given. Each time you hear a word, just repeat it. Repeat the words even if they sound very soft. You may have to guess, but repeat each word if you have any idea what it is. Are there any questions?

Based on investigation with normal-hearing subjects, Burke and Nerbonne (1978) suggest that the slight improvement observed when normal-hearing subjects guess at the correct response should be controlled during SRT tests by asking the patient not to guess. Because no data have surfaced that reveal the effects of guessing on patients with actual hearing losses, the practice will probably continue to encourage guessing and thus increase attentiveness to the test stimuli.

One reason for the selection of spondaic words for measuring SRT is that they are relatively easy to discriminate and often can be guessed with a high degree of accuracy. Once the threshold for spondees has been reached (50 percent response criterion), it does not take much of an increase in intensity before all the words can be identified correctly. This is illustrated by the curve in Figure 5.1, which shows the enhanced intelligibility of spondees as a function

FIGURE 5.1 Theoretical performance-intensity (PI) functions for spondaic and PB words. (1) Spondaic words. Note that, at about 5 dB above the 50 percent correct point, almost all of the words are intelligible. This shows an increase in recognition ability of approximately 10 percent per decibel for scores between 20 percent and 80 percent. (2) PB word lists. Note the more gradual slope for PB words than for spondees. The increase in intelligibility for the W-22 word lists averages about 2.5 percent per decibel. The normal increase in word-recognition scores with increased intensity is to a maximum of approximately 100 percent (suggesting normal hearing or conductive hearing loss). (3) PB word lists. Note the increase in word-recognition scores with increased intensity to a maximum of less than 90 percent (suggesting sensory/neural hearing loss). (4) PB word lists. Note the increase in word-recognition scores with increased intensity to a given level, beyond which scores decrease. This is the rollover effect, which occurs in some ears when there are lesions in the higher auditory centers (see Chapter 12).

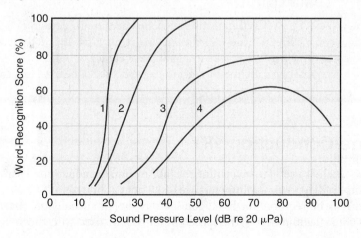

of increased intensity. As you view the video entitled Speech Recognition Threshold Testing note the carefully controlled presentation of words to attain equal stress on both syllables. SRT testing is routinely completed with monitored-live voice and care must be taken that the patient cannot see the examiner's face. In this video, the lights have been turned off on the examiner's side of the booth.

Recording SRT Results

After SRTs for each ear have been obtained, they should be recorded in the appropriate space on the audiometric worksheet (see the letter *p* in Figure 5.2). Many audiologists prefer to make routine measurements of the SRT binaurally or in the sound field. The audiometric worksheet used in this text does not provide for such notation, but many forms are available that do.

Relationship of SRT to SDT and the Pure-Tone Audiogram

The SRT is always higher (requires greater intensity) than the SDT. In the earliest years of the profession, Egan (1948) showed that the magnitude of the difference between the SRT and SDT does not normally exceed 12 dB. However, this difference may change with the shape of the pure-tone audiogram.

Different methods have been used for many years to predict the SRT from the pure-tone audiogram. Although some of these procedures have been quite elegant, most audiologists have agreed that the SRT can be predicted by finding the average of the lowest two thresholds at 500, 1000, and 2000 Hz (Fletcher, 1950). Carhart and Porter (1971) found that the SRT can be predicted from the pure-tone audiogram by averaging the thresholds at 500 and 1000 Hz and subtracting 2 dB. Although 500, 1000, and 2000 Hz have been called the "speech frequencies," Wilson and Margolis (1983) cautioned that such phrasing can be misleading if it is inferred that this narrow range of frequencies is all that is essential for the adequate discrimination of speech.

In some cases, the SRT may be much lower (better) than the pure-tone average (PTA), such as when the audiogram falls precipitously in the high frequencies. In other cases, the SRT may be higher (poorer) than even the three-frequency PTA, for example, with some elderly patients or those with disorders of the central auditory nervous system. The special significance of PTA-SRT disagreement regarding nonorganic hearing loss is discussed in Chapter 13.

Clinical COMMENTARY

The value of the SRT is frequently questioned because its determined level lends little to the diagnostic picture. Its true value lies in two areas. First, the SRT is useful as a comparative measure with pure-tone results to signal the accuracy of both tests. Second, the SRT may be used in counseling patients with regard to the degree of hearing loss they may have.

Bone-Conduction SRT

It is sometimes useful to determine the SRT by bone conduction. Because the bone-conduction circuits on diagnostic audiometers are often not calibrated for speech, some degree of manipulation may be required for bone-conduction speech audiometry (Barry & Gaddis, 1978). On most clinical audiometers, the speech input may be used with the bone-conduction output.

FIGURE 5.2 (A) The tabular worksheet has no space for notation of speech audiometrics. The audiologic evaluation form (B) shows spaces to record the items to be completed when performing speech audiometry as listed below the form.

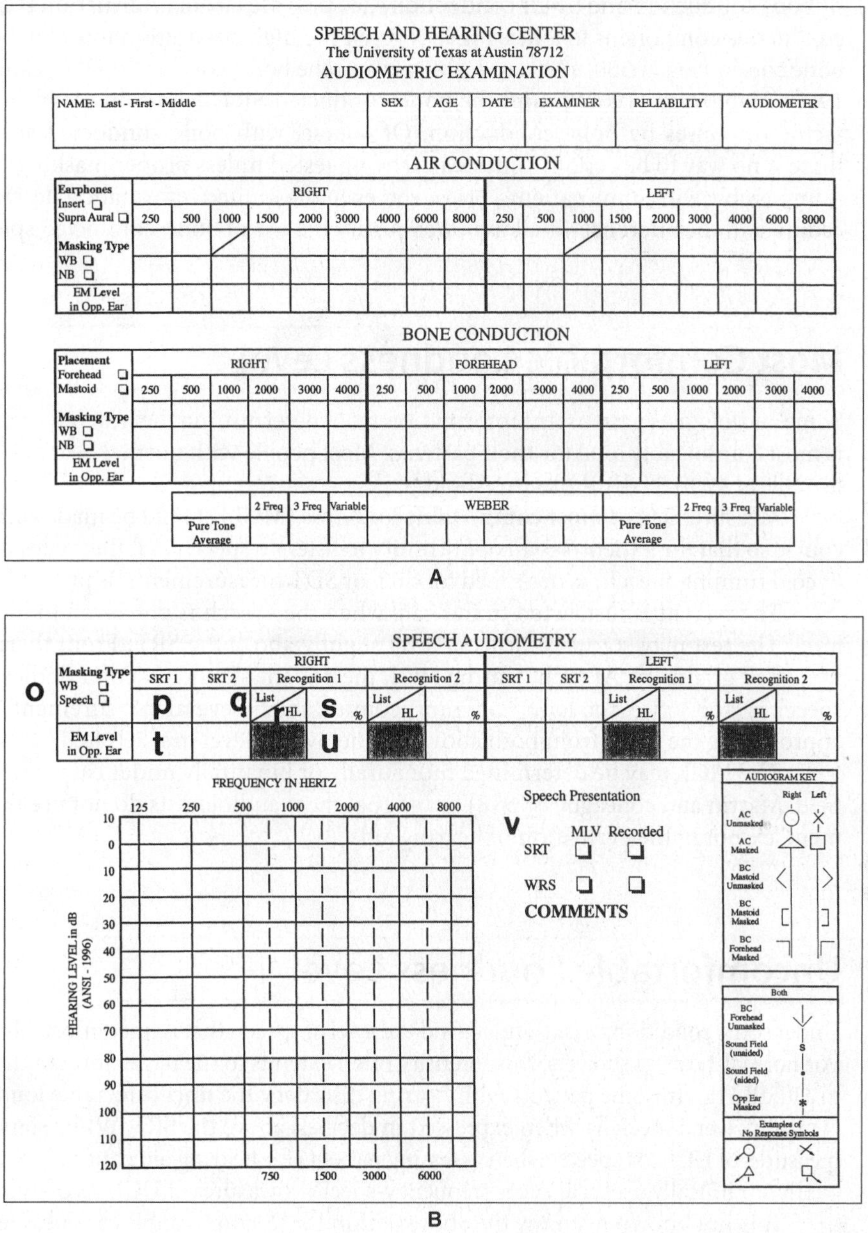

o. Masking type used in the nontest ear
p. SRT
q. Second SRT following re-instruction if required
r. Hearing-level setting for the WRS test
s. Word-recognition scores (WRS)
t. Effective masking level in the nontest ear used for SRT
u. Effective masking level in the nontest ear used for WRS
v. Presentation method for SRT and WRS testing

Bone-conducted SRTs are especially useful in testing children who will "play a game" with words but not with tones. A comparison between children's hearing thresholds for speech by bone conduction and by air conduction may provide useful information regarding a possible conductive component to a hearing loss given the high correlation found between the PTA by bone conduction at 500, 1000, and 2000 Hz and the bone-conducted SRT (Goetzinger & Proud, 1955). Hahlbrock (1962) found the bone-conducted SRT helpful in separating auditory from tactile responses by bone conduction. Of course, with bone-conducted speech audiometry, there is no way to be certain which ear is being tested unless proper masking is invoked, which is impossible with some patients. However, even the limited information derived from this procedure and the inferences it allows often justify the use of bone-conducted speech audiometry.

Most Comfortable Loudness Level

Some audiologists gain useful information from determining the hearing level at which speech is most comfortably loud for their patients. Most people with normal hearing find speech comfortable at 40 to 55 dB above threshold.

Measurement of **most comfortable loudness (MCL)** should be made with continuous discourse so that the patient has an opportunity to listen to speech as it fluctuates over time. The use of cold running speech, as described for SRT or SDT measurements, is practical for this purpose.

The patient is instructed to indicate when the speech is perceived to be at a comfortable level. The test may start at a hearing level slightly above the SRT. From there, the intensity is increased gradually. At each hearing level, the patient should respond, indicating whether the speech is "too soft," "too loud," or "most comfortable." Several measurements should be made, approaching the MCL from both above and below the level first selected.

The MCL may be determined monaurally or binaurally under earphones or in the sound field. Martin and colleagues (1998) found that most audiologists do not use the MCL measurement, except in the evaluation of hearing aids.

Uncomfortable Loudness Level

Under some conditions it is useful to find the level of speech that is uncomfortably loud for listeners. For normal-hearing subjects, this intensity often extends to the upper limit of the audiometer (100 to 110 dB HL). In some patients with hearing disorders, the **uncomfortable loudness level (UCL)** is much lower, especially when expressed in decibels above the SRT. While some audiologists use measures of UCL for speech when assessing patients for hearing aid candidacy, this measure is not nearly as clinically useful as more frequency-specific measures of UCL, as discussed in Chapter 14.

It is not known just how the abbreviation for uncomfortable loudness level became UCL because *uncomfortable* is one word, but these kinds of derivations are often obscure. Some patients find a given level of speech uncomfortable because of its loudness, others because of discomfort produced by the physical pressure of the sound. When possible, it is helpful to determine which effect is active in a given case. The UCL is also called the **threshold of discomfort (TD)**, the **tolerance level**, and the **loudness discomfort level (LDL)**.

Although there are better methods for ascertaining if amplification from hearing aids exceeds a patient's tolerance levels (see Chapter 14), some audiologists continue to measure aided UCL in the sound field. Testing materials used for the UCL can be identical to those used for the MCL. Patients should be instructed to signal, either verbally or by some other method, when the speech is uncomfortably loud. They should be reminded that the UCL may be considerably above the level at which they find the loudness of speech most enjoyable, but that they should signal only when exceeding a given level would be intolerable. Acoustic feedback can be a real problem when UCLs are measured in the sound field.

Clinical COMMENTARY

Clinicians need be aware that UCLs measured with speech stimuli reflect loudness perceptions based on hearing levels in the lower frequencies. Measures of frequency-specific acoustic tolerance levels yield more useful data for planning hearing loss rehabilitation.

Range of Comfortable Loudness

The **range of comfortable loudness (RCL)**, also known as the **dynamic range (DR)**, is the arithmetic difference between a threshold measure and the UCL. A normal-hearing person has an RCL of 100 dB or more for either speech or pure tones. The RCL determination is sometimes used in selecting hearing aids and in other rehabilitative measures. When an SRT cannot be obtained, the difference between the SDT and the UCL provides a reasonable estimate of the RCL for speech. When prescribing hearing aid settings, determining more frequency-specific RCL becomes more important.

Speech-Recognition Testing

Many patients report that the difficulties they have in understanding speech are solved when speech is made louder. This can be accomplished by decreasing the distance from the listener to the speaker, by having talkers increase their vocal output, or by using a system of sound amplification. Most patients with conductive hearing losses show improved speech recognition when loudness is increased.

A common complaint of many patients is difficulty in understanding what people are saying. Many individuals with sensory/neural problems, however, complain that even when sounds are made louder, they are not clearly recognizable. This difficulty in discriminating among the sounds of speech plagues many patients much more than a reduction in loudness. These are the patients who claim, "I can hear, but I can't understand."

Through the years, a number of different terms have been used to describe the measurement of speech discrimination. The expressions **speech-recognition score (SRS)** and **word-recognition score (WRS)** have appeared in the literature with increasing frequency and appear to be the current expressions of choice. Konkle and Rintelmann (1983) contend that the word *discrimination* in this context implies distinguishing among different stimuli, whereas recognition suggests the report of a patient on what has been heard after the presentation of a single item. For the most part, throughout this text, the term *speech-recognition score* replaces the older *speech-discrimination score (SDS)* to describe tests performed to determine an individual's understanding of speech stimuli. Use of the term *word-recognition score* is usually reserved for use when test materials are known to be words and not some other speech construct.

The development of test materials to assess speech-recognition ability has been arduous. For any test to be useful, it should be both reliable and valid. Reliability means that a test is able to reveal similar scores on subsequent administrations (test-retest reliability) and that different forms of the same test result in equivalent scores. The validity of any speech-recognition test relates to the following:

1. How well it measures what it is supposed to measure (a person's difficulties in understanding speech).
2. How favorably a test compares with other similar measures.
3. How the test stands up to alterations of the signal (such as by distortion or presentation with noise) that are known to affect other speech tests in specific ways.

The quantitative determination of a patient's ability to discriminate speech helps the audiologist in several ways:

1. It determines the extent of the speech-recognition difficulty.
2. It aids in diagnosis of the site of the disorder in the auditory system.
3. It assists in the determination of the need for and proper selection of amplification systems.

Several methods have been advanced for measuring speech recognition, including testing with nonsense syllables, digits, monosyllabic words, and sentences. Prerecordings of many of these are commercially available.[1] Procedures have included both open- and closed-response message sets. In the open-response format, the patient may select an answer from an infinite number of possible utterances. In a closed-response system, the patient must choose the correct response from a group of words, sentences, or pictures.

Egan (1948) showed a relationship between the number of sounds in a word and the ability to recognize that word. The more phonemes and the more acoustic redundancy contained in a word, the more easily it is recognized. Word recognition gets poorer as more and more high frequencies are eliminated from speech, which decreases intelligibility without affecting overall loudness very much. It has long been known that, as frequencies below about 1900 Hz are removed from speech, the effect on speech recognition is much less than when higher frequencies are removed (e.g., French & Steinberg, 1947). To hear how speech sounds to individuals with varying degrees of high frequency hearing loss, go to the **Simulated Hearing Loss** demonstration.

Phonetically Balanced Word Lists

Original attempts at speech-recognition testing (Egan, 1948) involved compiling **phonetically balanced (PB) word lists**, that is, lists that contain all the phonetic elements of connected English discourse in their normal proportion to one another. Egan's work at the Psychoacoustic Laboratories at Harvard University resulted in 20 lists of 50 words each. When these words are used, the word-recognition score is determined by counting the number of correctly identified words out of 50 and multiplying this number by 2 percent.

Hirsh and others (1952) eliminated most of Egan's original 1,000 words and added a few more for a total of 200 words, of which 180 were derived from Egan's list. These 200 words were divided into four lists of 50 words each, with each list scrambled into six sublists. The resultant PB word lists are known as CID Auditory Test W-22. Ross and Huntington (1962) found some slight differences among the W-22 word lists in terms of word-recognition scores, but the magnitude of the differences among lists is small enough that they may be used interchangeably in clinical practice.

Martin, Champlin, and Perez (2000) compared word-recognition scores using PB word lists and similar lists of words that were deliberately not phonetically balanced. They compared scores on subjects with normal hearing and those with sensory/neural hearing loss. The scores for the lists were almost identical, which brings into question whether the lists are, or need to be, phonetically balanced.

Because many of the words in adult word lists are unfamiliar to children, Haskins (1949) developed four lists of 50 words, all within the vocabularies of small children. The test may be presented by CD or other recorded input, or by monitored live-voice, and it is scored in the same way as word lists when adults or older children are tested. The test difficulty increases sharply for children younger than 3½ years of age (Sanderson-Leepa & Rintelmann, 1976).

Many clinicians erroneously refer to the test materials as "PB words." It must be remembered that it is the lists, and not the words themselves, that are purportedly balanced. This terminology is an old tradition and not likely to change, but it is inaccurate.

Consonant-Nucleus-Consonant Word Lists

The phonetic construction of the English language is such that there is no way to truly balance a list of words phonetically, especially a relatively short list, because of the almost infinite number of variations that can be made on every phoneme (allophones) as they are juxtaposed with other phonemes. Lehiste and Peterson (1959) prepared ten 50-word lists that were phonemically balanced, a concept they judged to be more realistic than phonetic balancing. Each monosyllabic word contained a consonant, followed by a vowel or diphthong, followed by another consonant. These were called **consonant-nucleus-consonant (CNC) words** and were scored the same way as the original PB word lists. Later, the CNC lists were revised (Lehiste & Peterson, 1962) by removing proper names, rare words, and the like.

Tillman, Carhart, and Wilber (1963) took 95 words from the CNC lists (Lehiste & Peterson, 1959) and added 5 of their own, thereby generating two lists of 50 words each. Tillman and Carhart (1966) later developed four lists of 50 words each (Northwestern University Test No. 6), which they found to have high intertest reliability. Each of the four lists is scrambled into four randomizations. Auditory test NU-6 and CID W-22 remain the most popular materials for word-recognition testing (Martin et al., 1998) and yield similar results on patients when testing in both quiet and with background noise, although scores are slightly higher on the NU-6 test. It is important to remember, however, that patients' responses to this test, as on other word-recognition tests, may change on the basis of a number of variables, not the least of them being differences among the talkers who make the recordings. This problem is increased when the test is performed in the presence of background noise. An obvious solution to this would be for all audiologists to test with commercially available prerecorded word lists.

High-Frequency Emphasis Lists

Gardner (1971) developed two lists of 25 words each, with each word carrying a value of 4 percent. The test used with these lists is designed to measure the word-recognition scores of patients with high-frequency hearing losses who are known to have special difficulties in understanding speech. Each of the words contains the vowel /I/ (as in kick) and is preceded and followed by a voiceless consonant. Gardner suggested that the test is more useful if the words are spoken by a woman with a high-pitched voice. A similar approach to high-frequency word lists was taken by Pascoe (1975).

Nonsense-Syllable Lists

Edgerton and Danhauer (1979) developed two lists, each with 25 nonsense syllables. Every item contains a two-syllable utterance, with each syllable produced by a consonant, followed by a vowel (CVCV). Carhart (1965) earlier suggested that nonsense words are too abstract and difficult for many patients to discriminate, and this is sometimes true of the CVCV test. It does have the advantage that each phoneme can be scored individually, thus eliminating the obvious errors in the all-or-none scoring used in word tests.

Testing Word Recognition with Half Lists

Time can be saved in word-recognition testing by limiting the test lists to 25 words, using one half of each list with a weight of 4 percent per word. Opposition to this procedure is based on the following arguments: (1) that one half of a list may produce fewer audible sounds than the other half, (2) that there may be some real differences in difficulty of discrimination between the two halves of a list, but primarily (3) that splitting the lists causes them to lose their phonetic balance (which is not truly obtainable). Tobias (1964) pointed out that phonetic balancing is unnecessary in a "useful diagnostic test" and that half lists do measure the same thing as full lists. Thornton and Raffin (1978) showed half lists to be as reliable as the full 50-word lists. Martin and colleagues (1998) found that most audiologists prefer to test with 25-word lists.

Short Isophonemic Word Lists

The Short Isophonemic Word Lists (Boothroyd, 1968) were designed to reduce word-recognition test time without sacrificing validity. Each of fifteen lists of 10 consonant-vowel-consonant words contains 30 phonemes. Rather than the traditional scoring of test words as correct or incorrect, each phoneme is scored individually, allowing for a potential of 30 speech-recognition errors per list. The time saved in administration of the isophonemic lists can be considerable when multiple word lists are employed for attaining word-recognition performance at a number of intensities. No significant differences were found between measures of word recognition utilizing the Short Isophonemic Word Lists and the more commonly employed CID W-22 test (Tonry, 1988).

Testing of Monosyllables with a Closed-Response Set

The closed-set paradigm for word-recognition testing followed the development of a rhyme test by Fairbanks (1958). House, Williams, Hecker, and Kryter (1965) developed the Modified Rhyme Test, in which the patients are supplied with a list of six rhyming words and select the one they think they have heard. Fifty sets of items are presented to the patient, along with a noise in the test ear. Half of the word sets vary only on the initial phoneme, and the other half differ in the final phoneme.

A test designed to be sensitive to the discrimination problems of patients with high-frequency hearing losses is the **California Consonant Test** (Owens & Schubert, 1977). One hundred monosyllabic words are arranged in two scramblings to produce two test lists. The patient, selecting from four possibilities, marks a score sheet next to the selected word. While normal-hearing individuals obtain high scores on this test, patients with high-frequency hearing losses show some difficulty.

The **Picture Identification Task (PIT)** was developed by Wilson and Antablin (1980) to test the word recognition of adults who could not produce verbal responses and had difficulty in selecting items from a printed worksheet. The CNC words are represented by pictures that are arranged into sets of four rhyming words. The developers of the PIT found that it provides good estimates of word recognition for the nonverbal adult population.

Recognizing the need for testing the word-recognition abilities of small children who are either unable or unwilling to respond in the fashion of adults, Ross and Lerman (1970) developed the **Word Intelligibility by Picture Identification (WIPI) test**. The child is presented with a series of cards, each of which contains six pictures. Four of the six pictures are possibilities as the stimulus item on a given test, and the other two pictures on each card (which are never tested) act as foils to decrease the probability of a correct guess. Twenty-five such cards are assembled in a spiral binder. Children indicate which picture corresponds to the word they believe they have heard. This procedure is very useful in working with children whose discrimination for speech cannot otherwise be evaluated, provided that the stimulus words are within the children's vocabularies. Incorrect identification of words simply because they are not known is common with children under 3½ years of age.

The **Northwestern University Children's Perception of Speech (NUCHIPS) test** (Elliott & Katz, 1980) is similar to the WIPI. The child is presented with a series of four picture sets, including 65 items with 50 words scored on the test.

Testing Speech Recognition with Sentences

A number of different sentence tests have been devised to measure speech recognition. Jerger, Speaks, and Trammell (1968) were among the first to object to the use of single words as a speech recognition test on the basis that they do not provide enough information regarding the time domain of speech. Normal connected speech consists of constantly changing patterns over time, thus necessitating the use of longer samples than single words can provide for a realistic test. Jerger and colleagues also iterated the problems inherent in testing with an open-message set. Criticisms of sentence tests include the effects of memory and learning, familiarity with the items as a result of repetition, and the methods of scoring. Much of the opposition to sentence tests is that their structure enables a listener who is a good guesser to make more meaning of a sentence than does another patient with similar speech-recognition abilities.

The test devised by Jerger and colleagues (1968) involves a set of ten synthetic sentences. Each sentence contains 7 words, with a noun, predicate, object, and so on, but carries no meaning. All words were selected from Thorndike's list of the 1,000 most familiar words. The sentences are recorded on CD and patients show their responses by indicating the number that corresponds to the sentence they have heard. Some sentences are more difficult than others. Because early experimentation showed that **synthetic sentence identification (SSI)** is not sufficiently difficult when presented in quiet, a competing message of connected speech is presented, along with the synthetic sentences, and the intensity of the competing message is varied.

Another sentence test, which continues in use, is the Central Institute for the Deaf (CID) Everyday Sentence Test (Davis & Silverman, 1978). Fifty key words are contained within ten sets of ten sentences each. The percentage of correctly identified key words determines the score.

Testing Speech Recognition with Competition

Many audiologists feel that speech-recognition tests carried out in quiet do not tax patients' speech-recognition abilities sufficiently to reflect the kinds of communication problems that are experienced in daily life. For this reason, a noise or other competing signal is often added to the test ear to make recognition more difficult. When this is done, the relative intensity of the signal (speech) and the noise is specified as the **signal-to-noise ratio (SNR)**. The signal-to-noise ratio is not a ratio at all, but rather the difference in intensity between the signal (that which is wanted) and the noise (that which is not wanted). See Table 5.1 for examples.

TABLE 5.1 Examples of Three Signal-to-Noise Ratios (SNRs)

Signal	Noise	SNR
50 dB HL	50 dB HL	0 dB
40 dB HL	50 dB HL	–10 dB
10 dB HL	0 dB HL	+10 dB

Signals used to help degrade performance have included modulated white noise; a mixture of noise in one or two speakers; a single talker or two-, three-, and four-talker combinations; and a multitalker babble. Speech has been shown to be a better competing signal than electronically generated noise with a spectrum that resembles speech.

Kalikow, Stevens, and Elliott (1977) developed a test made up of eight lists of 50 sentences each; only the last word in each sentence is the test item, resulting in 200 test words. The test items are recorded on one channel of a two-channel CD, and a voice babble is recorded on the second channel. In this way, the two hearing-level dials of an audiometer can control the ratio of the intensities of the two signals. This procedure, called the **Speech Perception in Noise (SPIN) test**, has undergone considerable modification (Bilger, Nuetzel, Rabinowitz, & Rzeczkowski, 1984). Schum and Matthews (1992) reported an interesting effect: A significant percentage of the elderly patients with hearing loss that they tested did not use contextual cues as effectively on the SPIN as did their younger counterparts.

The Quick SIN (Speech In Noise) test (Etymōtic Research, 2001) was designed to obtain an estimate of a patient's experienced difficulty hearing in noise that is representative of the patient's performance in the real world. The test is comprised of six sentences presented in the presence of a four-talker babble noise, with five key words per sentence (see Table 5.2). The sentences are presented at five prerecorded signal-to-noise ratios encompassing a range from normal to severely impaired performance in noise. The resultant score from the Quick SIN test represents a decibel increase in the signal-to-noise ratio required by someone with hearing loss to understand speech in noise with comparable performance to someone with normal hearing. The test takes only a minute to complete and can be used for counseling patients toward appropriate amplification options.

Another useful sentence-in-noise test is the **Connected Speech Test (CST)** (Cox, Alexander, & Gilmore., 1987; Cox, Alexander, Gilmore, & Pusakulich, 1988). The most recent version of the test is an audiovisual recording with a six-talker speech babble competition. The test may be given either audiovisually or audio only. Comprised of eight sets of six passages, the patient listens to each passage, given one sentence at a time, and is instructed to repeat as much of each sentence as he or she understands. Each passage contains 25 key words that are used for scoring, with intelligibility scores based on the number of key words repeated correctly.

The Hearing in Noise Test (HINT; Nilsson, Soli, & Sullivan, 1994) measures the listener's ability to hear sentences in quiet and in noise in the sound field. Speech noise is presented at 65 dB HL, and the intensity of the sentences is varied to find the hearing level required for 50 percent of a list of 10 sentences to be repeated correctly. The test score is given as the decibel difference between the background noise and the sentence level required to attain 50 percent. For example, a required hearing level of 70 dB HL for 50 percent correct sentence identification would result in a 5 dB SNR score (i.e., 70 dB [the level of the speech signal] minus 65 dB

TABLE 5.2 Practice Sentences from the Quick SIN Test

Sentences are presented in increasing levels of noise, with the first sentence presented at a 25 dB signal-to-noise ratio and the sixth sentence presented at a 0 dB signal-to-noise ratio. The test has a total of 18 equivalent lists.

1. The lake sparkled in the red hot sun.
2. Tend the sheep while the dog wanders.
3. Take two shares as a fair profit.
4. North winds bring colds and fevers.
5. A sash of gold silk will trim her dress.
6. Fake stones shine but cost little.

Source: © Etymotic Research, Inc. Used with permission.

[the level of the speech noise]). The higher the SNR, the more difficulty the listener has hearing in noise.

Recording Speech-Recognition Test Results

For the more commonly used speech-recognition tests, the results are recorded on the audiometric worksheet in terms of the percentage of correctly identified words. In addition, the clinician records the test or list number; the level at which the test was performed; and, if opposite-ear masking was used as discussed in Chapter 6, the effective masking level and the type of noise. If additional speech-recognition tests are carried out with a competing signal in the same ear, the SNR is indicated, along with results and other identifying information. Many audiologists routinely assess speech recognition binaurally to demonstrate the natural advantage of processing speech binaurally. The audiometric worksheet used in this text does not provide for notation of binaural tests, but many forms are available that do.

Clinical COMMENTARY

As described in Chapter 4, bone-conduction results are essential for determining the extent of sensory/neural involvement in a hearing loss. Some clinicians have found, however, that they do not need to test by bone conduction if speech-recognition scores are consistent with the degree of loss and if immittance results (see Chapter 7) show no evidence of conductive hearing loss.

Administration of Speech-Recognition Tests

In carrying out speech-recognition tests, audiologists must first help patients to understand what is expected of them, what the test will consist of, and how they are to respond. Audiologists must decide on:

1. The method of delivery of the speech stimuli (prerecorded material is recommended over monitored live-voice).
2. The type of materials to be used.
3. The method of response.
4. The intensity at which the test will be performed.
5. Whether more than one level of testing is desired.
6. Whether a competing signal is desired in the test ear (or loudspeaker) to increase the difficulty of the test and, if so, the intensity of the competition.
7. Whether masking of the nontest ear is necessary and, if so, the amount and type of noise to use.

Instructions to patients should be delivered orally, even if printed instructions have been read prior to the test. Gestures and pantomimes or the use of sign language may be necessary, although it is likely that any patient who is unable to comprehend oral instructions will be unable to participate in a speech-recognition test. If responses are to be given orally, patients should be shown the microphone and the proper response should be demonstrated. If the responses are to be written, the proper forms and writing implements, as well as a firm writing surface, should be provided. Determining that the patient understands the task may save considerable time by avoiding test repetition.

Selection of Stimuli, Materials, and Response Method

The presentation level of the stimuli should be properly controlled and monitored on the VU meter of the audiometer. If a recording is used, it must contain a calibration signal of sufficient duration for the gain control of the VU meter to be adjusted so that the needle peaks at zero VU. If monitored live-voice is used, proper microphone technique is very important. The audiologist should be seated in front of the microphone and should speak directly into its diaphragm. If monosyllables are being tested, a carrier phrase should be used to prepare the patient for the stimulus word. The last word of the carrier phrase should be at the proper loudness so that the needle of the VU meter peaks at zero, corresponding to the calibration signal. The test word should be uttered with the same monotonous stress and should be allowed to peak where it will because words vary in acoustic power. Test words are not normally expected to peak at zero VU. Sufficient time (about 3 to 5 seconds) should be allowed between word presentations to permit the patient to respond. Prerecorded test materials for speech-recognition testing are preferred over monitored live-voice (MLV) in almost all instances. Recorded speech-recognition scores reflect more accurately the difficulty patients experience because these scores are generally lower than scores obtained through MLV. The use of recorded material provides standardization to the test, allowing for greater comparisons of results on a single patient when the test is repeated by a different audiologist at a later date. If MLV is used, appropriate procedure is essential to ensure some validity to the results. For a demonstration of proper technique for MLV testing for word-recognition tests, see the video entitled Word-Recognition Testing.

Patients may respond by repeating the stimulus word, writing down their responses on a form (with 50 or 25 numbered spaces for standard word lists), circling or marking through the correct answer on a closed-message set, or pointing to a picture or object. It is difficult to gauge the criteria that patients use in determining their responses—that is, whether they are relatively strict or lax in expressing their recognition of specific items. Jerger and colleagues (1988) studied these criteria in elderly subjects and concluded that attempting to control for this variable is probably not essential.

Although no real satisfaction has been universally expressed for speech-recognition materials, audiologists have individual preferences. A survey on audiometric practices (Martin et al., 1998) showed the W-22 word lists to be most popular, with the NU-6 lists a close second. Clinical observations suggest that these two tests remain popular. It is probable that the sensitivity of these two tests in ferreting out true differences in hearing function is not as great as may be found with other tests (Wiley, Stoppenbach, Feldhake, Moses, & Thordardottir, 1994). Certainly, one type of test material may be preferred for routine hearing tests under earphones and another type for special diagnostic tests.

Performance-Intensity Functions in Speech-Recognition Testing

Many of the word lists currently used in speech-recognition testing were developed during World War II to test the efficiency with which electronic communications systems could transmit speech. Thus, the primary objective was to design military communication systems that would, while transmitting a minimum of acoustic content, enable the listener to understand the message. Hence, the term *articulation* was used to express the connection achieved between the listener and the speaker—that is, the joining together of the two by means of a communication system. Use of the word *articulation* in this context is sometimes confusing to students of speech-language pathology, who learn to use this word to mean the manner in which speech sounds are produced with structures such as the tongue, lips, palate, and teeth.

Research has been conducted to determine the articulation-gain functions of word-recognition lists—that is, the percentage of correct identifications of the words at a variety of sensation levels. As Figure 5.1 illustrates, for normal-hearing individuals, the maximum score (100 percent) is obtained about 35 to 40 dB above the SRT. For many people with sensory/neural hearing losses, the maximum obtainable score is below 100 percent regardless of presentation level. In deference to earlier research attempting to attain a phonetic balance to word lists, the highest word score obtainable, regardless of intensity, is often called the **PB Max** (Eldert & Davis, 1951). The term **performance-intensity function for PB word lists (PI-PB)** has replaced the old articulation-gain function terminology. In acknowledgment of the fact that performance-intensity functions can be completed with a variety of speech test materials, these functions may also be called *PI-SR functions,* or PI functions for speech recognition. These measures are discussed again in later chapters of this text in terms of their diagnostic value.

Test Presentation Level

Regardless of whether speech-recognition testing is done at a set sensation level (above the SRT) for each ear or a preset intensity that is the same in both ears, the amount of the audible signal in the ear varies depending on the degree of hearing loss and its configuration. If testing is done at only one intensity, there is no way to know that the speech-recognition score (SRS) represents the patient's maximum performance unless that score is 100 percent. Ideally, speech-recognition testing should be performed at a minimum of two levels. A good first level for testing SRS is a presentation level 5 to 10 dB above the patient's most-comfortable listening level. The MCL plus 5 to 10 dB usually affords an approximation of maximum performance, assuming most speech sounds are audible at this intensity. A second level of higher intensity (usually 90 dB HL) should then be used to reveal a possible rollover in performance (as illustrated in Figure 5.1), which is indicative of disorders beyond the cochlea. Other levels (higher or lower) may be tested at the audiologist's discretion in an attempt to more fully define the PI function. Testing at conversational levels (45 to 50 dB HL) may be done for counseling purposes to demonstrate difficulties experienced and the potential benefits from amplification.

Problems in Speech-Recognition Testing

Although the test-retest reliability of word tests is good for patients with normal hearing and conductive hearing losses, this consistency sometimes fails for patients with primarily sensory/neural impairments (Engelberg, 1968). Thornton and Raffin (1978) concluded that the significance of differences in speech-recognition scores for a given individual depends on the number of items in the test and the true score for that test. From a statistical viewpoint, the greatest variability in scores should be found in the middle range of scores (near 50 percent) and the smallest variability at the extremes (near 0 percent and 100 percent). Thornton and Raffin (1978) demonstrated that two speech-recognition scores in the mid-range obtained from the same patient may need to differ by more than 20 percent to be considered significantly different. In general, the variability may be assumed to decrease as the number of test items increases. Therefore, it is sometimes risky for audiologists to assume that an increase or decrease in a given patient's speech-recognition scores represents a real change in speech-recognition ability.

Attempts have been made to relate the results obtained on speech-recognition tests to the kinds of everyday difficulties experienced by patients. Statements such as "Our test shows you can understand 72 percent of what you hear," are oversimplified and naive because they ignore important real-world variables such as contextual cues, lipreading, ambient noise level, speaker intelligibility, and so on. Goetzinger (1978) compiled a general guide for evaluating speech-recognition scores, which is presented in Table 5.3. This table, though helpful, should not be interpreted rigidly. Many patients perform considerably better on speech-recognition tests than they do in daily conversation, and others not nearly as well. Speech-recognition tests are helpful in diagnosis, but they are far from perfect for predicting real-world communication.

Bone-Conduction Speech-Recognition Testing

In cases of severe mixed hearing loss, a patient's best possible speech-recognition score may not be attainable because of the severity of the air-conduction hearing loss. In many of these cases, it is possible to test speech recognition by bone conduction in the same way described earlier for testing SRTs. Speech-recognition testing by bone conduction has never become popular, but interest has been shown in this procedure from time to time.

Speech-Recognition, the Audibility Index, and Implications for Speech-Language Therapy

It is possible to estimate a person's speech-recognition ability based on the amount of the speech signal that is audible with a given hearing loss. Such estimations were originally referred to as the *articulation index* (the name came from the terminology used for articulation-gain function testing). Today, they are more frequently called the *audibility index*.

The computational steps proposed in the original articulation index formulas have been simplified for ease of comprehension of the resultant value (Clark, 1992; Killion, Mueller, Pavlovic, & Humes, 1993). Following these recommendations, the audibility index (AI) is computed by simply counting the number of dots below the hearing levels plotted on a count-the-dots audiogram (Figure 5.3). The value derived represents the percentage of conversational speech energy audible to the listener with a given hearing impairment at a distance of 3 to 6 feet.

Generally, as AI decreases, perceived hearing handicap increases (Holcomb, Nerbonne, & Konkle, 2000). Clinically, the AI should reflect the speech-recognition score for conversational speech intensity (approximately 45 to 50 dB HL). The count-the-dots audiogram can be useful as a visual tool when discussing the impact of a given hearing impairment or when comparing hearing levels with and without corrective amplification.

Plotting a patient's pure-tone test results on an audibility index audiogram is a quick means for the speech-language pathologist to see what frequency components of speech are audible to individuals in speech-language therapy. The voiceless consonants of human speech all lie at or above 1,500 Hz, with the acoustic energy of such consonants as *f, s,* and *th* lying primarily above 4,000 Hz. To concentrate on speech-discrimination training and speech-production

TABLE 5.3 General Guide for the Evaluation of Word-Recognition Tests (Based on Goetzinger, 1978)*

Word-Recognition Scores (in Percent)	General Word-Recognition Ability
90 to 100	Normal limits
75 to 90	Slight difficulty, similar to listening over a telephone
60 to 75	Moderate difficulty
50 to 60	Poor recognition; patient would experience marked difficulty in following conversation
<50	Very poor recognition; patient may be unable to follow running speech

Note caveats in text regarding a rigid interpretation of this guide.

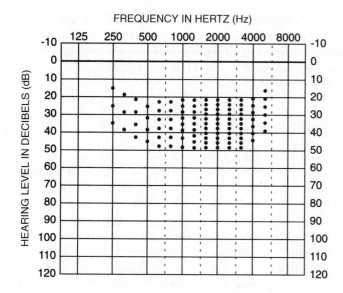

FIGURE 5.3 A count-the-dots audiogram. The number of dots above a patient's threshold is the audibility index, which reveals the percentage of conversational speech energy audible to the patient at a distance of 3 to 6 feet.

therapy through auditory-based approaches for a client who cannot fully perceive the targeted speech sounds even with properly fitting hearing aids rapidly becomes an exercise in futility. Determination of what sounds are audible to the client and which are inaudible can quickly guide the speech-language pathologist in the determination of the most efficacious approach to therapy. An alternate view of speech sound audibility is provided in Figure 5.4.

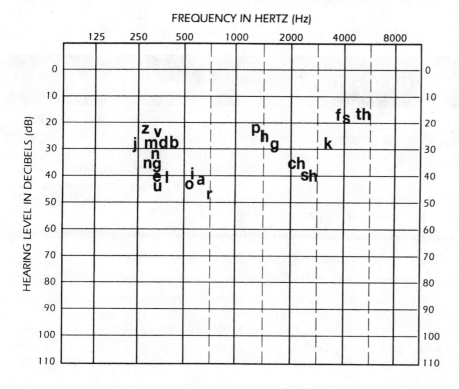

FIGURE 5.4 The Speech Sound Audiogram provides a quick visual depiction of the audibility of speech with a given hearing loss. In this audiogram, speech sounds of greater intensity than the hearing threshold are audible to the patient. High-frequency hearing loss diminishes the audibility of the higher-frequency sibilants and voiceless affricates, leading to the frequent patient complaint, "I can hear people, I just don't always understand what they are saying."

Understanding what speech energy is audible with and without hearing aids allows the speech-language pathologist to explain to classroom teachers, parents, or the significant others of adult clients what listening behaviors are expected. More discussion on the implications of speech understanding and the management of hearing loss is presented in Chapter 15.

Computerized Speech Audiometry

Speech audiometry, like any behavioral measurement, must at times be practiced as more of an art than a science. In a majority of cases, however, it is possible to carry out these measurements in a methodical, scientific manner, using the process of logical decision making. To illustrate this, over 40 years ago Wittich, Wood, and Mahaffey (1971) programmed a digital computer to administer SRT and SRS tests, including proper masking, to analyze the patient's responses and to present the results in an audiogram format at the conclusion of the test. Their results were compared to those of an experienced audiologist on a number of actual clinical patients, and very high correlations were observed. In addition, computerized speech audiometry can allow the flexibility of live-voice testing without its obvious limitations.

CHECK YOUR UNDERSTANDING

ACTIVITIES

Clinical COMMENTARY

As computer programs develop, a day may come in which many hearing tests are largely automated. While treatment cannot be initiated without hearing testing, some people erroneously believe that audiology is all about doing hearing tests. The freedom derived from automated testing would permit a greater concentration of effort toward audiology's larger goal of effective patient treatment.

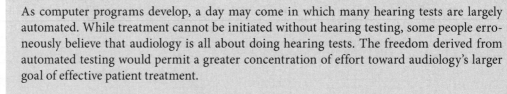

EVOLVING CASE STUDIES

In this section, you will attempt to calculate the results from basic speech audiometric tests described in this chapter. Before reading the case studies below, and based on the pure-tone results of Chapter 4 and what you now know about speech audiometry, propose the likely results of the following tests on the six theoretical case studies: speech recognition threshold (SRT), speech recognition score (SRS), most-comfortable loudness (MCL), and uncomfortable loudness (UCL). What hearing level(s) might you use for obtaining the SRS?

Case Study 1: Conductive Hearing Loss—Outer Ear Disorder

Even though the speech signals will be delivered to this child through air-conduction earphones, it is likely that the vibrations of these phones are actually generating a bone-conduction response. His SRTs should agree with his pure-tone averages of about 50 to 60 dB HL, and his speech recognition scores should be in the 90 to 100 percent range. His MCLs would probably be about 40 to 50 dB above his SRTs, and it is probable that uncomfortable loudness levels might not be reached. The sensation level for the SRS tests would be 30 dB. Given the caveat posed in the first sentence of this case study, it is unknown which ear is truly responding to the test signal regardless of which ear it was directed to. This will create a true masking dilemma, a topic addressed in Chapter 6.

Case Study 2: Conductive Hearing Loss—Middle Ear Disorder

The SRTs in both ears should be close to the two- or three-frequency pure-tone averages. In this case, this would be about 35 dB HL. Speech-recognition scores can be expected to be very high, probably at or close to 100 percent for each ear. The MCLs in conductive hearing loss cases are usually close to the same sensation levels as they are for those with normal hearing, in this case about 80 dB HL (approximately 45 dB HL). UCLs for either speech or more frequency-specific signals such as narrowband noise will probably be unreachable, even at the upper limits of the audiometer. A good starting sensation level for SRS testing would be 30 dB, although other levels may be useful as well. Certainly masking will be needed for this suprathreshold measure given the conductive hearing loss.

Case Study 3: Sensory/Neural Hearing Loss—Inner Ear Disorder

The SRTs for this patient should be close to either the two-frequency or three-frequency pure-tone averages, about 35 dB HL for each ear. In sensory/neural cases, the SRS is usually reduced, often in direct proportion to the degree of hearing loss. Scores of 70 percent to 80 percent would be reasonable for this patient. MCLs are usually reduced for most sensory/neural cases of cochlear origin and might be on the order of 25 or 30 dB SL or about 60 or 70 dB HL. Repeating SRS testing at a slightly higher level would ensure a better reception of the high-frequency components of the speech signal (see Figure 5.7) and may result in a higher SRS. Completing the SRS at conversational intensities (45 to 50 dB HL) may help demonstrate to the patient and his spouse the impact of the loss and the potential for benefit from amplification. Uncomfortable loudness would also be expected to be reduced and might be on the order of 80 to 90 dB HL. Administration of the SRS at a high intensity, such as 90 dB HL, can be of diagnostic value supporting the diagnosis of sensory (cochlear) hearing loss. The sensation level for SRS testing should be 30 dB SL for the first test (assuming this level permits audibility of the high-frequency components of the speech signal) and 90 dB HL for the second test.

Case Study 4: Sensory/Neural Hearing Loss—Auditory Nerve Disorder

It is expected that all the test results performed on this patient's right ear would be normal. That is, SRTs about 0 dB HL, SRSs close to 100 percent, MCLs about 40 to 50 dB HL, and UCLs near the intensity limits of the audiometer. Even though the left ear shows a very mild hearing loss with normal sensitivity in the low frequencies, there are some dramatic variations from the norm. Her SRTs might be normal, but her SRS will be reduced because of the distortion caused by damage to her auditory nerve, particularly when the tests are done at high intensities. MCL and UCL will probably appear close to the results in her right ear.

Case Study 5: Nonorganic Hearing Loss

Case Study 5 continues to be a challenge in testing. It is becoming more and more obvious that this patient is not complying with the request to indicate when a signal is barely perceptible. This will be manifested for speech in the same ways as it was for pure tones, probably resulting in a normal SRT, SRS, MCL, and UCL for the right ear and no response to any speech stimuli in the left ear. As in the case of pure tones, this total absence of response from the left ear is prima facie evidence of nonorganic hearing loss because a shadow response should have been observed at about 50 dB HL with supra-aural earphones or 80 dB HL for inserts. This behavior, if the patient is consistent in his perseverance at convincing you that he is, in fact, deaf in his left ear, will result in no response on tests of SRS, MCL, or UCL. While the diagnosis of nonorganic hearing loss is increasingly evident, the degree of hearing loss in the left ear, if any exists, is yet to be determined. More sophisticated tests will be necessary for this patient than have been described in this chapter, but they will be discussed in later chapters.

Case Study 6: Pediatric Patient

One of this child's problems is a delay in speech and language development, and she is increasingly giving the impression that she has a severe hearing loss, so it is unlikely that she will be able to participate in the tests described in Chapter 5. When working with children, it is almost always advisable to begin with the most adult-like procedures available and modify these as needed. The approach to speech audiometry for children described in Chapter 8 will probably have to be utilized in this case.

Summary

Speech audiometry includes measurement of a patient's thresholds for speech: speech-recognition threshold (SRT), speech-detection threshold (SDT), most comfortable loudness level (MCL), uncomfortable loudness level (UCL) or loudness discomfort level (LDL), range of comfortable loudness (RCL) or dynamic range (DR), and speech-recognition score (SRS) or word-recognition score (WRS). Measurements may be made either monaurally or binaurally under earphones, through a bone-conduction vibrator or in the sound field through loudspeakers. Materials for speech audiometry may include connected speech, two-syllable (spondaic) words, monosyllabic words, or sentences. The materials may be presented by means of a CD player, other recorded audio input or microphone (using monitored live-voice). At times the sensitivity of the nontest ear by bone conduction is such that it may inadvertently participate in a test under earphones. When cross hearing is a danger, a masking noise must be presented to the nontest ear to eliminate its participation in the test. Details of this procedure are explained in Chapter 6.

Measurements using speech audiometry augment the findings of pure-tone tests and help to determine the extent of a patient's hearing loss, loudness tolerance, and speech recognition. The knowledge gained from the use of speech audiometry is helpful in the diagnosis of the site of a lesion in the auditory system, as well as in audiological treatment.

The test results depicted in Chapter 4 illustrating normal hearing, conductive hearing loss, and sensory/neural hearing loss are repeated in Figures 5.5, 5.6, and 5.7. These figures show the probable results obtained during speech audiometry, including the use of masking, where indicated.

FIGURE 5.5 (A) Worksheet illustrating normal hearing in both ears. (B) Note that the two- and three-frequency PTAs, as well as the variable PTA, compare favorably with the SRTs. The WRS in each ear is very high at both 30 dB SL and 90 dB HL. Masking is needed only for the high-level WRS test, as will be discussed in Chapter 6.

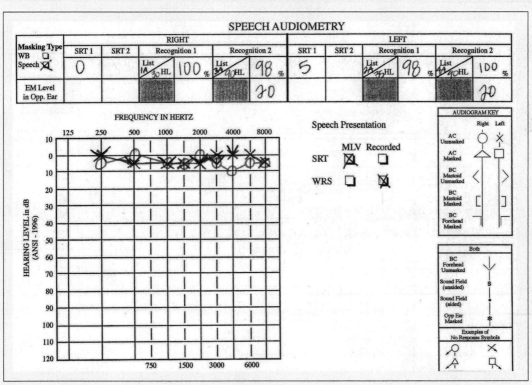

A

B

FIGURE 5.6 (A) Worksheet illustrating conductive hearing loss in both ears. (B) The PTAs are in close agreement with the SRTs. The WRSs are high in both ears, even at 90 dB HL. Masking was required for a number of the procedures used here and will be discussed in Chapter 6.

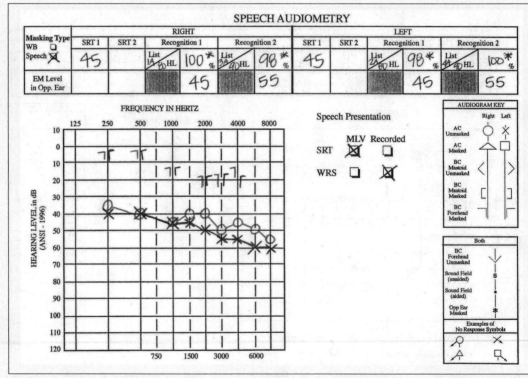

AIR CONDUCTION

Earphones Insert ☒ Supra Aural ☐	RIGHT									LEFT								
	250	500	1000	1500	2000	3000	4000	6000	8000	250	500	1000	1500	2000	3000	4000	6000	8000
Masking Type WB ☐ NB ☐	35	40	45/45	40	40	50	45	50	55	40	40	45/45	45	50	55	55	60	60
EM Level in Opp. Ear																		

BONE CONDUCTION

Placement Forehead ☒ Mastoid ☐	RIGHT						FOREHEAD						LEFT					
	250	500	1000	2000	3000	4000	250	500	1000	2000	3000	4000	250	500	1000	2000	3000	4000
Masking Type WB ☐ NB ☒	5*	5*	15*	20*	20*	15*	5	5	15	20	20	15	10*	5*	15*	20*	20*	20*
EM Level in Opp. Ear	40	40	45	50	55	55							45	40	45	40	50	55

	2 Freq	3 Freq	Variable	WEBER						2 Freq	3 Freq	Variable
Pure Tone Average	40	42	43	M	M	M	M	M	M	Pure Tone Average	43	45	50

A

SPEECH AUDIOMETRY

Masking Type WB ☐ Speech ☒	RIGHT				LEFT			
	SRT 1	SRT 2	Recognition 1	Recognition 2	SRT 1	SRT 2	Recognition 1	Recognition 2
	45		List 1A 80 HL 100 *%	List 3A 90 HL 98 *%	45		List 2A 80 HL 98 *%	List 4A 90 HL 100 *%
EM Level in Opp. Ear			45	55			45	55

FREQUENCY IN HERTZ

HEARING LEVEL in dB (ANSI - 1996)

Speech Presentation

	MLV	Recorded
SRT	☒	☐
WRS	☐	☒

AUDIOGRAM KEY

	Right	Left
AC Unmasked	○	✗
AC Masked	△	☐
BC Mastoid Unmasked	<	>
BC Mastoid Masked	[	]
BC Forehead Masked	⊐	⊏

Both

BC Forehead Unmasked	∨
Sound Field (unaided)	S
Sound Field (aided)	
Opp Ear Masked	*

Examples of No Response Symbols

B

FIGURE 5.7 (A) Worksheet illustrating sensory/neural hearing loss in both ears. (B) The two- and three frequency pure-tone averages agree closely with the SRTs, but because the audiogram falls in the high frequencies, the SRTs are lower than the variable pure-tone averages. WRSs show some word-recognition difficulties in both ears.

AIR CONDUCTION

Earphones Insert ☒ Supra Aural ☐	RIGHT									LEFT								
	250	500	1000	1500	2000	3000	4000	6000	8000	250	500	1000	1500	2000	3000	4000	6000	8000
Masking Type WB ☐ NB ☐	35	35	40/40	45	50	60	70	70	75	40	35	45/45	50	55	60	65	65	60
EM Level in Opp. Ear																		

BONE CONDUCTION

Placement Forehead ☒ Mastoid ☐	RIGHT						FOREHEAD						LEFT					
	250	500	1000	2000	3000	4000	250	500	1000	2000	3000	4000	250	500	1000	2000	3000	4000
Masking Type WB ☐ NB ☐							40	35	40	50	55	65						
EM Level in Opp. Ear																		

	2 Freq	3 Freq	Variable	WEBER							2 Freq	3 Freq	Variable
Pure Tone Average	38	42	53	M	M	M	M	M	M	Pure Tone Average	40	45	55

A

SPEECH AUDIOMETRY

Masking Type WB ☐ Speech ☐	RIGHT				LEFT			
	SRT 1	SRT 2	Recognition 1	Recognition 2	SRT 1	SRT 2	Recognition 1	Recognition 2
	35		List 16 /16 HL 78 %	List 36 90 HL 76 %	40		List 2 70 HL 80 %	List 36 90 HL 82 %
EM Level in Opp. Ear								

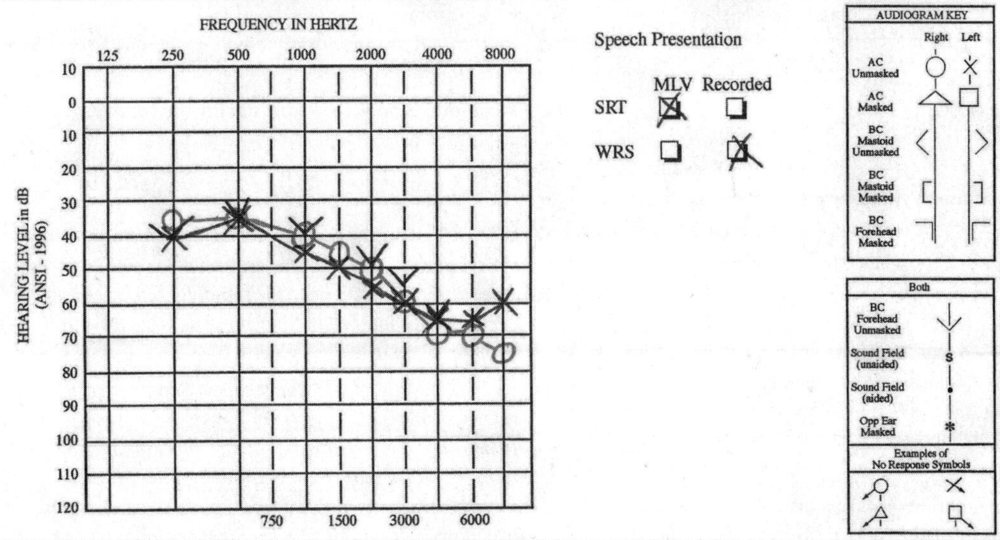

B

REVIEW TABLE 5.1 Summary of Tests Used in Speech Audiometry

Test	Purpose	Material	Unit
SRT	HL for speech recognition Verify PTA	Spondees; cold running speech	dB
SDT	HL for speech awareness	Cold running speech	dB
MCL	Comfort level for speech	Cold running speech	dB
UCL	Level at which speech becomes uncomfortably loud	Cold running speech	dB
RCL (DR)	Dynamic listening range for speech	Cold running speech	dB
SRS	Recognition of speech	PB words; CNC words; rhyming words; sentences	%

Frequently Asked Questions

Q In speech audiometry, what exactly does it mean to peak at 0 on the VU meter? What types of words are used for tests measuring SDT, SRT, and WRS?

A *Striking 0 dB on the VU meter ensures that the hearing-level dial reading on the audiometer is the actual intensity that reaches the earphone. The usual stimuli used are continuous discourse for the SDT, spondaic words for the SRT, and monosyllabic word lists for WRS.*

Q Does our uncomfortable loudness level (UCL) decrease or increase with age?

A *It surely does not increase with age but may or may not decrease depending on the presence of cochlear hearing loss with loudness recruitment.*

Q How much do audiologists have to practice before they can make their voices hit 0 on a VU meter?

A *This naturally varies from person to person, but most students find that with effort and some practice, this skill can be achieved in a relatively short time.*

Q Which is used more often when testing the WRS of children, an open- or closed-message test?

A *This depends on the age and maturity of the child. Younger children are usually tested with closed-message tests like the WIPI, and older children with PB word lists like the PBKs or even adult word lists.*

Q Why do audiologists not use MCL except in the evaluation of hearing aids?

A *Some audiologists do test MCL under earphones, but the majority of them do not, probably because it is not particularly useful in diagnosis. It can be useful, however, in patient counseling if the MCL is significantly greater than average with regard to conversational speech intensities (45 dB HL).*

Q What does the PI function graph tell us?

A *There are differences in the shape of the curve for conductive, cochlear, and retrocochlear hearing losses that may aid in diagnosis, particularly when a high rollover ratio is seen.*

Q Why do people with sensory/neural losses have speech recognition problems?

A *Damage to the sensory/neural system typically results in distortion of the speech signal so that, in many cases, just increasing the loudness of speech is not helpful in recognizing phonemes of speech.*

Q What is the signal-to-noise ratio?

A *It is not actually a ratio at all but rather a difference, in decibels, between the desired signal and the undesired signal (called noise). When the signal has greater intensity, the number is shown with a positive sign, and when the noise has greater intensity, the number is shown with a negative sign.*

Q If patients with conductive hearing loss have almost perfect word recognition scores, how do audiologists differentiate them, using word recognition tests, from patients with normal hearing?

A *That differentiation is made with threshold tests done with pure tones and speech.*

Q What exactly does the formula for the rollover ratio tell us about our patients' hearing?

A *A significant rollover ratio (greater than .25) suggests a retrocochlear lesion.*

Q Why are sentences instead of words used as stimuli for speech detection threshold testing?

A *The subject needs to hear the signal for a long enough period to assess its loudness. Single words are not audible long enough to make this judgment.*

Q Why is the spondee curve steeper than the curve for word-recognition tests?

A *It has long been known that the more phonemes and the more syllables that are contained in a word, the easier that word is to recognize. Spondees have two syllables, and words used for word recognition are single syllable.*

Q Which speech-recognition test was designed for patients with high-frequency loss?

A *A popular one is the California Consonant Test.*

Q Are all tests used for speech-recognition testing available in languages other than English and Spanish?

A *Yes, some tests are available in many languages.*

Q Has the reliability and validity of those tests been thoroughly examined?

A *More in some languages than in others.*

Q Why is the two-frequency pure-tone average the best predictor of hearing loss for speech?

A *This is often, but not always the best predictor of the SRT. There are many factors that may influence a patient's SRT. In many high-frequency hearing losses, patients gain cues from the low frequencies that help them to identify vowels and allow them to guess at spondaic words. For these high-frequency losses, the two-frequency pure-tone average is often the best predictor of hearing loss for speech.*

Q How do we know where to set the dB level to test WRS?

A *Some clinicians do speech recognition testing at a set sensation level above the SRT for each ear and others at a preset intensity equal in the two ears. Some clinicians find MCL and use that level. If testing is done at only one intensity, there is no way to know that the SRS represents the patient's maximum performance unless the score is 100 percent.*

Q If patients with conductive hearing loss have almost perfect word-recognition scores, how do audiologists differentiate them, using word-recognition tests, from patients with normal hearing?

A *That differentiation is made with threshold tests done with pure tones and speech.*

Q What exactly does the formula for the rollover ratio tell us about our patients' hearing?

A *A significant rollover ratio (greater than .25) suggests a retrocochlear lesion.*

Suggested Reading

McArdle, R., & Hnath-Chisolm, T. (2009). Speech audiometry. In J. Katz, L. Medwetsky, R. Burkhard, & L. Hood (Eds.), *Handbook of clinical audiology* (pp. 64–79). Baltimore: Lippincott Williams & Wilkins.

Endnote

1. Auditec of St. Louis (800-669-9065).

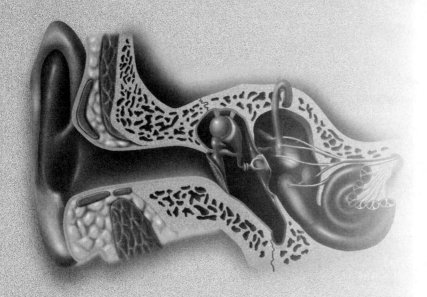

CHAPTER 6

Masking

LEARNING OBJECTIVES

This chapter describes the proper means of obtaining masked responses during audiometric testing when it is necessary to ensure that the patient does not respond to a signal received by the nontest ear. At the completion of this chapter, the reader should be able to

- Understand the concepts of cross hearing.
- Understand when masking signals should be employed.
- Describe the differences in determining the need to mask when testing pure-tone air conduction, pure-tone bone conduction, speech-recognition thresholds, and speech-recognition scores.
- Discuss the different masking methods for the above tests.
- Understand why different noise spectra are used for speech and pure-tone tests.

DURING VISION TESTING, ONE EYE is covered to make certain that the uncovered eye is the one taking the test. This cover is called a mask. Unfortunately, this simple solution is not available when testing hearing because covering the ear opposite the one being tested does not eliminate it from participation. In addition, in the case of some bone-conduction tests, covering the ear not tested actually makes the sound louder in the nontest ear and increases its participation. For this reason, masking for auditory tests requires that a noise be introduced into the ear not being tested to raise its threshold so that it cannot respond to a signal presented to the test ear. This is auditory masking, and the need for its use and its application vary depending on the kind of test performed.

Cross Hearing in Air- and Bone-Conduction Audiometry

It is logical to assume that if hearing sensitivity is considerably better in one ear than in the other (say, 50 dB to 70 dB), it is possible that, before the threshold of the poorer ear is reached, the intensity of the signal may be sufficient for the sound to escape from beneath a supra-aural air-conduction earphone or around the edges of an insert earphone into the room and be heard by the better ear. Resultant audiograms plotted when this happens have been called shadow-grams. However, it is more common for louder sounds introduced by air conduction to actually cross from one side of the head to the other, primarily by bone conduction (Chaiklin, 1967; Martin & Blosser, 1970). It is probable that whenever the intensity is raised to a high enough level, the supra-aural air-conduction receiver or insert receiver vibrates sufficiently to cause deformations of the skull, giving rise to bone-conducted stimulation. If the level of a tone thus generated is above the bone-conduction threshold of the nontest ear, the patient will respond, signaling that the tone has been heard before the auditory threshold of the test ear has actually been reached, assuming the test ear has sufficient hearing loss.

As sounds travel from one side of the head to the other, a certain amount of energy is lost in transmission. This loss of intensity of a sound introduced to one ear and heard by the other is called **interaural attenuation (IA)**. Interaural attenuation for air conduction varies with frequency and from one individual to another. Results of three studies of interaural attenuation using two different kinds of earphones are shown in Table 6.1.

The danger of **cross hearing** for air-conducted tones presents itself whenever the level of the tone in the test ear (TE) by air conduction, minus the interaural attenuation (IA), is equal to or higher than the bone-conduction threshold of the nontest ear (NTE). We can state this as a formula:

$$AC_{TE} - IA \geq BC_{NTE}$$

Because it is not possible to know in advance the interaural attenuation of a given patient, it is advisable to adopt a conservative approach and consider 40 dB to be the minimum possible value when using supra-aural audiometer earphones. Insert earphones provide more interaural attenuation than supra-aural phones, so 70 dB can be substituted for 40 dB in the formula, meaning that masking will be required much less frequently when using insert phones.

Because there is rarely a way of knowing for certain which cochlea has been stimulated by a bone-conducted tone regardless of where the vibrator is placed, cross hearing during bone-conduction tests is always a possibility. Therefore, the minimum IA for bone conduction should, for clinical purposes, be considered as 0 dB. There are many approaches to dealing with the problem of cross hearing, only one of which is discussed in this text.

From a practical clinical viewpoint, it seems important to ask, "Does it matter which ear has responded during pure-tone audiometry?" In the case of air conduction, the answer is an

TABLE 6.1 Minimum Interaural Attenuation for Pure Tones Using Supra-Aural Earphones According to (A) Coles and Priede (1968), (B) Zwislocki (1950), and (C) Sklare and Denenberg (1987)

	Interaural Attenuation		
Frequency in Hz	*(A) Supra-Aural Earphones*	*(B) Supra-Aural Earphones*	*(C) Insert Earphones*
250	61	45	89+
500	63	50	94+
1,000	63	55	81
2,000	63	60	71
4,000	68	65	77

emphatic yes because one must know for certain the hearing sensitivity of each ear. In the case of bone conduction, as was illustrated in Figures 4.13 (conductive loss) (see page 89) and 4.15 (mixed loss) (see page 91), the answer is also yes because the bone-conducted thresholds of each ear tell the amount of conductive involvement (by comparing them to air conduction) and the amount of sensory/neural involvement (by comparing them to 0 dB HL). If a bone-conduction response is obtained from the nontest ear, a completely incorrect diagnosis of the test ear may result. In the case of Figure 4.14 (page 90), however, it really does not matter which ear has responded to the bone-conduction signal because both ears show an absent air-bone gap, resulting in a diagnosis of bilateral sensory/neural hearing loss. Therefore, cross hearing in bone-conduction testing is of concern only when there is an air-bone gap in the test ear.

Masking

Whenever cross hearing is suspected, it is necessary to eliminate the nontest ear from the procedure to determine (1) whether the original responses were obtained through the nontest ear and, (2) if they were, what the true threshold of the test ear really is. The only way to accomplish masking for auditory signals is to deliver a noise to the nontest ear to raise its threshold, thereby removing it from the test.

The American Speech-Language-Hearing Association's (2005) most recent guidelines recommend that masking be used during bone conduction testing if the bone-conduction threshold in a given ear is better (lower) than the air-conduction threshold by 10 dB or more in the same ear. However, because there is a certain amount of normal variability between air- and bone-conduction thresholds, even among patients without conductive hearing losses, bone-conduction thresholds often appear to be slightly better (or even sometimes slightly poorer) than air-conduction thresholds. It seems practical, therefore, to consider air-bone gaps up to 10 dB to be insignificant. Thus, cross hearing for bone conduction should be suspected whenever an air-bone gap *greater* than 10 dB is seen in the test ear:

$$ABG_{TE} > 10 \text{ dB}$$

Clinical COMMENTARY

Masking must be undertaken whenever there is a possibility that unmasked test results may be derived from the nontest ear. In other words, one must mask whenever the use of masking may change the diagnosis of the type and/or degree of hearing loss at any frequency in either ear. After the air-conduction thresholds have been obtained, with proper masking when appropriate, the relationship between the thresholds by bone conduction and air conduction (the air-bone gap, the conductive component of the hearing loss) and between bone-conduction thresholds and normal hearing levels (the actual degree of sensory/neural hearing loss), become of paramount importance.

Many audiologists claim that, because they usually cannot be certain which ear has responded, they mask routinely for all bone-conduction tests (Martin, Champlin, & Chambers, 1998). This can be extremely time consuming and is often unnecessary and unpleasant for the patient. Other clinicians use interaural attenuation values, like 10 dB, to determine the possibility of cross hearing, but that is a passé notion because, as stated above, it must be assumed that there is no interaural attenuation for bone conduction.

The important question to ask is whether masking for bone conduction might result in a change in diagnosis from unmasked values. Using Table 6.2 as an example, four usual audiometric findings are demonstrated in terms of air-bone relationships in the same ear at any given frequency. What must be remembered is that, while masking may result in responses for bone-conduction thresholds remaining unchanged from unmasked values or may result in responses for bone-conduction thresholds becoming worse (poorer hearing), masking the nontest ear cannot cause thresholds to appear better.

If a split audiogram is used, there is no need to post the unmasked forehead bone-conduction responses on both audiograms. To determine if masking is needed for air-conduction testing, air-conduction thresholds for both ears must be compared to forehead bone-conduction results at all frequencies to show the potential for air-conduction crossover (remember $AC_{TE} - IA \geq BC_{NTE}$). When masking for bone conduction, it must be determined that there is a lack of air-bone gaps at each frequency and therefore that there is no need to mask (remember $ABG_{TE} > 10$ dB).

In the examples in Table 6.2, the similarity between normal hearing and sensory/neural hearing loss is that they both exhibit no significant air-bone gap; that is, there is no meaningful conductive component at the frequency tested. Therefore, opposite ear masking either leaves the threshold results unchanged or makes them appear poorer than air conduction. The conclusion that can be drawn is that masking cannot change the diagnosis in either of these cases, so there is no need to mask.

As shown in Table 6.2, conductive and mixed hearing losses both exhibit air-bone gaps; that is, there is some conductive component to the hearing loss. In either case, if the bone-conduction thresholds become poorer with masking, indicating that the initial results were obtained from the nontest ear, the diagnosis can change dramatically. In such cases, when the nontest ear received the signal, masking may reveal that either of those cases that appear to have conductive components may actually be sensory/neural, or the sensory/neural portion of the loss may be greater than what appeared without masking.

The alert audiologist will probably suspect the possibility of cross hearing more often than it actually occurs. This is good because it is better to mask unnecessarily than to fail to mask when a signal has been heard in the nontest ear. In clinical audiology the rule should be "When in doubt, mask."

Clinical COMMENTARY

Some experienced clinicians have noted that if mastoid bone-conduction testing is done, there is really no need to test from the second mastoid for those frequencies in which no air-bone gaps are observed. Air-conduction thresholds for both ears must, of course, be compared to the mastoid bone-conduction results. A notation must be made so that an interpreter of audiometric results will not believe that the second ear was not tested by bone conduction due to an oversight.

TABLE 6.2 Effects of Masking the Nontest Ear on the Diagnosis of True Bone-Conduction Thresholds

	Air Conduction	*Bone Conduction*	*Air-Bone Gap*	*Might Masking Change the Diagnosis?*
Normal	10	5	5	No
Sensory/neural	35	30	5	No
Conductive	35	5	30	Yes
Mixed	60	35	25	Yes

Noises Used in Pure-Tone Masking

The relative effectiveness of a noise in masking a pure tone is determined by several variables, including the spectrum of the noise, how the masking-level dial is calibrated, and the kind of earphone used to deliver the noise to the masked ear. When these variables are understood and controlled, the task of masking becomes considerably easier.

Several different kinds of masking noises are available on commercial pure-tone audiometers. Each noise has a characteristic spectrum and therefore provides a different degree of masking efficiency at different frequencies.

It is possible to generate a noise that has approximately equal energy per cycle and covers a relatively broad range of frequencies. Because of this analogy to white light, which contains all the frequencies in the light spectrum, this signal has been called **white noise.** White noise, which has also been called thermal and Gaussian[1] noise, sounds very much like hissing. Because the earphones accompanying many audiometers are not of very high quality, they do not provide much response in the higher frequencies and therefore limit the intensity of white noise above about 6,000 Hz. Hence, that which is labeled on the audiometer as white noise is more accurately termed broadband or wideband noise because it emanates from the earphone.

Because it has been proven that the masking of a pure tone is most efficiently accomplished by frequencies immediately surrounding that tone, the additional frequencies used in a broadband noise are redundant. They supply additional sound pressure and loudness to the patient, with no increase in masking effectiveness. Through the use of band-pass filters, it is possible to shape the spectrum of a broadband noise into **narrowband noise.** Modern digital technology now allows the generation of a digital noise that can be of any desired bandwidth and contain only the desired frequencies.

Surrounding every pure tone is a **critical band** of frequencies that provides **maximum masking** with minimum sound pressure. Narrowing the noise band to less than the critical bandwidth requires greater intensity to mask a given level of tone. Conversely, adding frequencies outside the critical band increases intensity (and therefore loudness) without increasing masking effectiveness. The narrow noise bands found in most audiometers are usually considerably wider than the critical band.

The earphones still frequently employed to deliver a masking noise during clinical pure-tone testing are the ones provided with most audiometers, the TDH-39, TDH-49, or TDH-50P earphones, with MX-41/AR (supra-aural) cushions. There are many reasons to prefer the use of insert earphones, which decrease the occlusion effect evident in bone conduction when an ear is covered (Dean & Martin, 2000) and therefore have an advantage in masking during bone-conduction testing. In addition, because they are coupled to a smaller area of the skull, insert receivers provide 70 to 100 dB of interaural attenuation. When the foam rubber surrounding the tubing at the end of an insert receiver is inserted deeply into the external ear, an additional 15 to 20 dB of interaural attenuation can be achieved (Killion, Wilber, & Gudmundsen, 1985).

Calibration of Pure-Tone Masking Noises

Just as with pure-tone test signals, electronic calibration must be completed annually to ensure that masking level intensities match the values chosen, that the signal increases and decreases in a linear fashion, and that the frequency spectrum selected for the signal is accurate. Surveys have shown that it is common practice for the decibel reference for masking to be in either sound-pressure level or hearing level. However, the concept of **effective masking (EM)** for clinical testing is very practical and easy to use once the audiometer has been properly calibrated.

Effective masking may be defined as the minimum amount of noise required to make a given signal inaudible. Thus, 20 dB EM at 1000 Hz is just enough noise to make a 20 dB HL, 1,000 Hz tone inaudible; 50 dB EM would just mask out a 50 dB HL tone, and so on. In the presence of 50 dB EM, a tone will not become audible until the tone reaches approximately 55 dB HL, regardless of an individual's hearing loss (assuming the hearing loss is less than 55 dB), because any hearing loss attenuates both the tone and the masking noise equally and because it assumes that the signal and the masker are both being heard *in the same ear* (as is the case when the test tone has crossed to the nontest ear, thus necessitating masking in the nontest ear).

The calibration of a noise in units of effective masking can be carried out using about a dozen normal-hearing subjects as follows:

1. Present a 1,000 Hz tone at 30 dB HL to one ear by air conduction. Pulse the tone on and off to minimize auditory fatigue.

2. Present a noise (preferably narrowband) to the same ear.

3. Raise the level of the noise in 5 dB steps until the 30 dB tone is no longer audible. The tone should be heard again at about 35 dB HL. Recheck several times for accuracy.

4. Take a mean value of the masking-level dial setting at which the 30 dB HL tone was just barely masked. Round this number to the closest multiple of 5 dB.

5. Add 10 dB as a safety factor to offset the normal dispersion seen around any mean. This is 30 dB EM at 1,000 Hz.

6. Subtract 30 dB from the above value. This is 0 dB EM at 1,000 Hz.

7. Repeat this procedure for all audiometric frequencies.

8. Post a correction chart on the audiometer showing the number of decibels that must be added to the hearing-level dial reading to reach 0 dB EM for each frequency.

A worksheet for determining effective masking is shown in Figure 6.1. For an example of how effective masking works, see Table 6.3. For most audiometers today, the audiometer's masking noise is fairly even across frequencies, resulting in very similar correction factors for all frequencies that rarely exceed 5 dB. Because this is not always the case, clinicians should complete a psychacoustic calibration of their own equipment.

Once calibration has been completed, any level at any frequency can be masked (in the same ear) up to the maximum masking limits of the audiometer simply by adding the determined correction factor to the threshold level of the ear to be masked. If, as in the example above, a +15 dB correction is needed for 0 dB EM, and a 40 dB tone is to be masked, the masking-level dial would be set to 40 dB EM, which is actually 55 dB HL: 40 dB for the tone to be masked plus a 15 dB correction, which includes the safety factor. The safety factor is therefore built into the correction, and it should not be added again when determining the need for individual masking levels.

Of course, when masking is done clinically, the masker is presented to the earphone *opposite* the test earphone. Using this procedure assumes that the test tone may have lateralized and is actually heard in the nontest ear, requiring this ear to be masked. Therefore, if the tone has indeed lateralized, introduction of an EM level into the nontest ear (equal to the threshold of the nontest [masked] ear plus the predetermined correction factor, which includes the safety factor) should render the tone inaudible if it has indeed crossed over to the nontest ear. At this point, the masking plateau process (to be described under *masking methods*) may begin. If the tone has not lateralized, introduction of that same level of masking into the nontest ear allows the tone to remain audible (because it is still being heard in the test ear), and the masking exercise is complete for the frequency tested.

FIGURE 6.1 Form for determining 0 dB of effective masking (EM) for pure tones and speech using a group of subjects with normal hearing. The following operations should be carried out for each column and the results from row G should be posted on the audiometer:

A	HL of Signal	30	30	30	30	30	30	30	30	30	30	30	30
B	Mean Noise Level												
C	Rounded to Multiple of 5												
D	Safety Factor												
E	Correction Factor (C + D)												
F	Subtract 30												
G	This is 0 dB EM (E − A)												
	Subject	125	250	500	750	1000	1500	2000	3000	4000	6000	8000	Speech
	1												
	2												
	3												
	4												
	5												
	6												
	7												
	8												
	9												
	10												
	11												
	12												

a. Present the signal and noise to the same ear at 30 dB HL for each frequency and for spondaic words.
b. Vary the intensity of the noise until the signal is barely masked out. Record the result in the appropriate cells for each subject in the desired columns. Record the mean value for each column at the top of the form in row B.
c. Round the numbers in row B to the closest multiple of 5 dB.
d. Add a safety factor of 10 dB to the numbers in row C.
e. This is 30 dB EM (row C + row D).
f. Subtract 30 dB from row E.
g. This is 0 dB EM (row F − row A). When masking during clinical tests, this value must be added to the threshold of the nontest ear to attain the initial EM for that threshold value.

Another example of correct masking protocols follows. Assume that a patient's thresholds (using insert earphones) are as follows:

Right ear AC 20 dB HL

Right ear BC 10 dB HL

Left ear AC 80 dB HL

When testing the left ear, criteria are met to mask the right (nontest) ear and retest the left (test) ear because cross hearing may have occurred (80 dB [test ear AC] −70 dB [IA] = 10 dB HL [nontest ear BC]).

TABLE 6.3 Example of Effective Masking*

1	2	3	4	5	6	7
Hearing Level of 1,000 Hz Tone	Hearing Level of Noise in Same Ear to Just Mask Out Tone	Difference	Safety Factor	Correction Factor to Be Applied to Reach 30 dB Effective Masking	Masking-Level Dial Reading for This Effective Masking Level	Effective Masking
30	35	5	10	+15	45	30
20	25	5	10	+15	35	20
10	15	5	10	+15	25	10
0	5	5	10	+15	15	0

Units are in decibels. Assume that the average for a dozen normal-hearing subjects shows that, at 1,000 Hz, a 30 dB HL tone is barely masked with a 45 dB HL masking noise.

The initial masking level would be 20 dB EM. The hearing-level dial to achieve 20 dB EM would be 35 dB HL, which is the threshold of the ear to be masked (20 dB HL) plus the predetermined correction factor of 15 dB, which includes the 10 dB safety factor. Stated as a formula:

$$EM = AC_{NTE} + CF$$

Central Masking

Decades ago, Wegel and Lane (1924) showed that a small shift is seen in the threshold of a pure tone when a masking noise is introduced to the opposite ear. This threshold shift increases slightly with increased noise but averages about 5 dB. It is believed that the elevation of threshold is produced by inhibition that is sent down from the auditory centers in the brain and therefore has been called **central masking.** Central masking must be differentiated from **overmasking (OM),** in which the masking noise is actually so intense in the masked ear that it crosses the skull and produces an undesired masking of the test signal in the test ear.

Masking Methods for Air Conduction

Masking must be undertaken whenever the possibility of cross hearing in air conduction exists. A survey of clinical audiologists on contemporary clinical practices (Martin et al., 1998) showed more disagreement on masking methods, and apparently greater insecurity, than on any other clinical procedure.

The "Shotgun" Approach

It is possible, in a large number of cases, for clinicians to mask by using some fixed or arbitrary level of noise in the masked ear, without really understanding what they are doing. In uncomplicated cases, the masking procedure often appears to be satisfactory. Because of insufficient feedback about their errors, some individuals fail to profit from their mistakes and continue with erroneous philosophies such as "Just use 70 dB of noise," with no recognition of the properties of the noise or of its effectiveness. Clinicians may be unaware of when they have used too little or too much masking noise.

The Minimum-Noise Method

Through calibration, it is possible to determine the minimum amount of noise necessary to mask a pure tone at a given intensity. There is no need to burden the patient with any more noise than is necessary to get the job done. As discussed earlier, the best way to do this is to regard the noise level in terms of decibels of effective masking.

Several time-consuming, and frequently clinically impractical, formulas have been developed over the years for the determination of the minimum and maximum amounts of effective masking to be used. Martin (1974) has shown that the different formula approaches yield the same noise sound-pressure levels as does a simple, direct approach, requiring almost no calculation. This simple approach is described in the following paragraph.

When test results suggest the possibility of cross hearing, they should be examined closely. Consider the example in Figure 6.2. The criteria for masking are met for the left ear by air conduction, assuming the use of supra-aural earphones, because the threshold (60 dB HL) minus minimal IA (40 dB) is greater than the bone-conduction threshold of the right ear (10 dB HL). Because the test was presumably performed carefully, we know that the 60 dB response was a threshold. However, here is the question that arises: "The threshold of which ear?" If the right (nontest) ear can be removed from the test by masking, and the threshold of the left (test) ear remains unchanged, this means that the original response was obtained through the test ear. If, however, eliminating the right ear from the test results in a failure of response at the left ear at the previous level (plus 5 dB for central masking), the right ear provided the hearing for the original response, and further masking is required to determine the true threshold of the left ear. It should be noted in this example that, had insert receivers been used, the entire issue of masking would have been averted.

The minimum amount of noise required for the threshold test described is an effective masking level equal to the AC threshold of the nontest ear plus the predetermined correction factor, and may be referred to as **initial masking (IM).** This is just enough noise to shift the threshold of that ear 5 dB, by both air conduction and bone conduction. If the threshold of the tone presented to the test ear was originally heard by bone conduction in the nontest ear, raising the threshold of the nontest ear with masking will eliminate the possibility of this response.

Maximum Masking

Just as a tone can lateralize from test ear to nontest ear, given sufficient intensity, so can the masking noise lateralize from masked ear to test ear, both by bone conduction. An individual's interaural attenuation cannot be less than the difference between the air-conduction level in

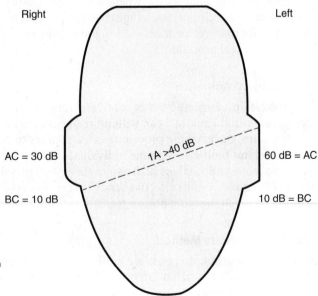

FIGURE 6.2 Illustration of the need to mask during air-conduction tests. Because the difference between the left-ear air-conduction threshold (60 dB HL) and the right-ear bone-conduction threshold (10 dB HL) exceeds the minimum possible interaural attenuation (40 dB, assuming supra-aural earphones were used), cross-hearing is a possibility. Note that the minimum interaural attenuation for this patient must be 50 dB (AC left minus BC right). Masking needed for the right ear is 30 dB EM.

Right   Left

AC = 30 dB   IA >40 dB   60 dB = AC

BC = 10 dB   10 dB = BC

the test ear and the bone-conduction level in the nontest ear at which threshold responses are obtained. For example, even though Figure 6.2 does not illustrate cross hearing per se, but rather the possibility of cross hearing, the interaural attenuation for the individual illustrated cannot be less than 50 dB for the test frequency (air-conduction threshold of the test ear minus bone-conduction threshold of the nontest ear).

Whenever the level of effective masking presented to the masked ear, minus the patient's interaural attenuation, is above the bone-conduction threshold of the test ear, a sufficient amount of noise is delivered to the cochlea of the test ear to elevate its threshold. This is over-masking (see Figure 6.3). The equation for overmasking for pure tones is:

$$EM_{NTE} \geq BC_{TE} + IA$$

Therefore, maximum masking is equal to the threshold of the test ear by bone conduction plus the interaural attenuation, minus 5 dB. When ears with large air-bone gaps are tested, mini-mum masking quickly becomes overmasking, sometimes making determination of masked pure-tone thresholds difficult. In such cases, audiologists must recognize the problem and rely on other tests and observations to make their diagnoses.

The Plateau Method

This text presents a modification of a popular masking method first reported more than half a century ago (Hood, 1960). By combining Hood's plateau method with the minimum-noise method, one begins with the initial masking level (the air-conduction threshold of the masked ear plus the predetermined correction factor). If the tone is no longer audible, the threshold for the tone is measured again in the presence of the contralateral masking noise. The noise level is then increased 5 dB, and the threshold is measured again. This often results in neces-sary increases in the tone level of 5 dB for every 5 dB increase in noise in order to keep the tone audible. The assumption is that the threshold of the tone in the test ear has not been reached (**undermasking**), and that both tone and noise are heard by the nontest ear (see Figure 6.4A). When the threshold of the tone for the test ear has been reached (see Figure 6.4B), the level of

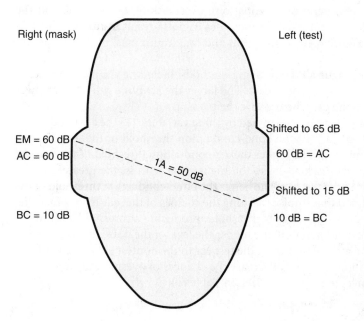

Right (mask)

Left (test)

EM = 60 dB
AC = 60 dB

IA = 50 dB

BC = 10 dB

Shifted to 65 dB

60 dB = AC

Shifted to 15 dB

10 dB = BC

FIGURE 6.3 Example of overmasking. The effective masking level in the right ear (60 dB) is decreased by the interaural attenuation (50 dB) so that 10 dB EM is received by bone conduction in the left ear. This shifts the bone-conduction threshold to 15 dB, plus any additional shift for central masking. Adding more noise to the right ear results in increased masking at the left ear, with further threshold shifts. In this case, the minimum amount of noise required to mask out the right ear produces overmasking.

FIGURE 6.4 The plateau method for masking. (A) Undermasking: The tone (by cross hearing) continues to be heard in the masked ear despite the noise because the tone level is below the threshold of the test ear. (B) The plateau: The tone has reached the threshold of the test ear. Therefore, raising the masking level in the masked ear does not shift the threshold of the tone. (C) Overmasking: The masking level is so intense that it crosses to the test ear, resulting in continuous shifts in the threshold of the tone with increases in the masking noise. Minimum (D) and maximum (E) masking are found at either side of the plateau.

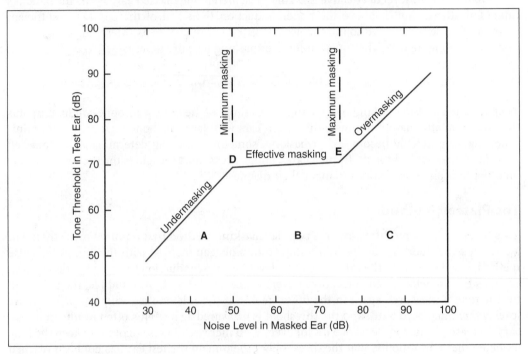

noise can be increased several times without affecting the level of tone that evokes a response. This is the **plateau.** If the noise level is raised beyond a certain point (the bone-conduction threshold of the test ear plus the interaural attenuation), overmasking takes place, and the tone and noise are mixed in the test ear. Further increases in noise result in further shifts in the threshold of the tone (see Figure 6.4C). Minimum and maximum masking are shown in Figures 6.4D and 6.4E.

Problems of overmasking plague all the masking methods, including the plateau system, whenever there are large air-bone gaps in both ears. The larger the air-bone gap, the narrower the plateau; the smaller the air-bone gap, the broader the plateau.

The width of the masking plateau is determined by three variables: (1) the air-conduction threshold of the nontest (masked) ear, (2) the bone-conduction threshold of the test ear, and (3) the patient's interaural attenuation. The higher the air-conduction threshold of the masked ear, the greater must be the initial masking level; the higher that level is, the greater are the chances that the noise will cross to the test ear. The better the bone-conduction threshold of the test ear, the greater is the likelihood that a noise reaching the cochlea of that ear from a masking receiver on or in the opposite ear will exceed its threshold, producing a threshold shift in the test ear. The smaller the interaural attenuation, the higher the level of the noise that reaches the test ear. By increasing interaural attenuation from the test ear to the nontest ear as well as from the nontest ear to the test ear, insert receivers decrease the chances of overmasking and widen the masking plateau. These concepts are summarized in Table 6.4.

TABLE 6.4 Factors That Influence the Width of the Masking Plateau

Factor	*Narrow Plateau*	*Wide Plateau*
AC threshold of masked ear	Higher	Lower
BC threshold of test ear	Lower	Higher
Interaural attenuation	Smaller	Larger

The time demands of routine audiological practice often make proper testing protocols difficult to employ. An excellent example is the need to remove air-conduction receivers; complete bone-conduction tests; and, when masking for air conduction is needed, reapply the receivers. Practicality and expediency cannot excuse a less-than-scientific approach to testing, but surely there are times when some procedures can be shortened. Table 6.5

TABLE 6.5 Examples of Seven Possible Sets of Pure-Tone Test Results That Can Indicate the Need to Mask for Air Conduction

Example	*AC Right*	*AC Left*	*BC Right*	*BC Left*
1	5	5	5	5
2	35	30	30	30
3	60 (60)	5	5 (5)	5
4	60	60	5 (5)	5 (60)
5	60	60	60	60
6	60	60 (60)	5	5 (35)
7	60 (NR)	60	5 (NR)	5 (5)

Example 1 Even without BC results, we can see that no masking is needed for AC for either ear. Many clinicians would not even perform BC in this case. The final diagnosis is obviously normal hearing in both ears.

Example 2 The air-conduction thresholds are not high enough, even using supraural earphones, to allow for cross hearing, even if the bone conduction thresholds turned out to be normal. The need for masking is not there. The final diagnosis is bilateral sensorineural hearing loss.

Example 3 Even without (before) performing BC, the need to mask the left ear is obvious because there is sufficient interaural difference to make cross hearing a possibility. After masking the left ear and retesting the air conduction for the right ear, the right BC will need to be carried out, and the need for masking the left ear becomes obvious. Final diagnosis is conductive loss in the right ear, normal hearing in the left ear, and cross hearing did not, in fact, take place.

Example 4 There is no obvious need to mask here until BC is carried out. Then AC and BC will need to be redone in both ears with masking to determine that the air-bone gap originally seen for the left ear was the result of cross hearing. The final diagnosis is sensorineural hearing loss in the left ear, conductive hearing loss in the right ear.

Example 5 The AC thresholds are the same as Example 4 and so there is no immediate need for masking. BC needs to be done to see if there is an air-bone gap in either or both ears. In this case, there is none. Final diagnosis is bilateral sensory/neural hearing loss with no masking required.

Example 6 As in Examples 3 and 4 there does not appear to be a need for masking. BC will need to be carried out before the need for masking can be determined. Final diagnosis is conductive loss in the right ear, mixed loss in the left ear. The original AC thresholds were correct.

Example 7 This is an unlikely but theoretically possible finding. Initial results show the same symmetrical pattern as in Examples 4, 5, and 6, but masking, following BC testing, reveals a totally deaf ear on the right side with a conductive loss on the left. This case would have been completely misdiagnosed had masking not been employed.

shows seven scenarios that may be encountered during routine audiometry. These examples assume the use of supra-aural earphones. Numbers in parentheses indicate the correct masked thresholds.

Only Example 3 of the seven listed in Table 6.5 clearly shows the need for masking before bone-conduction tests are completed. Examples 4 through 7 all show identical unmasked results, but when masking is used properly, the diagnoses are entirely different. In Examples 4, 6, and 7, the unmasked results would probably have been quite different had insert receivers been used, thereby increasing the interaural attenuation.

Clinical COMMENTARY

The significantly higher interaural attenuation (IA) with insert receivers makes masking considerably easier for the audiologist for two reasons. First, the need for masking is eliminated in many instances because the value for IA is placed at 70 dB in the formula that determines if masking is needed ($AC_{TE} - IA \geq BC_{NTE}$). Second, when masking is required, the chances of overmasking are greatly reduced because of the greater IA.

Masking Methods for Bone Conduction

Masking methods for bone conduction are very much the same as for air conduction, and their success depends on the training, interests, and motivation of the clinician. One problem in masking for bone conduction that does not arise for air conduction is the method of delivery of the masking noise. The matter is simple during air-conduction audiometry because both ears have earphones already positioned, and one phone can deliver the tone while the other phone delivers the masking noise. Because both ears are uncovered during bone-conduction testing, an earphone must be placed into or over the nontest ear without covering the test ear. The test ear must not be covered because this may further increase the occlusion effect created by the masking earphone. Figure 6.5 shows the proper positioning of supra-aural receivers (A) and insert receivers (B) for masking during bone conduction, with the vibrator on the mastoid and also on the forehead.

As just stated, when an earphone is placed over the nontest ear, an occlusion effect may be created in that ear. This means that the intensity of any cross-heard tones in the low frequencies is actually increased in the nontest ear. Of course, if the masked ear has a conductive hearing loss, no additional occlusion effect is evidenced, but it is not always possible to know whether there is a conductive component in the masked ear.

Because the masking earphone may make the bone-conducted tone appear louder in the masked ear, the initial effective masking level must be increased by the amount of the occlusion effect. Failure to do this results in undermasking in a significant number of cases. Therefore, the initial effective level for bone-conduction masking is the air-conduction threshold of the tone in the masked ear, plus the predetermined correction factor (CF), plus the occlusion effect (OE) for the tested frequency and can be expressed as:

$$EM = AC_{NTE} + CF + OE$$

FIGURE 6.5 Masking noise delivered to the nontest ear during bone-conduction audiometry performed from (A) the mastoid, using a supra-aural earphone, and (B) the forehead, using an insert earphone. (Commercial headbands for testing bone conduction on the forehead can be acquired through Audiology Incorporated.)

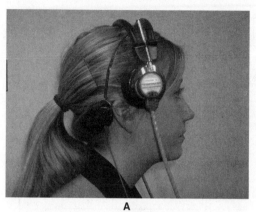
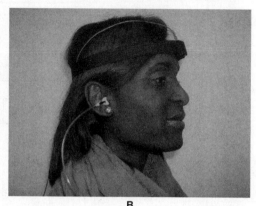

A   B

Of course, this increased amount of noise raises the chance of overmasking. In many cases it is advantageous to use insert receivers to deliver the masking noise because less noise needs to be delivered to offset the smaller occlusion effect. The increased interaural attenuation provided by these small phones further decreases the probability of overmasking.

Martin, Butler, and Burns (1974) suggest a simple method by which the occlusion effect of the patient's masked ear may be determined and added to the initial masking level for air conduction. The procedure takes only moments; it requires, after the need to mask for bone conduction has been determined, an audiometric version of the Bing tuning-fork test (described in Chapter 2) and is completed in three easy steps. (1) After the patient's unoccluded bone-conduction thresholds have been measured, the masking receiver is placed into or over the ear to be masked (no noise is presented). (2) With the nontest ear occluded, the thresholds at 250, 500, and 1,000 Hz are redetermined (the frequencies affected by the occlusion effect). (3) The occluded thresholds for each frequency are subtracted from the unoccluded thresholds. The difference is the patient's own occlusion effect. These differences should then be added to the initial masking levels determined for air conduction. The bone-conduction vibrator may be placed either on the forehead or on the mastoid.

Use of the audiometric Bing test results in little or no additional masking for conductive losses, where higher noise levels increase the danger of overmasking because there is no appreciable occlusion effect for conductive hearing loss. When increased masking is required to offset the effect of having occluded the masked ear, the precise amount of noise may be added rather than some average figure that may be more or less masking than required for the individual patient.

The form shown in Figure 6.6 is useful when performing the audiometric Bing test. The recorded results provide quantitative information about the amount of occlusion effect for each ear to be added to the initial effective masking level. In addition, the audiometric Bing test can be interpreted in the same way as the original tuning-fork test to assist in the diagnosis of conductive versus sensory/neural hearing loss.

FIGURE 6.6 Form for recording data obtained on the audiometric Bing test.

SPEECH AND HEARING CENTER
THE UNIVERSITY OF TEXAS AT AUSTIN 78712

Name: Last-First-Middle	Sex	Age	Examiner	Reliability	Date

	AUDIOMETRIC BING TEST					
	RIGHT			LEFT		
Frequency (Hertz)	250	500	1000	250	500	1000
1) Unoccluded						
2) Occluded						
3) Occlusion Effect (1-2)						

Plotting Masked Results on the Audiogram

Before any masked threshold data are entered on the audiometric worksheet for either air conduction or bone conduction, 5 dB may be subtracted from the values obtained with the nontest ear masked to compensate for central masking, assuming the originally measured threshold shifted when masking was introduced. The appropriate symbols to indicate air conduction or bone conduction with and without masking are shown on the audiogram. The graph should contain only symbols that represent accurate thresholds; otherwise, the audiogram appears cluttered and misleading. The plotting of unmasked response that later changed when masked is unnecessary because those responses can readily be seen by examining the numerical insertions at the top of the audiometric worksheet. Whenever the nontest ear is masked for pure-tone air- or bone-conduction testing, the level of effective masking should be indicated on the audiometric worksheet. In this way, if someone other than the examiner should review the test results, the precise effective masking level that was used in testing can be seen.

Figure 6.7 illustrates a case of normal hearing in the right ear with a sensory/neural hearing loss in the left ear. Note that the original unplotted test results recorded in the boxes suggest that the hearing loss in the left ear was conductive (compare the unmasked left ear thresholds to the unmasked forehead bone-conduction thresholds). The air-bone gaps in the left ear were closed when proper masking was applied to the right ear, indicating a sensory/ neural hearing loss.

Clinical COMMENTARY

As will be discussed in Chapter 7, results of immittance testing in the example shown in Figure 6.7 would have ruled out the possibility of a conductive component in the left ear without the need for bone-conduction testing.

FIGURE 6.7 (A) Worksheet showing normal hearing in the right ear and a sensory/neural hearing loss in the left ear. (B) Both the worksheet and the audiogram (B) illustrate that the original (unmasked) results by air conduction and bone conduction suggested a conductive hearing loss in the left ear because of the air-bone gaps. When proper masking was administered to the right ear, the bone-conduction thresholds shifted, proving absence of any air-bone gaps in the left ear. Tones on the Weber test, as noted on B, lateralize to the better-hearing right ear.

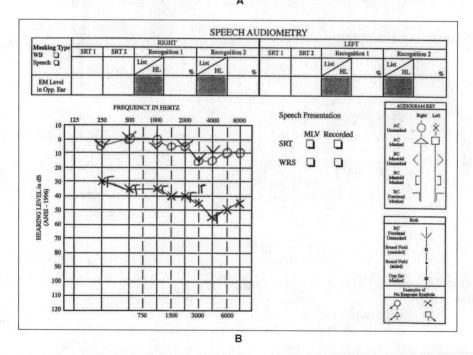

The unmasked results shown in Figure 6.8 suggest a conductive loss in both ears, with poorer hearing by air conduction in the right ear. Using the criteria described earlier in this chapter, masking was indicated for the right ear for air conduction and for both ears for bone conduction. Notice that the hearing loss in the left ear remains unchanged with masking, but the right ear actually has a severe mixed loss.

FIGURE 6.8 (A) Worksheet showing a mixed hearing loss in the right ear and a conductive hearing loss in the left ear. (B) Audiogram using the tabulated results in 6.8A. Unmasked results in both A and B showed conductive hearing losses in both ears. Masking was indicated for the right ear for air conduction, showing only slight threshold shifts. Masking for bone conduction was indicated for both ears, resulting in threshold shifts for the right ear. The Weber test refers consistently to the left ear, which has the better sensory/neural sensitivity. Note that no response is obtained in the right ear by air conduction at 6000 and 8000 Hz with masking in the left ear.

AIR CONDUCTION

Earphones Insert ☐ Supra Aural ☒	RIGHT									LEFT							
	250	500	1000	1500	2000	3000	4000	6000	8000	250	500	1000	1500	2000	3000	4000	6000	8000
Masking Type WB ☐ NB ☒	50	55	45/50	50	55	65	70	70	75	45	40	45/45	45	45	50	60	60	70
	55*	65*	70*	70*	75*	80*	85*	NR*	NR*									
EM Level in Opp. Ear	60	60	80	75	75	75	85	110	105									

BONE CONDUCTION

Placement Forehead ☒ Mastoid ☐	RIGHT						FOREHEAD						LEFT					
	250	500	1000	2000	3000	4000	250	500	1000	2000	3000	4000	250	500	1000	2000	3000	4000
Masking Type WB ☐ NB ☒	25*	35*	40*	45*	45*	50*	5	0	10	15	10	20	5*	0*	10*	15*	10*	20*
EM Level in Opp. Ear	75	85	85	85	95	100							55	65	70	75	80	85

	2 Freq	3 Freq	Variable	WEBER								2 Freq	3 Freq	Variable
Pure Tone Average	68	70	77	L	L	L	L	L	L	L		Pure Tone Average	43	43	50

A

SPEECH AUDIOMETRY

Masking Type WB ☐ Speech ☐	RIGHT						LEFT					
	SRT 1	SRT 2	Recognition 1		Recognition 2		SRT 1	SRT 2	Recognition 1		Recognition 2	
			List HL	%	List HL	%			List HL	%	List HL	%
EM Level in Opp. Ear												

B

Masking for the Speech-Recognition Threshold

Masking must sometimes be used in speech-recognition threshold (SRT) testing to eliminate the influence of the nontest ear and to ascertain the true threshold of the test ear when cross hearing is a possibility. As in pure-tone testing, the audiologist should suspect the need to mask more often than cross hearing actually occurs. Even in questionable cases, masking is a prudent practice.

The use of insert earphones can help to avoid some of the problems of overmasking for speech as it does for pure tones by increasing interaural attenuation to at least 70 dB. The recent emphasis on the use of insert earphones holds promise for solving many masking dilemmas encountered when using supra-aural earphones.

Cross Hearing in SRT Tests

Problems involving cross hearing exist for SRT measurements for the same reasons that they do for pure-tone air-conduction tests. In some cases the notion persists that there must be a significant difference between the SRTs of the two ears before suspicions of cross hearing arise (Martin et al., 1998). This action ignores the current knowledge that sounds contralateralize by bone conduction rather than by air conduction. Cross hearing is a danger whenever the SRT of the test ear, minus the interaural attenuation (conservatively set at 40 dB for supra-aural earphones and 70 dB for insert earphones), is greater than or equal to the bone-conduction thresholds of the nontest ear. Because speech is a complex signal and bone-conduction thresholds are obtained with pure tones, it must be decided which frequency to use in computation. Martin and Blythe (1977) found that frequencies surrounding 250 Hz do not contribute to the recognition of spondees presented to the opposite ear until levels were reached that considerably exceeded normal interaural attenuation values. Their research supports the recommendations later made by the American Speech-Language-Hearing Association (1988) that the SRT of the test ear should be compared to the lowest (best) bone-conduction threshold of the nontest ear at 500, 1,000, 2,000, or 4,000 Hz. The following formula reveals when cross hearing may occur and masking of the nontest ear must be used in the test:

$$\text{SRT}_{\text{TE}} - \text{IA} \geq \text{best BC}_{\text{NTE}}$$

Noises Used in Masking for Speech

The types of masking noises used for speech audiometry are more limited than those used for pure tones. Because speech is a broad-spectrum signal, speech-masking noises must consist of a broad band of frequencies. White noise is available on many diagnostic audiometers. Because it is a broad-spectrum noise, it masks speech satisfactorily, but it is slightly less intense in the low frequencies.

Speech noise is obtained by filtering white noise above 1,000 Hz at the rate of about 12 dB per octave. Speech noise provides more energy in the low-frequency spectrum than does white noise and is more like the overall spectrum of speech. Of the masking noises available on commercial audiometers, speech noise is usually preferred for masking speech.

Calibration of Speech-Masking Noises

All of the needs for adequate control of the masking system for pure tones are identical to those for speech. The linearity of the masking-level dial must be proved. If the masking circuit is calibrated in decibels of effective masking, procedures for masking speech can be carried out in the same way as those used for pure tones. Psychoacoustic calibration for effective masking may be carried out in the following fashion on a group of normal-hearing subjects:

1. Present a series of spondees at 30 dB HL.
2. Present a noise (preferably speech noise) to the same earphone.
3. Raise the level of the noise in 5 dB steps until subjects miss more than 50 percent of the words. Recheck this several times.
4. Obtain a mean for the dial reading on the noise attenuator that masked speech at 30 dB HL. This is 30 dB EM for speech.
5. Subtract 30 dB from what was determined in Step 4.
6. Add a safety factor of 10 dB to ensure masking effectiveness for most cases.
7. Post a correction chart showing the amount of noise that must be added to 0 dB HL (shown in Step 6). This is 0 dB EM for speech.

Once calibration is completed, speech at any level can be masked when an effective masking level equal to the SRT plus the predetermined correction factor is introduced into the same ear. In other words, to mask an SRT of 45 dB HL, the hearing level of the masker must be set at 45 dB plus the correction factor to reach a level of 45 dB EM. Of course, as with pure tones, when speech masking is done clinically, the masker is presented to the earphone *opposite* the test earphone. Using this procedure assumes that the test speech signal may have lateralized and is actually heard in the nontest ear, thus requiring this ear to be masked. Therefore, if the signal has indeed lateralized, introduction of an EM level into the nontest ear should render the speech signal inaudible if it has indeed crossed over to the nontest ear. At this point, the same masking plateau process described for pure-tone masking is used.

Central Masking for Speech

It has been demonstrated that threshold shifts for continuous discourse (Martin, Bailey, & Pappas, 1965) and for spondaic words (Martin, 1966) occur when a noise is presented to the nontest ear under earphones. Because the levels of noise need not be high enough to cause peripheral masking by cross conduction, it is assumed that the same central masking phenomenon exists for speech as for pure tones. Martin and DiGiovanni (1979) found smaller threshold shifts due to central masking than had been previously reported, but it should be expected that a threshold shift of about 5 dB will be seen for speech in the presence of a contralateral noise, even if that noise is of relatively low intensity (Konkle & Berry, 1983).

Masking Methods for SRT

Figure 6.9 illustrates the possibility of cross hearing for SRT. If we assume the use of supra-aural earphones, the difference between the SRT of the test ear (45 dB) and the minimal interaural attenuation (40 dB) exceeds the bone-conduction threshold (0 dB) of the nontest ear. In this example, no specific frequency is referred to in terms of the bone-conduction threshold. In actual clinical practice, the SRT of the test ear is compared to the best (lowest) bone-conduction threshold of the nontest ear at 500, 1,000, 2,000, or 4,000 Hz. If the nontest ear originally participated in the test, it should be removed by presenting an *initial* level of effective masking equal to the SRT of the masked ear plus the correction factor. If the SRT of the test ear does not shift by more than 5 dB (for central masking), the original threshold was correct as measured, and masking is completed. This is true because the nontest ear was rendered incapable of test participation. If the threshold shifted by more than 5 dB, the implication is that the nontest ear did, in fact, play a role in unmasked results by cross hearing. When original speech stimuli have been cross-heard, further testing using the plateau method is required.

Maximum masking for speech follows the same general rules noted previously for pure tones. If cross hearing has taken place, the patient's interaural attenuation is no greater than the SRT of the test ear, minus the lowest bone-conduction threshold of the nontest ear. When a level of effective masking, minus the *patient's* interaural attenuation, is equal to or above the lowest bone-conduction threshold of the test ear, overmasking (OM) has occurred. In equation form:

$$OM = EMN_{NTE} - IA \geq Best\ BC_{TE}$$

Plateau Method

The plateau method as described for pure tones can be used when measuring the SRT. If testing with the initial level of effective masking reveals that the SRT was obtained by cross hearing, the SRT is determined with that level of noise in the nontest ear. Then the intensity of the noise is raised 5 dB in the nontest ear, and spondaic words are again presented to the test ear. If fewer than three out of six words can be repeated correctly, the level of the words is raised 5 dB, and so forth. The true SRT is reached when the intensity of the noise can be raised or lowered at least three times in 5 dB steps without affecting the threshold for the words. As in the case of pure tones, the plateau for speech is influenced by the patient's interaural attenuation, the bone-conduction thresholds of the test ear, and the SRT of the masked ear.

FIGURE 6.9 Possible cross hearing during SRT testing. Both A and B show that the difference between the SRT of the test ear and the lowest bone-conduction threshold of the nontest ear exceed the minimum interaural attenuation found when speech sounds contralateralize (40 dB). Note that the SRT of the nontest ear in A is 0 dB HL and in B it is 30 dB HL. The SRTs of the nontest ears are unrelated to the danger of cross hearing for speech. The SRT of the test ear must be compared to the lowest bone-conduction threshold of the nontest ear. The initial effective masking level for the SRT is equal to the SRT of the nontest ear (i.e., 0 dB EM for A, 30 dB EM for B).

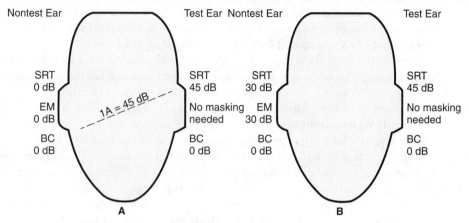

Recording Masked SRT Results

Before SRTs are recorded on the audiometric worksheet, a 5 dB correction for central masking should be subtracted from the SRT obtained with contralateral masking, assuming the initially measured SRT had shifted. The maximum level of effective masking required to obtain threshold must be recorded in the appropriate box below the SRT.

Cross Hearing and Masking in Speech-Recognition Score Testing

Given that speech-recognition tests are delivered at suprathreshold levels, the danger of cross hearing is even greater than during threshold tests. Because cross hearing of an air-conducted signal occurs by bone conduction, the likelihood of opposite-ear participation in a speech-recognition test increases as the level of the test signal increases. In addition, the better the bone-conduction threshold in the nontest ear, the greater is the probability that it will be stimulated by speech delivered to the test ear. In other words, whenever the hearing level of the stimuli minus the interaural attenuation equals or exceeds the lowest bone-conduction threshold of the nontest ear, cross hearing is a strong probability. Expressed as a formula, we have the following:

$$\text{SRSHL}_{\text{TE}} - \text{IA} \geq \text{best BC}_{\text{NTE}}$$

As in the case of the SRT, the interaural attenuation is considered to be as little as 40 dB for supra-aural earphones and 70 dB for insert earphones, and the bone-conduction threshold inserted in the formula is the lowest (i.e., the best) one obtained in the nontest ear at 500, 1,000, 2,000, or 4,000 Hz.

Whenever masking is needed during SRT testing, it will always be needed for speech-recognition testing for the same ear. Masking often becomes necessary, however, only when the level of speech is raised above the SRT for the speech-recognition test. Whatever masking noise is available for SRT should be used for finding the SRS. The noise should be calibrated as effective masking for speech, as discussed earlier. Although several masking methods have been suggested, the one described here has been found to be most useful (Martin, 1972). The effective masking level for the masked ear is equal to the hearing level at which the speech-recognition test is performed (HL), plus the correction factor (CF), minus 40 dB for interaural attenuation (70 dB if insert receivers are used), plus the largest air-bone gap in the masked ear:

$$EM = HL_{TE} + CF - IA + ABG_{NTE}$$

The effective masking level thus derived is just sufficient to mask speech at the nontest ear if the interaural attenuation is as low as 40 dB (or 70 dB if insert receivers are used), and it is more than enough noise if the IA is greater than these amounts (a probability). If the interaural attenuation can be computed on the basis of masking needs for SRT, the larger number should be used in the formula, which lowers the effective masking level and decreases the chance of overmasking. The interaural attenuation can never be less than the unmasked SRT of the test ear minus the lowest bone-conduction threshold of the nontest ear.

Insert receivers for speech-recognition testing have several distinct advantages over supra-aural audiometer earphones, and the two types of receivers may be used interchangeably for measuring SRS, assuming proper equipment calibration (Martin, Severance, & Thibodeau, 1991). Presenting speech through an insert receiver increases the interaural attenuation from the test ear to the nontest ear. For example, substituting 70 dB for 40 dB as the minimum amount of interaural attenuation in the formula shown previously for determining the need to mask during speech-recognition testing eliminates masking entirely for a large number of patients. When masking is required, and if it is delivered through an insert receiver, the possibility of overmasking is reduced or eliminated because the interaural attenuation of the masking noise from nontest ear to test ear likewise is increased. Finally, the attenuation of background noise that is provided by insert phones relative to supra-aural phones may result in improved speech recognition when testing is done at low sensation levels or when background noise is a problem.

Whenever the nontest ear is masked for speech-recognition tests, just as for other audiometric measures, the level of effective masking should be indicated on the audiometric worksheet. In this way, if someone other than the examiner should review the test results, the precise effective masking level that was used in testing can be seen.

Clinical COMMENTARY

As with pure-tone masking, the use of insert receivers can often completely eliminate the need for masking during speech audiometry, thereby simplifying testing. When masking is needed, problems of overmasking are far less common than when supra-aural earphones are used.

Compensation for Central Masking

CHECK YOUR UNDERSTANDING

If the SRT was obtained with contralateral masking, the central masking correction of 5 dB may have been subtracted before the result was recorded. This correction must be borne in mind when setting the hearing level for the speech-recognition test. If masking is required for finding the SRS, but not for determining the SRT, the clinician should assume that a 5 dB shift would have occurred if masking had been used when finding the SRT. In such cases, the hearing level should be increased for speech-recognition testing to compensate for the loss of loudness of the speech signal that results when noise is presented to the nontest ear.

Maximum Masking

ACTIVITIES

Just as the need for masking increases as the hearing level is increased for the test stimuli, so does the necessary masking level increase. The possibility of overmasking increases as the level of noise is raised in the masked ear. Rules for maximum masking and overmasking for speech are given in the section on speech-recognition threshold and should be scrutinized carefully when masking for suprathreshold speech-recognition tests.

EVOLVING CASE STUDIES

The six case studies followed in this text are examined here in terms of their need for masking during the tests performed. The precise methods for masking are dictated by the pathology and the results on pure-tone, speech, and other tests.

Case Study 1: Conductive Hearing Loss—Outer Ear Disorder

The complicating factor for this child is his lack of external auditory canals. Insert earphones cannot be used with this child for obvious reasons. Responses obtained with supra-aural earphones that are 40 dB HL or more above the unmasked bone conduction responses may be assumed to be heard through bone conduction. This greatly compromises testing with masking (delivered through supra-aural earphones) because it is not possible to determine which ear has received either the test or masking signal for either air- or bone-conduction testing. Interpretation of hearing levels, based on behavioral tests, must be based largely on conjecture utilizing what is known of unmasked results and the visual appearance of the ears and canal. Electrophysiological testing, as discussed in Chapter 7, may provide further insights.

Case Study 2: Conductive Hearing Loss—Middle Ear Disorder

When masking is needed, insert receivers are always the best choice because they limit the dangers of overmasking. If this patient's external auditory canals are dry and clear of infection or other debris, inserts should be used. Masking will probably be required at least for bone conduction but, depending on the differences between the pure-tone air-conduction thresholds and the contralateral bone-conduction thresholds, masking may also be required for SRT testing. It is likely that masking will also be needed when performing speech recognition tests because the intensity level of the test signal is higher.

Case Study 3: Sensory/Neural Hearing Loss—Inner Ear Disorder

The description of this patient's audiometric results suggests that there are no significant differences in hearing between the ears and no air-bone gaps. For this reason masking is probably not be needed except when determining speech recognition scores at high intensities if insert receivers are used.

Case Study 4: Sensory/Neural Hearing Loss—Auditory Nerve Disorder

The unilateral nature of this woman's hearing loss suggests that masking is required in the normal ear at least during bone-conduction and SRS testing. Whether it will be needed for pure-tone air-conduction and SRT tests is determined by the differences in decibels between the air-conduction thresholds in the poorer ear and the bone-conduction thresholds of the better ear.

Case Study 5: Nonorganic Hearing Loss

The likelihood is that routine tests will result in spurious responses. For this reason, the need for masking may not appear. If the nature of the loss, based on patient responses, suggests a unilateral loss, then it is essential that complete test results be obtained initially without masking to look for absent contralateral responses when they should logically appear. Repeat testing with masking does not provide valid, interpretable responses until such time that this patient provides true responses to unmasked testing.

Case Study 6: Pediatric Patient

The probability is that any test results on this child will be limited and that retesting may have to be performed a number of times before acceptable results are obtained. Therefore it is unlikely that masking will be indicated, at least initially. Masking is often confusing for children who are asked to ignore a loud sound and listen intently for a soft one. With patience, masked results can often be obtained once it is determined that they are needed.

Summary

When cross hearing occurs, proper masking procedures must be instituted. The approach for pure-tone air- and bone-conduction tests is very similar to that for the SRT. They involve using an initial effective masking level equal to the unmasked threshold of the nontest ear plus a predetermined correction factor. SRS tests are done at suprathreshold levels, so it is not necessary to determine unmasked results first. In fact, such results can be very misleading. The method used when masking for SRS involves more in the way of formulas and computations that are very practical for the clinical audiologist. These propositions are illustrated in Figure 5.5 (page 121), where masking was needed for the SRS test delivered at 90 dB HL, and Figure 5.6 (page 122) where masking was required for a number of tests.

REVIEW TABLE 6.1 Masking for Pure-Tone Hearing Tests*

Test	Air Conduction (AC)	Bone Conduction (BC)
When to mask	When difference between AC (test ear) and BC (nontest ear) exceeds minimal IA.	When there is an air-bone gap greater than 10 dB in the test ear.
How to mask	Initial masking: IM = AC of nontest ear. If tone not heard, plateau.	Same as AC plus occlusion effect in masked ear.
Overmasking occurs	When EM level in masked ear minus IA is equal to or greater than BC of test ear at same frequency.	Same as AC.

Minimal interaural attenuation is considered to be 40 dB for supra-aural earphones and 70 dB for insert earphones.

REVIEW TABLE 6.2 Masking for Speech Hearing Tests*†

Test	Purpose	Material	Unit	When to Mask	Initial Masking
SRT	HL for speech recognition Verify PTA	Spondees Cold running speech	dB	$SRT_{TE} - 40 \geq BBC_{NTE}$	$EM = SRT_{TE}$. If over 5 dB, shift plateau.
SDT	HL for speech awareness	Cold running speech	dB	$SDT_{TE} - 40 \geq BBC_{NTE}$	$EM = SDT_{TE}$
MCL	Comfort level for speech	Cold running speech	dB	$SDT_{TE} - 40 \geq BBC_{NTE}$	$EM = BBC_{TE} + 40$ dB
UCL	Level at which speech becomes uncomfortably loud	Cold running speech	dB	$UCL_{TE} - 40 \geq BBC_{NTE}$	$EM = BBC_{TE} + 40$ dB
RCL (DR)	Dynamic listening range for speech	Cold running speech	dB		
WRS	Recognition of speech	PB words; CNC words; rhyming words; sentences	%	$HL_{TE} - 40 \geq BBC_{NTE}$	$HL_{TE} - IA + ABG_{NTE}$

Minimal interaural attenuation is conidered to be 40 dB for supra-aural earphone and 70 dB for insert earphones.
†*CNC = consonant-nucleus-consonant; TE = test ear; NTE = nontest ear; PTA = pure-tone average; EM = effective masking; IA = interaural attenuation; BBC = best (lowest) bone-conduction threshold.*

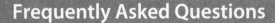

Frequently Asked Questions

Q Why is the occlusion effect absent in conductive hearing loss?

A *It has been stated that patients with conductive hearing losses have a built-in occlusion effect. Actually this is a misstatement of what happens. The occlusion effect is the result of bone-conducted sounds that produce acoustic energy in the external auditory canal (osseotympanic bone conduction) that impinges on the tympanic membrane, is conducted through the middle ear, and increases the energy that reaches the cochlea by acceleration of the head bone. Occluding the ear prevents sound from leaving the ear, so it moves toward the tympanic membrane. When there is a problem in the middle ear, the energy in the external auditory canal does not reach the cochlea and therefore does not increase the intensity of the sound that goes directly to the cochlea by distortional bone conduction.*

Q Why does interaural attenuation increase with the use of insert earphones?

A *When cross hearing occurs, the sound lateralizes by bone conduction when an air-conducted signal is so intense that the earphone actually sets the skull into sympathetic vibration. Because supra-aural earphones vibrate a larger area of the head than do insert earphones, it is easer for the former to generate this bone-conducted signal and so this occurs at a lower intensity than when insert earphones are used.*

Q Why can't the clinician just unplug the earphone on the nontest ear if she or he thinks it is affecting the test results?

A *This would have no effect because the signal is not coming from the earphone at the nontest ear. When cross hearing occurs, the signal is delivered to the test ear and may be heard in the nontest ear when circumstances are right for this to happen.*

Q How do you know when to mask?

A *The rules change depending on the kind of signal used (pure tones or speech) and whether air conduction or bone conduction is being tested. For details, refer to the discussion in this chapter (Chapter 6 of the text).*

Q What are the most common masking errors?

A *Failure to mask when necessary, undermasking (using too little noise so that the nontest [masked] ear is not effectively eliminated from the test), and overmasking (using too much noise so that the masker crosses the head and shifts the threshold of the test ear).*

Q How can you tell if a patient is cross-hearing in SRT testing? How do you know whether to mask?

A *These are basically the same question; that is, if cross hearing is a possibility, masking is needed. The determination is made by comparing the SRT in one ear to the lowest bone-conduction threshold in the opposite ear (excluding 250 Hz). If that difference exceeds 40 dB when using supra-aural phones or 70 dB when using insert phones, masking is indicated.*

Q What is the best way to avoid cross hearing in audiological testing?

A *Use insert earphones and follow the rules for when and how to mask.*

Suggested Reading

Ross, R. J., & Clark, J. L. (2007). Clinical masking. In R. J. Roeser, M. Valente, & H. Hosford-Dunn (Eds.), *Audiology diagnosis* (2nd ed., pp. 261–287). New York: Thieme.

Yacullo, W. S. (2009). Clinical masking. In J. Katz, L. Medwetsky, R. Burkard, & L. Hood (Eds.), *Handbook of clinical audiology* (6th ed., pp. 80–122). Philadelphia: Lippincott Williams & Wilkins.

Endnote

1. For Karl F. Gauss, German mathematician and physicist, 1777–1855.

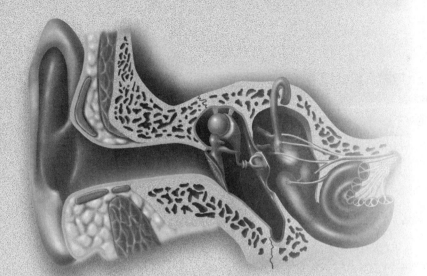

CHAPTER 7

Physiological Tests of the Auditory System

LEARNING OBJECTIVES

The purpose of this chapter is to discuss some of the electroacoustical and electrophysiological procedures that have been developed that serve both as indices of hearing sensitivity and as indications of the site of a lesion in the auditory system. These tests do not require behavioral responses from patients. At the completion of this chapter, the reader should be able to

- Discuss the purpose of acoustic immittance testing and, following supervised practice, perform tympanometry and acoustic reflex testing on a fellow student or friend.

- Describe the expected immittance results for several different ear pathologies.

- Define the differences among spontaneous, transient-evoked, and distortion-product otoacoustic emissions.

- Describe how evoked auditory potentials are measured and what these measures can reveal about hearing function and the site of lesion within the auditory system.

A T THIS POINT, THE READER should have a good grasp of the tests described earlier, as well as a general knowledge of how the ear is constructed and how it responds to sound. The comprehensive audiometric evaluation is defined by most insurance companies as administration of air- and bone-conduction pure-tone audiometry and speech audiometric measures comprising speech-recognition threshold and speech-recognition scores. While some of the tests described in this chapter have become routine within audiology clinics, others are reserved for more special occasions when additional diagnostic information is required. An understanding of the procedures to follow is essential to the study of clinical audiology. It will allow readers to comprehend more fully the examples of different hearing disorders caused by damage to different parts of the auditory system, which will be described in Chapters 9 through 12.

Diagnostic procedures beyond basic audiometrics can be separated into the categories of tests of function and tests of structure. Audiologists are concerned with the former, inferring specific lesions based on a constellation of test results. Modern medicine, with the development of imaging techniques, looks directly at the structure of, for example, specific areas within the auditory system. The development of these remarkable imaging procedures does not mitigate the importance of audiological procedures, but rather the two exist in a synergistic fashion.

The procedures described in this chapter require the use of specially designed equipment. With this equipment, audiologists can now accumulate valuable information for diagnostic purposes from a variety of procedures. These tests measure impedance and compliance in the plane of the tympanic membrane, tiny echoes whose presence can estimate the integrity of the inner ear and changes in the pattern of electrical activity in the inner ear and brain in response to acoustic stimuli. As a historical footnote, a brief review of earlier, behavioral site-of-lesion measures will be presented.

Combined Speech and Pure-Tone Audiometry with Immittance Measures

The immittance procedures to be discussed in this chapter are routinely combined clinically with those tests using pure tones (as described in Chapter 4) and speech (as discussed in Chapter 5). The union of these methodologies comprises the basic audiometric examination that is essential to diagnosis and provides the jumping-off point for advanced tests. When you view the video of the Audiometric Examination, note that acoustic immittance measures are completed first, which, if done with acoustic reflex testing, can often reduce the need for bone-conduction testing. The use of monitored live-voice for word-recognition testing that is demonstrated here is the most common approach to this portion of the audiometric examination. Given the greater test standardization obtained when using recorded materials, monitored live-voice testing for word-recognition tests is not the recommended protocol.

Acoustic Immittance

Measurements of acoustic **immittance** have become as routine in the audiological test battery as pure-tone and speech audiometry. Immittance measures guide the diagnostic audiologist in identifying abnormalities in the auditory system in a number of ways. The introduction of acoustic immittance measures more than three decades ago was a milestone in audiology, and most audiologists would agree that this procedure is basic to the test battery.

For a number of years, interest was directed toward the effects of various kinds of pathology on **acoustic impedance** in the plane of the tympanic membrane. Initially, most impedance measurements were made with mechanical devices too clumsy and too difficult to use routinely. A variety of commercial electroacoustic impedance meters (see, for example, Figure 7.1) are commonly used by audiologists today. Most devices measure **compliance,** which is related to the dimensions of an enclosed volume of air as expressed on a scale of different units of measurement. Examples of the different units are cubic centimeters (cm^3) or milliliters (ml) of an equivalent volume of air in the middle ear.

FIGURE 7.1 An electroacoustic immittance meter for the assessment of middle-ear function can measure the mobility of the tympanic membrane, the air pressure within the middle-ear cavity, and the presence of the acoustic reflex. Bluetooth wireless technology allows transmission of collected data to be sent to an office computer for storage and printing. (*Source:* GN Otometrics.)

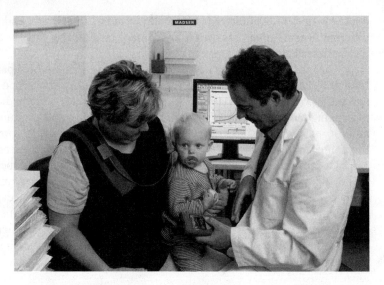

Several terms have been used to describe the various measurements made in the plane of the tympanic membrane. The word *immittance* is used as an all-encompassing term to describe measurements made of tympanic membrane impedance, compliance, or admittance. The American National Standards Institute (2007) has adopted a set of standards that define both the characteristics of instruments used in the measurement of acoustic immittance and the associated terminology.

Acoustic immittance measures have been called "impedance audiometry." Because audiometry per se is involved only with respect to the acoustic reflex, this term is not strictly accurate. Determinations of acoustic immittance are also frequently called "middle-ear measurements," which is also misleading because the measurements are not actually made of the middle ear. All determinations of middle-ear function are indirectly made by measurements made in the plane of the tympanic membrane.

Measurements Made on Acoustic Immittance Meters

Basically, three measurements are made in the plane of the tympanic membrane:

1. **Static acoustic compliance** (static acoustic admittance), which is the mobility of the tympanic membrane in response to a given value of air pressure in the external ear canal.

2. **Tympanometry,** which is a measurement of middle-ear pressure, determined by the mobility of the membrane as a function of various amounts of positive and negative air pressure in the external ear canal (the more positive or negative the air pressure in the external ear canal, the more the normal middle-ear system becomes immobilized, or "clamped").

3. Contraction of the middle-ear muscles, known as the **acoustic reflex,** in response to intense sounds, which has the effect of stiffening the middle-ear system and decreasing its static acoustic compliance.

These basic tests and their expected results on various pathologies are discussed in the appropriate portions of Chapters 10 to 12.

Factors Governing Acoustic Immittance

Recall from Chapter 3 that the impedance (Z) of any object is determined by its frictional resistance (R), mass (M), and stiffness (S). The effects of mass and stiffness are critically dependent on the frequency (f) of the sound being measured. The formula for impedance is stated as:

$$Z = \sqrt{R^2 + \left(2\pi fM - \frac{S}{2\pi f}\right)^2}$$

The combination of mass and stiffness (contained within the parentheses in the formula) is called complex resistance or **reactance.** Simple resistance is obviously independent of the rest of the formula, whereas mass reactance and stiffness reactance are inversely related to each other and are critically dependent on frequency. As frequency increases, the total value of the mass reactance factor also increases. Conversely, as frequency goes up, the effects of stiffness reactance diminish. Therefore, mass is the important factor in the high frequencies, and stiffness is the important factor in the low frequencies. As the stiffness of a system increases, it is said to become less compliant; that is, it becomes more difficult to initiate motion. Compliance, therefore, is the inverse of the stiffness factor of the formula.

The anatomy of the ear was described in a cursory fashion in Chapter 2. Details are brought out in Chapters 9 through 12, and the effects of various disorders on immittance are discussed. For the present, however, the following general assignments of values can be made: Resistance is determined primarily by the ligaments that support the three bones in the middle-ear cavity. The mass factor is determined primarily by the weight of these three tiny bones and the tympanic membrane. Stiffness is determined primarily by the load of fluid pressure from the inner ear on the base of the stapes, the most medial bone of the middle ear. The ear, therefore, is largely a stiffness-dominated system, at least in response to low-frequency sounds.

Clinical COMMENTARY

In pure-tone air- and bone-conduction testing, one finds that many conductive hearing losses have their greatest, or earliest, decrease in hearing for the lower frequencies. Because most conductive hearing losses tend to stiffen the middle-ear system, this finding would be expected from the impedance formula stated above as the effect of stiffness is lessened as frequency increases. There are many exceptions to this audiometric configuration, however, so it can be a dire mistake to diagnose a conductive loss, or any other kind of loss, based on the curve of the air-conduction audiogram.

Equipment for Middle-Ear Immittance Measurements

An electroacoustic immittance meter is diagrammed in Figure 7.2. Three small plastic or rubber tubes are attached to a metal probe, which is fitted into the external ear canal with an airtight seal. A plastic or rubber cuff, placed around the probe, can be varied in size to accommodate most ears. The three tubes are connected to (1) a miniature loudspeaker, which emits a pure tone, usually at 220 or 226 Hz (the incident wave), although a growing number of instruments have the capability of testing at higher-frequency probe tones as well; (2) a tiny microphone, which picks up the sound in the external ear canal (the sound comprising both the incident wave introduced to the ear from the speaker and the reflected wave as its returns from the tympanic membrane); and (3) an air pump, which can create either positive or negative air pressure within the canal. The air pump is calibrated in milliliters (ml), millimeters of water (mm H_2O), or dekapascals (daPa) (10 Pascals). The units of measurement are very

FIGURE 7.2 Diagram of an electroacoustic immittance meter showing its three primary components: a speaker to present a tone to the ear, a microphone to measure the intensity of the tone as it is reflected from the tympanic membrane, and an air-pressure pump to vary the pressure within the external auditory canal. (*Source:* Grason-Stadler Co.)

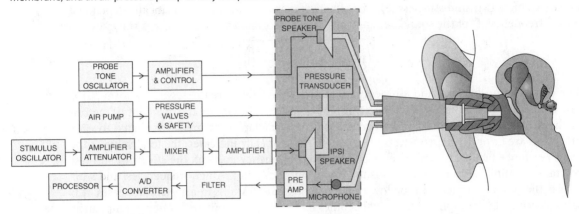

similar—1 daPa $=$ 1.02 mm H_2O, and 1 mm H_2O $=$ 0.98 daPa—when measurements are made at standardized conditions of temperature and pressure. The devices must be calibrated so that 0 daPa (or 0 mm H_2O, or 0 ml) is equal to atmospheric pressure at the site where measurements are to be made. The probe is attached to one side of a headset. An earphone connected to an acoustic reflex activator system is attached to the opposite side (see Figure 7.3) and functions as a built-in pure-tone audiometer.

FIGURE 7.3 Arrangements for acoustic immittance testing. (A) A subject configured with the probe assembly in the right ear and an insert earphone in the left ear. The shoulder harness kit is placed on the right shoulder. With this arrangement, tympanometry, static compliance, and ipsilateral acoustic reflexes can be tested in the right ear, and contralateral acoustic reflexes can be tested in the left ear. (B) The same subject configured with the probe assembly in the left ear and an insert earphone in the right ear. The shoulder harness kit is placed on the left shoulder. With this arrangement, tympanometry, static compliance, and ipsilateral acoustic reflexes can be tested in the left ear, and contralateral acoustic reflexes can be tested in the right ear.

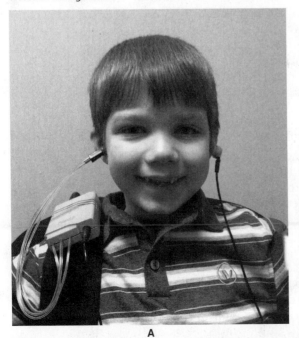

A

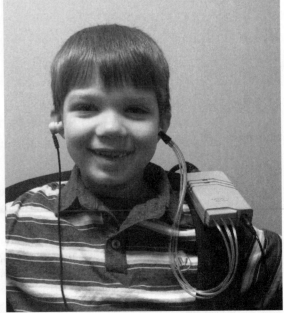

B

Measurement of Static Acoustic Compliance

For static acoustic compliance to be measured, the ear canal should first be cleared of any occluding earwax or other debris. Even the smallest amount of material in the ear canal may clog one of the tiny probe tubes and make measurements impossible or very misleading. The ear tip is pressed into the ear canal, a tight seal is obtained, and positive pressure is increased with the air pump. Observation of the meter indicates whether the necessary airtight seal has been obtained, or whether resealing, perhaps with a tip of a different size, is necessary. Once the seal is obtained, the pressure is increased to +200 daPa. On most instruments, the intensity of the probe tone is automatically adjusted until the desired sound-pressure level is obtained, usually 85 to 90 dB. The clinician can then determine the **equivalent volume** in cubic centimeters. Today's immittance meters make an automatic notation of this important first reading. This measurement, made with the tympanic membrane loaded with +200 daPa of pressure, is called c_1. Thus, this first measurement, c_1, is made with the tympanic membrane immobilized by positive air pressure, and it primarily represents the compliance of the outer ear.

Clinical COMMENTARY

The concept of equivalent volume in cubic centimeters for the c_1 reading gives a high clinical relevance to this first measure. The average volume of air in the human ear canal varies from approximately 0.5 cc in young children to 1.5 cc in adults. An important clinical observation in compliance measures rests on the fact that very high c_1 readings are indicative of even the smallest of perforations in the tympanic membrane. It should be noted, however, that a normal volume reading can be obtained in an ear with a tympanic membrane perforation in the presence of active middle-ear disease.

The second step in determining static acoustic compliance is attained when the pressure in the external ear canal is gradually decreased until the tympanic membrane achieves maximum compliance—that is, when pressures on both sides of the membrane are approximately equal. Another reading is taken, called c_2, which represents static acoustic compliance of the outer ear and middle ear combined. Many audiologists believe that c_2 should be measured with outer-ear pressure at 0 daPa (the ambient air pressure). The static acoustic compliance of the middle ear (c_x) can then be determined by working through this formula:

$$c_x = c_2 - c_1$$

During conditions for measurement of c_1, the tympanic membrane's relative immobility causes a good deal of energy to be returned to the probe, raising the sound-pressure level in the external ear canal. The membrane's increased mobility during the c_2 measurement allows more energy to be admitted to the middle ear, lowering the sound pressure between the tympanic membrane and the probe. The static acoustic compliance of the middle ear (ME) mechanism is the difference between these two conditions, which cancels the compliance of the external auditory canal (EAC). Stated as a formula:

$$c_x \text{ (ME)} = c_2 \text{ (EAC + ME)} - c_1 \text{ (EAC)}$$

Normal Values for Static Acoustic Compliance

Research over the years has not led to agreement on what values constitute normal static acoustic compliance. Studies have concluded that there are differences between adults and children and among the various probe-tone frequencies available. Most devices disregard the

TABLE 7.1 Normative Ranges for Static Admittance (Compliance), Tympanometric Width (TW), and Equivalent Ear Canal Volume (V_{ea})*

Age	Admittance/Compliance	TW (daPa)	V_{ea} (cm^2)
Children (3 to 10 years)	0.25 to 1.05	80 to 159	0.3 to 0.9
Adults (18 years and older)	0.30 to 1.70	51 to 114	0.9 to 2.0

*Data from Margolis & Hunter, 2000.

phase angle of the incident (original) and reflected waves in the ear canal. The fact that there is considerable variability for normal ears, often overlapping middle-ear conditions that cause high or low compliance, significantly reduces the value of this portion of immittance testing. Normative values of static compliance for children and adults are given in Table 7.1. The normal range is broad, and a patient's middle-ear compliance values really cannot be considered abnormal unless one of the extremes is clearly exceeded. Even in individuals with normal middle ears, the values of static compliance vary with both age and gender.

Recording and Interpreting Static Acoustic Compliance

Most modern clinics use devices that make these measurements automatically and provide a paper printout with the compliance values for each ear tested. Compliance values below the normal range suggest some change in the stiffness, mass, or resistance of the middle ear, causing less than normal mobility of the tympanic membrane. This may result from fluid accumulation in the normally air-filled middle ear or immobility of the chain of middle-ear bones. Reduced elasticity of the tympanic membrane may be due to age or caused by partial healing of a previous perforation. High compliance suggests some interruption in the chain of bones, possibly caused by disease or fracture, or by abnormal elasticity of the tympanic membrane. If static compliance values are determined manually, the data can be recorded on an immittance form (see Figure 7.4F).

Although static acoustic compliance measures are an integral part of any audiological workup, like any diagnostic test, they can be misleading. It is possible for different abnormalities of the ear to have opposing effects, resulting in what appear to be essentially normal immittance values (Popelka, 1983).

Tympanometry

The tympanic membrane vibrates most efficiently when the pressure on both sides is equal. This statement is basic to the understanding of tympanometry. As the membrane is displaced from its resting position by positive or negative pressure in the external ear canal, the vibratory efficiency of the membrane is decreased.

Tympanometry is performed by loading the tympanic membrane with air pressure equal to +200 daPa, measuring its compliance, and then making successive measurements of compliance as the pressure in the canal is decreased. After the pressure has reached 0 daPa (atmospheric pressure), negative pressure is created by the pump, and additional compliance measurements are made. The purpose of tympanometry is to determine the point and magnitude of greatest compliance of the tympanic membrane. Such measurements give invaluable information regarding the condition of the middle-ear structures. Performing tympanometry immediately after determining c_1 allows determination of both c_2 and the ear-canal pressure required for measuring acoustic reflex thresholds.

Tympanometry is generally conducted with a low-frequency probe tone of 220 or 226 Hz. The use of higher-frequency probe tones, or a succession of different frequencies, can modify results in a variety of ways, making this test more valuable diagnostically (Shanks, Lilly, Margolis,

FIGURE 7.4 Form for recording results of immittance measures: (a) acoustic reflexes obtained with the probe-tone and reflex-eliciting stimulus presented to the same ear; (b) contralateral acoustic reflex thresholds; (c) behavioral thresholds obtained during standard pure-tone audiometry; (d) sensation levels of the reflexes (b minus c); (e) the number of seconds required for the reflex to decay to half of its original amplitude; (f) static compliance; (g) graphs (the tympanograms) showing the pressure-compliance functions for both ears can be pasted here.

SPEECH AND HEARING CENTER
The University of Texas at Austin 78712

IMMITTANCE

NAME: Last - First - Middle		SEX	AGE	DATE	EXAMINER	INSTRUMENT

ACOUSTIC REFLEXES

		RIGHT				LEFT			
	Frequency (Hz)	500	1000	2000	4000	500	1000	2000	4000
a	Ipsilateral (Probe same)	▓▓			▓▓	▓▓			▓▓
b	Contralateral (Probe opposite)								
c	Audiometric Threshold								
d	Reflex SL								
e	Decay Time (Seconds)			▓▓	▓▓			▓▓	▓▓

STATIC COMPLIANCE RIGHT   LEFT $C_x = C_2 - C_1$

	Tymp. Width	M.E. Pressure	C_1 Volume	C_2	C_x Compliance	Tymp. Width	M.E. Pressure	C_1 Volume	C_2	C_x Compliance
f										

TYMPANOGRAMS

g   RIGHT   LEFT

Wiley, & Wilson, 1988). The difficulties encountered in the use of multifrequency tympanometry are mitigated by the newest generation of devices, which are microprocessor-controlled.

Recording and Interpreting Tympanometric Results

Compliance measurements are usually recorded directly and automatically on a graph called a **tympanogram,** which shows compliance on the y-axis and pressure, in dekapascals, on the x-axis. The results of this automatic printout may be appended to the form designed to record immittance measures (see Figure 7.4G).

Jerger (1970) has categorized typical tympanometric results into different types. This classical description of tympanometric shape is widely used despite the fact that shape classification is a qualitative assessment that lends a degree of clinical subjectivity to the measures. To facilitate direct comparison, all five classical tympanogram types are illustrated on the same form (see Figure 7.5).

Type A. Type A curves are seen in patients who have normal middle-ear function. The point of greatest compliance is at 0 daPa, and the curve is characterized by a rather large inverted V.

Type A$_S$. Type A$_S$ curves show the same characteristic peak at or near 0 daPa, suggesting normal middle-ear pressure; however, the peak is much shallower than that of the usual Type A. Type A$_S$ curves are often seen in patients in whom the stapes has become partially immobilized. The "S" may stand for "stiffness" or for "shallow."

FIGURE 7.5 Five typical tympanograms, labeled by their classical descriptions, illustrating various conditions of the middle ear. Type A shows normal pressure-compliance functions and is typical of normal middle ears. Type A$_S$ curves are like the A curves but are much shallower and are associated with stiffness of the stapes, the smallest of the middle-ear bones. Type A$_D$ curves are much deeper than the normal Type A curves and are symptomatic of interruptions in the chain of middle-ear bones or flaccidity of the tympanic membrane. Type B shows no pressure setting at which the tympanic membrane becomes most compliant, and suggests fluid in the middle-ear space. Type C shows the tympanic membrane to be most compliant when the pressure in the ear canal is negative, suggesting that the pressure within the middle-ear space is below atmospheric pressure.

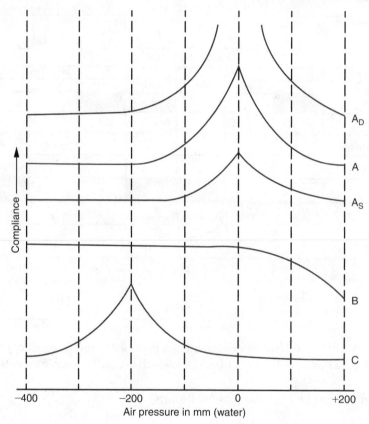

Type A$_D$. In some cases, the general Type A pattern is preserved; however, the amplitude of the curve is unusually high, or in some cases the positive and negative sides of the spike do not meet at all in Type A$_D$ curves. Such curves may be associated with flaccidity of the tympanic membrane or separation of the chain of middle-ear bones. The "D," therefore, may stand for "discontinuous" or for "deep."

Type B. Type B curves are seen when the middle-ear space is filled with fluid. Because even wide variations of pressure in the external ear canal can never match the pressure of fluid behind the tympanic membrane, the point of greatest compliance cannot be found. Type B curves may also be seen when a small amount of earwax or other debris occludes one of the tiny tubes within the probe, when a wax plug blocks the external ear canal, or when there is a hole in the tympanic membrane so that the meter measures the compliance of the rigid walls of the middle ear. Therefore, when Type B curves are evident, the clinician should make certain that these factors are not present.

Type C. In certain conditions, discussed in Chapter 10, the pressure in the middle ear falls below normal. In such cases, the tympanic membrane becomes most compliant when the pressure in the ear canal is negative, thus equaling the middle-ear pressure. When maximum tympanic membrane compliance occurs at a negative pressure of 200 daPa or greater, middle-ear pressure is considered to be abnormally negative.

At times, it may erroneously appear that a tympanogram is flat, missing a peak pressure point. This can be due to negative middle-ear pressure that is so extreme that the peak pressure point does not appear. In cases of flat tympanograms, it is often advisable to make immittance measures as low as 400 daPa. Such extremely negative middle-ear pressure may have significant medical effects on the patient, and such pressures should be pointed out to the physician managing the case, or a medical referral should be made.

On occasion, a peak pressure point is observed in patients at positive pressures greater than +50 daPa. This is sometimes seen in children who have been crying, patients who have blown their noses, and so on. It is likely that any such condition is short-lived, and normal middle-ear pressure will become restored in a short time. If positive peak pressure is observed for longer than a brief period, it might be advisable to ask for a medical consultation.

A number of factors may influence the outcome of tympanometry. When pressure is varied from positive to negative, the peak of the wave is lower than when pressure is changed from negative to positive, although this rarely affects the interpretation of results. Performing tympanometry with different probe tone frequencies and even multifrequency testing can yield different results.

As mentioned earlier, the classical tympanometric shape descriptions often lack the objectivity desired. The qualitative nature of this tympanometric shape classification can lead to some subjectivity in the differentiation of type A tympanograms from type A_S or type A_D. In the presence of an extremely shallow peak, classifying a tympanogram as type A_S or B can become a judgment call for many clinicians. While the classical descriptions of tympanometric shape will likely remain popular for some time, growing numbers of audiologists favor a more quantitative method of tympanometric classification that lends a greater objectivity to this important component of the overall hearing assessment. Such classification relies on measures of tympanometric peak pressure (TPP), tympanometric height (static **acoustic admittance** or compliance), and calculation of tympanometric width (TW), measures that are automatically calculated on most modern immittance meters (see Table 7.1).

Acoustic Reflexes

Definition of the Acoustic Reflex

Two small muscles, the **tensor tympani muscle** and the **stapedius muscle,** are involved in the operation of the middle-ear mechanism. The anatomy of these muscles is discussed in Chapter 10, but they are mentioned here because their action makes them an important part of the immittance battery. Although there is uncertainty about the role of the tensor tympani in response to sound in humans, it is generally accepted that the stapedius muscle contracts reflexively in response to intense sound, causing the tympanic membrane to stiffen. This has been called the acoustic reflex. Most normal-hearing individuals demonstrate a bilateral **intra-aural muscle reflex** when pure tones are introduced to either ear at 85 to 100 dB SPL (Gelfand, 2002).

Measuring the Acoustic Reflex

The immittance meter enables the clinician to present a signal to one ear and detect a decrease in tympanic membrane compliance in either that ear (the ipsilateral acoustic reflex) or the opposite ear (the contralateral acoustic reflex). The signal used to produce the acoustic reflex is called the **reflex-activating stimulus (RAS),** which can be any kind of sound, from a pure tone to a noise band. Normally, pure tones sampling the frequency range from 500 to 4000 Hz are used. A pure tone of the desired frequency should be introduced at 70 dB HL. If no compliance change is seen on the meter, the level should be raised to 80 dB, 90 dB, and so on, until a response is seen or the limit of the equipment is reached. Some commercial meters allow intensities up to 125 dB HL to be tested, but great care should be taken in introducing signals at such high levels. It is often inadvisable to exceed 115 dB HL.

If a response is observed, the level should be lowered 10 dB, then raised in 5 dB steps until the threshold can be determined. The tonal duration should be about one second, and measurements should be taken that sample the frequency range—for example, 500, 1000, 2000, and 4000 Hz; however, for no explainable reason, many normal-hearing individuals show no acoustic reflex at 4000 Hz. The lowest level at which an acoustic reflex can be obtained is called the **acoustic reflex threshold (ART).**

Criteria for the amount of compliance decrease that is required to constitute a response vary with different devices. At times, a very small compliance change is observed, and the audiologist may be uncertain whether a response has truly been obtained. In such cases, when the level is raised 5 dB, an unequivocal response is usually observed. Extraneous compliance variations sometimes occur as the patient breathes, or occasionally the very sensitive probe microphone picks up a pulse from a blood vessel near the external ear canal. Of course, the patient must be completely silent during these measurements lest vocalizations be picked up by the microphone, masking changes in compliance. Proper recording of the intensity required to evoke a contralateral acoustic reflex assists in appropriate interpretation of results (see Figure 7.4B).

Clinical COMMENTARY

While speech-language pathology and audiology are separate professions with independent scopes of practice, some services overlap between the professions. According to ASHA's Board of Ethics (American Speech-Language-Hearing Association, 2004), speech-language pathologists may screen for middle-ear pathology for the purpose of referral for further evaluation and management. A normal tympanogram accompanied by a present acoustic reflex indicates normal middle-ear function. According to ASHA's Board of Ethics, judgments and descriptive statements about immittance screening results should be limited to whether an individual has passed the screening.

Implications of the Acoustic Reflex

To understand the implications of acoustic reflex testing, it is important to have a basic knowledge of what is called the **acoustic reflex arc.** This pathway includes centers that are discussed in greater detail in Chapters 10 through 12 of this text, but they are mentioned here and diagrammed in Figure 7.6.

A sound presented to the outer ear is passed through the middle ear as mechanical energy, transduced to an electrochemical signal in the cochlea of the inner ear, and then conducted

RIGHT **LEFT**

FIGURE 7.6 Block diagram of the ipsilateral and contralateral acoustic reflex pathways.

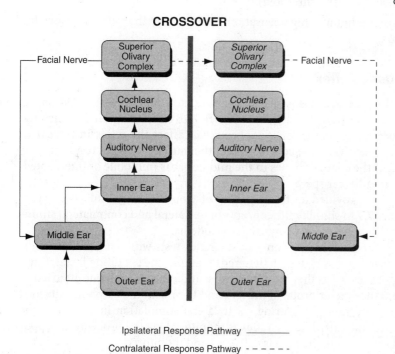

Ipsilateral Response Pathway ——————
Contralateral Response Pathway – – – – – –

along the VIIIth cranial (auditory) nerve to the brain stem. The impulse is received by the cochlear nucleus in the brain stem and is transmitted to the superior olivary complex. Here, some very interesting things occur: In addition to transmitting signals to higher centers in the brain (not shown in Figure 7.6), nerve impulses are sent from the superior olivary complex to the VIIth cranial (facial) nerve on the same side of the head, which in turn descends to innervate the stapedius muscle in the middle ear that originally received the sound, assuming that all systems are working properly. This is called the *ipsilateral response pathway*. In short, a sound presented to one ear can evoke an acoustic reflex in the same ear.

Almost simultaneously, neural impulses cross the brain stem to the opposite (contralateral) superior olivary complex, which in turn sends impulses by that facial nerve to the middle ear on the other side to evoke an acoustic reflex along the *contralateral response pathway*. Therefore, a stimulus presented to one ear evokes an acoustic reflex in the opposite middle ear as well as in the same ear. Although measurement of the acoustic reflex is made clinically in one ear at a time, in healthy ears, and in some pathological cases, responses occur in both ears in response to a stimulus presented to only one ear. Measurements are always made through the probe tip; however, the RAS may be presented through an earphone coupled to the ear opposite the probe assembly (the contralateral reflex), or through the probe tip itself (the ipsilateral reflex) (see Figure 7.3). The measurement of ipsilateral and contralateral reflexes is extremely valuable in audiological diagnosis.

There are four possible outcomes on an acoustic reflex test:

1. The reflex may be present at a normal sensation level (about 85 dB SL).
2. The reflex may be absent at the limit of the reflex activating system (usually 110 to 125 dB HL).

3. The reflex may be present, in the case of a hearing loss, but at a low sensation level (less than 60 dB above the audiometric threshold).

4. The reflex may be present but at a high sensation level (greater than 100 dB above the audiometric threshold).

Interpreting the Acoustic Reflex

Significance is placed on the presence or absence of the intra-aural muscle reflex and on the level of the RAS above the audiometric threshold (see Figure 7.4B and D) required to elicit the response. Of course, abnormalities in the muscles themselves affect the reflex in the ear to which the probe is affixed. In addition, the contraction of the muscles may not result in tympanic membrane stiffening if the chain of bones in the middle ear is immobile or interrupted, or if fluid is present in the middle-ear space.

The portion of Figure 7.4 provided for the recording of acoustic reflex results is exaggerated in the diagram in Figure 7.7 to simplify the concepts of ipsilateral and contralateral stimulation because these concepts are frequently confusing to students.

Table 7.2 illustrates theoretical findings on acoustic reflex tests with ten possible conditions of the auditory and related systems. In each (lettered) example, the condition is stated and the patients appear facing the reader as they would with the audiometer earphone attached to the right ear and the immittance meter probe in the left, and then with the earphone attached to the left ear and the probe in the right. During contralateral stimulation in each case, the earphone delivers the RAS to one ear while the reflex is monitored via the probe in the opposite ear. During ipsilateral stimulation, the RAS is delivered and monitored by the probe in the same ear. There are, of course, many other possibilities in addition to those shown below, and different constellations of responses may be attributed to a number of factors.

1. Middle-ear muscle reflexes are present at about 85 dB SL in normal-hearing individuals (see Table 7.2A).

2. The middle-ear muscle reflex is absent if the reflex-activating tone presented to the cochlea is not sufficiently intense. The intensity of the tone is attenuated if any of several types of hearing losses are present, especially those caused by conductive lesions (see Table 7.2B and C).

3. Sometimes the reflex appears in an ear with a hearing loss when the stimulus is presented at a fairly low sensation level. For example, a 50 dB hearing loss may show a reflex at 95 dB HL (45 dB SL). A precise explanation for low-sensation-level acoustic reflexes, which are associated with cochlear lesions, is lacking at this time (see Table 7.2D and E). Because behavioral auditory thresholds are not obtained through the probe of an immittance device, the sensation levels using ipsilateral stimulation cannot be determined. The examples in Table 7.2 are therefore hypothetical.

4. When a severe cochlear hearing loss exists in the ear that receives the RAS, there is often no response at the limit of the equipment (see Table 7.2F). This is because the intensity of the signal reaching the brain stem is insufficient to produce the reflex.

5. When there is damage to the auditory (VIIIth cranial) nerve, acoustic reflexes are frequently absent, they occur at higher-than-normal sensation levels, or the amplitude of the reflex is less than normal. This is probably due to alterations in the transmission of the RAS from the cochlea to the brain stem (see Table 7.2G).

6. The facial nerve supplies innervation to the stapedius muscle. If the facial nerve is in any way abnormal, the command supplied by the brain that mediates contractions may not be conveyed to the stapedius muscle. This occurs when the damage is on the side of the

FIGURE 7.7 The portion of the acoustic immittance form (see Figure 7.4) used for recording acoustic reflexes. Acoustic reflex thresholds (ARTs) obtained using pure tones as the reflex activating signals (RASs) as well as the sensation levels (SLs) of the ARTs are recorded as follows:

a. Right contralateral ARTs with the RAS presented to the right ear through an earphone placed on the right ear and the reflex monitored through the probe in the left ear. The SLs of the ARTs for the right ear are obtained by subtracting the voluntary audiometric thresholds obtained in the right ear from the right ear contralateral ARTs at 500, 1000, 2000, and 4000 Hz.

b. Left ipsilateral ARTs with the RAS presented to the left ear through the probe and the reflex monitored through the same probe. Frequencies tested are 1000 and 2000 Hz.

c. Right ipsilateral ARTs with the RAS presented to the right ear through the probe and the reflex monitored through the same probe. Frequencies tested are 1000 and 2000 Hz.

d. Left contralateral ARTs with the RAS presented to the left ear through an earphone placed on the left ear and the reflex monitored through the probe in the right ear. The SLs of the ARTs for the left ear are obtained by subtracting the voluntary audiometric thresholds obtained in the left ear from the left ear contralateral ARTs at 500, 1000, 2000, and 4000 Hz.

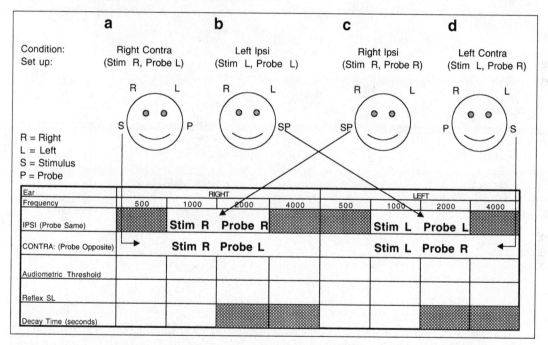

head to which the probe is affixed, regardless of whether the RAS is delivered ipsilaterally or contralaterally (see Table 7.2H).

7. Even if the ipsilateral acoustic reflex pathway is normal, but if damage occurs in the areas of the brain stem that house portions of the contralateral acoustic reflex pathway, ipsilateral reflexes may be present in both ears, but one, or more commonly both, of the contralateral reflexes are absent (see Table 7.2I).

8. Lesions in the higher centers of the auditory cortex usually produce no abnormalities in either contralateral or ipsilateral reflexes because these centers are above the acoustic reflex arc (see Table 7.2J).

The acoustic reflex portion of the immittance test battery can also serve as an important cross-check of findings in a pediatric evaluation or as an indication of normal hearing or potential hearing loss in otherwise difficult-to-test patients, as discussed in Chapter 12.

TABLE 7.2 Theoretical Examples of the Results of Ipsilateral and Contralateral Acoustic Reflex Testing for Ten Different Conditions*

		Right Contralateral *Phone Right* *Probe Left*	*Left Ipsilateral* *Phone Right* *Probe Left*	*Right Ipsilateral* *Phone Left* *Probe Right*	*Left Contralateral* *Phone Left* *Probe Right*
A	Right—Normal Hearing Left—Normal Hearing	Present at normal SL	Present at normal SL	Present at normal SL	Present at normal SL
B	Right—Normal Hearing Left—Conductive HL	Absent	Absent	Present at normal SL	Absent or present at high SPL
C	Right—Conductive HL Left—Conductive HL	Absent	Absent	Absent	Absent
D	Right—Normal Hearing Left—Cochlear HL (mild to moderate)	Present at normal SL	Present at low SL	Present at normal SL	Present at low SL
E	Right—Cochlear HL (mild to moderate) Left—Cochlear HL (mild to moderate)	Present at low SL	Present at low SL	Present at low SL	Present at low SL
F	Right—Cochlear HL (severe) Left—Cochlear HL (severe)	Absent	Absent	Absent	Absent
G	Right—VIIIth N. HL (mild to moderate) Left—Normal Hearing	Absent or present at high SPL	Present at normal SL	Absent or present at high SPL	Present at normal SL
H	Right—Normal Hearing (VIIth nerve lesion) Left—Normal Hearing	Present at normal SL	Present at normal SL	Absent	Absent
I	Right—Normal Hearing Left—Normal Hearing (brain-stem lesion)	Absent	Present at normal SL	Present at normal SL	Absent
J	Right—Normal Hearing (cortical lesion) Left—Normal Hearing	Present at normal SL	Present at normal SL	Present at normal SL	Present at normal SL

*HL = hearing loss, SL = sensation level, SPL = sound–pressure level.

This **sensitivity prediction from the acoustic reflex** test (Jerger, Burney, Maudlin, & Crump, 1974), based on a comparison of the acoustic reflex threshold (ART) for pure tones to the ART for broadband noise, does not reveal actual hearing thresholds, but it helps to categorize the patient as either having normal hearing or greater than a 30 dB sensory/neural hearing loss.

Acoustic Reflex Decay Test

When the stapedius muscle is contracted by an intense sound in normal-hearing individuals, it will gradually relax as it is constantly stimulated. This is called **acoustic reflex decay,** and it is normal in the higher frequencies; however, significant amounts of decay in the low frequencies are usually seen only in lesions of the auditory nerve and some parts of the brain stem. Reflex decay is measured by sustaining a tone at 10 dB above the ART and determining the number of seconds required for the amplitude of the reflex (the compliance change) to be reduced by 50 percent. The test is completed when the reflex has decayed to half its original amplitude or at the end of 10 seconds, whichever occurs first.

Recording and Interpreting Acoustic Reflex Decay Test Results

This test is scored according to the number of seconds required for the amplitude of the reflex to decay to half magnitude. Test results may be printed automatically on a graph, so that changes in the amplitude of the response can be observed as a function of time, or they may be recorded on a form such as the one shown in Figure 7.4E.

In subjects with normal hearing, there is some decay of the reflex at 2000 and 4000 Hz, but not at 500 and 1000 Hz, so this test is not performed in the higher frequencies. The slight decay sometimes evident in patients with cochlear hearing losses tends to occur more in the higher frequencies. Lesions in the auditory nerve cause decay to half the original magnitude of the reflex, often within three to five seconds, even at 500 Hz (Anderson, Barr, & Wedenberg, 1970) because the nerve cannot maintain its continuous firing rate. Because the primary innervation of contraction of the middle-ear muscles is by way of the descending tract of the facial nerve, damage to that nerve may also cause an absent acoustic reflex or an initial response followed by rapid acoustic reflex decay.

If contralateral acoustic reflexes and reflex decay are normal or provide information that confirms the audiometric findings, it is often unnecessary to perform ipsilateral reflex testing, although such elimination saves very little time. However, many times contralateral testing is inconclusive or cannot be carried out at all. In such cases, tests can be done ipsilaterally; however, it should be noted that slightly different results might be found (Oviatt & Kileny, 1984) for acoustic reflex decay. When abnormal patterns are observed, a comparison of ipsilateral and contralateral tests can help to isolate lesions in the ascending tract versus the descending tract (see Table 7.2).

Clinical COMMENTARY

Immittance measures should be among the first tests performed on a patient. Not only does this practice arm the audiologist with knowledge of what might be expected from pure-tone tests, under certain conditions bone-conduction audiometry may be unnecessary when acoustic immittance measures are viewed in light of other audiometric procedures. In the presence of normal hearing for pure tones, high word-recognition scores, normal tympanograms, and normal acoustic reflex thresholds, normal hearing may be diagnosed without performance of bone conduction. When air-conduction thresholds are depressed, tympanometry is normal, and acoustic reflexes are present, conductive hearing loss is eliminated as a possible finding, and bone-conduction audiometry will provide no further insights toward a diagnosis of sensory/neural hearing loss. If any signs of conductive loss, such as absent acoustic reflexes or abnormal tympanograms, do appear, bone-conduction audiometry must be carried out to ascertain the degree of any air-bone gap. Unfortunately, these are usually the times when bone-conduction measures are least straightforward due to complications presented by middle-ear artifacts and masking (i.e., in those with conductive and mixed hearing loss). For a demonstration of acoustic immittance with acoustic reflex assessment, see the video entitled Immittance.

Otoacoustic Emissions (OAEs)

The fact that many normal cochleas are capable of producing sounds in the absence of external stimulation came as a surprise to researchers and clinicians in audiology when it was first described by Kemp in 1979. These **spontaneous otoacoustic emissions (SOAEs)** occur in over half the population of persons with normal hearing as a continuous tonal signal that can be recorded in the external auditory canal. The typical frequency range of an SOAE is 1000 to 3000 Hz, although some have been reported well above and below this range. While there is considerable variation in the amplitude of an SOAE, it is often found to be between −10 and +10 dB SPL and is generally inaudible to the person in whom it is measured. It is possible to have more than one SOAE in a given ear and to have otoacoustic emissions in both ears. The physiological basis of these sounds is discussed in Chapter 11.

A second class of OAEs occurs either during or immediately following acoustic stimulation. These responses are called **evoked otoacoustic emissions (EOAEs),** and there are several types. The use of EOAE testing has come into clinical prominence in the differential diagnosis of sensory/neural hearing loss, hearing screenings of infants and other difficult-to-test patients, and the monitoring of outer hair cell function of patients particularly susceptible to the damaging effects of high-level noise exposure or ototoxic medications. In many places, application of EOAE has become the standard of care in pediatric practice (Lonsbury-Martin & Martin, 2003). In addition to the current uses of EOAE, we can expect the role of this measure to increase in the decades ahead as new protective and restorative treatments are developed for use with sensory/neural hearing impairment (Kemp, 2002). The two major types of EOAE are transient and distortion-product emissions.

Transient-Evoked Otoacoustic Emissions

Transient-evoked otoacoustic emissions (TEOAEs) are produced by brief acoustic stimuli, such as clicks or tone pips. Signal-averaging equipment, similar to that described in the section on auditory-evoked potentials (see page 14), must be used to separate the emission from ongoing noise in the ear. Anywhere from 260 to 500 stimuli are presented, and the waveforms of the responses are averaged, along with the ongoing noise in the ear, in order to improve the signal-to-noise ratio (SNR). Responses should be observable from nearly all individuals with normal outer, middle, and inner ears. As hearing loss due to cochlear damage increases, the amplitude of the response decreases until a hearing loss of about 40 dB is reached, where the response usually disappears altogether.

When a click stimulus is used, a wide area of the cochlea is stimulated and a broad range of frequencies is normally present in the TEOAE. If a broadband TEOAE can be observed, it may be inferred that the pathway up to the cochlea, the auditory periphery, is unimpaired. It cannot be known whether there is a disorder in the auditory nerve or other structures beyond the cochlea. Therefore, a normal TEOAE does not guarantee normal hearing. When a TEOAE is not seen, the suggestion is that a hearing loss is present, but it does not reveal whether the problem is in the conductive pathway or the cochlea. A commercial version of an OAE measurement device can be seen in Figure 7.8, and a typical response is shown in Figure 7.9. (Documentation of TEOAE results for a normal-hearing individual is shown in Figure 7.14.)

Distortion-Product Otoacoustic Emissions

When two "primary tones" that vary in frequency by several hundred hertz (F1 and F2, where F2 > F1) are presented to the ear, the normal cochlea responds by producing energy at additional frequencies. These are called **distortion-product otoacoustic emissions (DPOAEs).** By varying the primary-tone frequencies, responses are generated from different areas of the cochlea. Typically, the levels and the frequency ratio of the primary tones are not varied. These responses often compare favorably with voluntary audiometric results, provided that the hearing loss does not exceed 40 to 50 dB. As with TEOAEs, the conductive pathway must be normal to obtain DPOAEs.

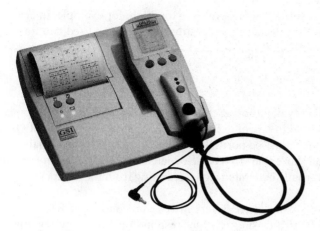

FIGURE 7.8 Commercial device for measurement of otoacoustic emissions, sounds generated by the cochlea indicative of cochlear function. (*Source:* Grason-Stadler Co.)

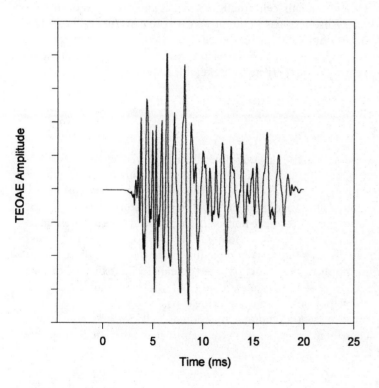

FIGURE 7.9 A typical transient-evoked otoacoustic emission.

Measuring OAEs

Advances in microcircuitry have allowed for accurate measurement of OAEs. A probe is placed in the external auditory canal that contains a miniature loudspeaker to present the evoking stimulus. A tiny microphone is also placed to pick up the emission and convert it from a sound into an electrical signal. The device that delivers the stimuli for DPOAE testing differs from the one for measuring TEOAEs because the probe that is fitted to the ear must have two openings (ports) that can deliver the two primary tones. Because DPOAEs are separate in frequency from the evoking stimuli, averaging background noise is less of a problem for measurement of DPOAEs than it is for TEOAEs, and fewer stimulus presentations are required, which may reduce test time slightly. Acoustic control of the test environment for OAE testing is less critical than might be imagined because the noise that must be averaged out is the noise contained in the ear of the subject. If subject noise levels are too high, for example, in crying babies, the noise may mask the emission because the sensitive microphone used cannot differentiate one acoustic signal from another.

Interpreting OAEs

Otoacoustic emissions reflect the activity of an intact cochlea, and a brief physiological explanation of this phenomenon can be found in Chapter 11 on the inner ear. For any type of OAE to be observed, the conductive pathway must be normal because the strength of a signal traveling from the inner ear to the outer ear canal may be attenuated by an abnormality of the middle ear in the same way as an externally generated signal traveling from the outer ear to the inner ear can be attenuated.

The presence of an EOAE suggests that there is very little or no conductive hearing loss caused by middle-ear abnormality. It further suggests that responding frequency regions of the cochlea are normal or exhibit no more than a mild hearing loss. If OAEs are present in sensory/neural hearing loss, then outer-hair-cell function is intact and the locus of the disorder is known to be retrocochlear. Absent OAEs in the presence of sensory/neural hearing loss confirm cochlear pathology but do not rule out the possibility of concomitant retrocochlear involvement. The result is that OAE measures allow for improved diagnostic differentiation among the different types of hearing losses (Prieve & Fitzgerald, 2009).

Clinical COMMENTARY

In the 1990s, otoacoustic emissions measures brought new insights and diagnostic capabilities to clinical audiology, just as the advent of acoustic immittance measures did in the 1970s. In addition to the use of transient-evoked otoacoustic emissions to help differentiate sensory from neural hearing losses, in the absence of peripheral pathology, distortion-product otoacoustic emissions can establish normal, or near-normal, hearing in a difficult-to-test child or a patient manifesting erroneous response behaviors (see Chapter 13). Otoacoustic emissions have found a prominent place in the hearing screening of newborns, as discussed in Chapter 8, and in the monitoring of cochlear function when potentially ototoxic medications are used to combat illness. As discussed in Chapter 12, research continues into the interactions of the TEOAE and stimulation of the contralateral ear with acoustic competition as potentially useful in assessment of central auditory function as well. For a demonstration of the performance of otoacoustic emissions, see the video entitled Otoacoustic Emissions.

Laser-Doppler Vibrometer Measurement

Just as acoustic immittance measures and otoacoustic emissions evolved from the research laboratory to regular clinical use, so may the use of Laser-Doppler Vibrometer (LDV) measurements. This promising tool measures the sound-induced velocity of the tympanic membrane near the umbo and may prove to be a sensitive tool for the differential diagnosis of ossicular disorders that surpasses the current utility of acoustic immittance (Rowsowski, Nakajima, & Merchant, 2008). This tool may also prove useful in differentiating between air-bone gaps secondary to ossicular fixations and the air-bone gaps that may be observed with some inner-ear malformations. While it may yet be a few years before this emerging tool is routinely used in audiology clinics, it holds promise for providing greater powers of noninvasive differential diagnoses for audiologists.

Auditory-Evoked Potentials

From the time acoustic stimuli reach the inner ear, what is transmitted to the brain is not "sound" but rather a series of neuroelectric events. For many years, there has been considerable interest in the measurement of the electrical responses generated within the cochlea to establish an objective measure of hearing sensitivity in infants and other persons who are unable to participate in behavioral audiometric tests. To this end, a procedure has evolved called **electrocochleography (ECoG).** Because hearing is a phenomenon involving the brain, it is only logical that whenever a sound is heard, there must be some change in the ongoing electrical activity of the brain. These electrical responses, which may be recorded from the scalp using surface electrodes, have been referred to by several names, but today they are commonly known as **auditory-evoked potentials (AEPs).** AEPs can be subdivided on the basis of where and when they occur. They are better understood with the background provided in Chapter 12, which briefly reviews the auditory nervous system. Before attempting to measure an AEP, much more auditory anatomy and physiology, as well as other aspects of neuroscience, should be known than can be presented in an introductory text.

In Chapter 2, some mention was made of the connections between the brain stem and the higher centers for audition in the cerebral cortex. These connections occur via a series of waystations, called nuclei, within the central nervous system. When a signal is introduced to the ear, there are immediate electrical responses in the cochlea. As the signal is propagated along the auditory pathway, more time elapses before a response occurs, and thus the signal can be recorded at each subsequent nucleus in the pathway. The term **latency** is used to define the time period that elapses between the introduction of a stimulus and the occurrence of the response. The term **amplitude** is used to define the strength, or magnitude, of the AEP.

Early AEPs, those that occur in the first 10 to 15 milliseconds after the introduction of a signal, are believed to originate in the VIIIth cranial nerve and the brain stem and are called the **auditory brain-stem responses (ABRs).** An AEP occurring from 15 to 60 milliseconds in latency is called the **auditory middle latency response (AMLR)** and originates in the cortex. Those called the **auditory late responses (ALRs),** or cortical auditory-evoked potentials, occur between 50 and 200 milliseconds and presumably arise in the cortex. Responses recorded between 220 and 600 milliseconds have been called **auditory event-related potentials (ERPs)** (or P300) because they are contingent on some auditory event occurring within a particular context of sound sequence and involve association areas in the brain.

An AEP is simply a small part of a multiplicity of electrical events measurable from the scalp. This electrical activity, which originates in the brain, is commonly referred to as electroencephalic and is measured on a specially designed instrument called an **electroencephalograph (EEG),** which is used to pick up and amplify electrical activity from the brain by electrodes placed on the scalp. When changes in activity are observed on a computer monitor or printout, waveforms may be seen that aid in the diagnosis of central nervous system disease or abnormality.

In coupling the EEG to a patient to observe responses evoked by sounds, the ongoing neural activity is about 100 times greater than the auditory-evoked potential and therefore obscures observation of the AEP. The measurement of AEPs is further complicated by the

FIGURE 7.10 Device used for recording auditory-evoked potentials, electrical responses to sound that are generated within the cochlea and measured through changes in the ongoing electrical activity of the brain. (*Source:* Natus Medical Incorporated.)

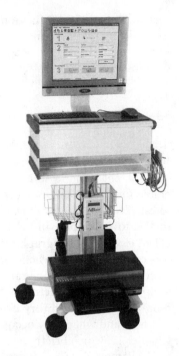

presence of large electrical potentials from muscles (myogenic potentials). These obstacles were insurmountable until the advent of averaging computers, devices that allow measurement of electrical potentials, even when they are embedded in other electrical activity. A commercial device for measuring AEP is shown in Figure 7.10.

To measure an AEP, a series of auditory stimuli is presented to the subject at a constant rate by a transducer (earphone, bone-conduction vibrator, or loudspeaker). Insert earphones are becoming the standard for AEP testing (as well as behavioral testing) because they are relatively comfortable to wear and help attenuate extraneous room noise. Also, their transducers are 250 millimeters from electrodes placed at the ear and therefore produce fewer electrical artifacts. The EEG equipment picks up the neural response, amplifies it, and stores the information in a series of computer memory time bins. Each bin sums neuroelectric activity that occurs at specific numbers of milliseconds after the onset of the stimulus. Of course, the computer is summing not only the response to the sound in any particular time bin, but also the random brain activity taking place at that precise moment. However, because the random activity consists of positive and negative voltages of varying amplitudes, summing reduces them to a value at or near zero. The polarity of the neural response is either positive or negative, but not both. Summing alone would cause the amplitude of the response to increase, but the waveform is then averaged by dividing the amplitude by the number of signal presentations. This decreases the summed response to the amplitude of the averaged response. While there is no increase in amplitude of the AEP, there is a decrease in the amplitude of the random noise as it is summed and averaged. It might be said that, as the summing and averaging process continues, the signal-to-noise ratio improves. Even though the amplitudes of the responses are extremely small, often on the order of 1 to 5 microvolts ($1\,\mu V$ is equal to one-millionth of a volt), they can nevertheless be detected and interpreted.

Electrocochleography

The procedure for measuring electrical responses from the cochlea of the inner ear is called electrocochleography (ECoG, or sometimes ECochG). An active electrode may be placed in one of several positions, ranging from surgical placement of the electrode on the promontory, the medial wall of the middle ear, to less invasive placements within the outer ear canal. The further the active electrode is from the inner ear, the smaller the amplitude of the response and, consequently, the greater the number of stimuli that must be summed before the response can be identified with confidence.

The decision on whether to use more- or less-invasive electrodes during ECoG is largely determined by the types of workplaces in which audiologists find themselves because all methods have their advantages and disadvantages (Ferraro, 1992). Transtympanic approaches, necessitating penetration of the tympanic membrane, are usually carried out in settings where physicians are on site because anesthesia is required. Extratympanic procedures, not requiring the risk or discomfort of minor surgery, can be performed in almost any audiological setting, although greater signal averaging is required to obtain a clear signal as the electrode is moved further from the promontory. Clinicians turned to the ABR as the electrophysiologic measure of choice in the mid-1970s largely because of the invasiveness of the conventional transtympanic electrode (Hall, 2007). The primary focus for ECoG testing has moved from the determination of auditory sensitivity in difficult-to-test individuals (Cullen, Ellis, Berlin, & Lousteau, 1972) to neuro-otological applications, such as monitoring the function of the cochlea during some surgical procedures; enhancing the results of other electrophysiological tests; and, probably most important, assisting in the diagnosis and monitoring of some conditions of the inner ear, such as Ménière's disease (see Chapter 11).

Auditory Brain-Stem Response (ABR) Audiometry

For measuring responses from the brain, electrodes are usually placed on the mastoid process behind the outer ear and the vertex (top of the skull), with a ground electrode placed on the opposite mastoid, the forehead, or the neck. Stimuli with rapid rise times, such as clicks, must be used to generate these early responses. Tone pips, or bursts, which provide some frequency-specific information, can be used. When a summing computer is used, seven small wavelets generally appear in the first 10 milliseconds after signal presentation. Each wave represents neuroelectrical activity at one or more generating sites along the auditory brain-stem pathway. The findings of Legatt, Arezzo, and Vaughan (1988) indicate the following simplified scheme of major ABR generators:

Wave Number	Site
I	VIIIth cranial nerve
II	VIIIth cranial nerve
III	Superior olivary complex
IV	Pons, lateral lemniscus
V	Midbrain, lateral lemniscus, and inferior colliculus
VI and VII	Undetermined

Routine ABR audiometry can be performed in several ways, only one of which is described here. The patient is first seated in a comfortable chair, often a recliner, which is placed in an acoustically isolated, electrically shielded room (see Figure 7.11). The skin areas to which electrodes will be attached are carefully cleansed, and a conductive paste or gel is applied to these areas. One electrode is placed on the vertex or the forehead and one on each earlobe or the mastoid process behind the external ear. An electrode opposite the ear being tested serves as a **ground electrode.** After the electrodes are taped in place, electrical impedance is checked with an ohmmeter. The impedance between the skin and the electrodes, and between any two electrodes, must be controlled for the test to be performed properly. An insert receiver is placed into the test ear, or a circumaural earphone is placed over the test ear, and the patient is asked to relax. The lights are

FIGURE 7.11 The ABR test can be completed with or without sedation. Here a patient is seated in a comfortable chair to encourage relaxation during ABR testing. (*Source:* Bio-logic Navigator® Pro AEP System photo courtesy of Natus Medical, Inc.)

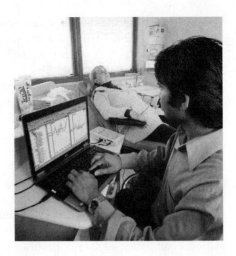

usually dimmed, and the chair placed in a reclining position. The ABR is not affected by sleep state; therefore, the subject may sleep while the responses are being recorded. This characteristic of the ABR is important because it allows anesthetized or comatose individuals to be evaluated.

One ear is tested at a time. A series of 1,000 to 2,000 clicks may be presented at a rate of 33.1 clicks per second. The click rate must not be one that is divisible by 1 with a resultant whole number in order to differentiate the real response from electrical artifacts in the room, such as the 60 Hz electrical current. The starting level is about 70 dB nHL (*n* is the reference to the normative group threshold for click stimuli).

In response to the stimulus, the ABR waveform appears as several narrow peaks and troughs within 1 to 10 ms of the signal onset. The main positive peaks are labeled, after Jewett (1970), in Roman numerals for Waves I, III, and V. If responses are not present, the intensity is raised 20 dB; if responses are present, the level is lowered in 10 or 20 dB steps until Wave V becomes undetectable. After the test has been completed, a hard copy may be printed out and these data may be summarized on a special form (see Figure 7.12). A complete ABR test provides the following information about each ear:

1. Absolute latencies of all identifiable Waves I to V at different intensities.
2. Interpeak latency intervals (i.e., I to V, I to III, III to V), or relative latencies.
3. Wave amplitudes (absolute and relative).
4. Threshold of Wave V if hearing threshold estimation was the purpose of the test.
5. A comparative response with a higher click rate (e.g., 91.1 clicks/second) if the ABR was for neurological assessment.

The ABR has developed into the most important test in the diagnostic site-of-lesion battery and has proven to be sensitive, specific, and efficient in detecting lesions affecting the auditory pathways through the brain stem. While the standard ABR protocol has proven useful in detecting medium and large VIIIth nerve tumors, it has been augmented by the development of a clinical procedure known as the **stacked ABR** (Don & Kwong, 2009; Don, Masuda, Nelson, & Brackmann, 1997), which allows for identification of even very small (<1.0 cm) acoustic neuromas. This procedure is based on a division of the standard ABR whole-cochlea response into five frequency bands by using a high-pass noise-derived-response technique. The amplitudes of the five narrowband responses are then "stacked," or added, to give a measure of whole-nerve activity. A tumor affecting any portion of the auditory nerve therefore yields a stacked ABR of smaller amplitude relative to the normal response. Thus, through the use of the stacked ABR procedure, auditory brain-stem response testing has become even more valuable to clinical audiology.

FIGURE 7.12 Form used for recording results of otoacoustic emissions tests and auditory brain-stem responses.

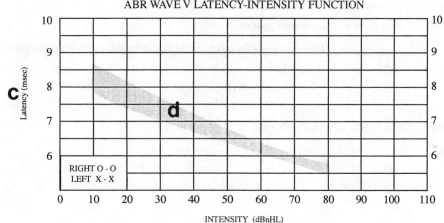

SPEECH AND HEARING CENTER
The University of Texas at Austin 78712

NAME: Last - First - Middle	SEX	AGE	DATE	EXAMINER	RELIABILITY	INSTRUMENT

OTOACOUSTIC EMISSIONS
(Present or Absent)

a ☐ TEOAE Level ____
☐ DPOAE Level F₁ ____ F₂ ____

	Right					Left			
500	1000	2000	4000	6000	500	1000	2000	4000	6000

b

AUDITORY BRAINSTEM RESPONSE
ABR WAVE V LATENCY-INTENSITY FUNCTION

c Latency (msec)

d

RIGHT O - O
LEFT X - X

INTENSITY (dBnHL)

SHADED AREA REPRESENTS Normal Wave V Range for patients older than 16 mos. for 30 clicks per second

EAR	nHL		Absolute Latency (ms) **g**			Interpeak Latency (ms) **h**			Latency Change w/ Increased Rate	**i**
	dB HL	Click Rate	I	III	V	I-III	III-V	I-V	V	Click Rate
RIGHT **e**		**f**								
LEFT										
Interaural Differences **j**										

k Amplitude Ratio (V same or > I)   R ____ L ____
l Estimated Air Conduction Threshold   R ____ L ____
m Estimated Bone Conduction Threshold   R ____ L ____

a. Type of otoacoustic emissions test performed.
b. Presence (P) or absence (A) of OAEs at five frequencies in each ear.
c. Latency-intensity functions of ABR.
d. Shaded area showing a normal distribution of Wave V latency values.
e. Intensity (in dB nHL) required to evoke the response.
f. Stimulus click rate.
g. Absolute latencies for Waves I, III, and V.

h. Interpeak latencies (in milliseconds) for Waves I–III, III–V, and I–V.
i. Wave V latency change (in milliseconds) due to increase in stimulus rate.
j. Differences between the right and left ears for g–i.
k. Amplitude ratio (Wave V same as or greater than Wave I).
l. Estimated air-conduction thresholds.
m. Estimated bone-conduction thresholds.

Interpreting the ABR

The ABR may be used as a test of audiological or neurological function. When testing to estimate behavioral hearing thresholds, as signal intensity decreases, the wave amplitudes become smaller and latencies increase. Because Wave V normally has the largest amplitude of the first seven waves, the ABR threshold is considered to be the lowest intensity at which Wave V can be observed. ABR threshold determinations can usually be ascertained to within 10 to 20 dB of behavioral thresholds. A comparison of ABR responses measured with air-conduction signals and bone-conduction signals is recommended when a conductive hearing loss is suspected.

The ABR may be used as a neurological screening test to assess the integrity of the central auditory pathway. The most significant finding in neurological lesions is an increase in the timing of one or more peaks in the response, indicating a slowing of the auditory response. This may be due to a tumor mass weighing on the nerve or nuclei, or possibly to other abnormal central-nervous-system disorders such as demyelinating diseases like multiple sclerosis. If Wave V can be observed at a slow click rate, for example, 11.1 clicks per second (often seen clearly at 70 dB nHL), a higher click rate may be presented, such as 89.1 clicks per second. An ABR is considered neurologically abnormal, indicating neuropathology affecting the auditory pathway of the brain stem, when any of the following occur:

1. Interpeak intervals are prolonged.
2. Wave latency is significantly different between ears.
3. Amplitude ratios are abnormal (normally Wave V is larger than Wave I).
4. Wave V is abnormally prolonged or disappears with high-click-rate stimulation.

Normal ABR results are shown in Figures 7.13 and 7.14. For a demonstration of patient preparation and recording of the ABR, see the video entitled Auditory Brainstem Response.

Auditory Steady-State Response

The **auditory steady-state response (ASSR),** also known as the steady-state evoked potential (SSEP), is another form of auditory-evoked potential and has proven useful in threshold determination for children. In addition, this procedure may prove to have certain advantages over tone-burst or click-evoked ABR.

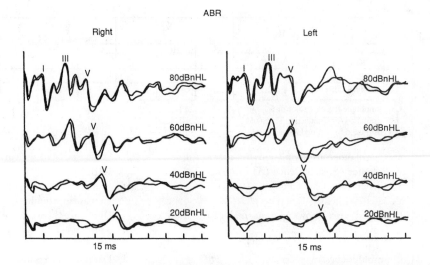

FIGURE 7.13 Auditory brain-stem response testing on a normal-hearing individual. Absolute latencies are shown in Figure 7.14.

FIGURE 7.14 Documentation of results of objective hearing testing on a normal-hearing individual. Latency-intensity functions for Wave V are derived from the auditory brain-stem response tracings shown in Figure 7.13. All the latencies are normal. Transient-evoked otoacoustic emissions are marked as present.

SPEECH AND HEARING CENTER
The University of Texas at Austin 78712

NAME: Last - First - Middle	SEX	AGE	DATE	EXAMINER	RELIABILITY	INSTRUMENT

OTOACOUSTIC EMISSIONS
(Present or Absent)

☑ TEOAE Level **80** dB Peak SPL
☐ DPOAE Level F₁ ____ F₂ ____

Right					Left				
500	1000	2000	4000	6000	500	1000	2000	4000	6000
P	P	P	P	P	P	P	P	P	P

AUDITORY BRAINSTEM RESPONSE
ABR WAVE V LATENCY-INTENSITY FUNCTION

RIGHT O - O
LEFT X - X

Latency (msec) vs INTENSITY (dBnHL)

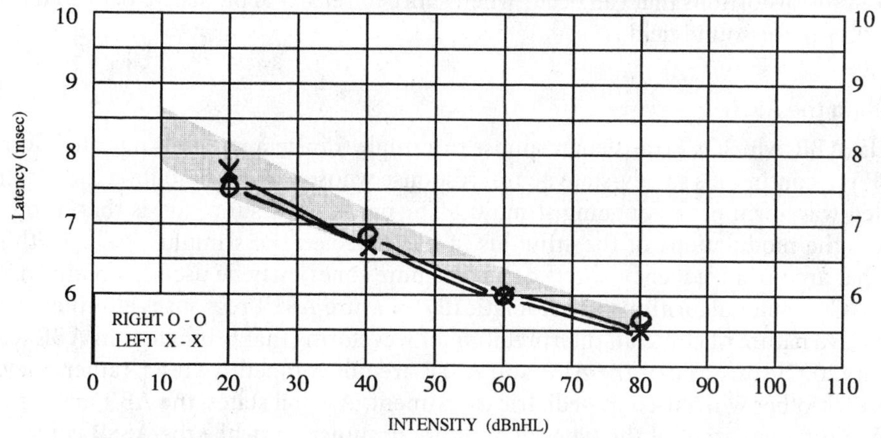

SHADED AREA REPRESENTS Normal Wave V Range for patients older than 16 mos. for 30 clicks per second

EAR	nHL		Absolute Latency (ms)			Interpeak Latency (ms)			Latency Change w/ Increased Rate	
	dB HL	Click Rate	I	III	V	I-III	III-V	I-V	V	Click Rate
RIGHT	80	33.1	1.8	3.75	5.7	1.95	1.95	3.9		
LEFT	80	33.1	1.6	3.62	5.6	2.02	1.98	4.0		
Interaural Differences										

Amplitude Ratio (V same or > I)   R **NL** L **NL**
Estimated Air Conduction Threshold   R ____ L ____
Estimated Bone Conduction Threshold   R ____ L ____

As discussed in Chapter 8, the age at which hearing loss in children is identified has dropped considerably in recent years. As the age of identification of hearing loss decreases, the need for accurate and objective measures of determining hearing thresholds for newborns increases. Individualized remediation is enhanced with the advent of means to uncover reliably the degree, configuration, and type of hearing loss. While the use of the sensitivity prediction from the acoustic reflex (SPAR) test discussed earlier can be useful in categorizing degree of hearing loss, the variability among results limits its usefulness in accurately predicting threshold and the frequency-specific configuration of hearing loss. Otoacoustic emissions can provide frequency-specific information on the status of outer-hair-cell function but provide little information on the degree of hearing loss. Tone-evoked ABR testing can yield frequency-specific estimates of hearing loss, including degree, configuration, and type (using bone-conduction ABR testing), but it can take considerable clinical time to complete. Reducing test time and obtaining the same results as the tone-evoked ABR may be possible using the ASSR technique. The ASSR is one of the latest tools to be added to the audiologist's arsenal to obtain reliable predictions of hearing sensitivity. While the tone-burst ABR and the ASSR provide similar estimates of behavioral pure-tone thresholds (Cone-Wesson, Dowell, Tolin, Rance, & Min, 2002), the investment of clinical time for testing can be considerably less for the ASSR. An important consideration is that the ASSR, like the ABR, is not affected by the patient's state of consciousness.

In addition to providing an estimate of auditory sensitivity, the ASSR can be employed to assess the efficacy of intervention through estimations of hearing thresholds in the sound field with and without hearing aids (Picton et al., 1998). These important measures for very young children who cannot overtly respond to test stimuli are not possible with tone-burst ABR measures given the distortions that can occur when short-onset signal bursts are delivered through loudspeakers in the sound field.

Interpreting the ASSR

Unlike the ABR, which is a transient response to a single transient stimulus repeated over time, the ASSR is a continuous steady-state neural response whose waveform follows the amplitude-modulated waveform of the ongoing stimulus. The operative assumption is that, if the brain can detect the modulations of the stimulus, it has detected the stimulus itself. In this way, stimuli that are most frequency-specific, such as pure tones, may be used to obtain threshold estimates. Computer algorithms to automatically measure ASSR responses eliminate some of the subjective nature of clinician interpretation of waveforms that is inherent in ABR testing.

Hall (2007) stresses that the ABR and ASSR are not competitive tests; rather, they complement each other when used in pediatric assessment. As Hall states, the ABR is the stronger measure in differentiation of the types of auditory dysfunction, while the ASSR is more valuable in estimating hearing for moderate to profound sensory/neural hearing loss. The ABR is accurate in establishing the presence of normal or mild-to-moderate hearing loss but not for losses of greater degree, while the ASSR may tend to overestimate hearing levels for those with normal hearing.

Auditory Middle Latency Response (AMLR) Audiometry

For some time it was uncertain whether the middle latency responses, which occur between 15 and 60 milliseconds after signal presentation, are myogenic (produced by changes in electrical potential generated in muscles on the scalp and behind the ear) or neurogenic (produced by electrical potentials in nerve units within the auditory pathways). It is now generally accepted that the AMLR has a neurogenic component. The AMLR reflects activity from the cortex and is therefore also called the early cortical auditory-evoked potential.

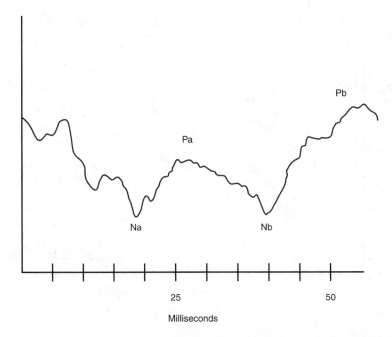

FIGURE 7.15 Auditory-evoked potentials showing the middle latency response providing information about hearing in the 2000 to 4000 Hz range.

Patient setup for measurement of the AMLR is essentially the same as for ABR. A major difference lies in the importance of keeping the patient awake because the amplitudes of the responses are reduced during sleep. As with the ABR and all other auditory-evoked potentials, it is important to keep the patient inactive to minimize myogenic artifacts. Patients must remain calm but alert. It may be necessary to average 500 to 1,000 responses to obtain a clear AMLR from clicks, filtered clicks, or tone bursts that may be delivered through an insert receiver or supraural earphone.

Interpreting the AMLR

The AMLR provides the same accuracy in frequency-specific threshold estimation as the ABR does. Indeed, the ABR and AMLR may be obtained simultaneously, giving the clinician more information about the auditory system in the same amount of time it takes to obtain one or the other response alone. The AMLR is also useful in the assessment of neurological function of the higher central auditory nervous system. Further refinement of AMLR measurement techniques will probably increase its use as a neurodiagnostic procedure. An AMLR response is shown in Figure 7.15.

Auditory Late Responses (ALRs)

The earliest work done on AEPs was on the late cortical auditory-evoked potential (CAEP), which includes those responses that appear at least 60 milliseconds after signal presentation (see Figure 7.16). Problems in interpreting ALR test results, along with improvements in microcomputers and averaging systems, led to a much greater interest in the earlier components of the evoked response (ABR and AMLR), but in subsequent years, renewed interest has been found in the later components. A major advantage of measuring the later responses is that it is possible to use frequency-specific stimuli, such as pure tones, as well as short segments of speech. The responses are considerably larger than the earlier waves and therefore can be tracked closer to the individual's behavioral threshold; however, unlike the ABR and

FIGURE 7.16 Auditory-evoked potentials showing the late evoked response. These responses depend on a state of wakeful consciousness and exhibit significant degradation when patients are sleeping.

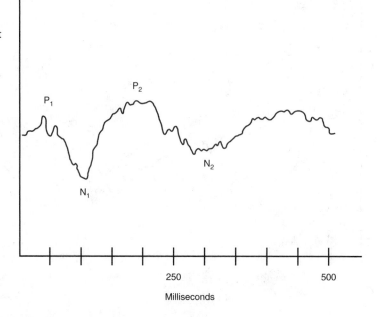

ASSR the responses are affected by a patient's attention, and therefore the ALR has limitations when used with children. These potentials depend on state of consciousness; that is, significant degradation occurs with sleep, whether natural or induced. Because it is possible to use frequency-specific stimuli, such as pure tones, the ALR can therefore be used for threshold estimation as well as speech-assessment procedures.

The first late response (P1) often occurs at a latency of approximately 60 milliseconds after stimulus onset for a moderately intense tonal or speech sound. P1 is followed by a series of negative (N) and positive (P) waves (N1, P2, N2) occurring between 100 and 250 milliseconds. At approximately 300 milliseconds, a larger (10 to 20 μV) positive wave is seen. This response has become known as P300 or the auditory event-related response. The amplitude of the P300 can be made to increase significantly by having the patient count the stimuli (one per second).

Another late evoked response, the **mismatch negativity (MMN),** has produced significant interest. This is a small negative electrophysiologic response using an oddball paradigm, for example, having "rare" stimuli at 2000 Hz presented 15 percent of the time along with "standard" stimuli like 1000 Hz presented 85 percent of the time (Kibbe-Michal, Verkest, Gollegly, & Musiek, 1986). Unlike with the P300, however, the subjects are instructed to ignore both the rare and standard stimuli, which may both be present in the same ear or presented individually to different ears. The greater negativity on the waveform in response to the "odd," or infrequently presented, stimuli compared to the response obtained to the standard, or frequent, stimuli reflects the neural response to a change in some physical attribute of the stimulus (e.g., pitch as in a 2000 Hz tone versus in a 1000 Hz standard tone). The effect is that different responses are evoked by the rare and standard signals, resulting in the acquisition of two different waveforms that are combined to obtain a different waveform containing the MMN. It is believed that the different responses to the rare and standard stimuli are due to the brain noticing a difference between the two stimuli, hence the term *mismatch* (Picton, 1995). The amplitude and latency of the MMN are related to the difference between the rare and standard signals rather than the absolute levels of these signals. The MMN is elicited in response to any change in auditory stimulation—frequency, intensity, rise time,

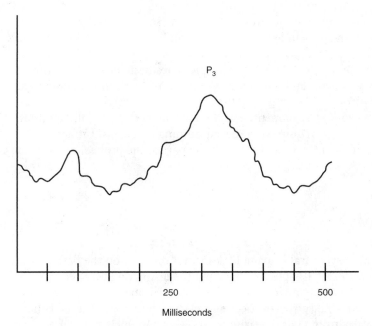

duration, etc.—although very small changes may not be recognized within the normal background electrical noise of brain activity. The MMN, whose multiple generator sites include the temporal cortex, holds great promise for understanding how the brain conducts its cognitive functions (Näätänen, 1995). In addition, it may prove useful in differentiating disorders of auditory perception from disorders involving higher levels of function, such as language, attention, and memory, or in demonstrating the effects of speech-sound-discrimination training.

Interpreting the Auditory Late Responses

Auditory late-evoked responses may aid in the estimation of threshold for pure tones over a wide frequency range and in the assessment of neurological function. Of course, if patients are awake and cooperative enough to allow late evoked responses, they can often be tested voluntarily. The P300 potential is called *event related* because it depends on discrimination of target stimuli by the listener (see Figure 7.17). For this reason, the P300 is thought to be related to the perception or processing of stimuli rather than to the mere activation of the auditory nervous system by a stimulus. Late-evoked, P300, and MMN responses offer great promise for practical applications in diagnosis of neurological disease and injury. In addition, measured changes in the P1, N1, and N2 responses and the MMN response may find utility in the documentation of the effects of training to maximize the use of residual hearing (Tremblay & Kraus, 2002; Tremblay, Kraus, Carrell, & McGee, 1997).

Intraoperative Monitoring

Improvements in equipment and procedures have also brought ABR testing into the operating room, where it is used to monitor responses from the brain during delicate neurosurgical procedures (Møller, 2000). Many of the electrical responses described above have been used for **intraoperative monitoring** of the physiological state of the patient. During these delicate operations, surgeons often require reports on the condition of the patient so that they may be alerted to possible damage to the auditory system before it occurs, thus averting both hearing loss and damage to other structures in the brain. Some operations that can benefit from this kind of monitoring include surgery on the auditory and facial nerves, as well as on the inner ear.

The modern operating room is filled with many people (anesthesiologists, technicians, and nurses) in addition to the surgeon and patient, as well as a lot of electrical equipment that can generate signals that can interfere with monitoring of neuroelectrical responses. The operating room is not an easy work environment, and the persons performing these duties, who increasingly include audiologists, require very special training and skills. Intraoperative monitoring usually involves ECoG and ABR and is becoming part of the professional role of many audiologists.

A Historical Note

Separating conductive from sensory/neural hearing losses is not difficult on the basis of the pure-tone and speech tests described in Chapters 4 and 5, but the distinction between sensory (cochlear) and neural (lesions beyond the inner ear, or retrocochlear) is more difficult to determine. Prior to the advent of today's electroacoustical and electrophysiological tests, behavioral measures to separate sensory from neural hearing losses were extremely popular among audiologists. As more objective measures became increasingly available, research has shown that the sensitivity and specificity of the behavioral site-of-lesion tests are not always high. It can be argued that the use of multiple weak tests do not necessarily combine to create a strong differential battery (Durrant & Collet, 2002). Despite the general absence of these behavioral measures in today's testing protocols, they do illustrate some important concepts in normal audition and diagnostic audiology and as such, a brief historical review of select behavioral measures is presented here.

Loudness Balancing

Loudness increases with intensity in a logical and lawful manner. That is, as the intensity of a sound is increased, so is the experience of loudness. An appreciation and understanding of the growth in loudness perception in impaired ears has important clinical utility in fitting hearing aids.

We expect that normal ears will show a logical progression of loudness as intensity is increased. This is also true of patients with conductive hearing loss, so that 50 dB above the threshold of a person with a 10 dB threshold (50 dB SL, 60 dB HL) is as loud as 50 dB above the threshold of a patient with a 40 dB hearing loss (50 dB SL, 90 dB HL). In patients with lesions in the cochlea, the loudness growth may be very rapid. Therefore, a patient with a threshold of 40 dB may experience a tone at 60 dB HL (20 dB SL) as being the same loudness that a person with a 0 dB threshold does at 60 dB HL (60 dB SL). This is called loudness **recruitment.** One can see that while the presence of recruitment is helpful in the diagnosis of a lesion site, it can present serious problems for some people in wearing their hearing aids.

Patients with retrocochlear lesions either demonstrate no recruitment or may show **decruitment,** which is a slower-than-normal increase in the loudness of a signal as intensity is increased. For example, a patient with a 40 dB hearing loss with decruitment might experience a tone at 60 dB HL (20 dB SL) as being as loud as a tone at 90 dB HL (50 dB SL). This is called loudness decruitment and is not always present with these lesions.

The best way to test for loudness recruitment in patients with unilateral hearing losses is by comparing the increase in loudness in the normal ear to the increase in loudness of the abnormal ear. This procedure is called the **alternate binaural loudness balance (ABLB) test.** While modern clinical audiometers still include circuitry for the administration of the ABLB, it is rarely performed by audiologists today (Martin, Champlin, & Chambers, 1998).

Clinical COMMENTARY

As was mentioned earlier, acoustic reflexes are often observed at low sensation levels in patients who have lesions of the cochlea. This has been interpreted by some audiologists as a manifestation of loudness recruitment, which occurs because a tone presented at, say, 45 dB SL appears to be very loud (as loud as a 95 dB HL tone for those with normal hearing). There is no evidence that recruitment per se produces an acoustic reflex at low sensation levels, although both phenomena are often found in the same patients.

The Short Increment Sensitivity Index

It has been known for some time that patients with lesions in the cochlea are able to detect extremely small changes in intensity. Jerger, Shedd, and Harford (1959) developed a test based on this principle called the **short increment sensitivity index (SISI).** The SISI is designed to test the ability of a patient to detect the presence of a 1 dB increment superimposed on a continuous tone presented at 20 dB SL. Twenty such increments are introduced, and patients with cochlear lesions are usually able to detect most of them, actually achieving scores at or close to 100 percent. Patients with retrocochlear and conductive loss, as well as those with normal hearing, do not have this ability and usually achieve scores close to 0 percent. Like the ABLB, modern clinical audiometers are still manufactured with circuit capability for administering the SISI test, although it is rarely performed today (Martin et al., 1998).

Tone Decay

In most cases, even among people with normal auditory systems, listening to sustained signals brings about a certain amount of shift in an individual's thresholds for those signals; that is, the tone appears to die away. For many years, it has been noted that patients with some forms of hearing disorder find it impossible to hear sustained tones for more than a brief time. To many of these patients, a tone heard clearly at a level 5 dB above threshold fades rapidly to inaudibility. If the level of the tone is increased, the tone may be heard again, only to disappear quickly to silence. This is called **tone decay.**

   People with normal hearing and those with conductive hearing losses show almost no tone decay. Those with cochlear lesions show some tone decay, perhaps up to 20 dB or so, but mostly in the higher frequencies (1,000 Hz and above). Patients with lesions on the auditory nerve often show dramatic tone decay at all frequencies, which may be a powerful diagnostic sign.

Clinical COMMENTARY

Compared to loudness balancing or the short increment sensitivity index, tone-decay testing has retained some clinical utility given its relatively high sensitivity, the limited clinical time required to administer it, and the absence of a need for any special equipment.

Békésy Audiometry

The use of a modern version of Békésy's automatic audiometer was once a popular audiological procedure that allowed patients to track their own auditory thresholds. During **Békésy audiometry,** the patient presses a button when a tone becomes audible in an earphone, keeps the button depressed as long as the tone is heard, and then releases it when the tone becomes inaudible. The tone is allowed to increase in intensity until the button is pressed again, which causes the tone to be attenuated. A pen, controlled by the attenuator of the audiometer, traces the level of the tone on an audiogram as a function of both time and either fixed or constantly changing frequency.

The initial report of Jerger (1960) led to the use of Békésy audiometry as a clinical tool in the differential diagnosis of **site of lesion.** Observations were made of responses to continuous and to pulsed tones. The result of these observations was a series of five different types of Békésy audiograms. Because of the significant clinical time investment to complete Békésy testing, coupled with the procedure's low test sensitivity, Békésy testing is rarely used in clinical practice today.

CHECK YOUR UNDERSTANDING

ACTIVITIES

EVOLVING CASE STUDIES

You will be asked to predict the results of the special tests described in this chapter on the six case studies that have been developed. These tests will include acoustic immittance, acoustic reflex thresholds (ARTs), otoacoustic emissions (OAEs), and auditory brain-stem responses (ABRs). The first two tests just named are performed routinely on patients who appear for audiometric evaluation. OAEs are obtained routinely in some clinics, but like ABR testing, they are usually reserved for special occasions when additional diagnostic information is required. For this exercise, predict the possible/probable results on all four types of tests. Because of the individual natures of the disorders in these case studies, you are asked to refer to other chapters where the pathologies are covered in greater detail for discussion of these tests.

Case Study 1 featuring a nine-year-old boy with a conductive hearing loss due to an outer ear disorder continues at the end of Chapter 9.

Case Study 2 about a 23-year-old woman with middle ear disorder continues at the end of Chapter 10.

Case Study 3 of a 79-year-old gentleman with an inner ear disorder resumes at the end of Chapter 11.

Case Study 4 featuring a 36-year-old woman with an auditory nerve disorder continues at the end of Chapter 12.

Case Study 5 involves a man with nonorganic hearing loss and continues at the end of Chapter 13.

Case Study 6 is a 3-year-old patient with delayed language development continues at the end of Chapter 8.

Summary

Acoustic immittance measurements give remarkably reliable information regarding the function of the middle ear. Both static compliance and tympanometry are measures of the mobility of the middle-ear mechanism. Distinctive tympanometric patterns, combined with other audiometric findings, can aid the clinician in determining the underlying pathology of a conductive hearing loss. The acoustic reflex and reflex decay give information regarding probable disorders of different areas of the auditory system. There is no doubt that the acoustic immittance meter has become as indispensable to the audiologist as the audiometer.

The introduction of otoacoustic emissions to the test battery is a giant leap in the direction of testing patients who cannot or will not cooperate during voluntary hearing tests. The advantages to using OAEs with children are obvious. This procedure is noninvasive and requires no patient cooperation, except to remain relatively motionless. Data-collection time has been estimated at 1 to 5 minutes per ear, which is very advantageous considering that children tend to be active. Otoacoustic emissions have added significantly to the battery of tests for site of lesion. OAEs may be used in combination with evoked potential measures to help differentiate sensory from neural lesions and may also be utilized as a cross-check of middle-ear status, as determined by acoustic immittance measures.

Auditory brain-stem response (ABR) audiometry has become an important part of the site-of-lesion test battery, and some of the other evoked potential techniques are becoming more valuable as they are improved. Using computer averaging techniques and a series of acoustic stimuli, it is possible to evoke responses on the basis of neuroelectric activity within the auditory system. By looking at the kinds of responses obtained during electrocochleography and auditory brain-stem response audiometry, along with the later components of electroencephalic audiometry, it is often possible to predict the site of lesion and estimate auditory threshold. Many of these tests are finding their way into the operating room for monitoring

REVIEW TABLE 7.1 Summary of Objective Tests

Test	Purpose	Measurement Unit
Tympanometry	Pressure-compliance function of TM	cm^3
Static compliance	Compliance of TM	cm^3
ART	Sensation level of acoustic reflex	dB
ABR	Latency-intensity function of early AEP	msec
OAE	Check cochlear function	dB

REVIEW TABLE 7.2 Typical Interpretations of Objective Tests

	Normal Hearing	Conductive Loss	Sensory Loss	Neural Loss
Tympanogram type	A	A_D, A_S, B, or C	A	A
Static compliance (cm^3)	0.3 to 1.6	<0.3 or >1.6	0.3 to 1.6	0.3 to 1.6
ART	Present at 85 to 100 dB SL	Absent or >100 dB SL	Present at <65 dB SL	Absent or >100 dB SL
ABR	Normal Wave V and interpeak latencies	All wave latencies prolonged	Slightly increased Wave V and interpeak latencies	Very increased Wave V and interpeak latencies
OAE	Present	Absent	Absent	Present

during neurosurgery. Although the ABR should be considered to be more a test of synchronous neural firings than of hearing per se, its value to diagnostic audiology and to neurological screening is well established.

Tests like the alternate binaural loudness balance test, SISI, tone decay, and Békésy audiometry have largely been replaced by the more objective procedures. Students interested in a more detailed presentation of behavioral site-of-lesion testing may consult Brunt (2002).

Frequently Asked Questions

Q Why are the acoustic reflexes of patients with cochlear hearing losses present at low sensation levels?

A *The answer to this question does not show agreement in the literature. Some people relate it to the presence of loudness recruitment in cochlear hearing losses. It is probably related to the stimulation of specific zones in the cochlea that respond to high-intensity stimuli.*

Q What type of tympanogram, showing the point of greatest compliance at 0 daPa, is seen in patients with normal hearing?

A *Type A is what is seen in patients with normal hearing, but it is seen in patients with sensory/neural hearing loss as well.*

Q What type of tympanogram is seen in patients with middle-ear fluid, showing no point of greatest compliance?

A *Type B is what is expected, but variations do occur.*

Q How are otoacoustic emissions produced?

A *They are considered to be produced by the distortion of the outer hair cells of the cochlea.*

Q As a signal travels to the brain, where does the first decussation in the waystations occur?

A *Although this is not universally agreed upon, it is generally acknowledged that the first decussation probably occurs from the ipsilateral cochlear nucleus to the contralateral superior olivary complex.*

Q Does a longer than normal latency period suggest damage or pathology of the middle ear, cochlea, or VIIIth cranial nerve?

A *Interpeak and overall latencies are pretty much the same in middle-ear disorders and normal ears. In cochlear lesions, the latencies are delayed at low intensities but may be normal at high intensities. In VIIIth nerve lesions, both interpeak and absolute latencies are delayed.*

Q What is the significance of observing two peaks of compliance in the tympanogram?

A *Observing two peaks of compliance in the tympanogram suggests the possibility of a healed perforation in the tympanic membrane, sometimes called a monomere. One peak shows the compliance of the entire TM, and the other peak shows the compliance of the thinner monomere.*

Q How are the components in the impedance formula related to each other?

A *Resistance increases impedance and is independent of the other impedance components and of frequency. Mass reactance is directly related to frequency, and stiffness reactance is inversely related to frequency.*

Q When do you perform the physical volume test (PVT)?

A *Perform the PVT whenever a perforation of the tympanic membrane is suspected.*

Q What is recruitment?

A *Loudness recruitment is an abnormally large increase in loudness as intensity is increased and is suggestive of a lesion in the cochlea.*

Q What is decruitment?

A *Decruitment is an abnormally gradual increase in loudness as the intensity of a signal is increased. It suggests a lesion on the auditory nerve.*

Q Why does the negative peak on a Type C tympanogram suggest a nonfunctioning eustachian tube?

A *The negative peak indicates less than normal air pressure in the middle ear. This, it must be assumed, is the result of a faulty eustachian tube.*

Q How does the probe measure acoustic reflexes in a contralateral test when the signal is presented to an earphone?

A *Unless there is some pathology to alter this, acoustic reflexes are bilateral. That is, a reflex-eliciting stimulus presented to one ear will cause almost simultaneous contraction of the muscles in both middle ears. The earphone placed in or on the ear opposite the probe can only present a sound, while the reflex is monitored in the ear with the inserted probe.*

Q What's the difference between a cochlear hearing loss and a sensory/neural hearing loss?

A *The term sensory/neural is used to describe those losses that are either sensory or neural. Therefore, a cochlear hearing loss is always sensory/neural but not all sensory/neural losses are cochlear.*

Q When testing the acoustic reflex, is the ear with the probe the ear that you are testing?

A *Terminology here gets confusing at times. It is least complicated to refer to the ear that receives the reflex-activating signal (RAS). Consider, for example, a patient with an earphone on the right ear and a probe in the left ear. If the RAS is delivered through the probe, this is clearly the left ipsilateral test. If the RAS is delivered through the earphone, this is the right contralateral test and the reflex is monitored via the probe in the left ear*

Suggested Reading

Clark, J. L., Roeser, R. J., Mendrygal, M. (2007). Middle ear measures. In R. J. Roeser, M. Valente, & H. Hosford-Dunn (Eds.), *Audiology diagnosis* (pp. 380–399). New York: Thieme.

Dhar, S., & Hall, J. (2009). *Otoacoustic emissions: Principles, procedures and protocols.* San Diego: Plural Publishing.

Hall, J. W. (2007). *New handbook of auditory evoked responses.* Boston: Pearson/Allyn & Bacon.

Musiek, F. E., & Baran, J. A. (2007). *The auditory system: Anatomy, physiology, and clinical correlates.* Boston: Pearson/Allyn & Bacon.

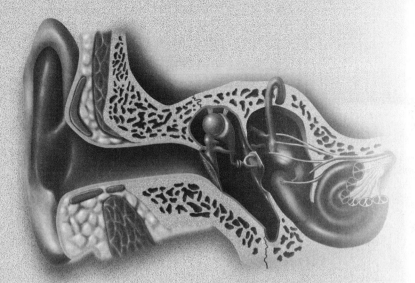

CHAPTER 8

Pediatric Audiology

LEARNING OBJECTIVES

This chapter presents information on early hearing-loss identification and a variety of techniques that have proved helpful in obtaining information about the auditory function of children who cannot be tested using usual audiometric procedures. Methods are described to determine the presence, type, and extent of hearing loss in children. At the completion of this chapter, the reader should be able to

- Describe the various responses that infants may give to auditory signals and how levels of sleep may affect these responses.
- List the components and goals of an early hearing detection and intervention program.
- Describe various test approaches with young children, providing discussion of what measures may be appropriate at different age levels and how the child may respond.
- Describe the components of a successful school hearing screening program, and the equipment and screening measures that would be employed for hearing screening in the schools.
- Discuss how special diagnostic difficulties may be presented by complications such as auditory processing disorders and nonorganic hearing loss.

OR A VERY LONG TIME children with hearing loss were denied the most basic of human rights. Those who reached adulthood could be denied the rights to marry, conduct business in their own names, and even to own property. Hearing loss was considered a major justification for infanticide, decisions about which were legally determined by the fathers and a policy that was not officially opposed until about 400 C.E. Unquestionably, the human race, for the most part, has come a very long way, although the means and motivation for pediatric audiology are not universally extant.

Most of the audiometric procedures described earlier in this text can be applied with great reliability to children beyond ages 4 or 5 years. In such cases, the examination is often no more difficult than it is with cooperative adults. However, in many instances, because of the level at which a particular child functions, special diagnostic procedures must be adopted. Because the average prevalence of hearing loss in children identified through newborn hearing screening programs is 1 per 1,000 infants screened and because up to 3.1 percent of children and youth have hearing loss in at least one ear (Mehra, Eavey, & Keamy, 2009), the need for pediatric audiology is self-evident.

Auditory Responses

It has been stated in this text that what is measured with hearing tests is not hearing itself, but rather a patient's ability and/or willingness to respond to a set of acoustic signals. Therefore, whatever determination is made about the hearing of any individual is made by inference from some set of responses. The hearing function itself is not observed directly.

The manner of a patient's response to some of the tests described earlier has not been considered to be of great concern. For example, it is not important whether the patient signals the awareness of a tone by a hand signal, by a vocal response, or by pressing a button. With small children, however, the manner and type of response to a signal may be crucial to diagnosis. It is also important to remember that most small children do not respond to acoustic signals at threshold; rather, sounds must be more clearly audible to them than to their older counterparts. Therefore, it is safe to assume that, during audiometry, small children's responses must be considered to be at their **minimum response levels (MRLs)**, which in some cases may be well above their thresholds (see Table 8.1).

Responses from small children may vary from voluntary acknowledgment of a signal to involuntary movement of the body, or from an overt cry of surprise to a slight change in vocalization. Response to sound may be totally unobservable, except for some change in the electrophysiological system of the child being tested. If a clear response to a sound is observed by a trained clinician, it may be inferred that the sound has been heard, although the sensation level of the signal may be very much in question. Conversely, if no response is observed, it cannot be assumed that the sound has not been heard.

TABLE 8.1 Typical Sound-Field Minimum Response Levels for Normal-Hearing Children from Birth to 24 Months of Age

Age (Months)	Noisemakers (dB HL)	Warble Tones (dB HL)	Speech (dB HL)
0–4	40	70	45
4–6	45	50	25
6–8	25	45	20
8–10	20	35	10
10–14	20	30	10
14–20	20	25	10
20–24	15	25	10

Source: Martin & Clark, 1996.

Obviously, a number of factors contribute to the responses offered by a child. Of primary concern is the physiological and psychological state prior to stimulation. Shepherd (1978) describes pre-stimulus activity levels as a range consisting of alert attentiveness, relaxed wakefulness, drowsiness, light sleep, and deep sleep. Students of audiology should spend time observing normal children to understand motor development, language and speech acquisition, and auditory behaviors.

Even though audiologists may have preferences for certain kinds of responses from a child, they must be willing to settle for whatever the child provides. Audiologists must also be willing to alter, in midstream, the kind of procedure used if it seems that a different system might be more effective. Modification of a procedure may be the only way to evoke responses from a child, and flexibility and alertness are essential. Response to a sound may appear only once, and it may be lost easily to the inexperienced or unobservant clinician.

Identifying Hearing Loss in Infants under 3 Months of Age

Speech and language are imitative processes, acquired primarily through the auditory sense. A hearing defect, either congenital or acquired early in life, can interfere with the development of concepts that culminate in normal communication. Of the 4 million babies born annually in the United States, it can be expected that about 1 to 3 per thousand will have some degree of hearing loss. In the absence of hearing screening at birth, many children with abnormal hearing proceed into the third year of life or beyond before a hearing problem is suspected. A hearing disorder in a child is often not detected because parents believe that, if their own child had a hearing loss, they would somehow know it because he or she would be obviously different from other children.

There has also been a mistaken notion that babies with hearing loss do not babble. It is probable that the act of babbling is a kind of vegetative activity that is reinforced by a child's tactile and proprioceptive gratification from the use of the mouth and tongue. Around the age of 6 months, children with normal hearing begin to notice that those interesting cooing sounds have been coming from their own mouths, and they begin to amuse themselves by varying rate, pitch, and loudness. Children with impaired hearing, who do not receive adequate auditory feedback, often gradually decrease their vocalizations. In contrast, children with normal hearing begin to repeat, in parrot-like fashion, the sounds they hear. Eventually, meaning becomes attached to sounds, and the projective use of words is initiated. Usually, the normal-hearing child is speaking well before the age of 2 years; the child with an auditory deficit is not.

The average age at which children with hearing losses were identified in the United States in the early 1990s was nearly 3 years of age (National Institutes of Health, 1993), whereas in Israel it has been between 7 and 9 months (Gustafson, 1989). This significant difference can be attributed primarily to the differences in the health-care delivery systems in the two countries and the auditory screening procedures used. With the knowledge that profound hearing loss in children is declining, whereas mild losses are on the increase, and that these mild losses produce more difficulties for children than had been supposed (Tharpe & Bess, 1991), it is generally agreed that early identification of hearing loss is of paramount importance. The earlier in the life of a child that specific educational and training procedures can be initiated, the greater the chance that they will be successful (Fulcher, Purcell, Baker, & Munro, 2012). There is, of course, no earlier time that testing can begin than immediately after birth. It is for these reasons that legislation for the implementation of universal infant hearing screening has been passed throughout most of the United States. Since the implementation of newborn hearing screening programs, an encouraging trend has been seen in the reduction of the age of hearing loss identification and subsequent intervention (Harrison, Roush, & Wallace, 2003). The purpose of early hearing detection and intervention (EHDI) programs is to identify children with hearing loss before they reach the age of 3 months.

A number of criteria must be met before newborn screening of any disorder can be justified, including (1) a sufficient prevalence of the disorder to justify the screening, (2) evidence that the disorder will be detected earlier than would be the case without screening, (3) the availability of follow-up diagnostics immediately after the failure of a screening, (4) treatment accessibility immediately following diagnosis, and (5) a documented advantage to early identification. All of these criteria are easily met in the argument for newborn hearing screening.

Infant Hearing Screening

Hearing screening procedures can be justified on several bases, including cost efficiency. When compared with other disorders for which screening is routine, such as phenylketonuria (PKU) or neonatal hypothyroidism, the yield is considerably higher for hearing loss. As a matter of fact, hearing loss of varying degrees has been ranked sixth in prevalence of chronic conditions in the United States (U.S. Department of Health and Human Resources, 1993). Within the general population, reported prevalence data vary because of differences among studies in screening procedures and definition of hearing impairment, but prevalence in some areas may be as high as six babies with significant hearing loss in every 1,000 births (Hayes & Northern, 1996). From a purely objective and financial viewpoint, the fact that hundreds of millions of dollars might be saved each year if early identification and habilitation of hearing impairments were in place seems to justify neonatal hearing screening, even if the obvious humanitarian aspects are ignored.

Apgar[1] (1953) developed a system for evaluating newborns that is used in many hospitals today. The procedure now utilizes an acronym based on her name: A (appearance), P (pulse), G (grimace), A (activity), R (respiration). Basically the **Apgar Test** score evaluates the normalcy of respiratory effort, muscle tone, heart rate, color, and reflex irritability. The evaluation of the newborn is usually carried out by trained nurses, who assign values of 0 to 10 at 1, 5, and 10 minutes after birth. These evaluations help to determine whether the child requires additional oxygen and whether there is a likelihood of central nervous system damage. Children with low Apgar scores should also be suspected of having sensory/neural hearing loss. Inexperienced audiologists enter their professional careers with little time spent in observing the behaviors of normal infants. Their initial professional experiences are often with children who have problems, which they must diagnose without a satisfactory standard for comparison. Learning the sometimes subtle differences in the appearance and behaviors between children with and without normal hearing is one of the vast benefits of clinical experience because diagnostic decisions are often based on subjective impressions.

Walker (2003) discussed the importance of early diagnosis of hearing loss as part of a "diagnostic imperative." There appears to be a biological relationship between newborn hearing loss and other conditions, including sudden infant death syndrome (SIDS). Both may be due to congenital deficiencies of important enzymes like biotin, which can lead to a wide variety of disorders of the auditory and other systems, including the heart, eye, and musculoskeletal system, as well as the predisposition to infection. Early detection of hearing loss may help lead to prevention or treatment of these other disorders. Walker considers "maladaptive parenting," along with these deficiencies, to be a major medical consideration for children. These findings add to the urgency of neonatal screening.

The History of Neonatal Hearing Screening

Wedenberg (1956) screened 150 infants between the ages of 1 and 7 days by hitting a cowbell with a hammer close to the child's head. Of the infants, 149 responded with an **auropalpebral reflex (APR)**, which is a contraction of the muscles surrounding the eyes.

Wedenberg subsequently used an audiometer, which powered a small loudspeaker positioned near a sleeping child's head. Testing with a variety of frequencies, he observed responses (in the intensity range from 104 to 112 dB SPL) from normal-hearing infants in light sleep. He noted that premature children do not respond well to external stimuli, and that arousal responses depend, to a large extent, on the sleep level of the child.

Downs and Sterritt (1967), using a specially designed device to produce a 3,000 Hz warble tone, found that they could observe responses of most infants at about 90 dB SPL. Responses consisted primarily of APRs, movement of the hands or head, or overall startle responses. These researchers tested about 10,000 infants using this procedure, with only 150 failing, 4 of whom were subsequently identified as having hearing losses.

For a time, these kinds of results suggested that screening the hearing of neonates before they leave the hospital might be the method by which early identification and follow-up could be achieved. There were, however, several problems. The training of the individual performing the test is of great importance. Attendance by a separate observer is often useful, but disagreements on acceptance of responses occur. Because a number of children with normal hearing may fail the screening, informing their parents of possible hearing loss may produce undue alarm and concern. Additionally, startle responses to high-intensity sounds may be observed from children with moderate hearing losses who show loudness recruitment. In large measure because of the lack of a sophisticated means to test the hearing of neonates, it looked for a time that the goal of large-scale screening, noble though it was, was just too impractical to implement.

A Joint Committee on Infant Hearing (JCIH) in 1994 outlined a **high-risk registry** containing a list of indicators of hearing loss for identifying newborns who should be screened for hearing loss. The JCIH later endorsed the goal of universal screening of all newborn children while maintaining a modification of the previously described high-risk registry for identifying children to be screened where universal screening of all newborns was not yet available (Joint Committee on Infant Hearing, 2000). Universal newborn hearing screening (UNHS) was recognized as the favored approach to the identification of hearing loss in newborns because the high-risk registry lacks the specificity required to find the majority of children at risk for hearing loss. In fact, Mehl and Thomson (1998) state that selective hearing screening based on high-risk criteria fails to detect at least half of all infants with congenital hearing loss. An obvious difficulty in using the high-risk registry lies in the fact that many hereditary hearing losses are of a recessive nature, and the genetic potential for hearing loss may exist without an obvious family history of this disorder.

At this time the JCIH (currently comprised of the American Academy of Audiology, the American Speech-Language-Hearing Association, the American Academy of Otolaryngology–Head and Neck Surgery, the American Academy of Pediatrics, the Alexander Graham Bell Association for the Deaf and Hard of Hearing, the Council on Education of the Deaf, and the Directors of Speech and Hearing Programs in State Health and Welfare Agencies) has fully endorsed UNHS through an interdisciplinary system of early hearing detection and intervention (Joint Committee on Infant Hearing, 2007, 2013). Although the cost per child for UNHS is significantly higher than screening tests performed on blood samples, the higher incidence of congenital hearing loss results in a comparable cost per case diagnosed. In fact, the incidence of bilateral congenital hearing loss discovered is many times greater than the combined incidence of all newborn screening tests currently conducted on blood samples (Mehl & Thomson, 1998).

Although successes of implementing UNHS are numerous, many who fail the screening still do not receive appropriate follow-up to confirm the presence of hearing loss or to institute early intervention. As a supplement to the Joint Committee on Infant Hearing 2007 position statement on early identification, the committee has published comprehensive guidelines for the establishment of strong early intervention systems for children who are deaf and hard of hearing (Joint Committee on Infant Hearing, 2013). A full accounting of risk indicators associated with permanent congenital, delayed onset, or progressive hearing loss in children as outlined by the Joint Committee on Infant Hearing (2007) includes caregiver concerns, family history, craniofacial anomalies, neurodegenerative disorders, and related syndromes, among other factors.

Because some losses are **hereditodegenerative hearing losses**, a child failing on the high-risk registry because of family history might pass an early screening, lulling the family into a false sense of security about the potential for later development of a hearing loss. Indeed, Mann, Cuttler, and Campbell (2001) report that one of the greatest weaknesses of any newborn hearing screening program is ensuring adherence to follow-up guidelines for those who pass the screening yet may be considered at high risk for hearing loss.

Neonatal Screening with ABR

Auditory brain-stem response (ABR) audiometry has become increasingly popular as a neonatal testing system (see Figure 8.1). Some of the disadvantages of this procedure have been discussed previously in Chapter 6, for example, the lack of frequency specificity evident when click stimuli are used. When testing infants on the high-risk registry, it is important to compare responses to norms that correspond to children's gestational ages, rather than to their chronological ages, because immaturity of the central nervous system in a premature child can have a profound effect on results and must be taken into account. Follow-up testing is essential when ABR results are either positive or negative for infants on the high-risk registry.

Equipment used for measuring ABRs in infants was initially rather costly and more sophisticated than that which was required in the neonatal nursery. Less expensive, dedicated units that have a higher degree of portability without sacrifice in quality have replaced this equipment. In recent years, automated systems have been developed that are easy to use; require little in the way of interpretation of results; and can be used by trained technicians, including volunteers. Electrodes and earphones are disposable and easy to apply and remove. Results with this kind of equipment have been very encouraging and can have a pronounced effect on lowering the cost of neonatal screening.

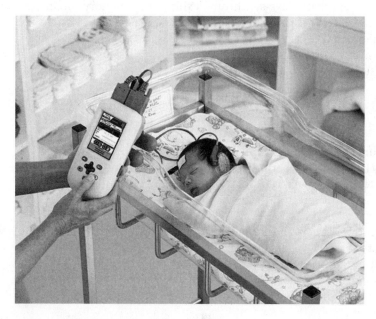

FIGURE 8.1 Auditory brain-stem response measurement is one method for screening neonatal hearing. (*Source:* ALGO® A3I Newborn Hearing Screener photo courtesy of Natus Medical Incorporated.)

Neonatal Screening with Otoacoustic Emissions

The use of otoacoustic emissions (OAE) as a neonatal screening method has emerged rapidly in recent years. The OAEs have been shown to be specific, sensitive, and cost-effective measures in infants (Dhar & Hall, 2011).

If all the requirements can be met, including a tightly fitting ear piece, quiet test environment, and so on, it can be assumed that infants whose ears produce evoked emissions have normal peripheral hearing, or no worse than a 30 dB hearing loss. The first few days of life are ideal for measuring OAEs because bodily movement makes it difficult to perform and evaluate, and neonates spend many hours each day in sound sleep. However, the presence of even a slight conductive hearing loss eliminates the measurable emission. Those who fail the OAE screenings should be followed up with ABR or other testing as deemed appropriate by the attending clinician.

As discussed in Chapter 7, the origin of the otoacoustic emission is the outer hair cells of the cochlea. If the cochlea is normal and a lesion exists in a retrocochlear area, there is a good chance for normal-appearing emissions to be evoked. This fact produces a cogent argument in favor of a combination of OAE and ABR testing. Some screening programs pass an infant when an ABR screen is passed following a failed OAE screen. Given that a failed OAE may signify outer-hair-cell damage, some have questioned if such practice might be missing an early predictor of late-onset progressive hearing loss in children if strict adherence to follow-up guidelines is not maintained (Mann et al., 2001). In spite of these concerns, an OAE screen followed by an ABR screen on those who fail has been reported to be successful both in enhanced identification and program cost reductions (Gorga, Preissler, Simmons, Walker, & Hoover, 2001). Hall, Smith, and Popelka (2004) recommend the use of essentially concurrent screenings of both OAE and ABR as a more effective screening approach than the use of either measure alone.

Auditory neuropathy/dys-synchrony (AN/AD) is often missed in newborn children because most hospitals screen using otoacoustic emissions. OAE tests for responses to sound by the outer hair cells of the cochlea but does not reveal how the brain responds. Therefore, a typical newborn hearing screening program may not identify a child with AN/AD. Some children have some abnormal cochlear function, which causes reduced OAE responses, in addition to AN/AD, that can be identified during newborn hearing screening.

Patients with auditory neuropathy/dys-synchrony exhibit no auditory brain-stem response (ABR), no middle-ear muscle response, and both normal otoacoustic emissions and normal cochlear microphonics. An absent or grossly abnormal ABR is not always associated with deafness. In contrast, a hearing loss of 30 dB or more usually predicts absent otoacoustic emissions, but normal emissions can be seen in some patients whose behavioral audiograms imply total deafness.

Meeting the Needs and Challenges of Newborn Hearing Screening

Approximately 4 million infants are born in the United States each year, creating a tremendous strain on personnel who may be qualified to perform newborn hearing screenings. Clearly there exists a need for supportive technicians who can work under the direction and supervision of audiologists so that the challenges of screenings can be successfully met. The use of support personnel for newborn screenings frees valuable time for the audiologist, whose efforts may be directed more meaningfully toward the provision of follow-up, diagnostic, and intervention services. Delineated duties of support personnel may include ensuring proper maintenance of screening equipment, operating screening devices in accordance with training received, disseminating information to appropriate personnel, cleaning and/or disposing of screening supplies, and completing records as required (American Academy of Audiology, 2004).

Beyond Early Identification

Any neonatal hearing-loss-identification program should be only a component part of a comprehensive program aimed at providing children with hearing loss the greatest chances possible for educational success and a subsequent entry into the mainstream of society. A comprehensive EHDI program has three components: a birth admission hearing screening, follow-up and diagnostic evaluations for infants who fail, and an intervention program with a goal of implementation before 6 months of age. Children identified and placed within an intervention program prior to 6 months of age exhibit significantly higher speech and language functioning compared to children identified after 6 months of age (Yoshinaga-Itano, Sedley, Coulter, & Mehl, 1998; Fulcher, Purcell, Baker, & Munro, 2012).

Objective Testing in Routine Pediatric Hearing Evaluation

Children may be referred to the audiologist for evaluation following neonatal hearing screening or subsequently due to parental or pediatrician concerns of auditory responsiveness or delayed speech and language development. Experienced audiologists do not launch quickly into hearing tests with small children. Even before beginning objective tests, they spend some time casually observing each child (see Tables 8.2 and 8.3). They should notice factors such as the children's relationships with the adults who have taken them to the clinic; their gaits, standing positions, and other indications of general motor performance; and their methods of communication. Compiling complete and detailed case histories is of paramount importance because they constitute a significant portion of the diagnosis. Special attention should be paid to noteworthy events during the prenatal, perinatal, and postnatal periods; family history; and any other such details. When dealing with families whose native language is not spoken English, the use of a translator is often essential.

TABLE 8.2 Childhood Communication Development Checklist*

Age	Behavior
Birth to 3 months	Child may startle or cry over loud noises; awakens to loud sounds; is soothed by caregiver's voice; listens to speech; smiles when spoken to; begins to repeat the same sounds (cooing).
4–6 months	Responds to "No," and changes in parental tone of voice; looks for the source of household sounds; notices toys that make sounds. Babbling begins to sound more speech-like, with a variety of sounds including bilabial consonants. Child may communicate by sound or gesture when he or she wants parent to do something again.
7 months–1 year	Recognizes common words like *cup, shoe,* or *juice.* Responds to requests such as "Come here," "Want more?" Turns when name is called and listens when spoken to. Enjoys simple games like pat-a-cake and peek-a-boo. Imitates different speech sounds. May have one or two words (although possibly not clear), i.e., *mamma, dada, bye-bye, no.* Pays attention to TV.
1–2 years	Will point to pictures in a book, or body parts, when named. Follows simple commands and understands simple questions ("Roll the ball." "Where's your shoe?"). Vocabulary is expanding each month. Begins to use one- or two-word sentences ("Where kitty?" "What that?" "No cookie." "More juice."). May repeat overheard words. Listens on the telephone.

(Continued)

TABLE 8.2 *Continued*

Age	Behavior
2–3 years	Understands differences in meaning (big–little, stop–go, up–down). Can follow two requests ("Get the ball and put it on the table."). Uses two- to three-word sentences and has a word for almost everything. Engages in pretend play. Parents can understand the child's speech most of the time.
3–4 years	Will answer simple "who," "what," "where," and "why" questions. Understands concepts of "same" and different." Talks about what he or she does at school or a friend's house. Says most sounds correctly except for later developing sounds like *r, l, th,* and *s*. People outside the family usually understand child's speech. Should be using a lot of sentences with four or more words.

*A wide range of normal developmental variability exists among children. Substantial deviation from expected norms may indicate a developmental lag.
Sources: www.cdc.gov/milestones; "Your Child's Speech and Hearing" developed by the Psi Iota Xi sorority and the American Speech-Language-Hearing Foundation; and www.preschoollearningcenter.org.

TABLE 8.3 Childhood Motor Developmental Checklist*

Age	Behavior
By 3 months	Can lift head when held on caregiver's shoulder. Child can raise head from a supine position. Looks at face when directly in front of him or her. Eyes follow a moving object. Wiggle and kick arms and legs
4–6 months	Can hold onto a rattle. Reaches for and grasps objects. Plays with toes. Pushes up on extended arms. Can turn over. Turns in response to sound. Sits with minimal support.
7 months–1 year	Bounces when held in a standing position. Drinks from a cup with help. Can move an object from hand to hand. Can sit alone momentarily. Can sit for several minutes without support. Can pull him- or herself up by holding onto things. Can move around the crib, or walk holding onto supports. Crawls on hands and knees.
1–2 years	Will wave good-bye or in response to others. Can walk with only one hand held. Can walk alone. Can balance three blocks together.
2–3 years	Can run. Can go up and down stairs. Can jump with both feet. Can stack six or more blocks together.
3–4 years	Can build a nine-block tower. Can copy a circle. Can kick a ball forward. Can throw a ball overhand.

*Significant deviation from normative values may warrant further evaluation. Prior to 2 years of age, the checklist should be adjusted for premature birth by subtracting the number of weeks of prematurity from the child's age.
Sources: National Network for Child Car (www.nncc.org); (American Academy of Pediatrics, New York Chapter, "Rapid Developmental Screening Checklist"; and www.preschoollearningcenter.org.

ASHA's most recent guidelines for pediatric hearing assessment (American Speech-Language-Hearing Association, 2004) recommend that testing include behavioral, physiologic, and developmental measures, with a corroboration of test results with the child's case history, parental reports, and the clinician's behavioral observations. The first measures in the pediatric hearing evaluation are often the objective measures of otoacoustic emissions and immittance testing, both of which are discussed more fully in Chapter 7. If present, otoacoustic emissions can quickly give the audiologist the knowledge that hearing is no worse than the level of a mild hearing loss. Tympanometry can determine a number of middle-ear disorders, including abnormal middle-ear pressure; eustachian tube dysfunction; effusion, mobility, and integrity of the middle-ear ossicles; thin or perforated tympanic membrane; and patency of pressure-equalization tubes. Additionally, the sensation level or absence of the acoustic reflex can give general kinds of information about a possible sensory/neural hearing loss. Subsequent pure-tone testing (preferably done with insert earphones to circumvent potential ear canal collapse from the pressure of supra-aural earphones) can yield meaningful results without the addition of bone-conduction measures if normal tympanograms and the presence of acoustic reflexes have ruled out a conductive component to any identified hearing loss.

A major problem with otoacoustic emissions and immittance tests with very small children results when children move about or cry. For a test to be accurate, the patient must be relatively motionless. Furthermore, any vocalizations—for example, crying—will be picked up by the probe microphone. An experienced team of clinicians can often work so efficiently that children are distracted and tested before they have time to object. At what point in the evaluation these measures are conducted with young children is often a judgment call. Infants and very young children usually accept administration of these measures with minimal objection while held in a parent's or caregiver's arms. The benefits of completing these tests at the outset of the evaluation may be outweighed by the advantage gained by building some degree of rapport with older children through the completion of other tests that may seem less frightening to some children. Sometimes a good time for these objective measures with small children is between speech and pure-tone testing.

Clinical COMMENTARY

Regardless of the age of a child, it is frequently prudent to begin testing with the measurement of otoacoustic emissions (OAEs). If emissions are normal, conductive hearing loss can be ruled out, and any possible sensory/neural hearing loss can be assumed to be no worse than a mild deficit. If emissions are absent, further testing is needed to illuminate both the type and degree of loss. OAEs do not depend on maturation of the auditory system and so can be performed as early in a child's life as is practicable. Distortion product otoacoustic emissions (DPOAEs) provide information in the frequency range between 500 and 4,000 Hz, so they can be especially useful in diagnoses when they can be obtained.

Immittance measures as the next test reveal additional information on a suspected conductive hearing loss when OAEs are absent. If OAEs were normal, suggesting normal middle-ear functioning, then tympanometry will be normal, and comparison of acoustic reflex thresholds for pure tones and broadband noise can help predict the degree of any existing loss. This knowledge can be helpful as the audiologist moves into behavioral assessment with the child. Often the usual probe-tone frequency of 220 Hz fails to elicit acoustic reflexes in infants, and a higher frequency of 660 Hz offers a higher yield of positive responses. Of course, if tympanometry is abnormal, precluding acoustic reflex measures, little can be said about hearing sensitivity, and without further testing, the examiner cannot rule out the possibility of a conductive hearing loss overlaying any potential sensory/neural hearing loss the child may have.

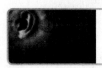

Behavioral Testing of Children from Birth to Approximately 2 Years of Age

It is unusual for a child to be seen for evaluation before 1 year of age unless the possibility of hearing impairment has been suggested through some means of newborn or infant hearing screening. At 1 year of age, the child with hearing loss may begin to lose the potential for normal spoken-language development. For this very reason, early screenings are of great importance. Lack of speech often brings a potential problem to the attention of the parents or other caretakers.

At 18 months, the normal child usually obeys simple commands. Speech tests are useful to evaluate children at this age because a child may give good responses to soft speech while apparently ignoring loud sounds. It is interesting that quiet-voiced speech sometimes elicits a response when whispered speech does not.

It has been frequently observed that, in general, the broader the frequency spectrum of a sound, the better it is at catching the attention of a small child. For this reason, many clinicians use speech or other broadband signals in testing. One of the great dangers of accepting an obvious response to a sound with a broad acoustic spectrum lies in the fact that many children with hearing loss have reasonably good sensitivity in some frequency ranges and impaired sensitivity in other ranges. Many children, for example, have sharply falling high-frequency hearing losses and respond quite overtly to sounds containing low-frequency energy, such as the clapping of hands or the calling of their names. In addition, there is a smaller but significant number of children who have congenital low-frequency sensory/neural hearing losses (Ross & Matkin, 1967).

Ewing and Ewing (1944), pioneers in the testing of young children, used a wide variety of noisemakers, such as bells, rattles, rustling paper, and xylophones, to elicit auditory responses. They advocated stirring a spoon in a cup, which produces a soft sound from a child's daily life that may evoke a response when a loud sound does not. Stress on using sounds that are meaningful to the child is most closely associated with the work of the Ewings, although such sounds elicit little in the way of frequency-specific information.

Many pediatric audiological procedures involve the child's response to a sound through auditory localization. During the first 6 to 8 months of age, a procedure now known as **behavioral observation audiometry (BOA)** is often employed with two clinicians working together. While one clinician may sit in front of the child, who may be seated on the parent's lap, to occupy the child's attention, the second clinician, located behind and to the side of the mother, presents a variety of sounds. Phonemes such as S, S, S, S or a variety of toys or noisemakers may be used. Crinkling cellophane or onionskin paper makes the sort of soft, annoying sound that is extremely useful in techniques such as these, but like most noncalibrated sounds, provides little or no information about the configuration of the hearing loss.

For a sound to be localized, hearing thresholds must be similar in both ears, although not necessarily normal. As a child's ability to localize sound matures, it progresses from eye and head movement seen horizontally, then vertically, then on an arc and finally in a direct line to the sound source (see Figure 8.2). If a child does not turn to locate a sound by the age of 8 months, it can be suspected that something is wrong, although not necessarily hearing loss. Mental disability and some childhood symbolic disorders may manifest themselves in a similar lack of response.

If a child cannot be tested by using formal methods, an imitation of vocalization can be tried. The clinician can babble nonsense syllables, without the child watching, to see if the child will imitate. If imitation does take place, it indicates that hearing is good enough to perceive voice. If no response is noted and the clinician babbles again in the child's line of vision,

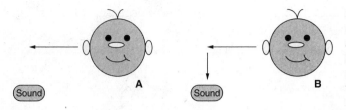

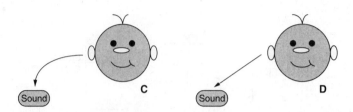

FIGURE 8.2 Development of auditory localization in infants. (A) At 3 months, the head moves somewhat jerkily along a horizontal plane. (B) At 5 months, localization is in straight lines, first horizontally and then vertically. (C) At 6 months, the head and eyes move in an arc toward the sound source. (D) At 8 months, the eyes and head move directly to the sound source.

the child with a severe hearing impairment may attempt to imitate, but may do so without voice. This is a most important diagnostic sign. In addition to being a strong indication of hearing loss, silent imitation indicates that the child's perceptual function is probably intact. If the child vocalizes, the voice quality can be evaluated. Although the vocal quality of individuals with hearing loss is sometimes different from that of individuals with normal hearing, it must be remembered that the voice of the very young child who has a hearing impairment frequently cannot be differentiated from that of the child with normal hearing.

It is possible to observe a child's reaction to the examiner's imitation of the child's sounds. In this case, the examiner gives a response to the child's babbling or other vocalizations. A child with normal hearing may cease vocalization and may sometimes repeat it. There are instances in which this procedure works when nothing else does, as the child may stop and listen, the interpretation being that the examiner's voice was heard.

Sound-Field Audiometry

Several approaches for the testing of infants use multiple loudspeakers in a sound-field situation. Recordings of animal noises and baby cries have been effective in eliciting responses, even when filtered into narrow bands. Although a sound such as a whistle, bell, drum, or some vocal utterance may appear subjectively to represent a specific frequency range, this often turns out not to be true. What may seem to be a high-pitched sound may have equal intensity in the low- and high-frequency ranges, as verified by spectral analysis.

Several kinds of responses may be observed when sounds are presented to a child from different directions in the sound field. The child may look for the sound source, cease ongoing activity, awaken from a light sleep, change facial expression, or offer a cry or other vocalized response. Once again, a response to sound has considerable significance, whereas a lack of response is not necessarily meaningful. A useful setup for sound-field localization is shown in Figure 8.3.

Frequently, children respond to the off-effect of a sound but not to the on-effect. Evaluation of responses to the cessation of sound often goes well with the use of noisemakers, but it can be adapted to sound-field audiometry. A high-intensity pure tone or narrow noise band can be introduced for a minute or so and then abruptly interrupted. This interruption may produce a response, whereas the initial presentation of the sound does not.

It is generally the case that at age 2 months, a soft voice begins to become a better stimulus than a loud voice. At 1 to 3 months, percussion instruments are best at eliciting APRs, startle

FIGURE 8.3 Diagram of a room useful for sound-field localization tests with small children. (*Source:* Adapted from F. N. Martin, *Hearing Disorders in Children*, p. 201, © 1991. Reproduced by permission of Pearson Education, Inc.)

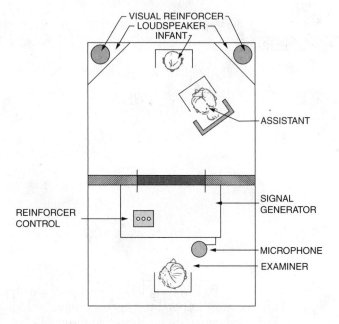

responses such as the **Moro reflex**,[2] and overall increases in activity or crying. At 4 months, percussion instruments are less successful than they were earlier, but the human voice gains in effectiveness. By 6 months of age, much reflex activity begins to disappear.

A potential problem, present whenever screening responses involving high-intensity stimuli are used, is the effect of loudness recruitment on startle responses. If recruitment is present, a child could conceivably respond to a sound as if it were loud, when in fact it might be only slightly above auditory threshold. If this occurs, a child with a cochlear hearing loss with loudness recruitment may pass early screening tests because of the very nature of the disorder. The criteria for minimum response level may be very different for children with hearing impairment. Certainly, if OAEs can be successfully attained, concerns such as this can be circumvented.

Relying on the localization ability of normal-hearing babies more than 4 months old, Suzuki and Ogiba (1961) developed a sound-field procedure called **conditioned orientation reflex (COR)**. A child is seated between and in front of a pair of loudspeakers, each of which holds an illuminated doll within the child's peripheral vision. Pure-tone and light introductions are paired; after several of these paired presentations, the child will begin to glance in the direction of the light source in anticipation of the light whenever a tone is presented. The introduction of the light may then be delayed until after the child has glanced at the speaker; this can serve as reinforcement for orientation to the signal. This procedure works well with some small children and has been modified in several ways, including the puppet in the window illuminated (PIWI) procedure (Haug, Baccaro, & Guilford, 1967).

Rewarding children's auditory responses with visual stimuli has led to the use of **visual reinforcement audiometry (VRA)** (Liden & Kankkonen, 1961). The reinforcer may be anything, including a light, a picture, or an animated toy, as long as it evokes the children's interest. Schmida, Peterson, and Tharpe (2003) report that projected video images may be one of the best reinforcers for sustaining localization responses. VRA works with earphones, if the children will tolerate them, as well as in the sound field, with or without hearing aids. Many young children will tolerate insert earphones much more readily than supra-aural earphones. Speech as well as tones may serve as signals. It can be expected that responses to VRA may be obtained from children whose corrected age (chronological age minus the estimated number of weeks of prematurity, if any) reaches 6 months (Moore, Thompson, & Folsom, 1992). A decrease in appropriate responses due to boredom can be avoided by changing the reinforcer as needed to hold the child's attention.

Sound-Field Test Stimuli

Audiologists do not completely agree on the best acoustic stimuli for testing small children. Many, but not all, authorities believe that pure tones are probably not the ideal stimuli because they are not meaningful to children. Pure tones have the obvious advantage of supplying information about children's hearing sensitivity at specific frequencies. If a child shows no interest in pure tones, however, other carefully controlled acoustic stimuli may be used.

The justification for narrowband filtering of a signal for a small child is obvious, and many clinicians use the narrowband noise generators on their clinical audiometers. The belief is that this provides specific frequency information if the child responds. Such an approach may be very misleading. The narrow bands on many audiometers are not very narrow at all, and they may reject frequencies on either side of the center frequency at rates as little as 12 dB per octave. This allows sufficient energy in the side bands to produce a response when a child has not heard the frequency in the center of the band. A variety of sound effects (e.g., cow mooing, bird singing, glass shattering) subjected to steep-slope filtering can be useful with very young children as well as older children and adults with special needs (Abouchacra & Letowski, 1999). It is obvious that audiologists must understand the nature of the equipment they use, and if they elect to test with narrow bands or filtered sounds, they should ascertain for themselves just what the bandwidths are.

Clinical COMMENTARY

Nearly 40 years ago, Jerger and Hayes (1976) advanced the need to cross-check results obtained in a pediatric evaluation with a separate independent measure. Interpretation of results of behavioral observation audiometry can be quite subjective, and clinical decisions on the validity of responses to VRA and COR testing may rely heavily on the clinician's judgment when frequent random movements are noted from an active child. It is the audiologist's role to provide an accurate assessment of a child's hearing status to avoid misdiagnosis and subsequent mismanagement of the child with hearing loss. Behavioral results should be consistent with cross-checks available from acoustic reflexes and OAEs. When they are not, further investigation is necessary. On occasion, these measures cannot be attained due to active middle-ear pathology or patent ventilation tubes. If the child's history or parental concerns raise suspicion of hearing loss, behavioral results that otherwise appear normal need to be repeated as soon as middle-ear function has been fully restored, or referral should be made for ABR testing. The cross-check principle mandates that no test, regardless of how reliable it is felt to be, should be relied on until it is substantiated by other tests.

Behavioral Testing of Children Approximately 2 to 5 Years of Age

At 2 to 3 years of age, children who have no problems other than hearing loss can often be taught to respond to pure tones, especially warble tones. For this reason, awareness tests with voice, whispers, pitch pipes, and other special stimuli may begin to take a back seat in the evaluation process as clinicians increasingly rely on test stimuli with greater frequency specificity and procedures that more closely approximate true threshold responses.

Early reports in the literature on testing children indicated that it was not possible to get pure-tone threshold responses from children under 5 years of age. It is now quite common to test children age 3 years or under. It is naturally necessary to work rapidly and smoothly to keep such a young child's attention and cooperation. A child with a "pure" hearing loss (i.e., no other significant problems) should be testable well before 3 years of age.

Speech Audiometry

In spite of the goal to obtain frequency-specific auditory responses, behavioral assessment with children frequently begins with speech audiometry. Speech audiometric procedures permit a greater interplay between the audiologist and child, allowing for the establishment of the requisite rapport needed for subsequent pure-tone testing. Some children do not respond to pure tones, and by their almost stoic expressions, it appears that they cannot hear. A large number of these children can be conditioned to respond to speech signals. If they possess the appropriate language skills, many children can point to parts of their bodies or to articles of clothing. If this kind of response can be obtained, the clinician can recite a list of items, to which the child points. The level of the signal can be raised and lowered until speech threshold is approximated.

Often even small children can be tested using adult-like stimuli. Sometimes only an estimate of speech-detection threshold (SDT) can be observed, but when this happens, interpretation must be made very judiciously. The normally expected difference of about 10 dB between the SDT and the speech-recognition threshold (SRT) may be exceeded in cases of precipitous high-frequency hearing loss, thereby underestimating a child's true hearing loss. Valuable time may be lost in correct diagnosis in such cases.

Pictures or objects that can be named with spondaic stress can be used to test children. A child can often point to a cowboy or hot dog. The clinician may first demonstrate the procedure and then reward the child's appropriate behavior with a smile, a nod, or a wink. SRTs can frequently be obtained with pictures by age 2 years. Speech-recognition tests designed for children, as described in Chapter 5, may be accomplished in the same way.

Speech audiometry is often possible with children, even when they have very severe hearing losses. Use of the Ling Six Sound Test (Ling, 1989; Ling & Berlin, 1997) can provide frequency-specific hearing-loss information even when reliable tonal responses cannot be attained. The six sounds /a/, /u/, /i/, /S/, /s/, and /m/ are representative of the speech energy contained within all the speech sounds of English. In particular, audibility of /a/, /u/, and /i/ indicates usable hearing through 1,000 Hz; audibility of /S/ suggests hearing through 2,000 Hz; and audibility of /s/ indicates hearing through 4,000 Hz. How well children can recognize those phonemes, and the formant frequencies they represent, can illustrate how well a hearing aid may meet their acoustic needs. At times the Six Sound Test is the only speech measurement that a child can or will perform. It is most useful when carried out in conjunction with other speech and pure-tone audiometric procedures.

The child may also be tested by asking such questions as "Where is Mommy?" or "Where are your hands?" The question "Do you want to go home now?" often evokes a clear response, but it should be reserved as a last resort because, if children do hear that question, it may become impossible to keep them longer. Often a whisper may cause 2- or 3-year-old children to whisper back. If they can hear their own whisper, this may indicate good hearing for high-pitched sounds.

Speech audiometry has revealed hearing abnormalities, or their absence, in children who were unable or unwilling to take pure-tone tests. This has resulted, in many cases, in a substantial savings of time in initiating remedial procedures. Of course, failure of children to respond during speech audiometry may occur because they do not know what the item (picture or object) is, rather than because they have not heard the word. The clinician should ask the adults accompanying their children to the examination whether specific words are in the children's vocabularies. It is essential to ensure that it is word-recognition ability and not receptive vocabulary that is being tested.

Pure-Tone Audiometry

Many times, in testing small children, the problem is to get them to respond. The ingenuity of the clinician can frequently solve this problem. For a child to want to participate, usually the procedure must offer some enjoyment. Some children, however, are so anxious to please that they deluge the clinician with many false positive responses on pure-tone tests, so that it is difficult to gauge when a response is valid. In such cases, slight modifications of adult-like tests may prove workable with some older children. A child may be asked to point to the earphone in which a tone is heard. The ears may be stimulated randomly, and in this way the appropriateness of the response can be determined. The same result may be achieved by using pulsed-tone procedures, asking the child to tell how many tones have been presented.

Operant Conditioning Audiometry

Many times it appears that no approach to a given child produces reliable results. This is particularly true of children with mental disability. However, Spradlin and Lloyd (1965) suggest that, given sufficient time and effort, no child is "untestable," and they recommend that this term be replaced by the phrase *difficult to test*.

In **operant conditioning audiometry (OCA)**, food is often used as a reward for proper performance. A child may be seated in the test room before a table that contains a hand switch. Sounds are presented either through the sound-field speaker or through earphones. The child is encouraged to press the switch when the sound, which can be either a pure tone or a noise band, is presented. If the child's response is appropriate, a small amount of food, such as a candy pellet, or a token is released from a special feeder box. Once children see that pressing the switch results in a reward, they will usually continue to press it in pursuit of more. It is essential that the switch that operates the feeder be wired in series with the tone-introducer switch so that no reward is forthcoming without presentation of the sound. In this way, the child gets no reinforcement for pushing the switch unless a tone is actually introduced and, presumably, heard. Signals that are thought to be above the child's threshold must be introduced first, after which the level may be lowered until threshold is reached. If severe hearing loss is suspected, a good starting point is 500 Hz at 90 dB HL because there is a strong likelihood of hearing at this frequency and level.

Operant conditioning audiometry requires much time and patience if it is to work. Often, many trials are required before the child begins to understand the task. As in other audiometric procedures, it is essential that the signals be introduced aperiodically because the child may learn to predict a signal and to respond to a sound that has not been heard. Often operant conditioning audiometry can be successful when other procedures have failed. The term **tangible reinforcement operant conditioning audiometry (TROCA)** was coined by Lloyd, Spradlin, and Reid (1968) to describe specifics of operant conditioning to audiometry.

For a number of years clinicians have been using *instrumental conditioning* in testing younger children—that is, teaching the children to perform in a certain way when a sound is heard. This requires a degree of voluntary cooperation from the children, but the clinician can select a method that evokes appropriate responses.

A number of devices for operant audiometry have been described in the literature dating back to the earliest years of audiology. The peep show (Dix & Hallpike, 1947) gives children the reward of seeing a lighted picture when they respond correctly to a tone presented through a small loudspeaker below the screen. The pediacoumeter (Guilford & Haug, 1952) works on a similar principle, except that the child may wear earphones to increase the accuracy of the test. If the child hears a tone and responds correctly by pushing a button, one of seven puppets pops up to startle and amuse. Similar approaches have been used with animated toys, pictures, slides, motion pictures, and computers.

Martin and Coombes (1976) applied the principles of operant audiometry to the determination of speech thresholds using a brightly colored clown whose body parts (e.g., hand, mouth, nose, leg) were wired to microswitches that triggered a candy-feeder mechanism. Children were shown how to touch a part of the clown. Reinforcement of the correct response was the immediate delivery of a candy pellet to a cup, which was momentarily lit in the clown's hand. Preprogramming of the proper switch on a special device in the control room ensured that false responses would not be rewarded. Speech thresholds were obtained on very young children in a matter of several minutes through this operant conditioning approach. Weaver, Wardell, and Martin (1979) found this procedure for obtaining speech thresholds useful with children with mental disability.

Play Audiometry

Often, using elaborate devices and procedures to test the hearing of young children is unnecessary. Many can simply be taught by demonstration to place a ring on a peg, a block in a box, or a bead in a bucket when a sound is introduced. The more enthusiasm the clinician shows about the procedure, the more likely the child is to join in. Children seem to enjoy the action of the game. Tones can be presented through earphones if children tolerate them, or through the sound-field speaker if they do not. Many children readily accept insert receivers because they are light and do not encumber movement. As has been discussed earlier, insert receivers increase interaural attenuation, which often decreases the need for masking and minimizes the possibility of overmasking in most cases. Any time testing is completed using sound-field speakers, the examiner cannot know which ear has responded.

One problem in using play audiometry is to find suitable rewards for prompting the children to maintain interest and motivation in the test. The premises underlying successful conditioning in audiometry stated by DiCarlo, Kendall, and Goldstein in 1962 have not changed and include (1) motivation, (2) contiguity (getting the stimulus and response close together in time and space), (3) generalization (across frequency and intensity), (4) discrimination (between the stimulus and any background activity), and (5) reinforcement (conveying to children that they are doing what is wanted).

The probable reason that some clinicians do not embrace play audiometric techniques is that they feel these techniques can easily become boring to children, and conditioning therefore extinguishes rapidly. This is probably a case of projection of adult values because many alert children can play the "sound game" for long periods of time without boredom. When asking children to move beads or other objects from one container to another, it is a good idea to have a large supply on hand. Many children refuse to play further once the first bucket has become empty, even if they have appeared to enjoy the game up to this point.

Clinical COMMENTARY

It often becomes apparent to a clinician that a limited amount of time is available to test a small child and that, even though some reliable threshold results are forthcoming, the test should best be abbreviated before the child ceases to cooperate. In such cases, it may be advisable to test one frequency in each ear by air conduction and, if immittance measures were not normal, by bone conduction. This provides information about the relative sensitivity of each ear and the degree of any conductive component revealed through immittance testing. If an SRT is obtained that suggests normal hearing, the frequency to be tested may be a higher one, say, 3,000 or 4,000 Hz, to make certain that the normal SRT does not mislead in cases of high-frequency hearing loss. If only three to six thresholds are to be obtained, it is often more meaningful to get readings at one or two frequencies in each ear by both air and bone conduction (assuming bone-conduction testing is being done due to abnormal immittance measures) than to obtain six air-conduction thresholds in one ear. Accurate threshold readings at only 500 and 2,000 Hz give some evidence of degree, configuration, and type of hearing loss.

Sometimes it is impossible, for a variety of reasons, to teach a child to take a hearing test in one session. In such cases, the child should be rescheduled for further testing and observation. It is often worthwhile to employ the talents and interests of the child's parents or other adults. They can be instructed in methods of presenting sounds and evoking responses. Children may also be more amenable to training in the comfort and security of their homes than in the strange and often frightening environment of sound-treated rooms. One parent may use a noisemaker, such as a bell, in full view of the child, while the other parent responds by dropping a block in a bucket or by some other enjoyable activity. Children can be encouraged to join in the game and, after beginning to participate by following the parents' lead, can be encouraged to go first. Once they participate fully, the sound source can be gradually moved out of the line of vision so that it can be determined that responses are to auditory, and not visual, stimulation. A few minutes a day of such activities may allow the audiologist at the next clinic appointment to use the same procedure, preferably with the same materials, which are already familiar to the child. After professional observation of the child's responses, the audiologist can substitute other sound stimuli in an attempt to quantify the hearing loss, if any. It has also been found useful to have the parents borrow an old headband and set of earphones to accustom the child to wearing them without fear. Similarly, parents can be given a set of foam-style noise reduction earplugs to use with the child at home so the child may become better acquainted with what insert receivers are like during subsequent testing.

Clinical COMMENTARY

Small children's failure to produce observable responses to intense sounds during informal testing may or may not be due to profound hearing loss. The lack of response during formal testing, such as pure-tone audiometry, may mean either that the children have not heard the sounds or that they have not responded correctly when they have heard them. Deciding between these two possibilities is often difficult. It is sometimes advisable to teach children to respond to some other stimulus, such as to a light, or to the vibrations of a hand-held bone-conduction vibrator set to deliver a strong low-frequency tone. If a child can be taught to give appropriate responses to one sensory input, the inference is that the child can be conditioned to respond, and thus lack of response to a sound probably means that it was not heard.

Electrophysiological Hearing Tests

It has been obvious for some time that objective tests for measuring hearing in young children are highly desirable. Thus, there has long been a search for a clear electrophysiological measure of hearing sensitivity to employ when other measures of hearing are inconclusive. Past electrophysiological tests have monitored changes in pulse rate, respiration, heart rhythm, and skin resistance. Procedural limitations and poor reliability have precluded these attempts at electrophysiological assessment from gaining popularity in the assessment of children.

Electrophysiological tests today for the assessment of hearing thresholds primarily involve auditory evoked potentials through auditory brain-stem response (ABR) audiometry and the auditory steady-state response (ASSR), as discussed in some detail in Chapter 7. A primary advantage to these objective measures is that the procedures are effective during sleep. Many small children will sleep naturally during ABR testing or may be anesthetized with no effects on test accuracy.

Clinical COMMENTARY

In all audiological measures, efficiency in test administration leads to the greatest degree of success. This may be especially true in ABR testing with young children because results must be attained before the child awakes from either natural or sedated sleep. An efficient ABR test protocol for children is to begin binaurally. If testing must end following determination of a binaural ABR threshold, one at least knows the threshold for the better-hearing ear. On the other hand, if one starts monaurally and happens to choose the poorer ear, approximation of the child's best hearing may not be attained if the child wakes before the other ear's testing is completed. Once a binaural threshold has been attained, testing can proceed at the observed response level in each ear individually. One of the advantages of ABR testing is the ability to differentiate the type of hearing loss; however, it is limited in threshold determination beyond approximately 80 dB HL. ASSR measures complement ABR testing when estimating thresholds for more severe hearing losses.

There is little doubt that continuing research brings us closer to the goal of an efficient and reliable index of auditory function in uncooperative children. Until that goal is reached, audiologists will still have to confirm their findings with behavioral tests, sometimes attained only through repeated attempts at testing. It should be assumed that the diagnosis is never complete until a voluntary hearing test is obtained from the child, although such is not always possible in cases of concomitant handicap. However, the absence of a full voluntary hearing test cannot be construed as reason to delay (re)habilitation when the presence of hearing loss has been determined through electrophysiological measures.

Clinical COMMENTARY

Most often the presence of normal OAE and normal immittance measures, even in the absence of a full behavioral audiogram, can eliminate referral for ABR/ASSR testing that may have otherwise been necessary. Such practice is not only more economical in time and testing expense, it circumvents the need to otherwise sedate a child whose ABR results would have proven normal. ABR and ASSR are special tests reserved for those instances in which the presence of hearing loss is suspected based on the objective measures of OAE and immittance, yet clear indications of hearing level cannot be ascertained through behavioral approaches.

Language Disorders

Small children are frequently seen in audiology centers because they show some deficiencies in the normal development of speech and language. Because language and speech depend on interactions between the peripheral and central nervous systems, a detailed history must be taken. Special attention should be paid to details such as onset of different kinds of motor development, the age at which meaningful speech or an alternative communication system was acquired, social development, communication of needs, and pre- and postnatal developmental factors. Pertinent data should also include prenatal diseases, the length of the pregnancy, difficulties at birth, and early distress—seen, for example, in cyanotic ("blue") babies, in babies with jaundice, and so on. Notations should be made of childhood illnesses, especially those involving high or prolonged fevers, and medications taken. Attention should be paid to any illnesses or accidents and any regressions in development associated with them. Some objective data may be obtained from tests of hearing, symbolic behavior, intelligence, and receptive and expressive language.

A young child's unwillingness to cooperate may be common to all sensory modalities and could indicate a disorder or combination of disorders other than hearing loss (e.g., mental disability or emotional maladjustment). If a child does not respond to visual stimuli such as lights or shadows or to touching or vibration, one might wonder whether the problem is in fact behavioral. However, if a positive response is obtained in one modality and a negative one in another, a certain pattern appears, which is more significant than a generalized response (or lack of response). Although long lists of possible causes for significant language delay have been postulated, such delay is usually produced by hearing loss, some congenital or early acquired symbolic disorders, attention deficit hyperactivity disorder (ADHD), mental disability, emotional disturbance, or **autism**. A common error committed by clinicians is to consider causes as an either-or condition and to attempt differential diagnosis to rule out all but one cause. The experienced clinician will have observed that the presence of one significant disorder increases, rather than decreases, the probability of another.

When a small child has a language disorder, and hearing loss cannot be eliminated as a possible causal factor, the resources and experience of the clinician are called on for an appropriate diagnosis. The behavioral characteristics of the clinical entities mentioned here can frequently be ruled out on the basis of observation of behavior and developmental history. The problem then remains to differentiate between the hard-of-hearing and the otherwise language-disordered child. Even though the child with brain injury is said to manifest such symptoms as impatience, hyperactivity, poor judgment, **perseveration**, and **dysinhibition**, often there is a symbolic disorder without the presence of bizarre behavior.

Audiologists frequently see children who are either believed to have hearing losses or whose auditory behavior is so inconsistent as to cast doubt on the presence of normal hearing. A parent or teacher may complain that a child's responses to sound are inconsistent, that performance is better when background noises or competing messages are at a minimum, and that it is possible that the child "just doesn't pay attention." Sometimes auditory test results appear normal on such a child, and the parents are mistakenly assured that all is fine. The audiologist must constantly be alert for auditory-processing disorders that can coexist with other learning and language disabilities. Screening tests are needed so that children with auditory processing disorders, however mild, will not be overlooked but will be correctly referred to the proper specialists, such as speech-language pathologists, for complete diagnosis and therapy (Martin & Clark, 1977). Many of the tests for auditory processing disorders, described in Chapter 12, can be performed accurately on children as young as 6 years old.

In the final analysis, the diagnosis of the "difficult case" must often be made subjectively by a highly qualified, experienced examiner. Despite the initial diagnosis, it must be remembered that, until peripheral hearing status has been deemed normal through behavioral or objective measures, hearing loss cannot be ruled out as a possible contributory element.

Auditory Processing Disorders

Recent years have brought a focus on an auditory disorder in children with otherwise normal hearing sensitivity or whose effective use of audition is impeded by more than the detrimental effects expected from peripheral pathology alone. The earlier term *central auditory processing disorder* has appropriately been replaced by the term **auditory processing disorder (APD)**, a term that may emphasize the interactions of disorders at both peripheral and central sites without necessarily attributing difficulties to a single anatomical locality (Jerger & Musiek, 2000). The term *auditory processing disorder* is often applied to children whose recognition or use of language is not age-appropriate and/or is inconsistent with their level of intelligence. Many of these children also have additional learning disabilities that prevent them from progressing normally in their education.

APD has been estimated to occur in 2 to 3 percent of children, with occurrence twice as likely in boys (Chermak & Musiek, 1997). Since APD has become recognized, it may be a favored diagnostic category, and there may be reason to be concerned that overdiagnosis of this condition may occur, leading to inappropriate educational methods. Accurate diagnosis of APD is based on a multifaceted, comprehensive assessment, which includes input from audiologists, speech-language pathologists, psychologists, and educators.

Children with APD, despite normal intelligence, often have poor listening skills, short attention spans, seemingly poor memories and reading comprehension, difficulty in linguistic sequencing, and problems in learning to read and spell. One of the most frequently reported dysfunctions is difficulty in recognizing speech in the presence of background noise. Deficits related to auditory processing difficulties contribute to delays in speech and language and to poor performance in school. As a result, these children may suffer from lowered self-esteem, which further complicates the disorder. Many children with auditory processing disorders make inappropriate social contacts because their failures with children in their age group lead them to seek playmates who are younger than they are. Often parents and other adults report that these children prefer to play alone.

Intervention is aimed at improving listening skills and spoken language comprehension through a multistrategy approach. This may include enhancement of the signal-to-noise ratio in the listening environment through preferential seating in the classroom, reduction of background noise and reverberation through acoustic modifications and often the use of FM systems (see Chapter 14), auditory skills training, and development of **metalinguistic training** and **metacognitive training** strategies (Musiek & Chermak, 2007). Additional discussion of APD management is found in Chapter 15.

For communicating with other professionals, such as teachers, technical diagnostic statements are less useful than those that describe the kinds of difficulties a child may have in learning and suggestions for specific remedies. Diagnostic entities such as APD, ADHD, dyslexia, emotional disturbance, and so on, may be more threatening than useful to professionals who must assist these children. Suggestions for a more structured learning environment can be a useful addendum to reports to the classroom teacher (Clark, 1980; Hall & Mueller, 1997).

Auditory Neuropathy in Children

Auditory neuropathy is probably rare in children, although this is controversial. Symptoms include mild-to-moderate sensory/neural hearing loss, abnormal or absent ABRs, absent or markedly elevated acoustic reflexes, and normal OAEs. The presence of OAEs strongly indicates that the lesion in these cases is medial to the cochlea. Amplification with hearing aids is met with mixed success, and many experts urge the use of signs for the teaching of language.

Psychological Disorders

Hearing loss that is congenital or acquired early in life can have an effect on social, intellectual, and emotional development, including "egocentricity, difficulty in empathizing with others, rigidity, impulsivity, coercive dependency, and a tendency to express feelings by actions rather than by symbolic communication" (Rose, 1983). As a child without normal hearing continues to develop, the normal parent–child relationship is invariably affected, lending further justification for intervention at the earliest possible time.

Developmental Disabilities

Children with developmental disabilities may include those with mental disability, cerebral palsy, epilepsy, autism, or a wide variety of physical or mental challenges. While a high percentage of children with developmental disability have cognitive impairments as well, many have normal or greater than normal intelligence. Hearing loss among these children may go undetected because behaviors of auditory inattention may be attributed to the child's more overt handicap.

Evaluation of children with developmental disabilities presents a true challenge to the audiologist. Responses from children who are profoundly multidisabled may be more reflexive than representative of true attention behaviors (Flexer & Gans, 1985). Such responses may be better evaluated in the context of the child's developmental age than his or her chronological age. Hearing may be considered normal if the development of auditory responses is generally consistent with the age level of the child's other developmental behaviors. This judgment becomes more difficult if the child's cognitive and developmental ages have not yet been determined.

The physiologic measures described in Chapter 7 provide a dimension to the evaluation of the difficult-to-test patient that was not available in the past. However, the sometimes ambiguous results of physiologic measures of hearing increase with central nervous system involvement, thereby increasing the value of any behavioral results that may be obtained (Martin & Clark, 1996).

Identifying Hearing Loss in the Schools

The exact number of school-age children who have hearing impairments is not known. Surveys that attempt to come up with figures are also confounded by factors such as geographic location and season of the year; there are more failures during cold weather. It is probable that more than 5 percent of the public school population has a hearing impairment at any given time. This does not count the students enrolled in residential and day schools for children with profound hearing impairments. Clearly, there is a need for screening methods that identify school children with hearing loss.

Equipment accuracy and the use of acceptable workspaces are mandatory in hearing-loss-identification programs. In addition to annual electroacoustic calibration of audiometers, it is frequently recommended that output levels be verified every few months. Of course, if an audiometer or its earphones are jarred or dropped, calibration should be checked before any additional hearing screenings are done. Listening checks should be performed at the start of every test day, with special attention to breaks in the receiver cords.

Hearing Screening Measures

Early school hearing screenings were conducted in groups, thereby decreasing the demands on personnel, space, and equipment. Problems arising from difficulties in maintaining equipment calibration, and from the many false positive responses from children striving to pass due to fear of nonacceptance, eventually led to discontinuation of group screening measures. School screenings are carried out today on an individual basis. They are usually done by fixing the intensity of the audiometer and changing frequencies. Obviously, screenings may be performed more rapidly if a restricted number of frequencies is sampled and screening is done at a level high enough to be attended to easily by young children. Some authorities have recommended screening only at 4000 Hz because this frequency is often affected by hearing loss. Other people believe that screening with immittance meters uncovers the major source of hearing disorders in the schools: otitis media. It is possible that this approach could catch middle-ear disorders in the early stages, perhaps averting any conductive hearing loss at all. The combination of tympanometry and ipsilateral acoustic reflex screenings is most useful for this purpose. Utilizing a pulsed tone to elicit the reflex has been demonstrated to increase significantly the utility of the ipsilateral acoustic reflex within a screening protocol (Sells, Hurley, Morehouse, & Douglas, 1997). Of course, middle-ear problems are not the only cause of hearing loss in school children.

In 1984, the American Speech-Language-Hearing Association published guidelines for hearing-loss identification in the schools. Updates of hearing screening guidelines that have since appeared (e.g., American Speech-Language-Hearing Association, 1993, 1997; American Academy of Audiology, 2011) state that the goals of such programs are to incorporate acoustic immittance measures with pure-tone audiometry to identify students who are in need of audiological and/or medical services. Patrick (1987) states that 80 to 90 percent accuracy is obtained when acoustic immittance is combined with pure-tone screenings, compared to 60 to 70 percent accuracy when pure tones are used alone. Automated, portable, easy-to-use immittance screening devices (see Figure 8.4) produce a tympanogram and screen for acoustic reflexes on each ear tested in a matter of seconds (see Figure 8.5). The most recent childhood hearing screening guidelines from the American Academy of Audiology (American Academy of Audiology, 2011) are summarized in Table 8.4.

Testing the Reliability of Screening Measures

For a hearing screening to be useful, it must be both sensitive and specific. The sensitivity of a test may be determined by dividing the number of children with hearing loss who fail the screening by the number who actually have a hearing loss. This yields the percentage of those who have been correctly identified as positive. The specificity of a screening procedure is calculated by dividing the number of children who pass the screening and do not have a hearing loss by the total number who do not have a hearing loss. This is the percentage of true negative results. A comparison of the sensitivity and specificity of a screening test to the overall population with hearing loss determines the predictive value of a screening procedure, which accounts for the inevitable over-referrals and under-referrals for follow-up.

FIGURE 8.4 Portable acoustic immittance device in use (A). Device holders can store and recharge the unit, and print the tympanogram and acoustic reflex results (see Figure 8.5). (*Source:* Clark Audiology, LLC, and Welch-Allyn, Inc.)

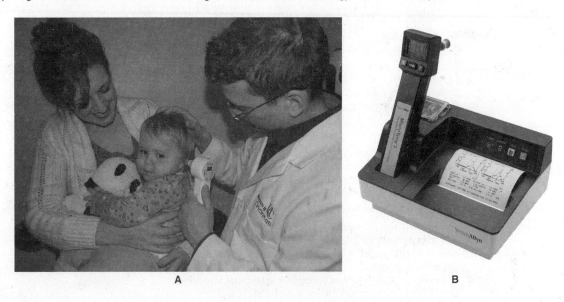

A   B

Any screening carries the danger of misclassification. No matter how cleverly a screening measure is designed, it is not possible to determine its shortcomings without submitting it to some empirical verification. A procedure described by Newby (1948) involves the use of a **tetrachoric table** and appears to serve this purpose well (see Figure 8.6). One hundred children who have taken the screening are selected at random and given threshold tests under the best possible test conditions. The threshold test serves as the criterion for the accuracy of the screening measure. Cells A and D in Figure 8.6 represent agreement between threshold assessments and screenings, showing correct identification of those children with and without hearing losses. Cells B and C represent disagreement between the two measures; the larger the number in those two cells, the poorer the screening is at doing its job. Cell C seems to be the biggest offender, passing children on screenings who fail the individual test, thereby missing their hearing losses. This suggests that

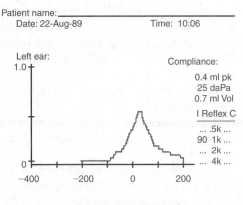

Patient name: _____
   Date: 22-Aug-89   Time: 10:06

Left ear:
1.0

Compliance:

0.4 ml pk
25 daPa
0.7 ml Vol

I Reflex C

... .5k ...
90 1k ...
... 2k ...
... 4k ...

0
−400   −200   0   200

American Electromedics Corp.
AE-106 Tympanometer Serial #360147
Calibration date: 30-May-89

Tester: _____
Comments:

FIGURE 8.5 Printout of a tympanogram and acoustic reflex screening done on a young child with normal hearing.

TABLE 8.4 Summary of American Academy of Audiology (2011) Childhood Hearing Screening Recommendations[*][†]

Targeted Grade Levels: preschool; kindergarten; and grades 1, 3, 5, and 7 or 9 at a minimum.

1. Pure-tone screening
   a. Screen frequencies 1000, 2000, and 4000 Hz at 20 dB HL. Present a tone at least twice but no more than 4 times if no response.
   b. Failure defined as a lack of response at any frequency in either ear. Rescreen immediately on failure, preferably with a different tester and different audiometer.
   c. Preschool, kindergarten, and grade 1 use tympanometry screening in conjunction with pure-tone screening.

2. Tympanometry screening
   a. To be used as a second-stage screening following failure of pure-tone or otoacoustic screenings.
   b. Failure set at tympanometric width >250 daPa (preferred criteria), <0.2 mmhos static compliance or negative pressure > −200 daPa to −400 daPa.

3. OAE screening
   a. Recommended only for preschool and school-age children when pure-tone screening is not developmentally appropriate (ability levels less than 3 years).
   b. Maintain primary DPOAE levels at 65/55 dB SPL.
   c. Select DPOAE or TEOAE cut-off values carefully as default settings (set for newborn screenings) may not be appropriate.
   d. Children who fail should be given a tymanometric screening.
   e. OAE screenings must involve an audiologist.

4. Rescreening
   a. Rescreen with tympanometry immediately following a pure-tone rescreening.
   b. Rescreen within 8 to 10 weeks for children failing pure-tone or OAE screening and tympanometry.
   c. Refer as failed is immediately required following failed pure-tone screening

[*]*Refer to the American Academy of Audiology (AAA) Guideline for greater details on these recommendations.*
[†]*Note: All referrals for hearing-impairment screening should ensure prompt completion of the diagnostic process and timely initiation of habilitative procedures. Screenings should be completed within acoustically appropriate settings as defined within the comprehensive guidelines with calibrated equipment. Screenings may be carried out by support personnel under the supervision of an audiologist.*

the criteria, such as the screening level, are too lax. A large number in cell B shows that time and energy are being wasted by identifying children with normal hearing as having hearing losses. In such cases, screening criteria may be too stringent, failing children who should have passed.

No matter how carefully a screening is conceived, the numbers in cells B and C will probably never reach the ideal of zero. If the criteria are so stringent that no child passes who should fail, the penalty is to retest a lot of children with normal hearing, or to make many over-referrals. On the other hand, decreasing the number in cell B at the expense of missing children with hearing losses seems unthinkable.

In the real world, the person in charge of any screening program must balance factors of money, personnel, and the number of children to be tested against the efficiency of the screening measure. There appears to be an inverse relationship between efficiency and accuracy in any screening if one defines *efficiency* in terms of the number of screenings performed with the least expenditure of time and money.

Public school environments for hearing screenings are often less than satisfactory. Often the testing is done in large rooms with poor acoustics and with considerable background noise. Many children may be tested before an audiometer calibration defect is detected. Unless all the criteria for adequate testing are met, the purpose of the procedure is defeated.

The desirability of any hearing screening procedure is obvious. However, screening procedures can be terribly misleading if the strictest criteria are not adhered to. Even at the time of this writing, the gold standard for determining hearing loss is the pure-tone audiogram.

FIGURE 8.6 Tetrachoric table used to validate the efficiency of a hearing screening measure. The children correctly identified as having hearing losses by the screening and verified by the threshold assessment are shown in cell A (true positive). Those properly identified as having no hearing loss are shown in cell D (true negative). Those children with normal hearing incorrectly identified by the screening as having hearing losses are shown in cell B (false positive). Cell C shows the children with hearing losses who were missed by the screening (false negative).

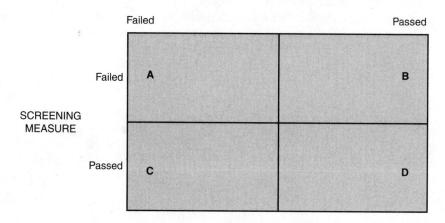

Procedures like the Calibrated Finger Rub Auditory Screening Test (CALFRAST) (Torres-Russotto et al., 2009) may be attractive as timesavers but such tests can easily miss hearing losses, especially losses in the high frequencies, and are not recommended.

Clinical COMMENTARY

Children with total or even partial unilateral hearing loss often go undiagnosed for long periods of time because they obtain their auditory information from their normal ear. Many of these children experience greater academic difficulties than has been previously thought.

Nonorganic Hearing Loss in Children

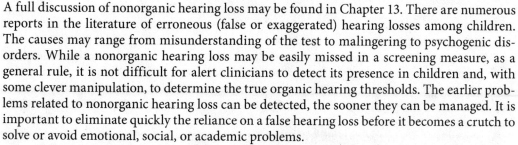

A full discussion of nonorganic hearing loss may be found in Chapter 13. There are numerous reports in the literature of erroneous (false or exaggerated) hearing losses among children. The causes may range from misunderstanding of the test to malingering to psychogenic disorders. While a nonorganic hearing loss may be easily missed in a screening measure, as a general rule, it is not difficult for alert clinicians to detect its presence in children and, with some clever manipulation, to determine the true organic hearing thresholds. The earlier problems related to nonorganic hearing loss can be detected, the sooner they can be managed. It is important to eliminate quickly the reliance on a false hearing loss before it becomes a crutch to solve or avoid emotional, social, or academic problems.

Children who exhibit nonorganic hearing loss typically do not appear to have hearing difficulty in normal conversation situations and often show normal speech thresholds, despite apparent hearing losses for pure tones. Within the pediatric population, prevalence of nonorganic hearing loss is generally less than 7 percent (Campanelli, 1963; Maran, 1966). Despite this relatively low prevalence, audiologists must recognize nonorganic hearing loss in children when they see it, know how to establish hearing levels, be prepared to talk with parents about the identified behavior, and know when and how to refer for additional psychological consultation (Clark, 2002). As Peck (2011) notes, it would be a mistake to assume that simply because organic thresholds may have been established, the underlying disturbance that manifested as nonorganic hearing loss has been resolved.

Among adults, the exhibition of nonorganic hearing loss may arise from a variety of origins, but it probably is most frequently rooted in a motivation based on anticipated financial gain. When nonorganic hearing loss appears in children, the underlying motivation is frequently much less apparent. In children, the reasons for displays of nonorganic hearing loss are typically an anticipated psychological gain and may be seen when parents divorce or are separated; when there is alcohol, substance, physical, or sexual abuse in the home; or when there is a sibling with hearing loss.

CHECK YOUR UNDERSTANDING

ACTIVITIES

Although many school children try diligently to pass their hearing tests, others manifest symptoms of nonorganic hearing loss. Ross (1964) has pointed out the dangers of reinforcing children's notions that they have a hearing loss. They may consciously or unconsciously see the advantages of hearing loss and may decide that the risk is worth the secondary gains to be realized in the forms of favors and excuses. Ross advised that children should not be referred to physicians for follow-up examinations unless the person in charge of the school tests is reasonably certain that a hearing problem exists. Most experienced audiologists can probably recall specific incidents in which a child has become committed to continued fabrication of a hearing loss, no matter how the problem got started.

EVOLVING CASE STUDIES

Only Case Study 4 is included here for obvious reasons. Look at the tests described in this chapter and determine which ones are indicated and best suited to this 3-year-old child. Project what might happen on behavioral tests, including speech audiometry, pure-tone audiometry, operant-conditioning audiometry (OCA), and play audiometry. Conjecture about what might be observed on objective tests that were discussed in Chapter 7, such as acoustic immittance, otoacoustic emissions (OAEs), and auditory brain-stem response (ABR). How would you deal with the obvious language disorder this child exhibits?

Case Study 4: Pediatric Patient

Inclusion of otoacoustic emissions testing has become a standard in pediatric assessments. Some children respond best if testing begins with the more interactive behavioral measures of hearing, but with a skilled and personable clinician, it is possible to begin with the more objective measures of OAE, acoustic immittance, and acoustic reflexes. If emissions are normal, conductive hearing loss is ruled out and no worse than a mild sensory/neural hearing loss is present. Given the negative history of middle-ear infections, Type A tympanograms would probably be evinced with essentially normal static compliance measures. Testing for acoustic reflexes (ipsilateral and contralateral) provides a cross-check with the results of behavioral measures as the diagnostic picture is formed for this child.

Behavioral testing may be addressed next using a team of two audiologists or, if necessary, employing a parent or caregiver as an assistant. Testing with earphones should be attempted, but if the child is at all fearful of these, initial testing should begin in the sound field and then transition to earphones if it appears likely that the child will accept them. In Chapter 4, it was suggested that parents be sent home with foam ear inserts to facilitate acclimation to insert earphones on the return to clinic. This can certainly facilitate success. Obtaining a reliable hand-raise response to pure tones in a young child is unlikely, so a technique such as conditioned play audiometry would probably be the best choice. If that fails, OCA could be employed. While it might take several sessions, fairly reliable results can probably be obtained and would most likely reveal a severe loss by air conduction of 70 to 90 dB HL with essentially absent bone-conduction responses. A finding of absent OAEs and absent acoustic reflexes would be consistent with these pure-tone findings. While this child has no language abilities, precluding administration of most speech audiometric measures, determination of speech awareness levels could be made in the same manner that pure-tone thresholds were obtained and should be in agreement with those. If behavioral testing fails, ABR might be necessary, which in this case would reveal absent responses. The auditory steady state response, which can provide responses for more severe and profound hearing losses, should be consistent with a 70 to 90 dB HL sensory/neural hearing loss.

Even if precise thresholds are not known for several frequencies in each ear, if there is a reasonable probability of hearing impairment, hearing aids should be introduced at the earliest possible time. Modern hearing instruments are extremely flexible and can be adjusted to suit the child's hearing loss as more details are obtained. The child should be entered in a language stimulation program, and the parents should be referred to a parent support group as soon as possible. Further testing is necessary to be certain of the accuracy of test results.

More discussion of the management of this little girl's case will be covered in ensuing chapters.

Summary

While pediatric audiology can be stimulating and rewarding, it can also be time-consuming and frustrating. Often clinicians do not have the feeling, as they have with most adults, of complete closure on a case at the end of a diagnostic session. Nevertheless, the proper identification and management of hearing loss in children is one of the most solemn responsibilities for the audiologist. Under ideal conditions, children with identified hearing loss should have their hearing tested every six months until stability of the loss is documented, and annually thereafter. Work with children is often carried out more as an art than a science, testing the cleverness and perseverance of clinicians, and calling on all their training and experience.

Pediatric audiology includes the use of those tests and diagnostic procedures designed especially for children who cannot be tested by conventional audiometry. Approaches vary with both the chronological and mental ages of children. Some tests, designed merely to elicit some sort of startle reaction, may be carried out on children as young as several hours of age. Other tests employ play techniques or use special rewards to encourage proper performance. Still other procedures involve measuring changes in electrophysiological states or electroacoustical properties in response to sound, or the detection of sounds emitted from the ear. With some children it is possible to test by making slight alterations in conventional audiometric techniques used with adults. Hearing testing is designed to determine the nature and extent of a child's communicative problem and is almost useless unless some (re)habilitative path is pursued, as discussed in Chapter 15.

REVIEW TABLE 8.1 Procedures Used in Pediatric Audiometry

Procedure	Age Group for Which the Procedure Is Most Suitable	Probability of Success
Warblet	Infants	Fair
Speech sounds	4 to 8 months	Good
COR, VRA	6 months to 2 years	Good
Imitation of vocalization	Under 1 year	Fair
Play audiometry	2 to 6 years	Good
Operant conditioning	2 to 5 years	Good
Noisemakers	Under 3 years	Fair
Pure-tone audiometry	Over 3 years	Good
AEP	All ages	Very good
OAE	All ages	Very good
Immittance measures	All ages	Very good

Frequently Asked Questions

Q What is the best procedure for screening a 2-year-old toddler for a hearing loss?

A *Some children at this age can be trained to respond to sounds using play techniques. ABR and OAE tests may also be used.*

Q Are different hearings tests available for children with special needs to better facilitate accurate results with these patients?

A *Yes, several different behavioral and electrophysiological tests are available.*

Q What extra measures should be taken when testing the hearing of children with disorders and special needs such as Down syndrome and autism?

A *Electrophysiological tests may be carried out using sedation if necessary. Under the proper conditions, behavioral audiometry may also be used, but results must be interpreted carefully.*

Q When testing a child's hearing, is it difficult to keep parents from disrupting the tests?

A *Parents should be included in the diagnostic procedures, at least as observers. This makes explanation of results much easier to convey. Disruption is rare and can be controlled with tact and diplomacy.*

Q Do hearing tests given to babies hurt the child?

A *They certainly should not.*

Q What is the best approach when testing a child for hearing loss?

A *This depends entirely on the chronological and mental ages of the child, the severity of the problem, and the existence of other disabilities.*

Q What warning signs for deafness in children should parents look for?

A *Obviously parents become concerned when a child fails to respond to environmental sounds. Delays in speech or language development also raise concerns.*

Q What more can audiologists do if a parent refuses to allow them to help a child who has a hearing loss?

A *There is very little that can be done beyond maintaining an interested and professional demeanor. Referring caregivers to others who have children with hearing loss sometimes helps.*

Q Once a child is placed on the high-risk registry, what are the procedures to follow?

A *The high-risk registry is rarely used since the advent of universal neonatal screening.*

Q What should be the first step taken in finding newborns with hearing loss?

A *Public awareness of hearing loss is essential, along with neonatal screening.*

Q Is hearing screening mandated for elementary-age children?

A *Yes, most states require some sort of hearing and/or tympanometric screening in the public schools.*

Suggested Reading

Bess, F., & Gravel, J. (2006). *Foundations of pediatric audiology.* San Diego, CA: Plural Publishing.

Seewald, R. & Tharpe, A. M. (Eds.) (2011). *Comprehensive handbook of pediatric audiology.* San Diego, CA: Plural Publishing.

Jackson, R. (2001). *Screening for hearing loss and otitis media in children.* San Diego, CA: Singular Publishing Group.

Northern, J. L., & Downs, M. P. (2002). *Hearing in children* (5th ed.). Baltimore, MD: Lippincott Williams & Wilkins.

Endnotes

1. Dr. Virginia Apgar, American anesthesiologist, 1909–1974.

2. Named for Ernst Moro, German pediatrician, 1874–1951.

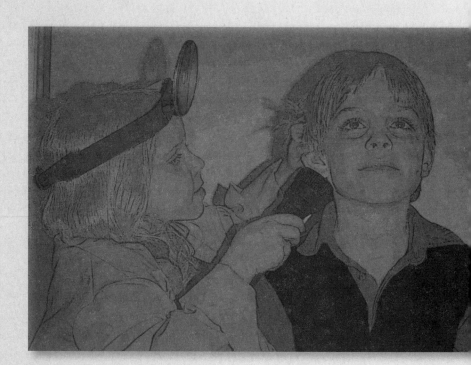

In Chapters 9 through 12, the description of the auditory system is divided into four separate parts for study of the outer ear, middle ear, inner ear, and auditory nerve and central auditory pathways. The anatomy and physiology are described, as well as different disease processes that produce auditory disorders, their causes, and appropriate treatments. Chapter 13 discusses patients who are either pretending to have a hearing loss or exaggerating the loss they do have for some special gain. Examples are given of actual and theoretical findings on a variety of auditory tests described in Chapters 5 through 8, so that each disorder is exemplified from a diagnostic point of view. Additional tests are described where appropriate.

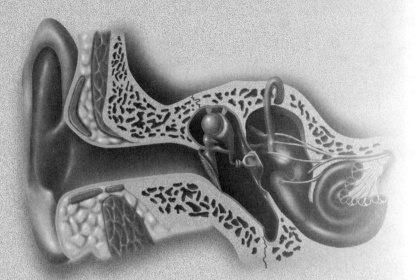

CHAPTER **9**

The Outer Ear

LEARNING OBJECTIVES

This chapter requires no previous knowledge of human anatomy, but it does assume an understanding of the physics of sound and the various tests of hearing described earlier. All the minuscule details of the anatomy of the outer ear are not provided here. These may be obtained readily from books on anatomy. At the completion of this chapter, the reader should be able to

- Discuss in basic terms the outer-ear anatomy and its purpose.
- List a variety of common disorders that may affect the outer ear.
- Describe how these disorders are caused and treated, and how they may manifest on a variety of audiometric tests.

WHEN LAYPERSONS THINK of the ear, it is the outer ear that comes to mind. The outer ear is responsible for gathering sounds from the acoustical environment and funneling them into the auditory mechanism. Some of the outer-ear structures found in humans are absent in animals such as birds and frogs, whose hearing sensitivity is nevertheless similar to that of humans. Of course, it is the outer ear of humans with which this chapter is concerned.

Anatomy and Physiology of the Outer Ear

The Auricle

The most noticeable portion of the outer-ear mechanism is the **auricle** or pinna (see Figure 9.1). The auricle varies from person to person in size and shape, and its funnel-like configuration plays a substantial role in gathering sound waves from the environment. The auricle is made entirely of cartilage, with a number of individually characteristic twists, turns, and indentations. The entire cartilage is covered with skin, which is continuous with the face. The bottommost portion of the auricle is the lobule, or ear lobe. Extending up from the lobule, the outer rim of the auricle folds over outwardly, forming the helix. Above the lobule is the antitragus. Another elevation running closer to the center of the auricle is the antihelix. A small triangular protrusion, which points slightly backward and forms the anterior portion of the auricle, is called the **tragus,** Latin for "goat's beard." The tragus is so named because, in older men, bristly hairs appear in this region. Depression of the tragus into the opening of the external ear canal is an efficient means of blocking sounds. This occlusion provides more efficiency than plugging the ear with a finger, clasping the hands over the auricle, or even using some earplugs specifically designed for sound attenuation. Although humans cannot voluntarily close off the tragus, as can some animals, vestiges of muscles designed for this purpose remain in the human ear.

The middle portion of the outer ear, just before the opening into the head, is called the concha because of its bowl-like shape. The concha is divided into two parts, the lower cavum concha and the upper cymba concha. This portion of the external ear aids in the human ability to localize the sources of sounds that come from in front of, behind, below, and above the head. The concha helps to funnel sounds directed to it from the surrounding air into the opening of the **external auditory canal (EAC),** or external auditory **meatus.** The anatomy of the auricle makes it more efficient at delivering high-frequency sounds than low-frequency sounds, and it helps in the localization of sounds delivered to the head.

The External Auditory Canal

In discussing this portion of the ear, it is important not to omit the word *external* to avoid confusion with the internal auditory canal, discussed in Chapter 12. The external auditory canal is a tube, formed in the side of the head, beginning at the concha and extending inward at a slight upward angle for approximately 1 inch (2.5 cm) in adults. Although it appears to be round, the EAC is actually elliptical and averages about 9 mm in height and 6.5 mm in width. It is lined entirely with skin (see Figure 9.2).

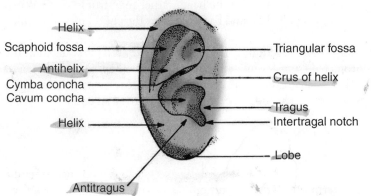

Helix —
Scaphoid fossa —
Antihelix —
Cymba concha —
Cavum concha —
Helix —
Triangular fossa
Crus of helix
Tragus
Intertragal notch
Lobe
Antitragus

FIGURE 9.1 The human pinna (auricle) and its primary landmarks.

FIGURE 9.2 Cross-section of the external ear.

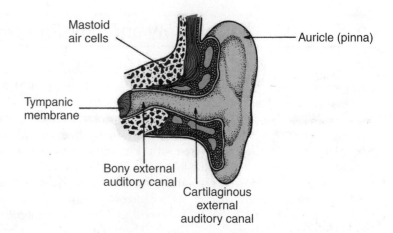

The outer portion of the EAC passes through cartilage. The skin in this area supports several sets of glands, including the sebaceous glands, which secrete sebum, an oily, fatty substance. The major product of these secretions is earwax, or **cerumen,** which is usually soft, moist, and brown, but can be light in color, flaky, and dry; if accumulated in the ear canal for a protracted period, it may become quite dark and hard. Cerumen exits the ear naturally when the walls of the EAC are distorted by movement of the jawbone during chewing or speaking. The outer third of the EAC contains a number of hair follicles. The combination of hairs and cerumen helps to keep foreign objects, such as insects, from passing into the inner two-thirds of the canal.

The inner area of the EAC passes through the tympanic portion of the temporal bone. There are no glands and no hair in this area. The two portions of the EAC meet at the osseocartilaginous junction. The **condyle,** a protrusion of the mandible (jawbone), comes to rest just below the osseocartilaginous junction when the jaw is closed. If the mandible overrides its normal position, as in the case of missing or worn molar teeth or a misaligned jaw, the condyle presses into the junction, causing pain. The term **temporomandibular joint (TMJ) syndrome** has been coined for this neuralgia. The TMJ syndrome produces a referred pain, perceived in the ear, which constitutes a significant amount of **otalgia** (ear pain) in adults.

The term *myofacial pain dysfunction (MPD) syndrome* is sometimes used to describe pain in the temporomandibular joint, along with headaches; grating sounds (crepitus); dizziness; and back, neck, and shoulder pain. At times, emotional stress and tension have been associated with MPD syndrome, and treatment has ranged from emotional therapy to biofeedback training, the use of prosthetic devices, and major maxillofacial surgery.

In infants and small children, the angle of the EAC is quite different from that in adults. The canal angles downward, rather than upward, and is at a more acute angle. For this reason, it is advisable to examine children's ears from above the head, rather than from below. When one looks into an ear, the adult pinna is pulled up and back, whereas the child's pinna is pulled down and back.

The EAC serves several important functions. The **tympanic membrane** is situated at the end of the canal, where it is protected from trauma and where it can be kept at constant temperature and humidity levels. The canal also serves as a filter to reduce low frequencies and as a tube resonator for frequencies between 2000 and 7000 Hz, thereby creating an efficient transfer of energy to the tympanic membrane.

The Tympanic Membrane

The external auditory canal terminates in a concave, disk-like structure called the tympanic membrane (see Figure 9.3). The term *eardrum* is commonly used to describe this structure, although properly speaking a drum would include the space below a vibrating membrane

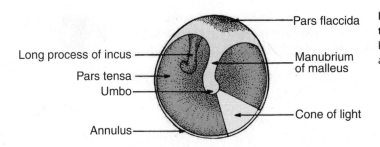

Pars flaccida

Long process of incus

Manubrium of malleus

Pars tensa

Umbo

Cone of light

Annulus

FIGURE 9.3 A right tympanic membrane as viewed through the ear canal. Note that the light reflex, known as the cone of light, appears in the inferior/anterior quadrant of the tympanic membrane.

(in this case the middle ear), and so the term *eardrum membrane* is more accurate. The tympanic membrane is discussed in this text along with the outer ear because it can be viewed along with the outer-ear structures. The tympanic membrane marks the border between the outer ear and the middle ear, however, so it is really a common boundary between both areas. Whether the tympanic membrane is thought of as part of the outer ear or the middle ear is not important as long as its structure and function are understood.

The total area of the tympanic membrane is about 90 mm² (Harris, 1986) and is constructed of three layers. The outer layer, as viewed from the external auditory canal, is made up of the same skin that is stretched over the osseous meatus. Below the skin is a layer of tough, fibrous, connective tissue, which contributes most to the membrane's ability to vibrate with impinging sound waves. Behind the tympanic membrane is the middle-ear space, which is completely lined with mucous membrane, including the third layer of the tympanic membrane.

The tympanic membrane is extremely thin, averaging about 0.07 mm. Harris describes it as "a little conical loudspeaker." It is an extremely efficient vibrating surface. Movement of one-billionth of a centimeter is sufficient to produce a threshold response in normal-hearing individuals in the 800 to 6000 Hz range. The entire area of the tympanic membrane has a very rich blood supply, which is why it appears so red when infection is present and blood is brought to the area.

Embedded in the fibrous portion of the tympanic membrane is the **malleus,** the largest bone of the middle ear (described in Chapter 10). The tip of the malleus ends in the approximate center of the tympanic membrane and angles downward and backward (see Figure 9.3). If an imaginary line is drawn through the tympanic membrane at a 180-degree angle to the handle of the malleus and that line is bisected through the center of the tympanic membrane at right angles, the two intersecting imaginary lines thus drawn conveniently divide the tympanic membrane into four quadrants: anterior-superior, posterior-superior, anterior-inferior, and posterior-inferior. A photograph of a normal right tympanic membranes can be seen in Figure 9.4.

The tip of the handle of the malleus is so poised as to cause the center of the tympanic membrane to be pulled inward, resulting in its concave configuration. The point of greatest retraction is called the **umbo.** To observe the tympanic membrane, it is necessary to direct a light, as from an **otoscope** (see Figures 9.5 and 9.6), into the external auditory canal.

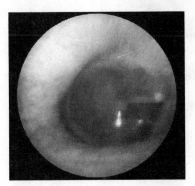

FIGURE 9.4 Normal right tympanic membrane (TM). Note that the cone of light is clearly visible. The manubrium of the malleus is also visible through the TM. (*Source:* Clark Audiology.)

FIGURE 9.5 One of a variety of hand-held otoscopes used for inspection of the outer ear, ear canal, and tympanic membrane. Many pathologies in the middle-ear cavity discussed in Chapter 9 may be evidenced by their effect on the appearance of the tympanic membrane. (*Source:* Welch-Allyn, Inc.)

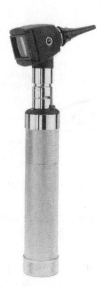

Because the tympanic membrane is semitransparent, such a light allows some of the structures of the middle ear to become visible. However, some of the light rays directed against the membrane are reflected and refracted. The concavity of the tympanic membrane usually causes the light reflex to appear in a cone shape directed inferiorly and anteriorly.

One of the many modern breakthroughs in medical instrumentation is the video otoscope (see Figure 9.7). It combines an otoscope with a separate light source, fiber-optic cable, video camera, and color monitor. Viewing of the tympanic membrane takes place, not through the

FIGURE 9.6 External inspection of the outer ear and ear canal is an important prerequisite to the hearing evaluation. Otoscopes are frequently inverted so that the otoscope handle can easily clear the patient's shoulder. The pinna is pulled upward and back (downward and back for infants) to better straighten the canal for a more direct view of the tympanic membrane, and the examiner's fingers brace the head to prevent injury to the ear canal if the patient should suddenly move. Pressing the pinna against the head while looking into the ear canal reveals any potential for ear canal collapse during testing with supra-aural earphones. (*Source:* Clark Audiology.)

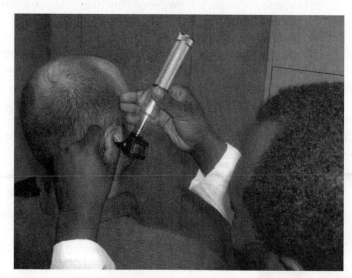

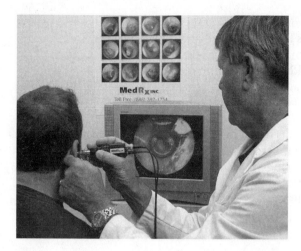

FIGURE 9.7 A video otoscope can display the structures of the ear on a video monitor visible to both the examiner and the patient. Here, a curette is used for cerumen removal instead of the standard speculum. (*Source:* MedRx, Inc.)

otoscope in conventional ways, but by watching the video monitor, where the structures can be seen by the examiner, the patient, and other interested parties. Attachments for the device allow for still photography or video recording for later viewing. When you watch the videos for use of the hand-held otoscope and the video otoscope, note the proper technique for use of these instruments and the relative advantages of each.

The tympanic membrane is held in position at the end of the EAC by a ring of tissue called the tympanic **annulus.** The slight stretching of the tympanic membrane into the middle ear results in its tension and conical appearance. The greatest surface area of the tympanic membrane is taut and is appropriately called the pars tensa. At the top of the tympanic membrane, above the malleus, the tissues are looser because they contain only the epidermal and mucous membrane layers, resulting in the name **pars flaccida.** The pars flaccida is also called **Shrapnell's membrane.**[1]

The auricle and external auditory canal provide a resonating tube through which sound waves may pass, and the tympanic membrane is the first mobile link in the chain of auditory events. Pressure waves, which impinge on the tympanic membrane, cause it to vibrate, reproducing the same spectrum of sounds that enters the external auditory canal. Movement of the tympanic membrane causes identical vibration of the malleus, to which it is attached. The further transmission of these sound waves is discussed in ensuing chapters.

Development of the Outer Ear

About 28 days after conception of the human embryo, bulges begin to appear on either side of the tissue that will develop into the head and neck. These are the **pharyngeal arches.** Although there may be as many as six arches, separated by grooves or clefts, significant information is available only about the first three: the mandibular arch, the hyoid arch, and the glossopharyngeal arch. These arches are known to have three layers, the **ectoderm,** or outer layer; the **entoderm,** or inner surface; and the **mesoderm,** or inner core. Each arch contains four components: an artery, muscle, and cartilage that come from the mesoderm, and a nerve that forms from the ectoderm.

The auricle develops from the first two pharyngeal arches. The tragus forms from the first arch, and the helix and antitragus form from the second arch. Development of the auricle begins before the second fetal month.

The external auditory canal forms from the first pharyngeal groove and is very shallow until after birth. A primitive meatus forms in about the 4th gestational week, and a solid core forms near the tympanic membrane in the 8th week. The solid core canalizes (forms a tube or canal) by the 28th gestational week, although the entire osseous meatus is not complete until about the time of puberty. Pneumatization of the temporal bone surrounding the external auditory canal begins in the 35th fetal week, accelerates at the time of birth, and is not complete until puberty.

The tympanic membrane annulus forms in the third fetal month. The outer layer of the membrane itself forms from ectoderm; the inner layer, from entoderm; and the middle layer, from **mesenchyme,** which is a network of embryonic tissue that later forms the connective tissues of the body, as well as the blood vessels and the lymphatic vessels. The tympanic membrane has begun formation by the beginning of the second embryonic month.

Hearing Loss and the Outer Ear

When conditions occur that interfere with or block the normal sound vibrations transmitted through the outer ear, conductive hearing loss results. Except in rare cases, the loss of hearing is rarely severe and never exceeds a 60 dB air-bone gap because, beyond that intensity, supra-aural earphones vibrate the skull and generate bone-conduction signals. Because some of the disorders alter the normal resonance frequency of the outer ear, or otherwise interfere with the osseotympanic mode of bone conduction, the bone-conduction audiogram may be slightly altered; however, this does not, in itself, suggest abnormality of the sensory/neural system.

Disorders of the Outer Ear and Their Treatments

Some abnormalities of the external ear do not result in hearing loss. They are mentioned, nonetheless, because of the audiologist's usual curiosity about disorders of the ear in general, and because abnormalities in one part of the body, specifically congenital ones, are frequently related to other abnormalities.

Disorders of the Auricle

Hearing tests performed with earphones ignore the auricle, so they do not reveal any effects it may have on hearing sensitivity, word recognition, and localization. For example, people who have had a portion or an entire auricle removed by accident or surgery, as in the case of cancer, appear to have no apparent hearing loss. At times, one or both ears may be of very small size (**microtia**), or the pinna may be very prominent and stand away from the head or be entirely absent (**anotia**). Congenital malformations of the auricle (see Figure 9.8) have also been associated with other disorders, such as **Down syndrome.**[2]

When the auricle protrudes markedly from the head, or when it is pressed tightly against the skull, a simple surgical procedure called otoplasty or pinnaplasty may be performed. This procedure may improve the patient's appearance, which often has a beneficial psychological effect. In cases of missing auricles in children, plastic surgery is often inadvisable because the scar tissue formed from the grafts does not grow as does normal tissue. Plastic auricles can be made that are affixed to the head with adhesive and are amazingly realistic. Hairstyles can be arranged to conceal malformed auricles entirely.

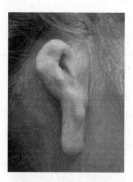

FIGURE 9.8 Microtia is a congenital deformity of the outer ear. Reconstructive surgery can often restore the appearance of a near normal ear. The accompanying atresia in this case signals the presence of substantial conductive hearing loss, which may include an absent middle ear cavity. When the hearing loss cannot be corrected surgically, the loss may be addressed through a bone-anchored hearing implant (see Chapter 14). (*Source:* Bechara Y. Ghorayeb, MD; from http://www.ghorayeb.com/Pictures.html.)

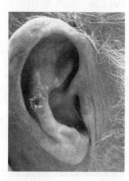

FIGURE 9.9 Basal cell carcinoma, the most common form of skin cancer, can appear on the ear following too much exposure to the ultraviolet light of the sun. (*Source:* Bechara Y. Ghorayeb, MD; from http://www.ghorayeb.com/Pictures.html.)

The most common form of skin cancer is the basal cell carcinoma, which begins in the top layer of the skin, or epidermis. Basal cell carcinomas occur on skin that has high exposure to ultraviolet radiation, which occurs from excess sun exposure, and the helix of the ear is a prime area for occurance. Most common in persons over 40 years of age, this slow-growing cancer is painless and may appear as a raised bump on the surface of the skin or as a sore that bleeds easily and does not heal. This form of cancer rarely spreads to other parts of the body and is cured when early treatment is sought. Audiologists are in a prime position to be early observers of basal cell carcinoma on the ear and should advise patients to seek immediate medical attention (see Figure 9.9).

Atresia of the External Auditory Canal

In some patients, the cartilaginous portion, the bony portion, or the entirety of the external auditory canal has never formed at all. Such congenital abnormalities may occur in one or both ears. This lack of canalization is called otic **atresia** and can occur in the EAC either in isolation or in combination with other anomalies. One inherited condition, Treacher Collins syndrome, involves the facial bones, especially the cheek and lower jaw; the auricle; and congenital atresia of the EAC. At times, patients with Treacher Collins syndrome present with preauricular tags, which represent incomplete embryological development and appear just in front of the auricle. These do not, in themselves, cause hearing difficulties. Sometimes these tags contain a core of cartilage and are large enough to be called accessory auricles. A number of abnormalities of the middle ear and temporal bone are seen with Treacher Collins syndrome, making surgical correction quite difficult.

The **CHARGE syndrome** is often first noticed in children because of the obvious anomalies of the pinna and external auditory canal. However, this condition can affect almost any part of the auditory system. This acronym stands for *coloboma* (a keyhole slot in the retina, iris, or optic nerve), *h*eart disorders, *a*tresia choanae (blockage of the respiratory passages), *r*etarded growth and development, *g*enitourinary abnormalities, and *e*ar anomalies. CHARGE is a genetic disorder that occurs in one out of every 10,000 to 15,000 births (Thelin & Swanson, 2006) and, because of the multiple disorders, presents major difficulties in habilitation to audiologists, speech-language pathologists, and physicians.

Not all closures of the external auditory canal are congenital; some may occur as the result of trauma or burns. Trauma to the outer ear may result in an unsightly blood blister, called a hematoma. Because the pinna protrudes from the side of the head, it can be damaged by sunlight or extreme cold. Frostbite can appear rather like a severe burn. Either condition can lead to loss of the pinna.

Sometimes when an ear is malformed in a small child, it is difficult to determine whether the condition is one of congenital atresia or a marked stenosis (narrowing) of the canal. Surgical procedures for correction of atresia of the EAC have improved in recent years, and surgeons have been assisted greatly by the advent of modern imaging techniques. Chances for success are better when only the cartilaginous canal is involved, and when the middle ear and tympanic membrane are normal. Drillouts of the bony canal have led to some serious after-care problems. Although in some cases it may appear that it is better to treat a child with a congenital external-ear-canal atresia with a hearing aid rather than with surgery, the ultimate decision on such matters is always left to the family in consultation with a physician.

Stenotic EACs do not produce hearing loss, as does atresia, although earwax or other debris can easily clog the very narrow lumen and thus cause a conductive problem. In cases of atresia of the canal, the hearing loss is directly related to the area and the amount of occlusion. The loss may be mild if only the cartilaginous area is involved, and certainly can be more severe if the bony canal is occluded. As stated earlier, a congenital anomaly in one part of the body increases the likelihood of another anomaly elsewhere. For this reason, when an atresia is seen, it must be suspected that the tympanic membrane and middle ear may likewise be involved. Figure 9.10A and B show the test results for a theoretical patient with atresia of both external ear canals. Notice that the conductive loss reaches near maximum (about 60 dB). In cases of atresia, the valuable information from measurements of acoustic immittance and otoacoustic emissions is unobtainable because the probes cannot be inserted into the EAC.

Collapsing External Auditory Canals

A conductive hearing loss sometimes appears during examination because the pressure of a supra-aural earphone causes the auricle to move forward, blocking the opening of the canal and attenuating sound entering it. Often the patient does not experience the loss subjectively. Inspection of the ear prior to testing can often prevent the finding of a false conductive hearing loss. When insert earphones, which circumvent the problem of earphone-induced canal collapse, cannot be used, a plastic tube can be inserted into the canal with a strong string attached for easy retrieval, or a wedge of foam rubber can be put behind the pinna before the headset is placed in position.

Collapsing external ear canals (see Figure 9.11) may occur in as many as 4 percent of a typical audiology caseload, with most incidences occurring at the extremes of the age spectrum. Among children, collapse is possible because the outer portion of the ear canal is less rigid before 7 years of age. Among the elderly, the greater elliptical shape of the canal coupled with the more flaccid nature of the cartilaginous outer portion of the canal can lead to collapse. The otoscopic examination should include inspection for canal collapse that may be induced by the pressure of supra-aural earphone cushions. The problems of collapsing ear canals during audiometric testing are completely circumvented with insert earphones.

FIGURE 9.10 (A) Worksheet used to determine the need for and determination of appropriate effective masking levels for the patient with a moderately-severe bilateral conductive hearing loss depicted in Figure 9.10B. (B) Audiogram showing a moderately-severe conductive hearing loss in both ears consistent with Treacher Collins syndrome. Because both external ear canals are atretic, insert earphones cannot be used, and the supra-aural receivers are placed where the external auditory canals would normally be found. Note the large air-bone gaps with essentially normal bone conduction. The SRTs and pure-tone averages are in close agreement, and the word-recognition scores are normal.

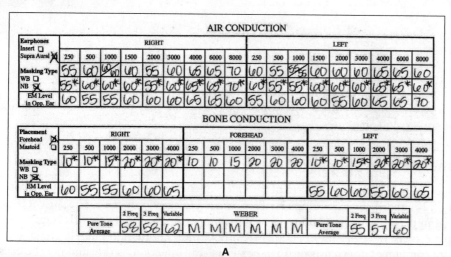

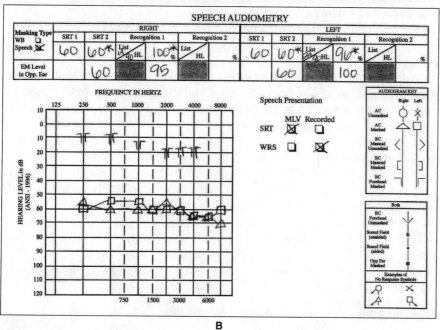

Foreign Bodies in the External Ear Canal

For unexplained reasons, children, and sometimes adults, place foreign objects, such as paper, pins, and crayons, into their mouths, noses, and ears. If the object is pushed past the osseocartilaginous junction of the external ear canal, swelling at the isthmus formed by this junction

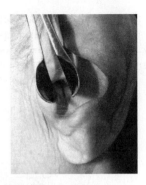

FIGURE 9.11 A collapsed left ear canal. A full collapse frequently only occurs with pressure against the ear canal with telephone use or when supra-aural earphones are used in an audiometric examination. When the canal is collapsed, the resulting test results will show a pseudo-conductive hearing impairment. Accurate testing may be best attained through the use of insert receivers to hold the canal open during testing. (*Source:* Bechara Y. Ghorayeb, MD; from http://www.ghorayeb.com/Pictures.html.)

may result. Although hearing loss may result from such an incident, it is of secondary importance to prompt and careful removal of the object, which may be a formidable task and may require surgery in some cases.

External Otitis

An infection that occurs in the skin of the external auditory canal is called **external otitis** (see Figure 9.12 A and B). The condition is often referred to as swimmer's ear because it frequently develops in people who have had water trapped in their ears. External otitis is quite common in tropical areas. External ear infections are often called fungus, although bacterial infections are more common. **Otomycosis** or fungal external-ear infection, is rare and may be caused by the overuse of eardrops. The natural defenses of the external auditory canal are often affected by excessive moisture or trauma. Avoidance of these common causes should be a primary goal in preventing this condition.

The external auditory canal is actually a cul-de-sac that is lined with skin, the only such structure in the human body, which makes it particularly susceptible to infection. It is an almost ideal environment for the development of bacterial growth because the skin is thin and the area is dark, warm, and often moist. Part of its natural defense is the cerumen, which contains certain bacteria-destroying enzymes and tends to reject the absorption of water. External otitis may originate from allergic reactions to earplugs, hearing aid earmolds, soap, or other allergens. **Furunculosis,** infection of hair follicles, may begin with infection of a single hair in the lateral third of the external auditory canal and spread to involve the entire area.

Systemic antibiotics are frequently unsuccessful in the treatment of external otitis because the pocket of infection may not be accessible through the bloodstream. External otitis can usually be treated with topical agents within eardrops, yet Halpern, Palmer, and Seidlin (1999) found that physicians used systemic antibiotics about 65 percent of the time.

FIGURE 9.12 A right ear external otitis with redness and crusted exudate (A). A close up of the same ear showing ear canal occlusion (B). External otitis can be very painful. (*Source:* Bechara Y. Ghorayeb, MD; from http://www.ghorayeb.com/Pictures.html.)

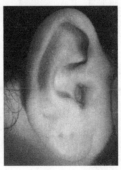

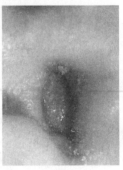

A   **B**

Itching is a common complaint in early or mild infections. Patients with more advanced infections are sometimes in extreme pain, especially upon touch to the infected area, which may become red and swollen and may produce a discharge. Often body temperature elevates. The condition may be successfully treated by irrigating the canal with warm saltwater, drying it carefully, and applying topical antibiotics. Sometimes a cotton wick saturated with antibiotic drops is inserted into the canal. The skin may be treated topically with steroids to curtail the inflammation.

Hearing tests often cannot be performed on patients with external otitis because the ear is too painful to allow the pressure of supra-aural earphones or the penetration of insert earphones. It is suspected that if the lumen of the canal is closed, either by the accumulation of infectious debris or by the swelling of the canal walls, a mild conductive loss is likely, as shown in Figure 9.13A and B and Figure 9.14. Some concern has been expressed by audiologists regarding the contamination by bacteria on supra-aural earphones and their rubber cushions. Large colonies of certain organisms may be found on earphone cushions (Kemp, Roeser, Pearson, & Ballachanda, 1995). These can often be controlled using ultraviolet light, but of course are avoided with the use of insert receivers.

Sometimes the tympanic membrane itself becomes inflamed, often in response to systemic viral infection. The patient may develop blood blisters on the surface of the tympanic membrane, which in turn produce fever and pain. Often these blebs must be carefully lanced to relieve the pain. Inflammations of the tympanic membrane are called **myringitis.**

Several forms of external otitis are considered particularly dangerous to the patient and require rather aggressive therapy. For example, necrotizing, or malignant, external otitis is often initially a routine infection of the skin of the external auditory canal. The condition is particularly threatening to diabetic and elderly patients, and may result in massive bone destruction in the external, middle, and inner ears. It can also result in **osteitis** and in **osteomyelitis** of the temporal bone. Patients suffering from this condition, which is often fatal, may be hospitalized and treated with systemic antibiotics. Surgery is sometimes required to stop the spread of infection through the bone.

Growths in the External Auditory Canal

Tumors, both benign and malignant, have been found in the EAC. Bony tumors, called osteomas, do not present hearing problems unless their size is such that the lumen of the canal is occluded and conductive hearing loss results; however, they may result in serious infection of the EAC. Some physicians believe that osteomas should be removed and biopsied to be certain they are not malignant.

Exostoses, the outward projections for the surfaces of bone, are sometimes seen in the ears of people who have done a great deal of swimming in cold water. To the untrained eye, such protrusions in the bony wall of the EAC may be confused with osteomas (see Figure 9.15). As with osteomas, exostoses require treatment only when their size produces a conductive hearing loss or when they block the normal cleansing action of the EAC, resulting in infection.

Earwax in the External Auditory Canal

In some cases, the wax glands in the EACs are extremely active, producing copious amounts of cerumen. When the canal is small, it may become blocked and cause a hearing loss. Even when a large amount of wax is found in the ear, hearing may remain fairly normal as long as there is a tiny opening between the tympanic membrane and the outside environment (see Figure 9.16A and B). Overzealous cleaning of the external ears, however, may result in cerumen being pushed from the cartilaginous canal into the bony canal, where natural cleansing cannot

FIGURE 9.13 (A) A worksheet used to determine the masking levels needed for bone conduction for the patient with a mild conductive hearing loss whose audiometric results are shown in Figure 9.13B. (B) A mild unilateral (left) conductive hearing loss due to external otitis. SRT and pure-tone findings are in close agreement, and word-recognition scores are normal. Masking is needed for the left ear for bone-conduction and higher-level WRS. The Weber results show lateralization to the left ear.

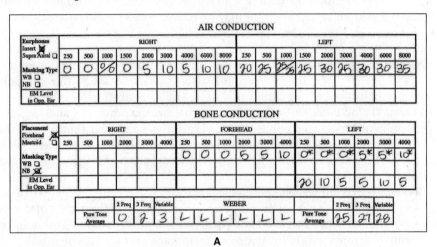

A

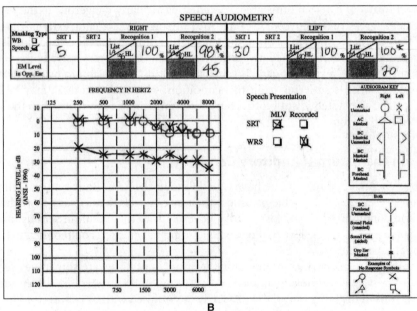

B

take place. Cotton swabs and wadded tissues are often used for such purposes, frequently by well-meaning parents on the ears of their children. As people age, the cartilage in the EAC begins to lose its support, narrowing the canal and thereby causing more problems with wax accumulation. This can be particularly annoying when water is trapped behind the wax.

Once the cerumen is deposited in the bony canal, it remains there until it is properly removed. Wax deposited in the bony canal becomes dry, causing itching, which encourages the individual to push still more wax from the cartilaginous canal by instruments such as cotton swabs. Sometimes water pressure during diving forces wax deep into the canal. As in the case of external otitis, the amount of hearing loss produced by impacted cerumen is directly related to the amount of ear canal occlusion, with hearing losses ranging from very mild to moderate.

FIGURE 9.14 Results on the audiometric Bing test for a patient with unilateral conductive hearing loss caused by external otitis (see Figure 9.13). Note the absence of the occlusion effect in the left ear on the Bing test.

SPEECH AND HEARING CENTER
THE UNIVERSITY OF TEXAS AT AUSTIN 78712

Name: Last-First-Middle		Sex	Age	Examiner		Reliability	Date

AUDIOMETRIC BING TEST						
	RIGHT			**LEFT**		
Frequency (Hertz)	**250**	**500**	**1000**	**250**	**500**	**1000**
1) Unoccluded	0	0	0	0	0	0
2) Occluded	-25	-15	-10	0	0	0
3) Occlusion Effect (1-2)	25	15	10	0	0	0

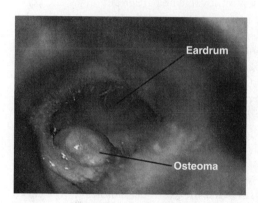

Eardrum

Osteoma

FIGURE 9.15 Slow-growing, benign bony growths may appear in the ear canal and often occur bilaterally. While there are clinical differences between exostoses and osteomas their removal is usually only necessitated if they become large enough to impede the natural outward migration of cerumen. Here an osteoma is seen in a patient's left external auditory canal. (*Source:* Bechara Y. Ghorayeb, MD; from http://www.ghorayeb.com/Pictures.html.)

FIGURE 9.16 Excess cerumen accumulation causes only minimal change in hearing until it reaches full occlusion. The degree of loss once occluded depends on the thickness of the plug (A). A "cerumen tunnel" (B) may be seen in a hearing aid user's ear. Cerumen may appear in various consistencies and can become quite hard with time. Cerumen can affect hearing test results, hearing aid performance measures, and hearing aid function. (*Sources:* (A) Clark Audiology, LLC; (B) Roy F. Sullivan, Ph.D. Audiology Forum: Video Otoscopy, www.rcsullivan.com.)

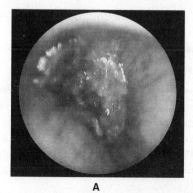

A

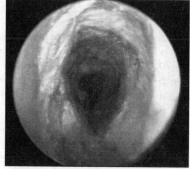

B

Because more and more audiological procedures—such as testing with insert receivers, immittance measures, electrocochleography, and the fitting of hearing aids—require patients' external ear canals to be clear, the role of the audiologist has changed concerning cerumen removal. The removal of cerumen by audiologists specifically trained in this procedure is included in the scope of audiological practice of both the American Academy of Audiology and the American Speech-Language-Hearing Association.

Prior to cerumen removal, a complete history must be taken to rule out possible tympanic membrane perforation, ear disease, or the presence of **pressure-equalizing (PE) tubes** (see Chapter 10). If anything in the history seems to contraindicate the audiologist's removal of the cerumen (e.g., diabetes, AIDS, previous ear surgery), the patient should be referred to a physician to have the wax removed.

Careful otoscopic examination must be performed, in part, to determine that it is cerumen and not some other substance or object occluding the canal. If the tympanic membrane can be seen, its integrity should be ascertained, which is often most efficiently done using tympanometry. In many older patients, the cartilaginous external auditory canal loses its firmness and partially collapses, narrowing the canal and making earwax removal more difficult.

To facilitate cerumen removal, an approved **cerumenolytic,** a chemical substance known to soften earwax safely, may be used. This substance should be placed into the ear at least an hour before removal is attempted; however, it is preferable for patients to use the substance several times a day for several days prior to cerumen removal. The harder and dryer the cerumen is found to be at examination, the longer the wax takes to soften, but when soft, the wax can often be simply suctioned out of the ear.

Although many audiologists use water irrigation to flush the cerumen from the external auditory canal, many others prefer the use of suction and curettes for mechanical removal. Of course, proper illumination is essential, as from a headlamp or, preferably, a surgical microscope or video otoscope. Audiologists must be careful whenever they insert any object or perform any procedure on a patient's external ear, and all procedures should be duly noted in the patient's chart.

An ancient technique purported to be effective for cerumen removal, which may go back nearly 5,000 years, is called ear candling. For this maneuver, a special hollow candle, usually 10 to 12 inches in length, is placed into the concha, and the opposite end is lighted. The purpose is to create a partial vacuum to remove earwax. Claims that the use of ear candles rid the ear of wax and provide a wide range of "cures" to human maladies are unsupported, and while there is no scientific evidence that there is any medical efficacy in this procedure (Shenk & Dancer, 2004), it remains extremely popular, most especially in third-world countries. In the United States, many thousands of these candles are sold annually, and they are frequently found in health-food stores. A variation of this procedure has been carried out by forming a sheet of paper into a cone, placing the narrow end into the external ear and lighting the more open end. There are no available data to support the use of ear candling, and it is obviously not free of the risk of mild to severe burns.

Perforations of the Tympanic Membrane

The tympanic membrane may become perforated in several ways. Excessive pressure buildup during a middle-ear disorder may cause rupturing of the membrane. Sometimes, in response to infection, usually in the middle ear, the membrane may become necrosed (dead) and perforate.

A frequent cause of perforation is direct trauma from a pointed object such as a cotton swab or hairpin. This may happen if patients are attempting to cleanse their own ears and either misjudge the length of the EAC or are jarred or startled while probing in it. Such accidents are

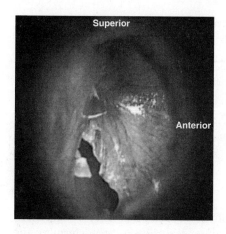

FIGURE 9.17 A dry right inferior tympanic membrane perforation as may be seen following a blow to the ear. The degree of conductive hearing loss secondary to a perforation is greatest in the lower frequencies and depends largely on the size of the perforation. (*Source:* Bechara Y. Ghorayeb, MD; from http://www.ghorayeb.com/Pictures.html.)

extremely painful, as well as embarrassing. The tympanic membrane may also be perforated from sudden pressure in the external ear canal, as created by a hand clapped over the ear or an explosion. The amount of hearing loss produced by a perforated tympanic membrane depends on several variables. The exact size and place of the perforation can cause variations not only in the amount of hearing loss but in the audiometric configuration as well (see Figure 9.17).

Because traumatic perforations alter what is essentially normal tissue, they tend to show spontaneous closure better than do perforations resulting from disease. Perforations in the inferior portion of the tympanic membrane heal more rapidly than those in the superior portion because the normal epithelium migration is more active inferiorly. Placing a thin piece of cigarette paper over the perforation has encouraged the migration of tissue. Often, when a perforation is thus healed, the mucosal and epidermal layers close off the opening but a thin area remains in the fibrous layer, which does not migrate as well. Such thin areas in the tympanic membrane lend themselves to easy reperforation, as from water irrigation of the external canal or even a strong sneeze.

Surgical repair of a perforated tympanic membrane is called **myringoplasty.** In early versions of myringoplasty, skin grafts, usually taken from the inner aspect of the arm, were placed over the perforation. Even though the grafts often "took" initially, they tended to desquamate (flake off), with consequent reperforation. Vein grafts, taken from the patient's hand or arm, later replaced skin grafts. Vein works well for this purpose because its elasticity is similar to that of the fibrous layer of the tympanic membrane; however, narrow veins are inadequate for large perforations. Most middle-ear surgeons today prefer to use fascia, the tough fibrous protective covering over muscle. Results with myringoplasty have been very gratifying.

Measurements on acoustic immittance meters are sometimes impossible because an airtight seal cannot be formed as a consequence of pressure leakage from the air pump of the meter through the perforation into the middle ear. The immittance meter can detect perforations that may not be readily visible with the naked eye because of their small size. If a seal can be obtained when there is a tympanic membrane perforation, the c_1 value will be very large because the air in the outer-ear cavity is continuous with the air in the middle-ear cavity.

Thickening of the Tympanic Membrane

Often, in response to infection, usually of the middle ear, the tympanic membrane becomes thickened and scarred. At times calcium plaques appear, adding to the mass of the tympanic membrane and interfering with its vibration but sometimes causing no appreciable hearing loss. Such conditions are called **tympanosclerosis,** and they do not respond well to medical or surgical treatment (see Figure 9.18).

FIGURE 9.18 Tympanosclerosis, a common abnormality also known as myringosclerosis, is a condition of calcification caused by either inflammation or infection, often following otitis media. Frequently there is no accompanying hearing loss unless the condition becomes more advanced. Tymanosclerosis is most clearly seen in the anterior/inferior quadrant of this right tympanic membrane. The lateral process of the malleus, or "elbow," is seen in the anterior/superior quadrant. (*Source:* Roy F. Sullivan, Ph.D. Audiology Forum: Video Otoscopy, www.rcsullivan.com)

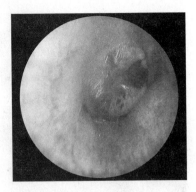

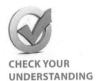

CHECK YOUR UNDERSTANDING

ACTIVITIES

Often the tympanic membrane can become quite thickened. The thickening can be coincidental with disorders of the middle ear, thus making it impossible to determine the amount of hearing loss each disorder contributes.

EVOLVING CASE STUDY

You were introduced to six theoretical case studies in Chapter 2. The next step is to predict, based on your reading of Chapter 9, what the results would be for Case Study 1 on a variety of tests (see the description of Case Study #1 at the end of Chapter 2 before reading the discussion below).

Case Study 1: Conductive Hearing Loss—Outer Ear Disorder

Supra-aural earphones were placed on this child's head, with the receivers positioned where his ears would normally be. He took a reliable hearing test and results showed large air-bone gaps in both ears, with air-conduction thresholds about 50 to 60 dB HL, similar to Figure 9.10. Bone-conduction thresholds were normal with the bone oscillator applied to the forehead. All of the masking (as described in Chapter 6) was accomplished with supra-aural earphones placed on the part of the skull where the external ears are normally situated. Because this child has no external auditory canals, it is impossible to do any tests of acoustic immittance or otoacoustic emissions. Results of ABR would probably result in normal waveforms, all of which are delayed. More testing is needed.

Summary

The outer ear, including the auricle, external auditory canal, and tympanic membrane, is the channel by which sounds from the environment are first introduced to the hearing mechanism. The auricle helps gather the sound, the external auditory canal directs it, and the tympanic membrane vibrates in sympathy with the airborne vibrations that strike it. When portions of the outer ear are abnormal or diseased, hearing may or may not become impaired, depending on which structures are involved and the nature of their involvement.

Abnormalities of the external ear do not affect the sensory/neural mechanism. However, alterations in the canal may cause a change in the osseotympanic mode of bone conduction, which may alter the bone-conduction curve slightly. Audiometric findings on word recognition and site-of-lesion tests are the same as expected for persons with normal hearing. Measurements on the acoustic immittance meter are frequently impossible in external-ear anomalies, by virtue of the disorders themselves.

Whenever an audiologist sees a patient with an external-ear disorder, an otological consultation should be recommended. If hearing is impaired and no medical therapy is available, audiological treatment options should be investigated, depending on the extent of hearing loss and the needs of the patient.

REVIEW TABLE 9.1 The Outer Ear

Anatomical Area	Disorder	Causes Hearing Loss?	Treatment
Auricle	Missing, small, or malformed	No	Plastic surgery
External auditory canal	Wax	Sometimes	Removal
	Infection	Sometimes	Medical treatment
	Atresia	Yes	Surgery
	Stenosis	Sometimes	Observation/surgery
	Foreign bodies	Sometimes	Removal
Tympanic membrane	Perforation	Yes	Surgery
	Thickening	Sometimes	Sometimes

Frequently Asked Questions

Q How does the concha aid in localization of sound?

A *The concha aids in funneling sounds into the external auditory canal. The entire pinna assists both in hearing and in sound localization.*

Q What is the difference between the pars tensa and the pars flaccida?

A *The pars flaccida contains only the epidermal and mucosal layers of the tympanic membrane and not the middle, fibro-cartilaginous layer that tenses the pars tensa.*

Q Can hearing loss due to atresia be helped with hearing aids?

A *Yes, children with atresia should be fitted with aids at the earliest possible time. Because the external auditory canal is closed in aural atresia, bone-conduction aids must be used.*

Q How does frequent swimming in cold water lead to exostoses?

A *Frequent swimming in cold water has been shown to be the cause of exostoses, but the precise reason is not entirely agreed upon.*

Q Are there any distinct characteristics that differentiate temporomandibular joint (TMJ) syndrome from something else?

A *Temporomandibular-joint neuralgia is a major cause of pain, which is referred to the ear in adults. An otolaryngologist usually makes this diagnosis after ruling out infection or other otic abnormalities.*

Q What exactly causes TMJ syndrome?

A *One major cause is malocclusion of the teeth caused by missing or ground down molars. Some cases are also congenital.*

Q What can be done to suppress or cure TMJ syndrome?

A *Some treatments include realignment of the jaw with braces, night guards to reduce bruxation (grinding of the teeth), tooth restoration, some exercises and occasionally maxillofacial surgery.*

Q How do auricle malformations affect the hearing of people with disorders and special needs such as Down syndrome?

A *If all the other ear structures are normal, malformations of the pinna, while they probably do cause sounds to be heard differently, have not been shown to cause hearing loss.*

Q Does ear piercing have any effect on hearing sensitivity?

A *Ear piercing affects hearing sensitivity only if an infection ensues that swells the external auditory canal so that sound cannot efficiently pass through.*

Q How do extremely cold temperatures affect the pinna and external auditory canal? What happens if the pinna has frostbite?

A *Because the pinna protrudes from the head, it is particularly prone to frostbite. Partial or complete amputation of the pinna may result. If the skin of the external auditory canal is affected by frostbite, it may flake off, blocking the canal. This condition is rare, however.*

Q Is it possible for an insect to enter the external auditory canal and perforate the TM?

A *Yes, this has been known to happen. Medical attention should be sought as soon as possible.*

Q Does the hair in the outer ear have a function?

A *It probably assists in keeping insects and other substances from entering the external auditory canal.*

Q Are there other symptoms of Treacher Collins syndrome that are unrelated to hearing?

A *These patients may manifest a number of unusual physical characteristics, including down-slanting eyes, a small and slanting mandible, malformed or underdeveloped pinnas, atresia of the external auditory canal, underdevelopment of the cheekbones and eye sockets, and notched lower eyelids.*

Q What is the best way to remove cerumen, including home remedies?

A *Some of the over-the-counter products for cerumen removal may be used safely, but the surest and safest way is in the hands of a professional trained in cerumen management. Otolaryngologists frequently use gentle suction and mechanical removal under the magnification provided by a surgical microscope. Most audiologists use mechanical removal, although some use suction as well.*

Q Is the cone of light the same in adults and children?

A *Yes.*

Q What is furunculosis?

A *Furunucolosis is the inflammation of a hair follicle.*

Q What is the auricle's function?

A *It helps to gather sound and funnel it into the external auditory canal.*

Q When can osteomas present hearing problems?

A *Osteomas can present hearing problems when their size is such that the lumen of the canal is occluded.*

Q Does stenosis cause hearing loss?

A *Stenosis cannot, by itself, cause hearing loss, but a narrow external auditory canal is more easily occluded by wax and other debris.*

Q How is the TM approached during myringoplasty?

A *The usual approach is via the external auditory canal.*

Q Is the umbo just the point of greatest retraction of the tympanic membrane or is it considered part of the anatomy of the tympanic membrane, or part of the anatomy of the malleus?

A *The umbo is the point of maximum retraction of the tympanic membrane and not an actual piece of anatomy.*

Q I read in my notes that osteomas are bony growths and that osteophytes are bony outgrowths, but I still don't understand the difference between the two.

A *Osteophytes may form in the ear but are not actual tumors, as are osteomas.*

Q The text says that TMJ causes perceived pain in the ear. Can other dental problems cause pain in the ear? For example, can people needing a root canal perceive the pain in their ears?

A *Referred pain is certainly possible in such cases.*

Q What is the difference between pinnaplasty and otoplasty?

A *Otoplasty is the general term for plastic surgery of the ear, while pinnaplasty is limited to the pinna.*

Q What is the name of the surgery for removal of middle-ear fluid?

A *Myringotomy.*

Q What is usually the best procedure when the middle ear is filled with pus?

A *Removal of the pus is commonly done with myringotomy rather than completely relying on antibiotics.*

Q What is the most popular surgical treatment for otosclerosis?

A *Today, it is stapedectomy or stapedotomy.*

Q Why is myringotomy performed?

A *Myringotomy is usually performed to drain fluid from behind the tympanic membrane.*

Q Is otitis media more common among males or females?

A *Like most conditions, it is more common in males.*

Q A common home remedy for curing otitis media is pouring warm olive oil into the ear. Can this remedy be damaging and cause more ear problems?

A *Warm oil is sometimes used as a palliative; that is, it may alleviate the symptoms, but it does not cure the condition. The warmth may be soothing to the aching ear, but oily substances in the external ear canal may collect dirt and create problems of their own. Of course, if the oil is too warm, it may burn the skin.*

Suggested Reading

Hirsch, B. E. (1996). Diseases of the external ear. In C. D. Bluestone, S. E. Stool, & M. A. Kenna (Eds.), *Pediatric otolaryngology* (pp. 378–387). Philadelphia: W. B. Saunders.

Kenna, M. A. (1996). Embryology and developmental anatomy of the ear. In C. D. Bluestone, S. E. Stool, & M. A. Kenna (Eds.), *Pediatric otolaryngology* (pp. 113–126). Philadelphia: W. B. Saunders.

Lipscomb, D. M. (1996). The external and middle ear. In J. L. Northern (Ed.), *Hearing disorders* (pp. 1–13). Boston: Allyn & Bacon.

Zemlin, W. R. (1998). *Speech and hearing science: Anatomy and physiology* (4th ed.). Boston: Allyn & Bacon.

Endnotes

1. For Henry Jones Shrapnell, nineteenth-century British anatomist, 1792–1834.

2. Named for John Langdon Haydon Down, British physician, 1828–1896.

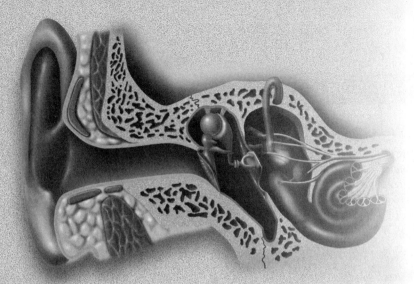

CHAPTER 10

The Middle Ear

LEARNING OBJECTIVES

At the completion of this chapter, the reader should be able to

- Describe the anatomy and physiology of the middle ear.
- Recognize some of the etiologies and treatments of common disorders that produce conductive hearing loss.
- Predict the typical audiometric results for middle-ear pathologies discussed in this chapter.
- Make a reasonable attempt at stating the etiology of a conductive hearing loss based on audiometric and other findings.

THIS CHAPTER ASSUMES a basic understanding of hearing loss as introduced in Chapter 2, the physics of sound in Chapter 3, and the details of hearing tests and their interpretation in Chapters 4 through 7. Oversimplifications of the anatomy of the middle ear and its function, provided as an introduction earlier in this text, should be clarified. The development of the middle ear was no doubt one of evolution's most splendid engineering feats. The middle ear carries vibrations from the outer ear to the inner ear by transferring the sound energy from the air in the outer ear to the fluids of the inner ear. The middle ear overcomes the loss of energy that results when sound passes from one medium (in this case, air) to another medium (fluid).

Anatomy and Physiology of the Middle Ear

An average adult middle ear is an almost oval, air-filled space of roughly 2 cm^3 (about one-half inch high, one-half inch wide, and one-quarter inch deep). The roof of the middle ear is a thin layer of bone, separating the middle-ear cavity from the brain. Below the floor of the middle ear is the **jugular bulb,** and behind the anterior wall is the **carotid artery.** The labyrinth of the inner ear lies behind the medial wall, and the **mastoid process** is beyond the posterior wall. The lateral portion of the middle ear is sometimes called the membranous wall because it contains the tympanic membrane. The space in the middle ear above the tympanic membrane is called the **epitympanic recess.**

As is shown in Figure 10.1, the middle ear is separated from the external auditory canal by the tympanic membrane. The middle ear is connected to the **nasopharynx,** that area where the back of the throat and the nose communicate, via the **eustachian tube,** which is also called the **auditory tube** or **pharyngotympanic tube.** The eustachian tube and middle ear form the **middle-ear cleft.** The entire middle-ear cleft, including the surface of the tympanic membrane that is within the middle ear, is lined with **mucous membrane,** the same lining found in the nose and paranasal sinuses. Much of this mucous membrane is ciliated; that is, the topmost cells contain **cilia,** small hairlike projections that provide a motion similar to that of a wheat field in the wind. The motion of the cilia creates a wiping action that helps to cleanse the middle ear by moving particles down and out of the eustachian tube.

The Eustachian Tube

The eustachian tube[1] enters the middle ear anteriorly at a 30 degree angle in adults and passes down into the nasopharynx for a distance of about 36 millimeters. The tube is lined with ciliated epithelium, and the underlying tissue is bone in the superior one-third and cartilage in the inferior two-thirds. In adults, the tube is normally kept closed by the spring mechanism of cartilage and is opened by the action of four sets of muscles at the orifice of the tube in the nasopharynx. These muscles are the levator veli palatini and the salpingopharyngeus, both of which are innervated by the vagus nerve (cranial nerve X), and the tensor tympani and tensor veli palatini, both of which are innervated by the mandibular portion of the trigeminal nerve (cranial nerve V).

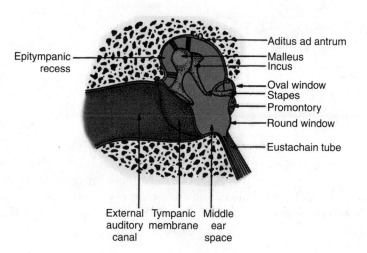

Epitympanic recess

External auditory canal

Tympanic membrane

Middle ear space

Aditus ad antrum
Malleus
Incus
Oval window
Stapes
Promontory
Round window
Eustachain tube

FIGURE 10.1 The human middle ear in cross section.

Opening of the tube occurs during yawning, sneezing, or swallowing, or when excessive air pressure is applied from the nose. While we are awake, our eustachian tubes open about once per minute; during sleep, on an average of once every five minutes. In infants, the eustachian tube is shorter and wider in relation to its length and in a more horizontal plane than it is in adults. The orifice of the eustachian tube in the nasopharynx tends to remain open in infants until the age of about 6 months.

The air pressure of the middle ear must match that of the external auditory canal to keep the pressure equal on both sides of the tympanic membrane to maximize its mobility. The absorption of air by middle-ear tissues is the major reason for the need for a pressure-equalization system. The only way for this pressure equalization to be maintained is through the eustachian tube. At one time or another, most people have had the experience of fullness in the ear—for example, when flying or driving to a higher or lower elevation. During ascension, this fullness results when the air in the external ear canal becomes rarefied (thin), while the middle ear remains at ground-level pressure. The sense of fullness occurs when the tympanic membrane is pushed outward by the greater pressure from within the middle ear. Upon descent, the pressure in the middle ear may be less than in the external ear canal, so that the tympanic membrane is pushed in. The sensations are the same whether the tympanic membrane is pushed in or out. The simple solution is to swallow, yawn, or otherwise open the eustachian tube so that the pressure may be equalized. Because the normal function of the tube is to replenish air pressure, moving from lesser to greater air pressure is more traumatic. At extreme pressures, the eustachian tube locks shut, making pressure-equalization impossible and great pain and tympanic-membrane rupture likely. A type of earplug has been developed for people who experience eustachian-tube difficulties during flying. The plugs are flanged and gradually release pressure during ascent and descent, providing decreased discomfort for many flyers.

Clinical COMMENTARY

Air-pressure differentials between the ambient pressure and that within the middle ear created during air travel can be quite painful for some passengers. The following clinical advice is often given by physicians and may prove helpful to these persons:

1. Take an over-the-counter decongestant one hour prior to takeoff.
2. One-half hour prior to takeoff, spray the nose with a nasal decongestant.
3. One-half hour prior to landing, repeat Step 2.
4. Chew gum and pop the ears, particularly while landing.

The Mastoid

Figure 10.1 shows that some of the bones of the skull that surround the ear are not solid but rather are honeycombed with hundreds of air cells. Each of these cells is lined with mucous membrane, which, though nonciliated, is similar to that of the middle-ear cleft. These cells form the **pneumatic mastoid** of the temporal bone. The middle ear opens up, back, and outward in an area called the **aditus ad antrum** to communicate with the mastoid. The bony protuberance behind the auricle is called the mastoid process.

Windows of the Middle Ear

A section of the bony portion of the inner ear extends into the middle-ear space. This is caused by the basal turn of the cochlea, which is described in Chapter 11. This protrusion is the **promontory** and separates two connections between the middle and inner ear. Above the promontory is the **oval window** and below it the **round window,** both of whose names are derived from their shapes. The round window is covered by a very thin, but tough and elastic, membrane. The oval window is filled by a membrane that supports the base of the stapes, the tiniest bone in the human body.

Bones in the Middle Ear

To accomplish its intended function of carrying sound waves from the air-filled external auditory canal to the fluid-filled inner ear, the middle ear contains a set of three very small bones called **ossicles.** Each of these bones bears a Latin name descriptive of its shape: **malleus, incus, and stapes** (the mallet, anvil, and stirrup, respectively).

The **manubrium** (handle) of the malleus is embedded in the middle (fibrous) layer of the tympanic membrane; it extends from the upper portion of the tympanic membrane to its approximate center (the umbo). The head of the malleus is connected to the body of the incus, and this area of connection extends upward into the aditus ad antrum (or epitympanic recess). Details of the anatomy of the malleus are shown in Figure 10.2. The incus (see Figure 10.3) has a long process, or **crus,** which turns abruptly to a very short crus, the lenticular process. The end of the lenticular process sits squarely on the head of the stapes. As is shown in Figure 10.4, the stapes comprises a head, neck, and two **crura** (plural of crus). The posterior crus is longer and thinner than the anterior crus to aid in its rocking motion. The base, or **footplate,** of the stapes occupies the space in the oval window.

Because the malleus and incus are connected rather rigidly, inward and outward movement of the umbo of the tympanic membrane causes these two bones to rotate, thus transferring this force to the stapes, which in turn results in the inward and outward motion of the oval window. Each of the ossicles is so delicately poised by its ligamental connections within the middle ear that the collective function is unaltered by gravity when the head changes in position. The photograph in Figure 10.5 illustrates the very small size of the ossicles.

FIGURE 10.2 Anatomy of the human malleus.

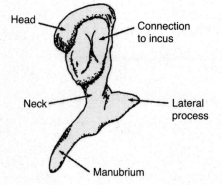

FIGURE 10.3 Anatomy of the human incus.

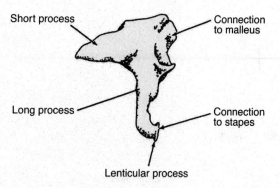

FIGURE 10.4 Anatomy of the human stapes.

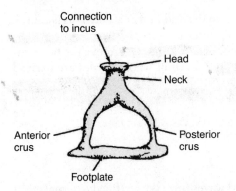

Connection
to incus

Head

Neck

Anterior
crus

Posterior
crus

Footplate

FIGURE 10.5 Three human ossicles shown against a penny to illustrate their small size.

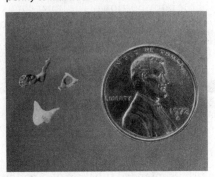

Vibrations of the tympanic membrane are conducted along the ossicular chain to the oval window. The chain (2 to 6 mm in length) acts much like a single unit when transmitting sounds above about 800 Hz. The action of these ossicles provides the energy transformation for which the middle ear is designed.

The Middle-Ear Impedance Matcher

Fish have an organ called the lateral line that is similar in some ways to an unrolled version of the cochlea of the inner ear of humans. As its name implies, this fluid-containing structure runs along the sides of the fish's body. The water in which the fish swims conducts waves that distort the membranes covering the lateral lines, setting the fluids within them into motion. This leads to perception in the fish's brain, the nature of which is not understood. Fish have no need for an impedance matcher.

The average adult tympanic membrane is 85 to 90 mm^2, but the effective vibrating area is only about 55 mm^2. This vibrating area is 17 times that of the oval window. Therefore, the sound pressure collected over the larger area of the tympanic membrane is concentrated on the oval window, which increases the sound pressure in the same way that a hose increases water pressure when a thumb or a finger is placed over the opening. What results is not a greater volume of water but greater pressure. The drawing in Figure 10.6 illustrates this action.

FIGURE 10.6 Sound pressure collected over the surface area of the tympanic membrane is concentrated on the (smaller) surface area of the oval window, thus increasing the pressure.

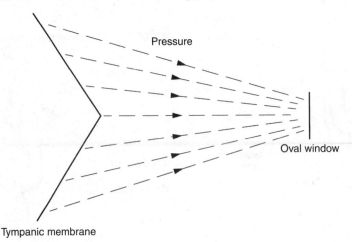

Pressure

Oval window

Tympanic membrane

Despite the exquisite engineering of the middle ear, all sound pressure delivered to the tympanic membrane is not made available to the inner ear because the middle-ear mechanism is not 100 percent efficient as an impedance-matching device.

The mass of the ossicular chain (malleus = 25 mg, incus = 25 mg, stapes = 2.5 mg) is poised to take advantage of the physical laws of leverage. Figure 10.7 illustrates this simple principle. Through leverage, the force received at the footplate of the stapes is greater than that applied at the malleus. In this way, the ratio of tympanic membrane displacement to oval window displacement is increased by about 1.3:1. The ossicular chain actually rocks back and forth on an axis, and the action of the stapes in the oval window is not that of a piston but rather that of a pivot.

The combined effects of increased pressure and the lever action of the malleus result in a pressure increase at the oval window 23 times what it would be if airborne sound impinged on it directly. This value is equivalent to approximately 30 dB, remarkably close to the 28 dB loss that would be caused by the air-to-fluid impedance mismatch without the ossicular chain. The fact that the tympanic membrane is conical, rather than flat, assists slightly in the process of impedance matching by increasing the force and decreasing the velocity because the handle of the malleus does not move with the same amplitude as the tympanic membrane.

FIGURE 10.7 Demonstration of the advantage of lever action. Note that the advantage is increased in B when the fulcrum is moved closer to the mass to be lifted.

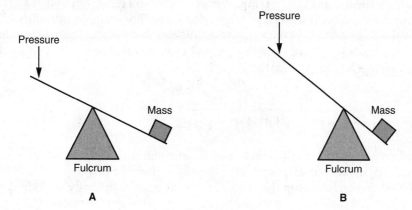

Nonauditory Structures in the Middle Ear

The middle ear contains several structures that are unrelated to hearing. The **fallopian canal,** containing a portion of the facial (VIIth cranial) nerve, passes through the middle ear as a protrusion on its medial wall. The fallopian canal is a bony channel covered with mucous membrane. The **facial nerve** runs beside the auditory (VIIIth cranial) nerve as the two travel to the brain stem, about which more is said in Chapter 12.

The **chorda tympani nerve** is a branch of the facial nerve that passes through the middle-ear space. This nerve carries information about the sensation of taste from the anterior two-thirds of one side of the tongue. Unfortunately, the chorda tympani frequently acts as an obstruction during middle-ear surgery. Sometimes the nerve is accidentally or intentionally sacrificed to increase visibility of the operative field. Taste changes caused by surgical severance of the chorda tympani nerve frequently disappear after several months.

Two muscles, the primary functions of which continue to be debated, are active in each middle ear. It has been thought that contractions of these muscles may serve a protective function for the inner ear by stiffening the ossicular chain and attenuating loud, and therefore potentially damaging, sounds that enter it. It is known, however, that the latency of the reflex is too long to protect the inner ear from impulsive sounds such as gunshots. Contraction of these muscles may additionally serve to decrease the loudness of sounds generated within the head, for example, by chewing or speaking.

The **stapedius muscle** (length 7 mm, cross section 5 mm^2) originates in the posterior (mastoid) wall of the middle ear. The stapedius tendon emerges through a tiny hole in the mastoid wall, but the muscle itself is in a canal beside the facial canal. The tendon attaches to the posterior portion of the neck of the stapes. When the stapedius muscle is contracted, the stapes moves to the side and tenses the membrane in the oval window, reducing the amplitude of vibration. It is possible that contraction of the stapedius muscle may help to improve speech recognition in noise by attenuating the low-frequency components of the noise. The stapedius muscle is innervated by a branch of the facial nerve. In addition to its function of attaching the stapedius muscle to the stapes, the stapedius tendon also supplies blood to the lenticular process of the incus.

The **tensor tympani muscle** (length 25 mm, cross section 5 mm^2) is also encased in a small bony cavity. The tendon from this muscle inserts into the manubrium of the malleus and, upon contraction, moves the malleus so that the tympanic membrane becomes tense. The innervation of the tensor tympani is from the **trigeminal nerve** (Vth cranial nerve).

Both the stapedius and tensor tympani muscles respond reflexively and bilaterally, but in humans only the stapedius is thought to respond to sound. For example, introduction of a loud sound into the right ear causes both stapedius muscles to contract. The tensor tympani can be caused to contract by a jet of air in the external auditory canal or the eye and by changes in temperature or touch in the external auditory canal.

Development of the Middle Ear

During embryonic or fetal development, specific anatomical areas form, or differentiate. Like the outer ear, the middle ear and eustachian tube form from the pharyngeal arch system, limited to the first two arches. As in the outer ear and all areas of the body, developmental milestones are somewhat variant and at times should be viewed as approximate.

Both the middle-ear space and the eustachian tube form the first pharyngeal pouch, which is lined with entoderm. During gestation, the middle-ear space is filled with mesenchyme (a diffuse network of cells forming the embryonic mesoderm) as the ossicles are developing. The ciliated epithelium that lines these spaces also arises from the entoderm. The oval window is formed by about the 47th gestational day.

The ossicles first form as cartilage of the first and second pharyngeal arches. The superior portions of the incus and malleus, which form the incudomalleal joint, come from the first arch. The lower parts of the incus and malleus, and the superstructure of the stapes, come from the second arch. The base of the stapes forms from the otic capsule.

At about 29 to 32 days, tissue forms that will become the malleus and incus. By the 12th fetal week, the ossicles differentiate and are fully formed by the 16th week as cartilaginous structures begin to ossify. Almost total ossification of the malleus and incus has taken place by the 21st week. The 24th week shows rapid ossification of the incus and stapes. The middle-ear muscles derive from mesenchyme, the tensor tympani from the first arch, and the stapedius from the second arch.

Hearing Loss and the Middle Ear

Abnormalities of the middle ear produce conductive hearing losses. The air-conduction level drops in direct relationship with the amount of attenuation produced by the disorder. Theoretically, bone conduction should be unchanged from normal unless the inner ear becomes involved; however, our knowledge of middle-ear anatomy and physiology should make our understanding of the effects of inertial bone conduction even clearer. Conductive hearing losses produced by middle-ear disorders may show alteration in the bone-conduction thresholds without sensory/neural involvement. The amount of sensory/neural impairment in mixed hearing losses may be exaggerated by artifacts of bone conduction. These facts were demonstrated in a report by Orchik, Schumaier, Shea, and Xianxi (1995), where, in one case, the bone-conduction thresholds were significantly altered by a displacement of a prosthetic device used in middle-ear surgery.

Disorders of the Middle Ear and Their Treatments

Negative Middle-Ear Pressure

Many, although not all, middle-ear disorders arise from poor function of the eustachian tube. Eustachian tube function may fail for a number of reasons. Two of the most common causes are edema of the eustachian tube secondary to infection or allergy and blockage of the orifice of the eustachian tube by hypertrophied (overgrown) adenoids. Structural abnormalities of the mechanism responsible for opening the tube are sometimes also present.

Any condition that interferes with the eustachian tube's function of equating air pressure between the middle ear and outer ear may result in a drop in pressure as the air trapped within the middle ear becomes absorbed by the tissues that line it without normal replenishment through the eustachian tube. When this absorption occurs, the greater pressure in the external auditory canal causes the tympanic membrane to be retracted (Figure 10.8). The retraction from eustachian-tube dysfunction (ETD) interferes with the normal vibration of the tympanic membrane and may produce a slight conductive hearing loss.

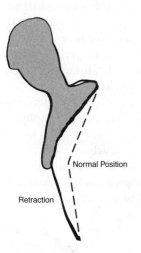

FIGURE 10.8 Retracted tympanic membrane caused by negative middle-ear pressure.

A method has been developed to use an immittance meter to test eustachian-tube function, if the tympanic membrane is intact, by using a pressure swallow technique (Williams, 1975). The patient is asked to swallow normally, after which a tympanogram is run. Then +400 daPa of pressure is applied to the membrane, and the patient is asked to swallow four times; a second tympanogram is then run on the same graph. Pressure is returned to 0 daPa, and the patient swallows again to equalize middle-ear pressure. Finally, the patient is asked to swallow four times with −400 daPa in the external auditory canal, and a third tympanogram is run. If the eustachian tube is normal, the peaks of the three tympanograms differ by at least 15 daPa. Differences smaller than this suggest dysfunction because the tube cannot equalize the middle-ear pressure.

When a retracted tympanic membrane is diagnosed and no infectious fluids are present in the nose, the otologist may elect to pressurize the middle ear through a process called **politzerization.**[2] One nostril is held closed while an olive tip, connected to a tube or nebulizer, is held tightly in the other nostril. The patient elevates the soft palate by saying "k-k-k" and then swallows; the otologist, meanwhile, observes the movement of the tympanic membrane during this process. In this fashion, tympanic membrane perforation or eustachian tube failure may be diagnosed.

The patient may autoinflate the eustachian tube by increased pressure on forced expiration with the nostrils held shut, a maneuver called **Valsalva**[3] that must be performed by divers as they descend or surface. Patients are often taught the Valsalva maneuver following middle-ear surgery. The **Toynbee maneuver**[4] accomplishes eustachian tube opening when the patient closes the jaw, holds the nose, and swallows.

Figure 10.9A and B illustrate a mild conductive hearing loss in the left ear. The bone-conduction results are essentially normal, as are word-recognition scores. Results on all site-of-lesion tests are expected to suggest conductive hearing loss. Acoustic immittance measurements show normal compliance in both ears, with a Type C tympanometric function in the left ear typical of negative middle-ear pressure (see Figure 10.10). All of these findings are produced by the partial vacuum set up within the left middle-ear space.

Suppurative Otitis Media

One of the most common disorders of the middle ear causing conductive hearing loss is infection of the middle-ear space, or **otitis media.** Otitis media is any infection of the mucous-membrane lining of the middle-ear cleft. It is seen in nearly 70 percent of children born in the United States before they are 2 years old, with more than half of these children experiencing further episodes. The common cold is the only illness seen more frequently in children (Brooks, 1994). Otitis media is more common in children than adults because their eustachian tubes are horizontal and shorter, making the entrance of bacteria to the middle ear easier. The diameter of the tube is also smaller in children, thus making fluid drainage more difficult. Children are also prone to respiratory infections because their immune systems are still developing.

Recent years have seen a dramatic increase in pediatric ear, nose, and throat infections (most frequently ear infections) caused by the difficult-to-treat methicillin-resistant staphylococcus aureus (MRSA) bacteria (Naseri, Jerris, & Sobol, 2009). MRSA is a strain of staph infection found to be highly resistant to broad-spectrum antibiotics. MRSA, which may be related to large-scale inappropriate use of antibiotics, can lead to dangerous, life-threatening invasive infections. Once limited mostly to nursing homes and healthcare settings, MSRA is frequently contracted within the community through direct skin-to-skin contact or contact with surfaces that have been contaminated with germs from cuts or open wounds.

Factors that predispose an individual to otitis media include poorly functioning eustachian tubes, **barotrauma** (sudden changes in air pressure, as when flying or diving), abnormalities in the action of the cilia of the mucous membranes, anatomical deformities of the middle

FIGURE 10.9 (A) Worksheet showing the need for and use of masking the right ear during bone-conduction tests on the left ear with the forehead as the oscillator placement site. The result is a mild conductive loss in the left ear. (B) Audiogram illustrating a mild conductive hearing loss in the left ear produced by a retracted tympanic membrane. The right ear is normal. Masking was required for bone-conduction and word-recognition tests for the left ear. The Weber lateralizes to the left ear at all frequencies.

AIR CONDUCTION

Earphones Insert ☒ Supra Aural ☐	RIGHT									LEFT								
	250	500	1000	1500	2000	3000	4000	6000	8000	250	500	1000	1500	2000	3000	4000	6000	8000
Masking Type WB ☐ NB ☐	5	0	5/5	5	0	5	10	10	5	15	20	20/20	15	15	20	15	15	15
EM Level in Opp. Ear																		

BONE CONDUCTION

Placement Forehead ☒ Mastoid ☐	RIGHT						FOREHEAD						LEFT					
	250	500	1000	2000	3000	4000	250	500	1000	2000	3000	4000	250	500	1000	2000	3000	4000
Masking Type WB ☐ NB ☐							0	5	0	0	0	5	5*	5*	5*	0*	0*	5*
EM Level in Opp. Ear													30	10	20	0	5	10

	2 Freq	3 Freq	Variable	WEBER							2 Freq	3 Freq	Variable
Pure Tone Average	0	2	5	L	L	L	L	L	L	Pure Tone Average	18	18	18

A

SPEECH AUDIOMETRY

Masking Type WB ☐ Speech ☒	RIGHT				LEFT			
	SRT 1	SRT 2	Recognition 1	Recognition 2	SRT 1	SRT 2	Recognition 1	Recognition 2
	0		List 1A 30HL 100 %	List 1B 40HL 98 *%	15		List 2C 45HL 98 %	List 4D 60HL 100 *%
EM Level in Opp. Ear				40				25

FREQUENCY IN HERTZ

Speech Presentation

	MLV	Recorded
SRT	☒	☐
WRS	☐	☒

AUDIOGRAM KEY

B

ear and eustachian tube, age, race, socioeconomic factors, and the integrity of the individual's immune system. This last fact suggests that the growing epidemic of acquired immune deficiency syndrome (AIDS) will probably increase the incidence of otitis media. External factors associated with otitis media include exposure to cigarette smoke or other fumes. A link has been found between otitis media and Haemophilus influenza in the nasal passages of children. There is apparently also a gene that is linked to otitis media, and so both treatment and avoidance techniques may change dramatically in the not-too-distant future.

FIGURE 10.10 Typical results on immittance tests performed on a patient with a normal right-ear (Type A) and left negative middle-ear pressure (Type C). Static compliance is within the normal range for both ears. The right ipsilateral acoustic reflex threshold is normal, and the left ipsilateral acoustic reflex is absent. When the reflex-activating signal is introduced to the (normal) right ear (contralateral right stimulation), the acoustic reflex is shown here as present but may, in such cases, be absent. The hearing loss in the left ear causes the contralateral reflex to be absent when the RAS is presented to the left ear.

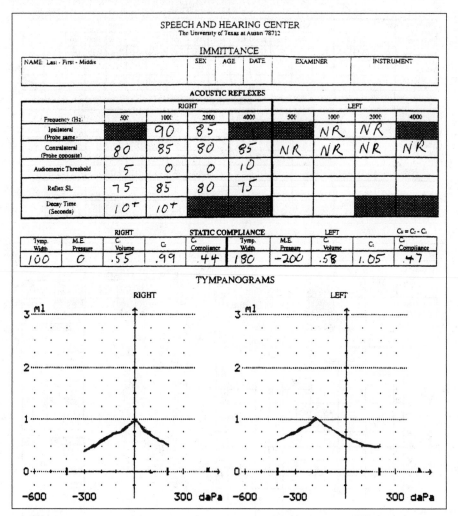

Although otitis media is primarily a disease of childhood, it can occur at any age. There are clear seasonal effects (otitis media is most common in the winter months), but it is less clear why the disease is more common in males than in females. Also difficult to explain are the differences in incidence among racial groups. Otitis media is most common in Eskimos and Native Americans, less common in whites, and least common in blacks (Giebink, 1984). The interrelationships among socioeconomic, anatomical, and genetic differences are unclear.

As a rule, organisms gain access to the middle ear through the eustachian tube from the nasopharynx. They travel as a subepithelial extension of a sinusitis or pharyngitis, spreading the infection up through the tube. Often the infection is literally blown through the lumen of the tube by a stifled sneeze or by blowing the nose too hard. In general, it is probably a good idea not to teach small children to blow their noses at all. They should also be encouraged to minimize pressure through the eustachian tube when sneezing by keeping their mouths open. Infection may also enter the middle ear through the external auditory canal if there is a perforation in the tympanic membrane. Bloodborne infection from another site in the body may occur, but this source of middle-ear infection is less common.

As stated earlier, infection usually begins at the orifice of the eustachian tube and spreads throughout the middle-ear cavity. When the tube is infected, it becomes swollen, interfering with its middle-ear pressure-equalization function. Also, when the tubal lining becomes swollen, the cleansing action of the cilia is compromised, and the infection is spread to adjacent tissues. A major contributing cause of otitis media, especially in children, is exposure to tobacco smoke. One study shows that in households in which more than three packages of cigarettes are smoked in a day, the risk to children of otitis media and other respiratory infections is four times more than it would be without such exposure (Kraemer et al., 1983).

Parents often report that as little as several hours may elapse between the appearance of initial symptoms and a full-blown infection in their children. In such rapidly progressing cases, it is probable that fluids that functioned as a culture medium for **purulent** (pus-producing) organisms had previously been deposited in the middle ear, perhaps from an earlier bacterial or viral infection. The rate of spread is also related to the virulence of the organisms.

In cases of otitis media, medical treatment is imperative. Proper diagnosis of the several usual stages can result in appropriate therapy. In the initial stage of eustachian tube swelling, causing occlusion of the tube, negative middle-ear pressure may be set up. The tympanic membrane may appear to be retracted (sucked in). Often audiometric examination reveals normal hearing on all tests. The tympanometric function may appear as a Type C, suggesting that the pressure within the middle ear is lower than that of the external auditory canal.

Before the actual accumulation of pus in the middle ear, the tympanic membrane and middle-ear mucosa may become very vascular. This inflammation produces the so-called red ear described by many physicians. If the condition is allowed to continue beyond this stage, suppuration (production of pus) may result. Enzymes are usually produced by bacterial infections, some of which have a dissolving effect on middle-ear structures. In **suppurative** otitis media, the mucosa becomes filled with excessive amounts of blood, the superficial cells break down, and pus accumulates. Patients complain of pain in the ear, their pulse rates and body temperatures become elevated, and they are visibly ill. If pressure from the pus goes up, there is compression of the small veins and capillaries in the middle ear, resulting in **necrosis** (death) of the mucosa, submucosa, and tympanic membrane. If the condition continues even further, the tympanic membrane may eventually rupture. Pus that cannot find its way out of the middle ear may invade the mastoid. The resulting **mastoiditis** causes a breakdown of the walls separating the air cells. Untreated mastoiditis can result in meningitis and sometimes death.

Before the development of antibiotics, mastoiditis, secondary to otitis media, was often uncontrolled and was a common cause of death. Often the trigeminal nerve (cranial nerve V) became involved, causing retro-orbital pain and involvement of the abducens (cranial nerve VI) and leading to paralysis. Patients complained of photophobia (light sensitivity) and excessive lacrimation (tearing), along with fever and pain. It is disappointing to note that even in modern times, because of inadequate medical care, entire communities manifest these symptoms, along with headaches, fever, paralysis of the muscles of mastication (chewing), double vision, and hearing loss.

The general category of suppurative otitis media is frequently dichotomized by the terms **chronic** and **acute.** As a rule, the chronic form implies a condition of long standing. Symptoms of acute otitis media generally develop rapidly and include swelling, redness, and bleeding. Bleeding in the middle ear may also be caused by barotrauma, when there is a sudden pressure change, causing the blood vessels in the lining of the middle ear to rupture. Bleeding in the middle ear from any cause is called **hemotympanum.**

Audiometric Findings in Suppurative Otitis Media

Otitis media results in the typical audiogram of conductive hearing loss (see Figure 10.11A and B). Generally, the amount of hearing loss is directly related to the accumulation of fluid in the middle ear. The audiometric contour is usually rather flat, showing approximately

FIGURE 10.11 (A) Worksheet for a moderate bilateral conductive hearing loss. Masking was required for both ears during bone-conduction tests, with the forehead as the oscillator site. Masking for air-conduction was not necessary because insert earphones were used for testing, thereby increasing the interaural attenuation. They would have been required if supra-aural phones had been used. (B) Audiogram illustrating a moderate conductive hearing loss in both ears. The contour of the audiogram is relatively flat and fairly typical of otitis media. Word-recognition scores are excellent. Note that masking is not necessary for air conduction or SRT because insert receivers are used and they provide significant interaural attenuation. Masking is required for bone-conduction tests and word-recognition testing.

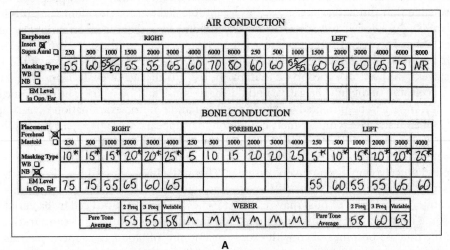

A

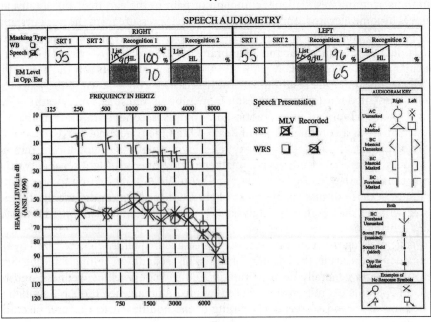

B

FIGURE 10.12 Typical results on immittance tests performed on a patient with bilateral otitis media or serous effusion (see Figure 10.11). Note that the tympanogram is Type B, the tympanometric width is high, the static compliance is low, and acoustic reflexes are absent in both ears.

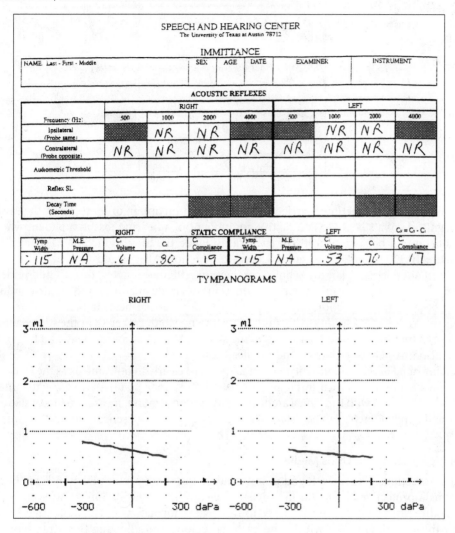

equal amounts of hearing loss across frequencies. Word-recognition scores are generally excellent, although proper masking must often be instituted to ensure against cross hearing. Bone-conduction results are usually normal.

Measurements of static compliance show lower-than-normal values. The tympanometric function is a Type B (see Figure 10.12) suggesting the presence of fluid behind the tympanic membrane. Acoustic reflexes cannot be elicited in either ear because the intensity of each reflex-activating stimulus, even at maximum levels of the immittance meter, is below the acoustic reflex threshold. Additionally, abnormalities of the middle ear cause increased impedance of the ossicular chain, which resists movement in response to contraction of the stapedius muscle. Figure 10.13 shows that the latencies of all the waves resulting from ABR testing are increased at all sensation levels. No otoacoustic emissions can be evoked (see Figure 10.14).

FIGURE 10.13 Results of auditory brain-stem response testing on the patient with a bilateral conductive hearing loss caused by otitis media (see Figure 10.11).

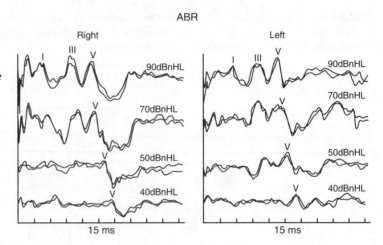

ABR testing is sometimes carried out by bone conduction in order to verify the existence and magnitude of a suspected conductive component of a hearing loss in a patient who cannot cooperate on behavioral tests. In such cases, while the air-conduction ABR would look like Figure 10.13, results of the normal bone-conduction ABR would look like Figures 7.13 and 7.14. If audiologists plan to do bone-conduction ABR audiometry, they should remember to norm their equipment using a bone-conduction oscillator in addition to an air-conduction receiver because the correction factors are different for normal-hearing persons. It must also be remembered that for testing ABR on infants, the mastoid, rather than the forehead, is the preferred testing site because the sutures in the skull may not be closed, creating a larger-than-normal disparity between mastoid and forehead results.

Many or all of the audiometric results that point so clearly to otitis media as the cause of the conductive hearing loss shown in Figures 10.11 and 10.12 may be unattainable in the infant or small child. However, with a minimal amount of patient cooperation, measurements of static compliance and tympanometry can be obtained and may suggest the presence of middle-ear infection.

Antibiotic Treatment of Otitis Media

Bacterial infections, like those found in otitis media, survive by multiplication. Each bacterial cell forms a protective capsule around itself to ensure its survival. Some antibiotics kill the bacteria directly. Other antibiotics serve to inhibit the formation of the protective covering, thereby limiting the growth within the bacterial colony and allowing the white blood cells to surround and carry off the bacteria. When a substantial pocket of infection exists, as in suppurative otitis media, the mass of bacteria, by virtue of numbers alone, may resist a complete bacteria-killing action. Different drugs are specific to different organisms, and unless the appropriate drug is prescribed, the action may be less than useful. Modern laboratory facilities allow for culturing the organism causing the infection, so that the physician may take advantage of the specificity of a given antibiotic. One problem in using antibiotics when a pocket of infected fluid exists in any part of the body is that the antibiotics travel through the bloodstream and have difficulty passing from the bloodstream to the site of the infection.

When the middle ear is filled with pus, produced by the body to carry cells to the area to ingest the bacteria, frequently the best procedure is to remove the pus, rather than to rely completely on the effects of antibiotics. As long as the tympanic membrane remains intact, antibiotic drops in the external ear canal can have no therapeutic effect in cases of otitis media because the drops cannot reach the infection.

FIGURE 10.14 Objective hearing test results showing absent otoacoustic emissions because of a conductive hearing loss (see Figure 10.11). Latency-intensity functions for wave V are shown as derived from the auditory brainstem response tracings shown in Figure 10.13 on the patient with a bilateral conductive hearing loss. The latencies of all waves are increased at all levels tested.

SPEECH AND HEARING CENTER
The University of Texas at Austin 78712

NAME: Last - First - Middle	SEX	AGE	DATE	EXAMINER	RELIABILITY	INSTRUMENT

OTOACOUSTIC EMISSIONS
(Present or Absent)

☑ TEOAE Level **80** dB Peak SPL
☐ DPOAE Level F₁____ F₂____

	Right						Left		
500	1000	2000	4000	6000	500	1000	2000	4000	6000
A	A	A	A	A	A	A	A	A	A

AUDITORY BRAINSTEM RESPONSE

ABR WAVE V LATENCY-INTENSITY FUNCTION

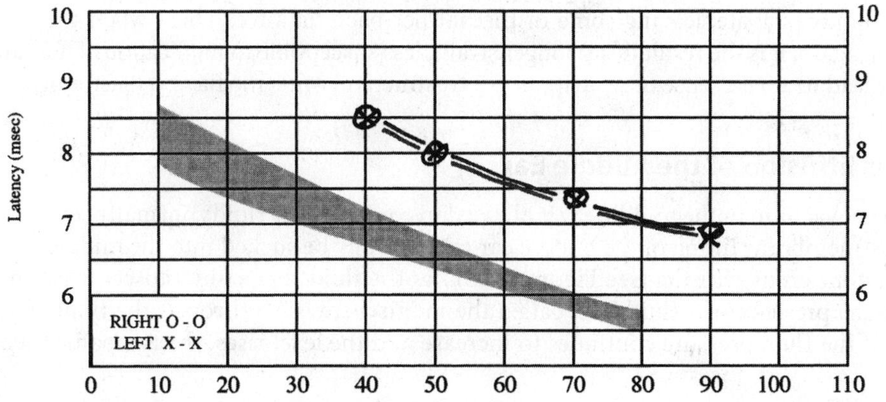

RIGHT O - O
LEFT X - X

Latency (msec) / INTENSITY (dBnHL)

SHADED AREA REPRESENTS Normal Wave V Range for patients older than 16 mos. for 30 clicks per second

EAR	nHL		Absolute Latency (ms)			Interpeak Latency (ms)			Latency Change w/ Increased Rate	
	dB HL	Click Rate	I	III	V	I-III	III-V	I-V	V	Click Rate
RIGHT	90	33.1	2.7	5.1	6.85	2.4	1.75	4.15		
LEFT	90	33.1	2.8	5.0	6.8	2.2	1.8	4.0		
Interaural Differences										

Amplitude Ratio (V same or > I) R _NL_ L _NL_
Estimated Air Conduction Threshold R≤ _90_ L ≤ _40_
Estimated Bone Conduction Threshold R ____ L ____

The American Academy of Pediatrics revised the guidelines for treating acute otitis media (Lieberthal et al., 2013). Acute otitis media presents as a rapid onset of inflamation of the middle ear. The revised guidelines were designed in part to reduce the overuse of unnecessary antibiotics, which leads to antibiotic-resistant bacteria. The guidelines recommend limiting prescription of antibiotics to those children with severe ear infection, defined as significant pain or fever of 102.2 degrees or higher. Less severe infection tends to clear on its own with physician monitoring and medication to relieve pain. Children whose infection persists for 72 hours are given antibiotics.

It should be noted that chronic otitis media can place a child at risk for the development of a high-frequency sensory/neural hearing loss secondary to the long-standing infection. In some cases of chronic otitis media, toxins in the middle ear can pass through the round window membrane, leading to both outer and inner hair cell damage within the basal turn of the cochlea (Cureoglu et al., 2004).

Dormant Otitis Media

The introduction of antibiotics at the close of World War II drastically altered the treatment of otitis media. Although antibiotics have dramatically decreased the number of serious effects of otitis media, they have also had some undesirable side effects. Unless the proper type and dosage of antibiotics are used, the disease may go not to resolution but to a state of quiescence. Because the overt symptoms may disappear, both the physician and patient may assume a complete cure. Several weeks later, the patient may experience what seems like a whole new attack of otitis media, which is in reality an exacerbation of the same condition experienced earlier but was allowed to lie dormant. Many patients discontinue their own antibiotic treatments when their symptoms abate, leaving some of the hardier bacteria alive. Then, when the condition flares up again, it is the result of a stronger strain, less susceptible to medication. Thus, antibiotics may lead to a false sense of security in the treatment of otitis media and mastoiditis.

Serous Effusion of the Middle Ear

If a partial vacuum in the middle ear is allowed to continue, the fluids normally secreted by the mucous-membrane lining of the middle ear may literally be sucked into the middle-ear space, resulting in serous effusion (see Figure 10.15). As the fluid level rises, otoscopic examination reveals the presence of a fluid line, called the **meniscus,** visible through the tympanic membrane. If the fluid pressure continues to increase and the level rises, the tympanic membrane

FIGURE 10.15 A left serous otitis media showing a retracted tympanic membrane and air-fluid levels (meniscus) in the middle ear. (*Source:* Bechara Y. Ghorayeb, MD; from http://www.ghorayeb.com/Pictures.html.)

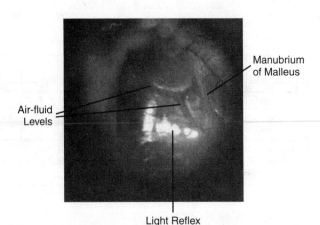

may return to its normal position when the meniscus rises above the superior margin of the tympanic membrane. At this stage, the condition is sometimes difficult to diagnose visually.

When fluid fills the middle-ear space, a Type B tympanometric function results (Figure 10.12). This function occurs because no amount of air pressure delivered to the tympanic membrane from the pump of the immittance meter can match the pressure on the middle-ear side of the tympanic membrane. Because a serous accumulation in the middle ear affects the mass of the system, it is expected that the audiogram will initially show a greater loss for higher- than for lower-frequency sounds (Figure 10.16A and B). It is likely that the slightly depressed

FIGURE 10.16 (A) Worksheet showing the need for and use of masking for bone-conduction tests in both ears at all frequencies, with the forehead as the oscillator placement site. The result is a bilateral conductive hearing loss. (B) Audiogram illustrating conductive hearing loss in both ears produced by serous effusion. Note that masking was needed at all frequencies for bone conduction and word recognition. Speech recognition is normal, the Weber does not lateralize, and the audiogram falls noticeably in the higher frequencies.

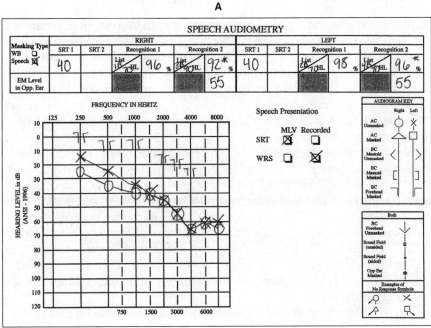

A

bone-conduction thresholds in Figure 10.16B are artifacts produced by the fluid in the middle ear. Post-treatment audiograms would probably show a disappearance of the air-bone gap and some improvement in the bone-conduction thresholds.

Because serous effusion is often secondary to a poorly functioning eustachian tube, drug therapy, including decongestants or decongestant–antihistamine combinations, has long been used to restore normal middle-ear pressure and to help clear the tube of secretions. However, decongestants are now believed to be almost useless for this purpose in infants and small children, whose eustachian tubes are less efficient than those of adults. Because the middle ear may not be actively infected during serous effusion, antibiotics are not frequently indicated. However, some physicians prescribe antibiotics prophylactically because the fluid, though sterile, may serve as a culture base for bacterial infection. There is evidence that the three organisms most associated with otitis media in children have become resistant to the most commonly used antibiotics (Brooks, 1994). Even if antibiotics destroy the organisms causing the condition, they cannot eliminate the fluids that have formed in the middle-ear space.

Clinical COMMENTARY

Decongestants are frequently prescribed in cases of middle-ear fluid to promote drainage through the eustachian tube. In young children, such treatments may be less successful because the eustachian tube is relatively horizontal compared to the steeper angle attained by age 6 or 7 years. The slight angle of the eustachian tubes of young children leads to a greater propensity for fluid accumulation in their middle ears.

Surgical Treatment for Middle-Ear Fluid

In the days predating antibiotics, therapy for otitis media was primarily surgical. Today surgery is still required in many cases. The primary purpose of surgery for patients with infection in the middle ear is to eliminate disease. Reconstructing a damaged hearing apparatus is an important but secondary goal.

If the fluid pressure continues to build within the middle ear, perforation of the tympanic membrane becomes a threat. If perforation appears imminent or disease-laden fluids are present in the middle ear and must be removed, the otologist may elect to perform a *myringotomy*, or *myringostomy* (incision into the tympanic membrane) to relieve the fluid pressure and suction out the remaining fluid. Frequently, a plastic **pressure-equalizing (PE) tube**, or tympanostomy tube, is inserted through the incision in the tympanic membrane to keep the middle ear patent. Figure 10.17 shows a myringotomy incision and a PE tube in position. A photograph of one kind of PE tube is shown in Figure 10.18. The derivation of the word *myringotomy* is from *myringa*, modern Latin for "drum membrane," and *tome*, Greek for "cutting." It is also called *myringocentesis, tympanotomy, tympanostomy,* or *paracentesis of the tympanic membrane.* Myringotomy is frequently performed as a simple office operation, but at times, especially with some small children, it requires brief hospitalization. An incision is made with a special knife, generally in the inferior-posterior quadrant of the tympanic membrane. As in the discussion of serous effusion, the fluids are removed by a suction tip placed through the incision. If myringotomy is performed on small children while they are awake, they must be immobilized sufficiently so that any sudden movement does not redirect the action of the knife, which could possibly cause damage to the middle ear. As a rule, children are lightly anesthetized for the procedure.

Wilder and colleagues (2009) have reported a possible association between repeated surgical procedures with anesthesia prior to 4 years of age and the development of learning disabilities. It remains uncertain whether anesthesia was the determining factor in learning

FIGURE 10.17 (A) A myringotomy incision in the same ear as Figure 10.16. The air-fluid meniscus is still present prior to aspiration of the middle ear effusion. (B) A pressure-equalizing tube positioned through the tympanic membrane to allow for middle-ear ventilation. (*Source:* Bechara Y. Ghorayeb, MD; from http://www.ghorayeb.com/Pictures.html.)

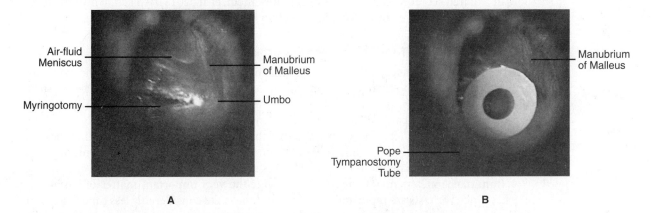

A   B

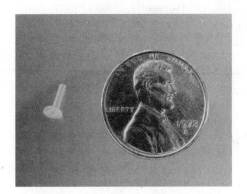

FIGURE 10.18 A pressure-equalizing (PE) tube shown next to a penny to illustrate its small size.

disabilities in the children studied or whether the condition requiring surgical intervention with anesthesia is a marker for unidentified contributing factors to the development of learning disabilities, so this is a subject requiring further inquiry.

Many individuals believe that the purpose of the PE tube is to permit fluid drainage from the middle ear. The actual function of the tube is to allow for direct ventilation of the middle ear, and it functions as an artificial eustachian tube to maintain normal middle-ear air pressure. The plastic tube provides a second vent to the middle ear, which acts much in the same way as the second hole punched in the top of a can of liquid. Air may enter the middle ear via the tube, allowing drainage down the eustachian tube. The tubes may remain in position from several weeks to several months, after which time some types extrude naturally and fall into the external auditory canal. In the interim, the eustachian tube problem should be appropriately handled when possible through adenoidectomy, allergic desensitization, or whatever medical means seem to be indicated.

To avoid multiple myringostomies in patients with unresolving eustachian tube problems, a tube has been developed that can stay in position almost indefinitely. Although surgical insertion is more complicated and lengthy than with the traditional PE tubes, the clinical experience with these Teflon-lined tubes holds promise for better long-term relief (Jahn, 1993).

Some otologists have found that tubes remain in position longer if they are placed in the superior-anterior quadrant of the tympanic membrane because there is less migration of epithelium in this area than in the larger inferior quadrants. Positioning the tube in this superior area requires the use of a surgical microscope. Failure to resolve the eustachian tube difficulty frequently leads to a recurrent attack of serous effusion. Recent guidelines address issues of patient selection as well as surgical implications for the use and management of tympanostomy tubes in children six months to 12 years of age (Rosenfeld, et al., 2013). An actual myringotomy (myringostomy) with tube insertion can be seen in the video titled Myringostomy.

Immittance Testing for Tube Patency and Eustachian Tube Function

Acoustic immittance meters can be very useful in diagnosing perforations of the tympanic membrane, even those too small to be seen with an ordinary otoscope (Chapter 7). The **physical-volume test (PVT)** can be used in the same way to test the patency of pressure-equalizing tubes placed through the tympanic membrane. If the clinician observes that c_1 is an unusually large value, in excess of 5 cm^3, it may be assumed that this measurement is of a cavity that includes both the outer-ear canal and the middle ear. Of course, many patients, especially children, have tympanic membrane perforations or open PE tubes and show less than 4 cm^3 as the c_1 value.

Immittance meters may be used to determine the very important matter of eustachian tube function. The tests are rapid and objective, and they take considerably less time than more elaborate methods. The patient is instructed to prevent eustachian tube opening during the test by not swallowing and by remaining as motionless as possible. The test is designed for patients with tympanic membrane perforations or with patent pressure-equalization tubes in place.

The first step is to establish a pressure of +200 daPa and to have the patient open the tube by swallowing or yawning. If the tube opens, pressure equalization takes place in the middle ear and the manometer indicates a shift toward 0 daPa. Eustachian tube function has been qualified by Rock (1974) as "good," "fair," or "poor," depending on the degree to which the pressure is reduced by this maneuver. According to Gladstone (1984), the eustachian tube function test must be performed with positive air pressure in the external auditory canal because negative pressure could cause the tube to "lock" shut rather than be forced open.

Mucous Otitis Media

At times, thick mucoid secretions, often forced through the eustachian tube by sneezing or excessive pressure when blowing the nose, accumulate in the middle ear. If these secretions are allowed to remain, they may become dense and darken in color. This condition, which has been referred to as glue ear, produces the same kind of audiometric results as suppurative otitis media. After some period of time, however, the hearing loss is not reversible by simple myringotomy. Even after the inflammatory process has been removed, imperfect healing of the tissue may leave scars. The tissues forming these scars may be fibrous in nature, resulting in a network or web of adhesions. These adhesions cause particular difficulty because they may bind any or all of the ossicles. In addition to the adhesions in the middle ear, calcium deposits sometimes form on the tympanic membrane, resulting in a condition called **tympanosclerosis.** Surgical dissection of adhesions in the middle ear may be fruitless because they tend to recur, causing conductive hearing loss. According to Meyerhoff (1986), mucous otitis media is more common in younger children, whereas serous effusion is more common in older children.

Cholesteatoma

Whenever skin is introduced to the middle-ear cleft, the result may be a pseudotumor called **cholesteatoma** (see Figure 10.19). Cholesteatomas form as a sac, with onionlike concentric rings made up of keratin (a very insoluble protein) mixed with squamous (scaly) epithelium and with fats such as cholesterol. In patients with perforated tympanic membranes, the skin may enter the middle ear through the perforations. This invasion produces a secondary

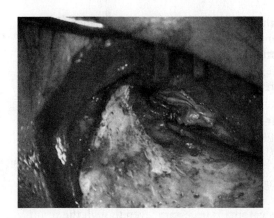

FIGURE 10.19 Surgical removal of a cholesteatoma. This erosive pseudotumor has begun eroding the epithelium of the attic of the middle ear and the canal wall. (*Source:* Jeffery Kuhn, M.D.)

acquired cholesteatoma. A primary acquired cholesteatoma may occur without a history of otitis media if the epithelium of the attic of the middle ear becomes modified. This alteration may occur if the pars flaccida of the tympanic membrane becomes sucked into the middle ear through negative pressure and then opens, revealing the skin from the outer portion of the tympanic membrane to the middle ear.

Cholesteatomas may also enter the middle ear in several other ways. In any case, they may be extremely dangerous. They have been known to occupy the entire middle ear and even pass down through the opening of the eustachian tube into the nasopharynx or up into the brain cavity. They are highly erosive and may cause destruction of bone and other tissue.

Although antibiotics may arrest otitis media, and even mastoiditis, the best treatment for cholesteatoma is still surgery. The condition spreads rapidly, and the surgeon must be absolutely certain that all the cholesteatomatous material has been removed because if even a small amount remains, the entire condition may flare up again in a short period of time. Most ears with cholesteatomas are secondarily infected and produce foul-smelling discharges that drain from the ears (**otorrhea**).

Mastoidectomy

Even with modern drug therapy, sometimes the only treatment for mastoiditis is a surgical procedure called **mastoidectomy,** usually performed under general anesthesia. In earlier days, the incision was made behind the auricle, and the bone in the mastoid process was scraped until all the infection was removed. This technique frequently resulted in a large concavity behind the ear. The surgically created mastoid bowl required cleaning for the rest of the patient's life and was in itself a breeding ground for infection.

The modern surgical approach to mastoidectomy is to avoid creating a mastoid cavity whenever possible. When a mastoid cavity does exist, it can often be obliterated by using portions of the temporalis muscle and/or bone chips taken from the patient. The obliteration of the mastoid cavity may be done at the time of initial surgery, or it may be staged at a later date, depending on the disease process found in the mastoid. Mastoidectomies are also performed sometimes in the absence of actual infection to repair paralyzed facial nerves. This procedure has been found to be very gratifying in recent years.

Tympanoplasty

Surgical reconstruction of the middle-ear auditory apparatus is called **tympanoplasty.** The simplest form of tympanoplasty is myringoplasty, or repair of the tympanic membrane, which was described in Chapter 9. Many surgical approaches have attempted to substitute metal or plastic prosthetic devices for damaged or missing ossicles. These attempts have met with limited success because the body tends to reject foreign materials. In recent years, tympanoplasties have been performed by attaching existing middle-ear structures together. This attachment may mean the loss of the function of one or more ossicles. The surgeon may place the tympanic membrane directly on the head of the stapes to restore a remnant of ossicular chain function.

Hearing improvement following tympanoplasty varies considerably, depending on the preoperative condition of the middle ear and, to a great extent, on the functioning of the eustachian tube. If the tube fails to function properly, and the middle ear is not normally pressurized, the surgical procedure is almost certainly doomed to failure.

Sometimes, though rarely, a patient's hearing may be poorer following surgery. The surgeon may have found, for example, that the long process of the incus is necrosed, but instead of there being a hiatus between the body of the incus and the stapes, the gap has been closed by a bit of cholesteatoma. Removal of the cholesteatoma is necessary, even though the result is interruption of the ossicular chain and increased hearing loss. Patients to whom this has happened may be difficult to console.

Audiograms of patients with interrupted ossicular chains show all the expected findings consistent with conductive hearing loss. The compliance of the tympanic membrane in such cases is unusually high because it has been decoupled from the stapes. The expected pressure-compliance function is a Type A_D (see Figure 10.20).

Although static-compliance values may not in themselves determine the presence of a conductive problem in the middle ear, comparison of c_X in the right and left ears of the same patient may be extremely useful. De Jonge and Valente (1979) suggest that when the static-compliance difference between ears exceeds 0.22 cm^3, a conductive problem may exist in one ear, even if both values fall within the normal range. However, differences exceeding this value can certainly exist in patients with normal hearing.

Anderson and Barr (1971) reported on high-frequency conductive hearing losses that may result from **subluxations** (partial dislocations) in the ossicular chain. When a portion of one of the ossicles is replaced by soft connective tissue, the elasticity of this connection, acting as an insulator against vibrations, transmits low frequencies more easily than high frequencies. Hearing losses caused by this condition are usually mild and result in an elevated acoustic reflex threshold.

Facial Palsy

In some cases of chronic otitis media, the bony covering of the fallopian canal becomes eroded, exposing the facial nerve to the disease process. Damage to the facial nerve may result in a flaccid paralysis of one side of the face. Appropriate treatment often includes middle-ear surgery.

At times, unilateral facial paralysis results when no other clinically demonstrable disease is present. Although there are several theories about why the paralysis, called **Bell's palsy,**[5] occurs, the reason is probably related to the blood supply to the nerve or to viral infection. A diagnosis of Bell's palsy is made by ruling out any other causative lesion in a patient with a flaccid facial paralysis. Bell's palsy resolves spontaneously in the majority of cases.

Patulous Eustachian Tube (PET)

There are some individuals in whom the eustachian tube is chronically patent (open), which often results in the sensation of **autophony,** the "head-in-a-barrel" feeling. As a result, their own voices are perceived as loud. This condition is observed more often in females than in males and has been associated with pregnancy. Some patients have claimed that their distorted autophony causes an echoing effect that interferes with their speech production. Other

FIGURE 10.20 Typical results on immittance tests performed on a patient with right ossicular chain discontinuity. Note that the tympanogram is Type A$_D$ (normal middle-ear pressure but extremely compliant tympanic membrane); the static compliance is high; and contralateral reflexes are absent in both ears, as is the right ipsilateral reflex. The left ear is normal in this case.

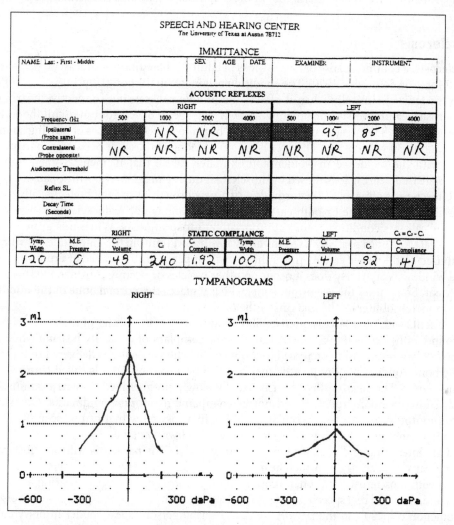

annoying effects of patulous eustachian tube include the sound of breathing and noises during chewing as the sound travels up the tube. Causes ascribed to this condition include the hormonal changes brought on by pregnancy or the use of some birth control pills, sudden changes in body weight, the use of decongestant medications, temporomandibular joint syndrome, and stress (O'Conner & Shea, 1981).

The problem of patulous eustachian tubes is more widespread than many people realize, and the incidence may go as high as 30 percent of people with otherwise normal ears (Kumazawa, 1985). Ten percent of a group of women studied had patulous eustachian tubes during pregnancy (Plate, Johnsen, Pederson, & Thompsen, 1979). Misdiagnosis is common because patients' complaints often make the condition sound like **serous effusion** or a blocked eustachian tube, resulting in completely inappropriate treatment.

If the patient suffers from a chronically patent eustachian tube and exhibits a Type A tympanogram, a simple test can verify the problem. Tympanic membrane compliance is observed during nasal breathing, oral breathing, and momentary cessation of breathing. If the tube is open, the compliance will increase during inhalation and decrease during exhalation. Interruption in breathing stops the changes in compliance. Henry and DiBartolomeo (1993) found tympanometry to be a useful tool in the diagnosis of patulous eustachian tube.

Otosclerosis

Otosclerosis, a common cause of hearing loss in adults, is hereditary in at least 70 percent of all cases (Morrison & Bundey, 1970). The condition originates in the bony labyrinth of the inner ear and is recognized clinically when it affects the middle ear, causing conductive hearing loss. Otosclerosis is a progressive disorder, with a varying age of onset from mid-childhood to late middle-adult life. The great majority of patients begin to notice some loss of hearing soon after puberty, up to 30 years of age. Otosclerosis is rare among children. It occurs primarily among whites, with the incidence in women approximately twice that in men. Women frequently report increased hearing loss caused by otosclerosis during pregnancy or menopause.

Otosclerosis appears as the formation of a new growth of spongy bone, usually over the stapedial footplate of one or both ears. Because the bone is not really sclerotic (hard), some clinicians call this condition (more appropriately) **otospongiosis.** When this growth occurs, the footplate becomes partially fixed in the oval window, limiting the amplitudes of vibrations transmitted to the inner ear. At times the growth appears on the stapedial crura or over the round window. Very rarely does it occur on other ossicles or occupy considerable space in the middle ear. Sometimes the abnormal bone, which replaces the normal bone of the middle ear, may completely obliterate the margins of the oval window.

Patients with otosclerosis often exhibit a bluish cast to the whites of their eyes, similar to that found with certain other bone diseases. They complain of difficulty hearing while chewing, probably a result of the increased loudness of the chewing sounds delivered to their inner ears by bone conduction. Frequently, they are also bothered by sounds called **tinnitus** in the affected ear(s). The hearing loss itself is usually slowly progressive. Physical examination of the ear shows normal structures and normal tympanic membrane landmarks. Occasionally, the promontory becomes very vascular, resulting in a rosy glow that can be seen through the tympanic membrane. This glow is referred to as the **Schwartze sign.**

One interesting and peculiar symptom of otosclerosis is **paracusis willisii.** Most patients who are hard of hearing claim they hear and understand speech better in quiet surroundings. Patients with otosclerosis (and often those with other forms of conductive hearing loss), on the other hand, may find that speech is easier to understand in the presence of background noise. This phenomenon results from the fact that normal-hearing persons speak louder in noisy environments. This increase in vocal loudness, something we have all experienced, is called the **Lombard voice reflex.** Because these patients' hearing losses attenuate the background noise to some degree, such people are able to enjoy the increased loudness of speakers' voices with less distracting noise.

Audiometric Findings in Otosclerosis

Carhart (1964) showed that the first symptom of otosclerosis is the appearance of a low-frequency air-bone gap. He also found that alterations in the inertia of the ossicular chain, produced by even partial fixation, alter the normal bone-conduction response. This artifact varies significantly from patient to patient, but on average, it causes the bone-conduction readings to appear poorer than the true sensory/neural sensitivity by an average of 5 dB at 500 Hz, 10 dB at 1000 Hz, 15 dB at 2000 Hz, and 5 dB at 4000 Hz, although the frequency with the greatest bone-conduction suppression is not always 2000 Hz. This anomaly of bone conduction is called the **Carhart notch** (Carhart, 1952) and probably occurs as a mechanical artifact because of the loss of the inertial mode of bone conduction and a shift in the normal resonant frequency of the middle ear, which ranges from 630 to 2000 Hz (Margolis & Goycoolea, 1993), all produced by the immobility of the oval window. The Carhart notch is also seen in some cases of middle-ear fluid.

Figure 10.21A and B illustrate results typical of early otosclerosis. Contrary to the typical audiometric contour in serous effusion, the otosclerotic patient shows a drop in hearing sensitivity in the low-frequency areas first, which is consistent with what is known of the effects of stiffness on impedance. As the principal site of otosclerosis increases in size, the hearing loss becomes greater

FIGURE 10.21 (A) Worksheet used for a patient with a mild conductive hearing loss. Results indicated that masking was required only for bone conduction at two frequencies in each ear. (B) Audiogram illustrating early otosclerosis in both ears. The loss appears first in the low frequencies because of the increased stiffness of the ossicular chain. A small air-bone gap is present. Word-recognition scores are normal, and the Weber does not lateralize. Masking was used for bone conduction only at 250 and 500 Hz, and for word-recognition testing. Note the early appearance of the Carhart notch.

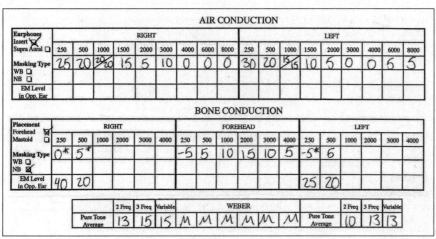

A

B

(see Figure 10.22A and B). Later in the disease, when the stapes has become more completely fixed, the mass effect becomes apparent, causing a reduction of sensitivity in the high frequencies, thus flattening the audiogram. With complete fixation, the entire mass of the skull is in fact added to the stapes. All auditory tests for site of lesion remain consistent with conductive hearing loss.

The pressure-compliance function remains normal in otosclerosis, except that the point of greatest compliance is shallower compared to the normal tympanogram. Jerger (1970) has called

FIGURE 10.22 (A) Worksheet used for a patient with a moderate bilateral conductive hearing loss. Because insert earphones were used for air-conduction testing, the interaural attenuation was increased so that masking was not required for this test, but it was required for bone conduction at all frequencies. (B) Audiogram showing a moderate loss of hearing in both ears caused by otosclerosis. The audiometric configuration is fairly flat, showing the combined effects of stiffness and mass. Bone conduction is normal except for the Carhart notch. Bone-conduction and WRS tests required masking.

AIR CONDUCTION

Earphones: Insert ☒ Supra Aural ☐	RIGHT									LEFT								
	250	500	1000	1500	2000	3000	4000	6000	8000	250	500	1000	1500	2000	3000	4000	6000	8000
Masking Type: WB ☐ NB ☐	45	50	40/40	40	40	35	40	40	35	50	50	45/45	40	40	40	45	45	40
EM Level in Opp. Ear																		

BONE CONDUCTION

Placement: Forehead ☒ Mastoid ☐	RIGHT						FOREHEAD						LEFT					
	250	500	1000	2000	3000	4000	250	500	1000	2000	3000	4000	250	500	1000	2000	3000	4000
Masking Type: WB ☐ NB ☒	0*	10*	15*	20*	15*	5*	0	10	15	20	15	5	0*	10*	15*	25*	15*	0*
EM Level in Opp. Ear	50	50	45	40	40	45							45	50	40	50	35	50

	2 Freq	3 Freq	Variable	WEBER							2 Freq	3 Freq	Variable
Pure Tone Average	40	43	43	M	M	M	M	M	M	Pure Tone Average	43	45	47

A

SPEECH AUDIOMETRY

Masking Type: WB ☐ Speech ☒	RIGHT						LEFT					
	SRT 1	SRT 2	Recognition 1		Recognition 2		SRT 1	SRT 2	Recognition 1		Recognition 2	
	45		List 1A / 75 HL	100 %*	List 3A / 90 HL	100 %*	45		List 2A / 75 HL	96 %*	List 4A / 90 HL	98 %*
EM Level in Opp. Ear				50		65				45		60

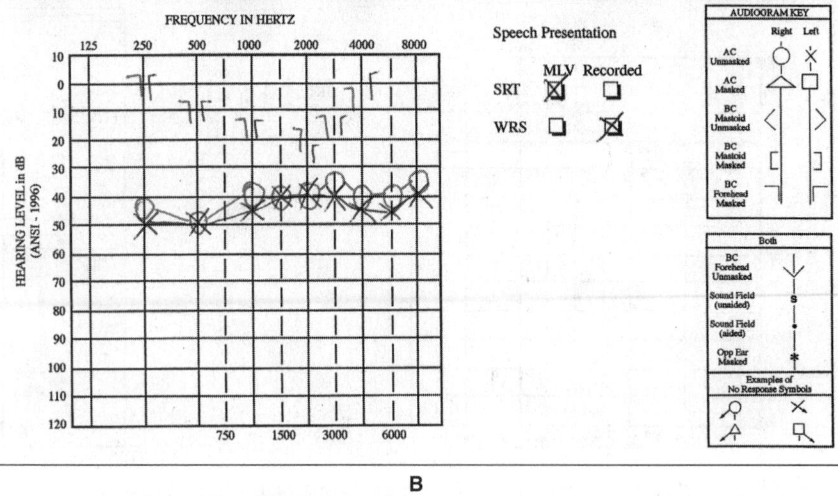

B

this type of tympanogram (see Figure 10.23) a Type A_S (stiffness). The A_S tympanogram appears in many, but not all, cases of otosclerosis. The acoustic reflex disappears early in otosclerosis, even in unilateral cases. When the tone is delivered to the involved ear, the hearing loss attenuates even a very intense sound so that the reflex is not triggered. When a tone is delivered to a normal ear opposite the one with otosclerosis, the reflex measured from the involved ear does not register because the stapes is incapable of movement, even though it is pulled by the stapedius tendon. In otosclerosis, the acoustic impedance may be expected to be high and the compliance low.

Treatment of Otosclerosis

Interest in the surgical correction of otosclerosis dates back many years. Even in fairly recent times, surgical relief of otosclerotic hearing loss met with failure, primarily for two reasons. First, before the introduction of antibiotics, postoperative infection caused severe

FIGURE 10.23 Results on immittance test performed on a patient with bilateral otosclerosis (Figure 10.21). The tympanogram is Type A_S, the static compliance is low, and the acoustic reflexes are absent in both ears.

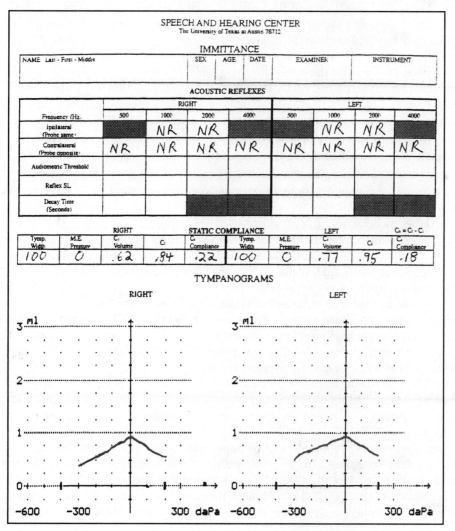

complications. Second, until the development of the operating microscope, middle-ear surgeons could not clearly see the very small operative field of the middle ear.

Because early attempts to free the immobilized stapes resulted in failure, often in the form of fractured crura, attention was turned to bypassing the ossicular chain. A new window was created in the lateral semicircular (balance) canal of the inner ear so that sound waves could pass directly from the external ear canal to the new window. This procedure was conducted as a two-stage operation until the one-stage **fenestration** was developed by Lempert (1938).

Fenestration surgery resulted in considerable hearing improvements for many patients with otosclerosis; however, it was recognized early that complete closure of the preoperative air-bone gap was impossible as a result of loss of the sound-transmission advantage of the tympanic membrane and the ossicular chain. A 25 dB conductive component to the hearing loss usually remained following even the best fenestration. Many people found no improvement in their hearing, and a number showed a considerable drop in their sensory/neural sensitivity. Some individuals with poor fenestration results even had total loss of hearing or were bothered by vertigo and increased tinnitus, as well as by poorer word-recognition scores and occasional facial paralysis. Hearing-aid use was sometimes obviated in the operated ear by a combination of poor speech discrimination and the large ear cavity created during surgery. Even if some patients were happy with the hearing results of their surgery, they were bothered by the constant after-care required to clean the cavity.

While palpating a stapes on a patient preparatory to performing a fenestration, Rosen (1953) managed to mobilize the stapes, breaking it free and restoring the sound vibrations into the cochlea. This happenstance led to a completely new introduction, the **stapes mobilization** procedure.

Advantages of mobilization over fenestration were manifold. Patients could be operated on using local anesthesia, eliminating some of the side effects of general anesthesia. Because the ossicular chain remained intact, the patient's potential for postoperative hearing could be fairly well predicted by the preoperative bone conduction. Of great importance was the fact that no after-care was required for mobilizations because no mastoid cavity was created during surgery.

In stapes mobilization, the ear canal is carefully cleansed and dried. The skin near the tympanic membrane is then anesthetized to deaden the area. A triangular incision is made in the skin, and the tympanic membrane reflected, exposing the middle ear. The surgeon then places a right-angle hook against the neck of the stapes, determines that it is fixed, and then rocks it until it is freed.

In spite of a number of variations of Rosen's operation, it was found that a great number of those patients whose hearing originally improved failed to retain this improvement after one year. The regression in hearing resulted from refixation of the stapes as new otosclerotic bone was laid down over the footplate. Refixation appears to be a greater problem for young patients, in whom the otosclerosis is more active, and for males.

Refixation following stapes mobilization led Shea (1958) to revive an operative procedure that had been described more than a half century earlier. This technique is called **stapedectomy,** which means "removal of the stapes," and is undoubtedly the procedure of choice for otosclerosis today.

The approaches to the middle ear for stapedectomy and mobilization are identical. After fixation has been determined, the incudostapedial joint is interrupted, the stapedius tendon is cut, and the superstructure of the stapes and remainder of the footplate are removed. In the original procedure, a vein graft, taken from the patient's hand or arm, was placed over the open oval window and draped on the promontory and over the facial ridge to obtain adequate blood supply. A hollow polyethylene strut was pulled onto the lenticular process of the incus, and the opposite end, which was beveled for a better fit, was placed in the oval window niche on the vein graft. In this way the polyethylene tube replaced the stapes.

In some cases, the polyethylene-with-vein procedure, though very popular, resulted in fistulas (leaks of inner-ear fluids into the middle ear), perhaps as a result of the sharp end of the strut resting on the vein. Testing for a **fistula** can be accomplished with the pressure portion of an immittance meter and an electronystagmograph (ENG) (see Chapter 11). Positive pressure is delivered to the middle ear by increasing the output of air pressure from the meter to 400 daPa. This may be accomplished whether or not a perforation of the tympanic membrane exists. If a fistula is present, the increased pressure within the middle ear may result in vertigo and an increase in rapid eye movement, called nystagmus, which can be monitored on the ENG.

In recent years, a number of modifications of the original Shea stapedectomy have been introduced. Different materials have been used as the prosthesis: stainless steel wire, stainless steel pistons, Teflon pistons, combinations of steel and plastic, and so on. Some surgeons have used fat plugs from the tragus of the pinna and some **fascia** (the tough protective layer over muscle) to cover the oval window and support the prosthesis. Use of the patient's own tissue (autologous grafts) obviously works best in avoiding rejection. Although the success of stapedectomy has been substantial, and many patients with unsuccessful mobilizations have been reoperated with great improvements in hearing, some adverse reactions can and do occur, including further loss of hearing and prolonged vertigo.

To reduce risk in stapedectomy, many middle-ear surgeons today prefer to use a small fenestra and avoid the trauma to the inner ear of complete removal of the stapedial footplate. Small fenestra stapedectomies have been referred to as **stapedotomies** (Bailey & Graham, 1984). One such procedure is illustrated in Figures 10.24 to 10.29. After the ear has been locally anesthetized, and the tympanic membrane elevated from its sulcus, exposing the middle ear, the operation is begun. It should come as no surprise that there is a relationship between the experience of the surgeon and the success rates of stapedotomies. Experience plays a primary role in the two most delicate parts of the operation, which are the actual fenestration of the

FIGURE 10.24 The proper length for the prosthesis is determined by measuring the distance from the undersurface of the incus to the footplate. A special measuring rod is used. (*Source:* Arkansas Otolaryngology Center.)

FIGURE 10.25 A small control hole is made in the center of the footplate; the hole is then enlarged with a pick or hand drill. (*Source:* Arkansas Otolaryngology Center.)

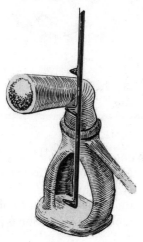

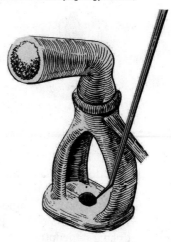

FIGURE 10.26 The crura are weakened and fractured, the incudostapedial joint is separated, and the stapedial tendon is severed with microscissors. (*Source:* Arkansas Otolaryngology Center.)

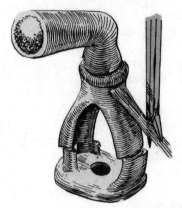

FIGURE 10.27 The superstructure of the stapes is removed. (*Source:* Arkansas Otolaryngology Center.)

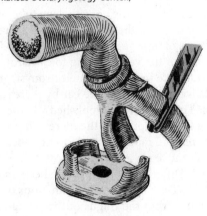

FIGURE 10.28 The prosthesis is carefully positioned, the wire hook is placed over the long process of the incus just above the lenticular process, and the hook is crimped snugly into position with a special crimping instrument. (*Source:* Arkansas Otolaryngology Center.)

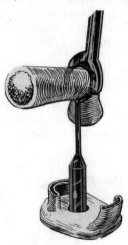

FIGURE 10.29 Superficial fascia from the temporalis muscle is placed around the end of the prosthesis, where it enters the footplate, to seal the inner ear. (*Source:* Arkansas Otolaryngology Center.)

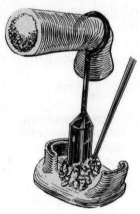

stapedial footplate and the crimping of the prosthesis onto the long process of the incus. As further modifications of the stapedectomy procedure continue to be perfected, such as the use of an argon laser, some form of stapedectomy will surely remain popular. Fisch (1982, 2009) states that results from both the use of a laser and mechanical creation of the hole in the stapes during stapedotomy yield similar results, while manual footplate perforation is probably more common because of the availability of equipment.

Other Causes of Middle-Ear Hearing Loss

Middle-ear abnormalities occur in isolation or in association with other congenital anomalies. Some cases of stapedial fixation appear purely on a genetic basis. A number of congenital middle-ear disorders were found in the offspring of mothers who took the drug thalidomide during pregnancy. Such conditions as fixation of the incudomalleal joint have been associated with atresias of the external auditory canal and microtias of the auricle. Other ossicular abnormalities have been associated with syndromes of the cheek, jaw, and face. Congenital malformations of the middle and outer ears are often seen together because these areas arise from the same embryonic tissue. Meyerhoff (1986) recommends delaying surgical repair in these situations until the child is 4 to 6 years old to permit the mastoid air-cell system to enlarge, allowing better surgical access.

CHECK YOUR UNDERSTANDING

Skull fractures have been known to result coincidentally in fractures or interruptions of the ossicular chain. Ossicular interruption has been reported in cases of skull trauma, even without fracture. An ossicle may also be damaged by a foreign object during traumatic perforation of the tympanic membrane, as with a cotton swab or bobby pin.

ACTIVITIES

Tumors, both benign and malignant, may form in the middle ear. They may take the form of polyps, vascular tumors, and granulomas in response to middle-ear infections, or, in rare cases, cancer of the squamous cells of the middle ear.

EVOLVING CASE STUDIES

In this chapter, we look at the case study (Case Study 2) that results in the diagnosis of otitis media. Consider the special diagnostic tests you might do and their probable results. In addition to pure-tone and speech audiometry, the basic workup should include immittance measures. It would probably not be necessary to perform otoacoustic emissions (OAEs) or auditory brain-stem response (ABR), but it would be interesting to speculate about how those results would turn out.

Case Study 2: Conductive Hearing Loss—Middle Ear Disorder

You have already been advised that audiometric findings for this patient would be comparable to what is observed in Figure 4.13. A similar, typical example in this chapter is shown in Figure 10.11. Note that there is a moderate hearing loss by air conduction for both ears and that the bone-conduction thresholds are normal. Speech audiometry shows good agreement between the pure-tone averages and the SRTs, and the speech-recognition scores are high. These tests confirm the diagnosis of conductive hearing loss in both ears but do not indicate the etiology (origin) of the hearing loss, or the part of the auditory system that is involved. The history of ear infections can be suggested as the cause, but this awaits further support by further testing.

Because the otologist reports that the tympanic membranes are intact, immittance measures (and your otoscopic examination) should confirm this. If it turns out that a seal cannot be obtained for immittance testing, the possibility of perforation should be explored again. A retracted tympanic membrane would result in a tympanogram Type C (see the left ear in Figure 10.10). If there is fluid in the middle ear, the tympanogram will be fairly flat, which is a Type B (see Figure 10.12). Because this hearing loss is a long-standing problem, it is possible that the incus in one or both ears may be eroded, which would cause a Type A$_D$ (see the right ear in Figure 10.19). Any of these etiologies would result in the loss of all acoustic reflexes.

If OAE and ABR testing were completed, there would almost certainly be no OAEs present. ABR findings would show a delay of all waves, as demonstrated in Figure 10.13. In cases such as this, medical reversal of the hearing loss is always the first avenue considered. Several different procedures of this type are described in this chapter. Failing improvement in hearing, the rehabilitation will be of an audiological nature and is discussed further in Chapters 14 and 15.

Summary

The middle ear is an air-filled space separating the external auditory canal from the inner ear. Its function is to increase sound energy through leverage, the step-down size ratio provided by the ossicular chain, and the area ratio between the tympanic membrane and the oval window.

Abnormalities of the structure or function of the middle ear result in conductive hearing losses, wherein the air-conduction thresholds are depressed in direct relationship with the amount of disease. Bone-conduction thresholds may deviate slightly from normal in conductive hearing losses, not because of abnormality of the sensory/neural mechanism, but because of alterations in the middle ear's normal (inertial) contribution to bone conduction. Alterations in the pressure-compliance functions give general information regarding the presence of fluid or negative air pressure in the middle ear, stiffness, or interruption of the ossicular chain. Measurements of static compliance may be higher or lower than normal, and acoustic reflex thresholds are either elevated or absent. Auditory brain-stem responses show increased latencies for all waves, and otoacoustic emissions are usually absent. Results on word-recognition tests are the same as for those with normal hearing. Although seldom completed today, results of the behavioral site-of-lesion tests discussed in Chapter 7, such as short increment sensitivity index (SISI), alternate binaural loudness balance (ABLB), and tone-decay, would also be the same as those with normal hearing.

Remediation of middle-ear disorders should first be concerned with medical or surgical reversal of the problems. When this fails, must be postponed, or is not available, careful audiological counseling should be undertaken, and treatment avenues, such as the use of hearing aids, investigated. Provided they have no medical contraindications to hearing-aid use and no planned medical or surgical intervention, patients with conductive hearing losses are excellent candidates for hearing aids because of their relatively flat audiometric contours, good word recognition, and tolerance for loud sounds.

REVIEW TABLE 10.1 Conductive Hearing Loss in the Middle Ear

Etiology	Degree of Loss	Audiometric Configuration	Static Compliance	Tympanogram Type
Suppurative otitis media	Mild to moderately severe	Flat	Normal to low	B
Tympanic membrane perforation	Mild	Flat	Not testable Large equivalent volume	Not testable
Ossicular chain discontinuity	Moderate	Flat	High	A$_D$

(Continued)

REVIEW TABLE 10.1 (*continued*)

Etiology	Degree of Loss	Audiometric Configuration	Static Compliance	Tympanogram Type
Serous effusion	Mild to moderate	Flat or poorer in high frequencies	Normal to low	B
Negative middle-ear pressure	Mild	Flat	Normal	C
Otosclerosis	Mild to moderately severe	Flat or poorer in low frequencies	Low	A_S
Congenital disorders	Mild to moderately severe	Varies	Varies	Varies

Frequently Asked Questions

Q Can PE tubes be placed in adults or are they used only in children?

A *PE tubes are used in adults as well as children when the need arises, which is far more frequent in children.*

Q How are the ossicles connected? Do they merely rest against each other or is there some kind of joint between them?

A *Like other connected bones, the ossicles are held together by a band of fibrous tissue called a ligament. These connections form joints.*

Q What causes the natural negative pressure of the middle ear?

A *The mucous membrane lining of the middle ear is very similar to the lining of the lungs. The gases present in the middle ear are absorbed by the small blood vessels in the mucosa so the air pressure drops, to be replenished when the eustachian tube opens. Failure of the eustachian tube to function properly results in negative middle-ear pressure and a retracted tympanic membrane.*

Q What is the size relationship between the TM and the oval window?

A *About 22 to 1.*

Q Why does the stapes rock against the oval window rather than push against it?

A *This is part of nature's design to take advantage of the lever action of the malleus.*

Q What can parents do to reduce the occurrence of otitis media?

A *Good hygiene and proper diet can be effective in preventing any disease. Of course, these approaches do not work in every case.*

Q How is the physical volume test (PVT) performed?

A *During tympanometry, when the c_1 value is large (greater than 5 cm^2), it is suspected that a perforation exists in the tympanic membrane and that this is the combined volumes of the outer and middle ears.*

Q How can you diagnose serous effusion rather than suppurative otitis media?

A *The two are similar on audiological tests. The medical history is helpful but, in the final analysis, a physician must diagnose this condition.*

Q What is an ear candle?

A *These are slender hollow candles made of bee's wax or tallow that are held in the ear canal and the opposite end is lighted. They are supposed to create a negative pressure to draw unwanted substances out of the external auditory canal, and a large number of other unsubstantiated claims have been made for their use. These are very popular in some third-world countries and even in the United States, although none of the claims has proven to be true.*

Q What are the symptoms of mastoiditis?

A *Mastoiditis is a very serious condition usually accompanied by fever and pain.*

Q Why might a person experience taste changes after a middle-ear surgery?

A *The chorda tympani nerve passes through the middle-ear space and is responsible for the sense of taste on the anterior two-thirds of each side of the tongue. If it is stretched or severed during surgery, taste changes are likely, although some of these are temporary.*

Q Why does the acoustic reflex disappear early in otosclerosis?

A *Even slight immobility of the stapes does not allow the stapedial tendon to be pulled to the side when the stapedial muscle tries to contract.*

Q What is the most common disorder of the middle ear?

A *The most common disorder of the middle ear is otitis media.*

Q How do bacteria and other organisms gain access to the middle ear?

A *Bacteria and other organisms may literally be blown up through the eustachian tube or result from infection that spreads up the lining of the tube. Less frequently they are carried by the bloodstream. A perforation in the tympanic membrane allows easy access to the middle ear.*

Q Why do patients with conductive hearing loss often experience difficulty hearing when chewing?

A *The combination of the hearing loss and the masking noise set up by bone conduction raises the patient's auditory thresholds. This is called deprecusis.*

Q Let's say that a child suffers multiple episodes of otitis media accompanied by TM perforations as a result of the infections. At what point will the child experience a permanent conductive loss?

A *This varies depending on a number of circumstances. Some patients experience multiple episodes of otitis media with no permanent hearing loss, while others may develop a permanent loss after one episode. Hereditary predispositions and a host of other factors contribute to these differences.*

Q Why is the incus the most frequent site of erosion in the ossicular chain?

A *Of all the ossicles, the incus is the one with the poorest blood supply.*

Q Is it possible to have worse hearing after a middle-ear surgery?

A *Many things can go wrong in any kind of surgery and may not be the fault of the surgeon. For example, sometimes there is an interruption of the ossicular chain that is bridged by a small amount of cholesteatoma. All cholesteatomatous material must be removed, of course, and when this is done, the ossicular chain is interrupted.*

Q If someone received improper water irrigation treatment for impacted cerumen in the external auditory canal, could it interrupt the ossicular chain?

A *A wide range of damage has been reported after improper irrigation of the external auditory canal. Both the tympanic membrane and the ossicles are at risk when excessive pressure is used.*

Q Is it possible for the stapedius and tensor tympani to contract so violently (as with exposure to high voltage) that they can break or completely displace the ossicular chain?

A *We have not heard such reports.*

Q When it comes to the phenomenon of paracusis willisii, who talks louder in a noisy environment, the person with normal hearing or the person with a conductive hearing loss?

A *Normal-hearing people talk louder in noisy places (the Lombard effect) because their normal auditory feedback has been masked. People with conductive hearing losses hear their voices better because they hear less of the noise than those with normal hearing do and their signal-to-noise ratios are improved.*

Q Can Bell's palsy cause a hearing loss? If so, which type of hearing loss is more prevalent?

A *Bell's palsy results from irritation of the VIIth (facial) nerve, which is not part of the auditory system.*

Q How does the aditus ad antrum communicate with the mastoid?

A *The aditus is in the superior portion of the middle-ear space and is separated from the mastoid air cells by a thin bony plate. If that plate erodes because of a middle-ear infection, those infectious materials may be introduced into the mastoid.*

Suggested Reading

Clark, J. G., & Jaindl, M. (1996). Conductive hearing loss in children: Etiology and pathology. In F. N. Martin & J. G. Clark (Eds.), *Hearing care for children* (pp. 45–72). Boston: Allyn and Bacon.

Kenna, M. A. (1996). Embryology and developmental anatomy of the ear. In C. D. Bluestone, S. E. Stool, & M. A. Kenna (Eds.), *Pediatric otolaryngology* (Vol. 1, pp. 113–126). Philadelphia: W. B. Saunders.

Lipscomb, D. M. (1996). The external and middle ear. In J. L. Northern (Ed.), *Hearing disorders* (pp. 1–13). Boston: Allyn and Bacon.

Sandridge, S. (2009). *Ear disorders.* (CD-ROM). San Diego: Plural Publishing.

Endnotes

1. For Bartolommeo Eustachio, sixteenth-century Italian anatomist, 1524–1574.
2. For Adam Politzer, Hungarian otologist, 1835–1920.
3. For Antonio Maria Valsalva, Italian anatomist, 1666–1723.
4. For Joseph Toynbee, British otologist, 1815–1866.
5. For Sir Charles Bell, Scottish physiologist, 1774–1842.

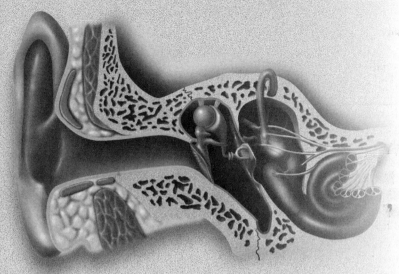

CHAPTER 11

The Inner Ear

LEARNING OBJECTIVES

This chapter describes the inner ear as a device that provides the brain with information about sound and the body's position in space. At the completion of this chapter, the reader should be able to

- Identify the anatomical landmarks of the inner-ear mechanism.
- Briefly describe the contributions of the inner ear to hearing and spatial orientation.
- List a variety of disorders that affect the inner ear and give their causes, stating whether they would be prenatal, perinatal, or postnatal in origin.
- Discuss the probable results on auditory tests described earlier in this text as they may relate to inner-ear disorders.

THE ANIMAL BRAIN cannot use sound vibrations in the form described in Chapter 3, so the function of the inner ear is to **transduce** the mechanical energy delivered from the middle ear into a form of energy that can be interpreted by the brain. In addition to information about hearing, the inner ear also reports information regarding the body's position and movement in a bioelectrical code. The inner ear is extremely complicated, with literally thousands of moving parts, but it is so tiny that it has been compared to the size of a small pea. Because of its similarity to an intricately winding cave, the inner ear has been called a **labyrinth.**

Anatomy and Physiology of the Inner Ear

The footplate of the stapes fits neatly into the oval window, so called because of its shape. The oval window is the separation between the middle ear and the inner ear. The immediate entryway is called the **vestibule;** it is an area through which access may be gained to various chambers of the inner ear, just as the vestibule in a house is a space that may communicate with several different rooms. The vestibule is filled with a fluid called **perilymph.** The organs of equilibrium are housed within the vestibular portion of the inner ear. The connections between the balance (vestibular) and auditory (cochlear) portions of the inner ear are considered separately here for ease of learning, but they are intricately connected both anatomically and physiologically (see Figure 11.1).

The Vestibular Mechanism

As in many animals, the human ability to maintain balance depends on information from several body systems, interactions among which are controlled in the **cerebellum.** These systems include visual, proprioceptive, and vestibular input. The visual system provides direct information from surrounding objects on the orientation of the body and depends on the ability of the eyes to see and the presence of sufficient light to make surroundings visible. Proprioception concerns **somatosensory** stimuli received in tissue from supporting structures, such as the muscles and tendons of the body. These stimuli allow the perception of body-part positioning. The vestibular system relies on the forces of gravity and inertia.

Within the vestibule are membranous sacs called the **utricle** and the **saccule.** Both sacs are surrounded by perilymph and contain another fluid, very similar in constitution, called **endolymph.** The saccule is slightly smaller than the utricle. The end organ for balance within the utricle *(macula acoustica utriculi)* is located at the bottom, and the end organ within the saccule *(macula acoustica sacculi)* is located on the side.

Arising from the utricle are the superior, lateral, and posterior **semicircular canals,** which are also membranous; they contain endolymph and are surrounded in a larger bony cavern by perilymph. Each of the three canals returns to the utricle through enlarged areas called *ampullae.* Each **ampulla** contains an end organ *(crista)* that provides a sense of equilibrium. The semicircular canals are arranged perpendicularly to one another to cover all dimensions in space. With any angular acceleration, at least one semicircular canal is stimulated.

FIGURE 11.1 Anatomy of the human inner ear.

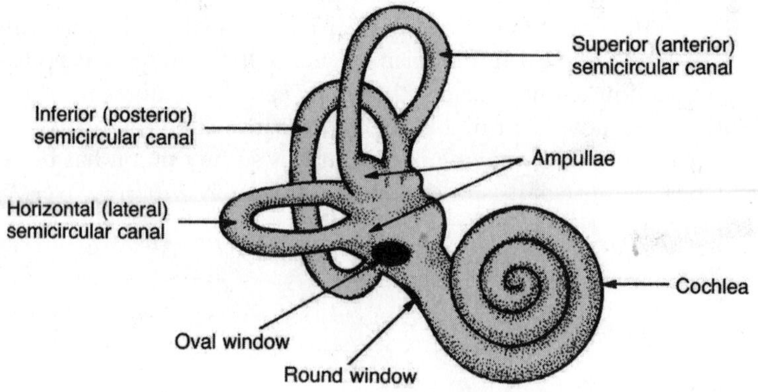

Superior (anterior) semicircular canal

Inferior (posterior) semicircular canal

Horizontal (lateral) semicircular canal

Ampullae

Cochlea

Oval window

Round window

When the head is moved, the fluids in the vestibule tend to lag behind because of their inertia. In this way the fluids are set into motion, which stimulates the vestibular mechanism. The utriculosaccular mechanism is responsible for interpreting *linear acceleration,* and it is through this mechanism that we perceive when an elevator or automobile is picking up speed or slowing down. The utricle and saccule are stimulated by the rate of change of linear velocity, which can be measured in centimeters per second squared. The semicircular canals are the receptors for *angular acceleration,* or the rate of change of angular velocity. These receptors report, for example, the increase or decrease in the number of revolutions per minute that the body is turning. Thus, angular acceleration can be measured in degrees per second squared.

When vestibular mechanisms become damaged or diseased, a common symptom called **vertigo** results. Patients with vertigo are truly ill because they experience the sensation of whirling or spinning. Because of connections in the brain between the vestibular portion of the auditory nerve and the oculomotor nerve, a rapid rocking movement of the eyes, called **nystagmus,** frequently occurs. Nystagmus always comes about with vertigo, regardless of whether one can see it, and it may occur spontaneously in cases of vestibular upset. It is important to differentiate true vertigo from dizziness, light-headedness, or falling tendencies, which do not result in the sensation of true turning.

Tests for Vestibular Abnormality

For some time, attempts to determine the normality of the vestibular system have centered on artificial stimulation. In one test, the patient is placed in a chair capable of mechanically controlled rotation. Following a period of rotation, the eyes are examined for nystagmus. The presence, degree, and type of nystagmus are compared to the examiner's concept of "normal."

A considerably easier test to administer in the otologist's or audiologist's office is the **caloric test.** Stimulation of the labyrinth is accomplished by "washing" cold or warm water or air against the tympanic membrane, with temperatures actually varying only slightly below or above normal body temperatures. The result of using cold water or air in patients with normal vestibular systems is a nystagmus with rapid eye movement away from the irrigated ear and slow movement back. When warm water or air is used, the direction of nystagmus is reversed. The acronym COWS (cold—opposite, warm—same) is a useful mnemonic. Interpretations of responses as normal, absent, hyperactive, or hypoactive are highly subjective and vary considerably among administrators of this test.

There is a difference in electrical potential between the cornea (positive charge) and the retina (negative charge) of the eye. Knowledge of this fact led to the development of a device called the **electronystagmograph (ENG)** to measure the changes in potential produced by nystagmus and to increase the objectivity of vestibular testing. This equipment allows for measurement of the rate and direction of nystagmus, which can be displayed on a paper chart as a permanent recording or exhibited on a computer terminal and saved and/or printed. Most commercial ENGs heat and cool the water for irrigation to precise temperatures (30° and 44°C) and eject the proper amount (250 milliliters) over a prescribed period of time (40 seconds). A slightly longer irrigation is required for air calorics. All this automaticity has considerable advantage over manual methods of testing, but most important is the fact that a permanent and accurate result is available. The use of microcomputers in vestibulography allows for better quantification of the eyebeats resulting from caloric testing through better control of the stimuli and resolution of the responses. A variety of tests is currently available, and software is constantly being upgraded. Computers have allowed for the reintroduction of **rotary chair testing** as a means of assessing the functions of the vestibular system, including those of children.

FIGURE 11.2 Specialized goggles allow for the observation and video recording of eye movement while testing the dizzy patient or while performing vestibular rehabilitation. (*Source:* Micromedical Technologies, 10 Kemp Drive, Chatham, IL 62629.)

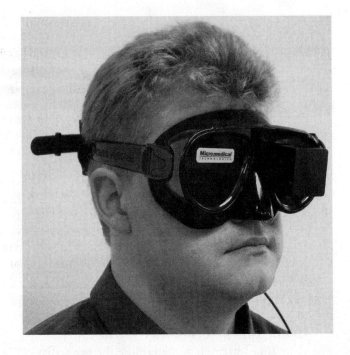

The use of strategically placed electrodes around the eyes for measurement of electrical potential changes in eye movement—with their calibration, physiologic noise, and other problems—has largely been replaced with an infrared video system that uses tiny cameras to track eye movements in response to vestibular tests (see Figure 11.2). The area inside the goggles is dark, which allows patients to keep their eyes open during testing because the infrared light is invisible to them. The absence of electrodes makes testing easier, and eye movements can be viewed on a video monitor or video-recorded for later review.

Before the advent of computerized vestibulography, ENG testing on infants and small children was difficult, if not impossible. Cyr and Møller (1988) recommend that children be tested for vestibular dysfunction if (1) they show delayed or abnormal motor function, (2) they take ototoxic medications, (3) they have a spontaneous nystagmus, or (4) there is suspected neurological disease. It would probably be advisable to carry out vestibular testing on children with sensory/neural hearing loss whenever possible because many of them apparently suffer from significant vestibular abnormalities (Brookhouser, Cyr, & Beauchaine, 1982).

Until recently, vestibulography was limited to the vestibulo-ocular reflexes, the connections between the balance and visual systems in the brain. There are new pursuits of other central nervous system interactions, including **computerized dynamic posturography (CDP),** that assess the ability to coordinate movement by measuring vestibulospinal reflexes. Many of the tests now available are directly related to the introduction of computers for the measurement of vestibular function. While measuring patients' postural compensations as the platform on which they are standing is rotated at various angles, CDP provides a quantitative assessment of upright balance through simulation of conditions encountered in daily life (see Figure 11.3). By isolating the sensory, motor, and biochemical components that contribute to balance, CDP analyzes a patient's ability to use these components individually and in combination to maintain balance.

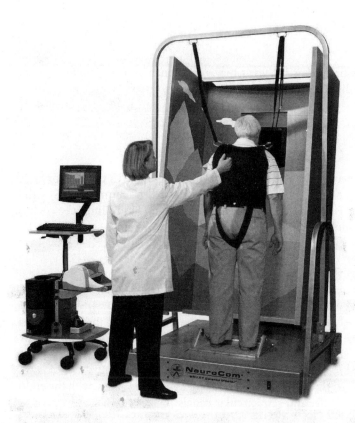

FIGURE 11.3 Computerized dynamic posturography provides a quantitative assessment of upright balance by measuring postural compensations as the platform on which a patient stands is rotated at various angles. (*Source:* Neurocom® International, Inc.)

While some of the test protocols within CDP provide insights on a patient's functional capacity for a variety of daily life tasks, others help to localize the cause of a balance disorder (Nashner, 1993). CDP test results can aid in the diagnosis of specific underlying disease processes.

The **vestibular-evoked myogenic potential (VEMP)** can also shed light on the status of a patient's vestibular system. The VEMP is a **sound-evoked muscle reflex** believed to be generated from acoustical stimulation of the saccule, one of the vestibular end organs that sense linear acceleration. The purpose of this reflex may be to stabilize the head in response to unpredictable movements. Measured through evoked-potential techniques, the response may be recorded from a variety of muscles, including the **trapezius muscles** or **sternocleidomastoid muscles,** when an acoustic stimulus is presented to one ear while the patient sharply turns his or her head in the direction opposite the stimulated ear. Asymmetries in response between the two sides of the head may shed clinical insights into cases of perilymphatic fistula (a pathologic communication between the normally fluid-filled inner ear and the air-filled middle ear typically at either the oval or round window) or patients who yield normal results on conventional measures of peripheral vestibular function, such as caloric or rotary-chair tests yet report abnormal sensations of linear acceleration.

Computerized dynamic posturography, vestibulography, and vestibular-evoked myogenic potentials are lending innovative and exciting aspects to the diagnosis of diseases of the inner ear and central nervous system. However, balance function tests must be considered along with the medical history, medical examination, and audiometric findings, and the extent to which audiologists should be clinically involved in such procedures continues to be debated.

Clinical COMMENTARY

The assessment of vestibular disorders has become a major component of many audiologists' professional responsibilities. As discussed in Chapter 14, in addition to assessment, audiologists' services also encompass rehabilitative interventions for the balance problems of their patients.

The Auditory Mechanism

The vestibular portions of the inner ear were shown in Figure 11.1, along with the auditory portions. Notice that the vestibule, the area just past the oval window, also communicates with a snail-like shell called the **cochlea.** For clarification, teachers are fond of "unrolling" the cochlea (see Figure 11.4), an act that is graphically advantageous but physically impossible because the cochlea is made up of a twisting bony shell about 1 cm wide and 5 mm from base to apex in humans.

Beyond the oval window within the cochlea lies the **scala vestibuli,** so named because of its proximity to the vestibule and its resemblance to a long hall. At the bottom of the cochlea, the **scala tympani** is visible, beginning at the round window. Both of these canals contain perilymph, which is continuous through a small passageway at the apex of the cochlea called the **helicotrema.** For frequencies above about 60 Hz, there is little fluid movement through the helicotrema because energy is transmitted through the fluids of the cochlea by the movement of the membranes.

Between the two canals just described lies the **scala media,** or **cochlear duct.** This third canal is filled with endolymph, which is continuous through the **ductus reuniens,** with the endolymph contained in the saccule, utricle, and semicircular canals. The scala media is separated from the scala vestibuli by **Reissner's membrane**[1] and from the scala tympani by the **basilar membrane.** When the cochlea, which curls about two and a half turns, is seen from the middle ear, the large turn at the base forms the protrusion into the middle ear called the **promontory.**

Along the full length of the scala media lies the end organ of hearing, the **organ of Corti,**[2] which resides on the basilar membrane, one of the three walls of the scala media. The other two walls are made up of Reissner's membrane and a bony shelf formed by a portion of the bony labyrinth. From this shelf extends the **spiral ligament,** support for the scala media, and also the **stria vascularis,** which produces the endolymph and supplies oxygen and other nutrients to the cochlea. The blood supply and nerve supply enter the organ of Corti by way of the **modiolus,** the central core of the cochlea around which it is wound. A cross section of the cochlea is shown in Figure 11.5. Much of what is known of the anatomy and physiology of the inner ear has been advanced in recent years with the introduction of electron microscopy.

FIGURE 11.4 Diagram of an "unrolled" cochlea, showing the relationships among the three scalae.

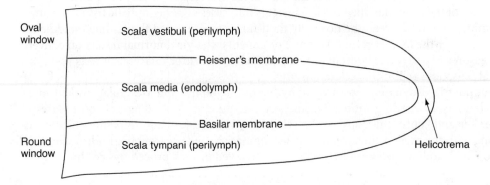

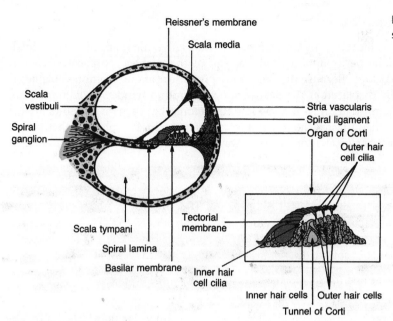

FIGURE 11.5 Cross
section of the cochlea.

Basilar Membrane

The basilar membrane is about 35 mm long and varies in width from less than 0.1 mm at the basal turn to about 0.5 mm at the apical turn, quite the reverse of the cochlear duct, which is broad at the basal end and narrow at the apex. Situated on the fibrous basilar membrane are three to five parallel rows of 12,000 to 15,000 outer hair cells and one row of 3,000 inner hair cells. The outer and inner hair cells are separated from each other by **Corti's arch.** The auditory nerve endings are located on the basilar membrane. Some of these nerve fibers connect to the hair cells in a one-to-one relationship, while others make contact with many hair cells. The hair cells themselves are about 0.01 mm long and 0.001 mm in diameter. Located on top of each hair cell are hair-like projections called **stereocilia.** The direction in which they are bent during stimulation is of great importance. If the cilia bend in one direction, the nerve cells are stimulated; if they bend the other way, the nerve impulses are inhibited; and if they bend to the side, there is no stimulation at all. A flow diagram of cochlear function is shown in Figure 11.6.

FIGURE 11.6 The functions of the cochlea.

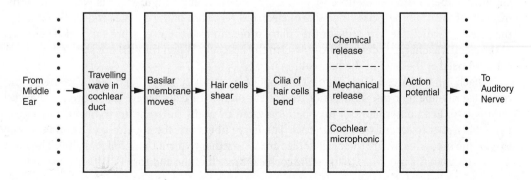

Physiology of the Cochlea

When the oval window is moved in by the stapes, the annular ligament around the footplate stretches and displaces the perilymph at the basal end of the cochlea, propagating a wave toward the apex of the cochlea. Because the fluids of the inner ear are noncompressible, when these fluids are inwardly displaced at the oval window the round window membrane must yield by moving into the middle ear. It may be said, therefore, that the two windows are out of phase–when one is pushed inward the other must move outward. It is obvious that, if they were in phase, a great deal of cancellation of sound waves would take place within the cochlea, just the opposite of the desired effect.

Sound vibrations that are introduced to the scala vestibuli are conducted into the cochlear duct by the yielding of Reissner's membrane. The endolymph is thereby disturbed, so the vibrations continue and the basilar membrane is similarly displaced, resulting in the release of the round window membrane. Therefore, sounds introduced to the inner ear cause a wavelike motion, which always moves from the base of the cochlea to the apex. This is true of both air- and bone-conducted sounds. Given areas along the basilar membrane show greater displacement for some frequencies than for others. Tones of low frequency with longer wavelengths show maximum displacement near the apical end, whereas tones of high frequency with shorter wavelengths show maximum displacement near the basal end.

The basilar membrane reacts more to vibrations of the inner ear than do most of the other structures. Because the organ of Corti resides on this membrane, the vibrations are readily transmitted to it. The stereocilia on the tips of the outer hair cells are embedded in the **tectorial membrane,** a gelatinous flap that is fixed on its inner edge and, according to some researchers, on its outer edge as well. When the basilar membrane moves up and down in response to fluid displacement caused by the in-and-out movement of the stapes, the hair cells are sheared (twisted) in a complex manner. Part of this shearing is facilitated by the fact that the basilar membrane and the tectorial membrane have slightly different axes of rotation and slide in opposite directions as they are moved up and down.

The three rows of outer hair cells are responsible for "sharpening" the fluid-borne wave within the cochlea, thereby enhancing frequency discrimination. Outer-hair cell damage, which occurs in many cochlear hearing losses, reduces this sharpening, with a resultant decrease in speech-recognition abilities, especially in background noise. The outer-hair cells also enhance the reception of sound by the inner hair cells by shortening themselves, thereby bringing the inner hair cells into contact with the tectorial membrane. Without this assistance from the outer hair cells, the inner hair cells are limited to stimulation from the motion of the endolymphatic fluid within the scala media and thus respond only to sounds above about 40 to 60 dB SPL. Hearing loss below these levels would be attributed primarily to outer-hair cell damage. Greater degrees of hearing loss would imply damage to both the outer and inner hair cells.

The mechanics of the organ of Corti are very complex, resulting from motion of the basilar membrane in directions up and down, side to side, and lengthwise, as well as an active motility of the outer hair cells. The size of electrical response of the cochlea is directly related to the extent to which the hair cells, or the ciliary projections at their tops, are sheared. The source of the electrical charge is derived from within the hair cell. When the cilia are sheared, a chemical is released at the base of the hair cell.

Each inner hair cell of the cochlea is supplied by about 20 nerve fibers, and each nerve fiber contacts only one hair cell. This is not true of the outer hair cells, where the neuron-to-hair cell ratio is 1:10. Each outer hair cell may be innervated by many different nerve fibers, and a given nerve fiber goes to several outer hair cells. The nerve fibers exit the cochlea and extend centrally toward the modiolus, where their cell bodies group together to form the spiral ganglion. The nerve fibers pass from the modiolus to form the cochlear branch of the auditory (VIIIth cranial) nerve.

The Auditory Neuron

The human cochlea contains about 30,000 afferent (sensory) **neurons** and about 1,800 efferent neurons. A neuron is a specialized cell designed as a conductor of nerve impulses. It is comprised of a **cell body,** an **axon,** and **dendrites** (see Figure 11.7). The axon and dendrites are branching systems. The dendrites, which consist of many small branches, receive nerve impulses from other nerve cells. The axon transmits the impulses along the neurons, which vary dramatically in length. The afferent neurons carry impulses from the cochlea to the central auditory nervous system and have their cell bodies in the spiral ganglion in the modiolus. As Figure 11.7 shows, auditory neurons are bipolar, in this case having one dendritic projection to the hair cells and another axon projecting to the sensory cells in the brain stem. The efferent axons project from the superior olivary complex in the brain stem and contact the hair cells both directly and indirectly.

Electrical impulses travel along the entire length of the axon. The stimulus is received by the dendrites, which conduct it to the cell body and then to the axon. The electrical power of the neuron is derived from the axon, which generates its voltage chemically from its surroundings. Connections between neurons are called **synapses.** Once the electrochemical threshold has been reached, a neuron always responds with its maximum charge, regardless of the stimulus intensity. This has been called the all-or-none principle.

The act of conveying information between neurons is called **neurotransmission.** At one end of each nerve cell, connections are made with other nerve cells, either through their dendrites or directly with their cell bodies. Chemical substances, called **neurotransmitters,** that cause activation or inhibition of adjacent neurons are released at these junctions.

The Fluids of the Cochlea

Although similar, the constituents of the perilymph and endolymph are different in ways essential to the physiology of hearing. Endolymph is high in its concentration of potassium ions and low in sodium, whereas the reverse is true of perilymph. Another way in which the two fluids are dissimilar is in their DC (direct current) potentials (voltages). Endolymph exhibits a strong positive potential, averaging about 80 millivolts (mV), which is

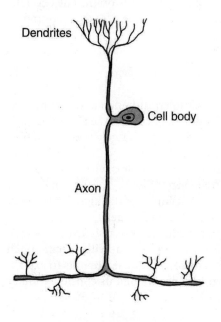

Dendrites

Cell body

Axon

FIGURE 11.7 Diagram of a bipolar sensory neuron, such as those seen in the cochlea.

caused by its high potassium concentration, compared to the perilymph of the scala tympani. The perilymph in the scala vestibuli demonstrates a positive, but much smaller, potential of about 3 mV when compared to the perilymph of the scala tympani. The remainder of the cochlear structures exhibits a negative DC potential. All of these potentials fluctuate.

The Cochlear Microphonic

The cochlea is the transducer that converts sound waves into an energy form useful to the auditory nerve. Because of its resemblance to the action of a microphone, which converts the pressure waves issuing from a speaker's mouth into an alternating electrical current, this action has been named the **cochlear microphonic (CM).** The cochlear microphonic is probably the result of changes in polarization caused by the bending back and forth of the hair cell cilia. For every up-and-down cycle of the basilar membrane, there is one in-and-out cycle of the stereocilia of the outer hair cells, causing them to become alternately depolarized and hyperpolarized. The size of the cochlear microphonic has been measured by placing pickup electrodes over the round window and, in some cases, within the cochlea.

The Action Potential

At the moment that auditory neurons are stimulated by the hair cells that rest on them, a change in the electrical potential occurs on the surface of each neuron. This is called the **action potential (AP).** Increases in the intensity of the auditory input signal to the cochlea result in increased electrical output from the hair cells. This stimulation causes increased electrical activity in the neuron, although each individual neuron continues to follow the all-or-none rule.

The Efferent System of the Cochlea

We tend to think of our sensory systems as being entirely **afferent,** carrying messages only from the sense organs, like the ear, to the brain for analysis. However, it is clear that the cochlea contains an efficient **efferent** system, receiving impulses from the brain. The relationship between afferent and efferent fibers is delicately balanced to provide a feedback, or monitoring, system for the cochlea.

Theories of Hearing

To this day, the precise means by which we hear remains unknown, although underlying mysteries continue to be resolved. Early theories that attempted to explain how the ear utilizes the mechanical energy delivered to the cochlea from the middle ear were largely theories of how we perceive pitch.

Helmholtz's[3] **resonance theory of hearing** stated that the structures within the cochlea consist of many tiny resonators, each tuned to a specific frequency. While his notions of hearing have since been disproved, he was the first to describe the placement of the higher-frequency fibers at the basal end of the cochlea and the lower frequencies near the apex.

A logical early belief was that every tone that could be heard was assigned to its own specific place within the cochlea, much as the keys of a piano are laid out with specific pitch representation. This **place theory of hearing** begins to break down when it attempts to explain why pitch discrimination is so poor close to auditory threshold, although its consideration as an incomplete theory of pitch perception may be viable.

While the place theories attributed analysis of pitch to the cochlea, several frequency-based theories, including the **volley theory of hearing** and the **resonance-volley theory,** attempted to place this analysis in a **retrocochlear** area. It was not until the middle of the 20th century that Békésy[4] (1960) described what he called the **traveling wave theory,** which put forth the explanation recognized today as the basis for cochlear pitch perception.

The traveling wave theory explains that, for each inward and outward movement of the footplate of the stapes, there is a downward and upward movement of the basilar membrane, produced by disturbance of the endolymph. The wave moves down the cochlear duct from base to apex, with the maximum amplitude of the wave occurring at the basal end of the cochlea for high-frequency tones and at the apical end of the cochlea for the low frequencies. The outer hair cells function to sharpen the wave for greater frequency discrimination. Although high frequencies excite only the fibers in the basal turn of the cochlea, the low frequencies excite fibers all along the basilar membrane. The input frequency, then, determines not only the distance the traveling wave moves before it peaks, but also the rate of basilar membrane vibration. The frequency of basilar membrane vibration is directly related to the perceived frequency.

The place theories, including the traveling wave theory, explain loudness in terms of the amplitude of movement of the basilar membrane; that is, a louder sound creates greater amplitude of basilar membrane movement than a softer sound. This greater amplitude increases the number of impulses transmitted by the nerve fibers. The frequency theories explain loudness in terms of the amount of spread along the basilar membrane. The greater the amplitude of the input signal, the larger the surface area of the basilar membrane that is stimulated, and the greater the number of nerve fibers that are firing, both at the peak of the traveling wave and on both sides of it. Although intensity coding is extremely complicated and poorly understood, it is generally agreed that as the intensity of a signal is increased, neurons in the brainstem fire at higher rates, resulting in greater loudness of the signal.

Hypotheses for Hair Cell Transduction

It is still not entirely understood how the mechanical motion of the hair cells (shearing) converts a sound source into a form of energy that can be transmitted by the auditory nerve. The *mechanical hypothesis* assumes that the pressure that moves the hair cells stimulates the nerve endings directly. The *chemical hypothesis* assumes that when the hair cells are deformed, a neurotransmitter substance is released that stimulates the nerve endings. The *electrical hypothesis* assumes that the cochlear potential stimulates the nerve endings. The conversion of acoustic energy into a neural impulse is a combination of an electrochemical response to the mechanical motion of the hair cells in the inner ear.

Otoacoustic Emissions

A great deal of thinking about the way the inner ear works has changed because of the remarkable discovery by Kemp (1978) that the cochlea, previously believed to be an organ that responds only to sounds entering the inner ear from the middle ear, in fact, generates sounds of its own. Acoustic emissions had been observed in previous research, but they were ignored and considered to be experimental artifacts. What Kemp discovered, through miniature microphones sealed in the external ear canals of human subjects, was an actual, weak acoustic signal, probably generated by the motility of the outer hair cells. The discovery now allows for study of these **otoacoustic emissions (OAEs)** in the cochlear function in humans and animals alike (Allen & Lonsbury-Martin, 1993) and adds credence to the theory of the cochlear amplifier.

Spontaneous otoacoustic emissions (SOAEs), which can be detected without external stimulation, occur in 40 to 60 percent of normal ears (DeVries & Decker, 1992; Probst, Lonsbury-Martin, & Martin, 1991). In some cases, they are audible to the subjects themselves at very low sensation levels. SOAEs may be understood on the basis of several generally accepted facts about the cochlea, specifically that the normal cochlea is very sharply tuned and processes sound nonlinearly. Damage to outer hair cells usually causes the emission to disappear.

Outer hair cell movement appears to generate waves that are conducted along the basilar membrane; through the intracochlear fluids; toward the basal end of the cochlea; then via the ossicular chain to the tympanic membrane, which acts as a loudspeaker in delivering a weak sound into the external auditory canal. It is known that the emissions are present in one or both ears of some humans (more often in right ears than in left ears, and more often in females than in males), but not of others, and that they are often absent in people with cochlear hearing loss. Any conductive hearing loss attenuates the intensity of the sound traveling outward from the cochlea and generally makes the emissions unrecordable.

Hypotheses that the phenomenon of OAEs arises from something other than a cochlear event (such as a muscular contraction or a sound generated in the middle ear) have been systematically eliminated. The relationship between these emissions and cochlear tinnitus (ringing, roaring, or other noises in the ears) has been studied (e.g., Kemp, 1981), but at present, emission behavior cannot explain this symptom in most patients with cochlear impairments.

A signal is now known to emanate from the cochlea between 5 and 20 milliseconds after the presentation of a stimulus introduced into the external ear, and it typically does not exceed 30 dB SPL, regardless of the intensity of the evoking stimulus (Whitehead, Lonsbury-Martin, & Martin, 1992). This signal is called the **transient-evoked otoacoustic emission (TEOAE).** These so-called Kemp echoes are generally described as being in the frequency range between 500 and 4,000 Hz. Additionally, when brief pure tones are used as stimuli, the emissions are close to the frequency of the evoking stimulus. To separate the TEOAE from ambient noise in the ear, a number of stimuli are presented and the response waveforms are computer-averaged.

The discovery of OAEs is providing a new way of understanding how the auditory system functions, a new means of identifying hearing loss, and another method for determining the site of auditory lesions. Some of the clinical applications of OAEs are discussed in Chapters 7 and 13.

Frequency Analysis in the Cochlea

The frequency response of the nerve cells of the cochlea is laid out in an orderly fashion, with the lowest frequencies to which the ear responds (about 20 Hz) at the apical end. The spacing between the nerve fibers is not equal all along the basilar membrane. Fibers for the frequencies between 2,000 and 20,000 Hz (the highest frequency to which the ear responds to air-conducted sounds) lie from the midpoint of the basilar membrane to the basal end of the cochlea near the oval window. Fibers for frequencies below 2,000 Hz are contained on the other half of the basilar membrane.

Humans are capable of excellent frequency discrimination, in part because auditory nerve fibers are sharply tuned to specific frequencies. The frequency that can increase the firing rate of a neuron above its spontaneous firing rate is called its characteristic frequency or best frequency. Békésy (1960), who was among the first to study the tuning mechanism of the cochlea, observed that the tuning becomes sharper (narrower bandwidth) as frequency is increased (traveling wave peak closer to the basal end of the cochlea), although it is less sharply tuned than the auditory nerve. The slope of the tuning curve is much steeper above the stimulating frequency than below it.

The concept of the **psychophysical tuning curve (PTC)** (e.g., Pick, 1980) has been used to attempt measurements of the cochlea's frequency-resolving abilities. It seems apparent that when the cochlea becomes damaged, its frequency-resolving power may become poorer, but this is not evident in all cases. Preservation of the normal psychophysical tuning curve contributes to the ear's ability to resolve complex auditory signals, such as speech. Conversely, widening the PTC in damaged ears may help to explain the kinds of speech-recognition difficulties characteristic of patients with cochlear impairment.

Development of the Inner Ear

Differentiation of the inner ear begins during the third week of gestation, and it reaches adult size and configuration by the sixth month. Placodes form early in embryonic life as thickened epidermal plates. The **auditory placode** infolds to form a pit, which closes off to form a capsule. This capsule divides to form a saccular division, from which the cochlea arises, and a utricular division, which forms the semicircular canals and probably the endolymphatic duct and sac. The vestibular portions of the inner ear develop earlier than the auditory portions.

The inner ear springs primarily from entoderm, although the membranous labyrinth is ectodermal in origin. The structure forms initially as cartilage and then changes to bone, usually by the 23rd gestational week. The cochlea and vestibule reach full size in their primitive form by the 20th week.

The cochlear turns begin to develop at about the sixth week and are complete by the ninth or tenth week. This is a particularly active time of embryogenesis of the inner ear because the endolymphatic sac and duct and the semicircular canals are also forming, and the utricle and saccule are clearly separated. The utricle, saccule, and endolymphatic duct form from the **otocyst,** the auditory vesicle, or sac, that begins its formation at the end of the first month of gestational age.

By the middle of the eighth week, the scalae are forming, and the semicircular canals reach adult configuration, including the ampullae with the cristae forming inside. The maculae are also forming within the utricle and saccule, as are the ducts that connect the saccule with the utricle and cochlear duct.

Between the 10th and 12th weeks, the organ of Corti has begun to form. By the 18th week, adult configuration of the membranous labyrinth has been reached, and by 25 weeks, the inner ear has fully formed.

Clinical COMMENTARY

The fact that fetal development takes place so rapidly probably accounts for the observation that interruption of normal development, as by a maternal disease in early pregnancy, can have such dire consequences for the inner ear. **Sensory/neural hearing loss** is the expected result of abnormality of the cochlea. In such cases, air- and bone-conduction sensitivity should be equally depressed in direct relationship to the severity of the disorder. The reasons that air-conduction and bone-conduction results may not be identical in cases of pure sensory or neural hearing loss were discussed in Chapter 4, and some variations should be expected, even though the inner ear theoretically contributes the pure distortional mode of bone conduction.

Hearing Loss and Disorders of the Inner Ear

Disorders of hearing produced by abnormality or disease of the cochlea probably constitute the largest group of hearing losses called sensory/neural, and these would clearly be sensory in nature. Much of cochlear hearing loss originates with pathology at the level of the hair cells. Promising research, based on early studies on the inner ears of birds and continuing with studies on mammalian ears, is ongoing for possible treatment of damaged hair cells or the regeneration of lost hair cells (Pirvola et al., 2000; Ryals, 2000). The current research on animals offers the greatest promise through the use of gene therapy and stem cells, both of which may bode well for future research on humans.

From a lay perspective, persons often think of hearing loss solely in terms of various levels of impairment. In reality, loss of hearing sensitivity can be quite complex, with areas of normal-hearing sensitivity and areas of profound loss coexisting in a single ear. One fact generally agreed on is that, as damage or abnormality occurs in the cochlea, loss of hearing sensitivity is not the only symptom. Indeed, a common complaint of patients with sensory or neural hearing loss is not so much that they cannot hear, but that they have difficulty understanding speech. This speech-recognition problem has been called **dysacusis,** to differentiate it from **hypacusis,** which suggests merely a loss of sensitivity to sound. Dysacusis probably results from a combination of frequency and harmonic distortion in the cochlea. As a general rule, patients with greater cochlear hearing losses have more dysacusis. Many patients with unilateral hearing losses indicate that a pure tone of a given frequency has a different pitch in each ear, a phenomenon known as **diplacusis binauralis.** At times, patients perceive that a pure tone lacks the musical quality we associate with it and that it sounds like a musical chord or a noise instead. This has been described as sounding like bacon frying. Such a lack of perception of tonal quality for a pure tone is called **diplacusis monauralis.**

Causes of Inner-Ear Disorders

Alterations in the structure and function of the cochlea produce more hearing losses than do abnormalities in other areas of the sensory/neural system. Hearing losses may result from either **endogenous** or **exogenous** causes and are significantly more frequent among men than among women (Ciletti & Flamme, 2009). For purely arbitrary reasons, this chapter examines cochlear hearing losses as they relate generally to the patient's age at onset.

Prenatal Causes

Prenatal causes are those that have an adverse effect on the normal development of the cochlea. It is difficult to know, in cases of congenital hearing loss, the extent of genetic versus environmental factors, or their possible interrelationships in a given patient. It has been known for some time that some forms of hearing loss tend to run in families. Some patients are born with the hearing loss, and others inherit the tendency for abnormalities to occur after birth. This latter form has been called **hereditodegenerative hearing loss.**

All hereditary information is incorporated in a molecule called **DNA** (deoxyribonucleic acid) and is contained in **genes,** which are the blueprints for the hereditary code. The physical manifestation of a trait is called a **phenotype,** and the actual genetic makeup that results in that trait is called a **genotype.** All of the approximately 30,000 genes are strung in a beadlike fashion along **chromosomes,** of which there are 23 pairs: 22 pairs of **autosomes** (nonsex chromosomes) and one pair of sex chromosomes. One chromosome from each pair is inherited from each parent and is randomly selected. Different forms of a gene are called **alleles.** If an allele is inherited from both parents, that trait is said to be **homozygous** (pure); if the alleles are different, this is called **heterozygous** (mixed).

Hereditary disorders can take a variety of forms. When a gene from only one parent is required for a trait to be shown, that allele is said to be dominant. If the allele from both parents is required for a trait to be shown, it is called recessive. **Autosomal dominant** hearing losses are often expected because each child has a 50 percent chance of inheriting the disorder, and a family pattern can be observed. In some cases, the dominant gene is not penetrant; that is, it does not show up phenotypically, and the hearing loss appears to skip one or more generations. Further complicating this matter is the factor of **variable expressivity,** which means that not all the signs of a hereditary condition may appear phenotypically.

Autosomal recessive inheritance accounts for about 80 percent of profound genetic hearing impairments, about half of which are associated with syndromes. Children with autosomal recessive hearing loss usually have two parents with normal hearing who are **carriers** of the recessive gene, resulting in a 25 percent chance of that gene being passed on with each pregnancy to the child, who would manifest the hearing loss, and each normal-hearing child having a two in three chance of being a carrier.

Although both of a female's sex chromosomes (labeled X) carry considerable genetic information, called **X-linked,** the male sex chromosome (which is smaller and labeled Y) contains only the information required to produce the male sex. Many recessive alleles for hearing loss are X-linked, so that a female child receiving an allele for hearing loss from one parent does not show the trait; but a male child, not having the corresponding normal gene, will probably develop the hearing loss. A female who is heterozygous for an X-linked recessive hearing loss does not have a genetic hearing loss but is a carrier and produces sons, each of whom has a 50 percent chance of having the hearing loss, and daughters, each of whom has a 50 percent chance of being a carrier. Males with X-linked hearing loss have sons who do not show the trait and daughters who are carriers. Multifactorial hereditary disorders are the result of **multifactorial genetic considerations,** combinations of hereditary and environmental factors.

Cases of hereditary hearing loss have been documented in patients with no associated abnormalities, as well as in association with external ear, skull, and facial deformities; cleft palate; optic disorders; changes in eye, hair, and skin pigmentation; thyroid disease; disorders of the heart; musculoskeletal anomalies; mental retardation; difficulty with balance and coordination; and other sensory and motor deficits. Whenever a group of symptoms is considered together for the diagnosis of a particular disorder, such a combination of signs is called a **syndrome.** At times, portions of the chromosomes are missing, or extra material is found. In some cases, an extra (third) chromosome is present; this is called **trisomy.** In cases of chromosomal disorders, the parents may be perfectly normal, but the fetus may have difficulty in surviving the pregnancy or may be severely impaired. For reasons not entirely understood, women above the age of 40 show an increased risk of bearing children with trisomic chromosomal disorders, such as Down syndrome.

The argument over the influences of heredity versus environment has gone on for a very long time and is probably counterproductive. Those who favor the former adopt a philosophy of "biological determinism" and tend to ignore the numerous environmental factors that influence all aspects of the human condition, not the least of which are the functions of the inner ear and the brain. The wide variety among humans cannot be explained on the basis of genes alone. As a matter of fact, the Human Genome Project revealed that of the 30,000 human genes, there is a difference of only one gene between humans and chimpanzees and only several hundred differences between humans and mice.

It is unknown how many disorders are determined primarily by heredity, but it is likely that genetics plays a major role in many conditions. As researchers perfect the science of gene mapping, the potential for altering the course of future diseases of all kinds brings an understandable excitement. Nevertheless, some medical ethicists fear that knowledge of an individual's susceptibility to a variety of conditions may carry with it a number of sociological dilemmas.

Different audiometric configurations have been suggested as *typical* of a given cause. There is no unanimity, however, on hereditary hearing loss, and clearly some cases may be moderate to severe bilateral losses with flat audiograms (see Figure 11.8) or predominantly high-frequency or low-frequency patterns. Some losses have been described as typically unilateral.

Problems associated with the Rh baby have become fewer in recent years as physicians have learned to predict and prevent the disorders with maternal immunization and infant

FIGURE 11.8 Audiogram showing a moderate sensory/neural hearing loss in both ears. The contour of the audiogram is relatively flat and reveals approximately equal hearing loss at all frequencies. The SRTs and the two-frequency and three-frequency pure-tone averages are in close agreement, and the word-recognition scores show some difficulty in understanding speech.

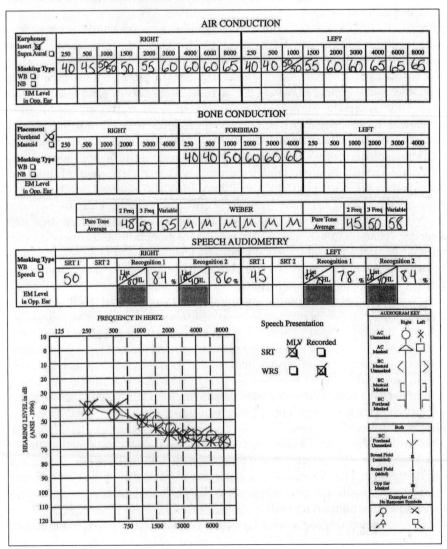

blood transfusion immediately after birth. The danger presents itself when a fetus whose blood contains the protein molecule called the **Rh factor** (rhesus factor) is conceived by a mother in whom the factor is absent. The mother's body produces antibodies for protection against the harmful effects of the Rh factor, and this antibody count is increased with succeeding pregnancies. Usually by the third pregnancy, there is a sufficient number of antibodies so that the developing red blood cells of the fetus are damaged to the extent that they cannot properly carry oxygen to essential body parts, including the cochlea. In addition, the blood of the newborn child may carry bilirubin (a component of liver bile) in increased concentration so that it may become deposited in the cochlea and produce a sensory hearing loss.

In addition to hearing loss, Rh incompatibility can result in a number of abnormalities in the newborn, including **cerebral palsy.** Cerebral palsy may be defined as damage to the brain, usually congenital, that affects the motor and frequently the sensory systems of the body. Cerebral palsy has many causes, many of which are associated with sensory hearing loss. Athetotic cerebral palsy, or **athetosis,** wherein the patient exhibits an uncontrolled writhing or squirming motion, has long been associated with hearing loss. Years ago it was assumed that, because cerebral palsy is the result of brain damage, the hearing loss is also produced by damage in the central auditory nervous system. There is evidence that, in many cases, the damage is cochlear. Because the hearing loss that accompanies athetotic cerebral palsy is often in the high frequencies, it may escape detection for years, masked by the more dramatic motor symptoms and often mental retardation.

In the 1960s, thalidomide, a tranquilizing drug first used in Europe, was introduced to pregnant women. The drug was allegedly free from unwanted complications, but this lack of side effects was more apparent than real, as evidenced by the number of children born with horrible birth deformities to mothers who had taken the drug. The most dramatic symptom was missing or malformed arms and legs; in addition, although it was not generally known, disorders of hearing also afflicted a large number of the thalidomide babies. Because large quantities of drugs, both legal and illegal, are being consumed by women of child-bearing age, it is probable that future research will disclose that many of these also contribute to congenital hearing loss.

Although a pregnant woman must always be fearful of contracting a viral disease, the fear is greatest during the first trimester (three months) of pregnancy, when the cells of the inner ear and central nervous system are differentiating most rapidly. For many years, probably the most dreaded viral infection was rubella, or German measles, because it is one of the few viruses that cross the placental barrier. Although this disease was known to be mild, or even asymptomatic in the patient, the effects on the fetus may be devastating.

The latest major rubella epidemic was seen in 1964 and 1965, with a reported 12.5 million cases and 20,000 infants born with congenital rubella syndrome (CRS). The introduction of a vaccine in 1969 reduced the number of reported cases drastically; however, there have been several resurgences through the years, mostly among the poor and religious groups that forbid vaccination. Statistics in developing countries are not readily available, so CRS continues to be a health threat.

Rubella babies tend to be smaller at birth and to develop more slowly than normal infants. They are shorter, weigh less, and have head circumferences that are less than normal. Common results of maternal rubella are brain damage, blindness, heart defects, mental retardation, and sensory hearing loss. The rubella hearing-impaired child presents special difficulties in habilitation and education because of the probability of multiple disorders.

Viral infections may actually kill or destroy cells, or they may slow down the rate at which each cell can divide and reproduce by mitosis. The rubella baby has normal-size cells, but fewer of them. It is not always clear whether the virus has affected the fetus by crossing the placental barrier or by contagion during the birth process. As the maternal body temperature increases in response to a viral or other infection, the oxygen requirement of the fetus increases dramatically. Oxygen deprivation is called **anoxia** and may result in damage to important cells of the cochlea.

Of all the congenital abnormalities produced by maternal rubella in the first trimester of pregnancy, hearing loss is the most common (Karmody, 1969). The main development of the cochlea occurs during the 6th fetal week and of the organ of Corti at the 12th week, making these critically susceptible times.

It is highly likely that the virus enters the inner ear through the stria vascularis, which would explain why the cochlea, rather than the vestibular apparatus, is usually affected. Alford (1968) has suggested that the rubella virus remains in the tissues of the cochlea even after birth. If destruction of cochlear tissue continues, the child may experience a form of progressive hearing loss that might not be associated with a prenatal cause and may elude early identification through newborn screening.

For about three decades there has been a major focus on the **acquired immune deficiency syndrome (AIDS)** and on the **human immunodeficiency virus (HIV)** found in those with AIDS. Mothers with HIV have a 50 percent chance of delivering a baby with the disease (Lawrence, 1987). How HIV affects the cochlea and the incidence with which this occurs are not known, although long-term treatment with corticosteroids has resulted in the reversal of some hearing losses and the arrest of the progression of others. Viral infections in the unborn are far more likely to occur when the mother suffers from a disease-causing deficiency in her immune system.

Probably a major cause of prenatal sensory hearing loss is **cytomegalovirus (CMV),** a seemingly harmless and often asymptomatic illness that is a member of the herpes group of viruses. The cause of the problem is an infection called cytomegalic inclusion disease (CID). When the developing fetus is infected, a variety of physical symptoms may be present, in addition to hearing loss. About 31 percent of infants infected with CMV have a serious hearing loss (Johnson, Hosford-Dunn, Paryani, Yeager, & Malachowski, 1986).

Cytomegalovirus may be transmitted from mother to child in several ways:

1. Prenatally: It may be transmitted through the placenta.
2. Perinatally: The infant may contract the virus from the cervix of an infected mother during the birth process.
3. Postnatally: The virus may be transmitted in the infected mother's milk.

Because CMV is potentially so devastating, it is curious to note that there is little active pursuit of neonatal screening for this disease. This would require only a simple test because the virus is present in the urine of all infected newborns. As a harbinger of potential acquired hearing loss, early detection of CMV can be beneficial from any point of view.

When CMV is acquired perinatally or postnatally, there are usually no serious side effects in the child. Unlike rubella, CMV does not warn an expectant mother with a telltale rash or other symptoms. Another difference is that, while investigation continues, at present there is still no vaccine to prevent CMV.

Perinatal Causes

Perinatal causes of hearing loss are those that occur during the process of birth itself. Such causes frequently produce multiple handicaps.

A common cause of damage both to the cochlea and to the central nervous system is anoxia, deprivation of oxygen to important cells, which alters their metabolism and results in damage or destruction. In the newborn, anoxia may result from prolapse of the umbilical cord, which cuts off the blood supply to the head; from premature separation of the placenta; or from a wide variety of other factors.

Accumulations of toxic substances in the mother's bloodstream may reduce the passage of oxygen across the placenta, which also results in anoxia. The fetus may also suffer from damage produced by the toxic substances themselves. For this reason, pregnant women should cautiously avoid exposure to contagious diseases such as hepatitis.

Prematurity is determined by the weight of the child at the time of birth, and not necessarily by the length of the pregnancy, as the word itself suggests. When infants weigh less than 1,500 grams (3.5 pounds) at birth, they are considered premature. Prematurity is often associated with multiple births, and both are associated with sensory hearing loss.

It is common practice to place premature infants in incubators so that, at least for the early days of life, their environments can be carefully controlled. Care must be taken not to overadminister oxygen because this produces retinal defects. At one time some motors operating incubators were found to produce extremely high noise levels (up to 95 dB SPL). Hearing losses in children thus treated may have been produced by noise, rather than, or in addition to, the results and causes of prematurity.

Trauma to the fetal head, either by violent uterine contractions or by the use of "high forceps" during delivery, may also result in damage to the brain and to the cochlea. It is possible that the head trauma itself does not produce the damage; instead, the initial cause of the difficulty in delivery may be the cause of the hearing loss.

Postnatal Causes

Postnatal causes of cochlear hearing loss are any factors occurring after birth. An often-named cause is otitis media. The toxins from the bacteria in the middle ear may enter the inner ear by way of the round or oval window, or pus may enter the labyrinth from the middle ear or from the meninges, the protective covers of the brain and spinal cord. Bacterial **meningitis,** inflammation of the meninges, may cause total deafness because, if the labyrinth fills with pus as healing takes place, the membranes and other loosely attached structures of the labyrinth are replaced by bone. Early treatment with corticosteroids may arrest the hearing loss before it becomes severe. If the enzymes produced by the infectious process enter the cochlea by diffusion through the round window, a hearing loss surely results. Often, patients with primarily conductive hearing losses produced by otitis media begin to show additional cochlear degeneration, resulting in **mixed hearing loss** (see Figure 11.9A and B).

Some viral infections have definitely been identified as the causative factors in cochlear hearing loss. These infections include measles, mumps, chickenpox, influenza, and viral pneumonia, among others. The two most common are measles (rubeola) and mumps (parotitis). Rubeola, the 10-day variety of measles, carries a significantly greater threat to the patient than does rubella. Rubeola can involve much more than the rash with which it is associated and can take a terrible toll on the patient. In addition to hearing loss, rubeola can cause heart defects, disorders of the central nervous system, and even death in severe cases. Rubeola may cause a sudden hearing loss that may not begin until some time after the other symptoms disappear. Mumps is an inflammation of the parotid (salivary) gland located on either side of the neck near the ear. When the salivary duct becomes blocked because of the viral infection, the result is the familiar lump in the neck, but neither the side of the neck most swollen, nor the degree of swelling has an effect on the degree of hearing loss that results. Both measles and mumps may be increasing in occurrence, in part due to complacency involving vaccination of small children.

Most virus-produced hearing losses are bilateral, but some viral infections, notably mumps, are associated with unilateral losses as well. Everberg (1957) estimates an incidence

FIGURE 11.9 (A) Worksheet showing a bilateral mixed hearing loss. The need to mask for air-conduction tests was averted through the use of insert receivers, which increased the interaural attenuation. Masking was required at all frequencies by bone conduction because of the large air-bone gaps. (B) Audiogram showing a mixed hearing loss in both ears. The impaired word-recognition scores reflect the sensory/neural component of the loss.

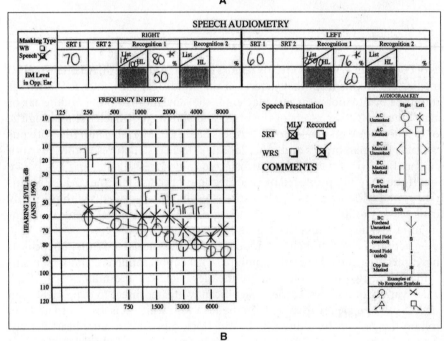

of hearing loss from mumps at 0.05 per 1,000 in the general population. Although the precise mechanism producing hearing loss from mumps is not clear, it seems likely that the route of infection is the bloodstream. Other theories, such as general infection of the labyrinth, would not explain why vestibular symptoms are frequently absent.

A disease once thought to be on the decrease, but now recognized as quite the opposite, is syphilis. This disease may be prenatal or acquired, and it often goes through three distinct but overlapping stages. Because its symptoms may resemble those of a number of different systemic diseases, it has been called the "great imitator." Brain damage is a frequent sequela of syphilis, but the cochlea may also be involved. A number of bizarre audiometric patterns have been associated with syphilis, and the variations are so great that a typical pattern does not emerge.

Infections of the labyrinth are called **labyrinthitis** and may affect both the auditory and vestibular mechanisms, producing symptoms of hearing loss and vertigo. The causes of labyrinthitis are not always known, and the condition is frequently confused with other causes of hearing loss; however, tuberculosis, syphilis, cholesteatoma, or viral infection may be implicated.

The body's natural response to infection is elevation of temperature. When the fevers become excessive, however, cells, including those of the cochlea, may become damaged. Sometimes children run high fevers with no apparent cause, but with ensuing hearing loss. When such histories are clear-cut, it is tempting to blame the fever, even when it would be logical to suspect the initial cause of the fever, such as a viral infection, as the real cause. In many cases, diagnosis of the primary cause of a hearing loss is mere speculation.

Infections of the kidneys may result in the deposit of toxic substances in the inner ear. Kidney disease may prevent medications from being excreted, thereby raising their levels in the blood abnormally high and producing ototoxicity. Other illnesses, including diabetes, have also been directly linked to cochlear damage.

Toxic Causes of Cochlear Hearing Loss

It has been said that progress has its side effects. This is notably true of the side effects of antibiotics, the wonder drugs that have saved many lives in the last seven decades. Most noted among the drugs that are cochleotoxic (i.e., cause hearing loss) are dihydrostreptomycin, viomycin, neomycin, and kanamycin. Because hearing losses ranging from mild to profound may result from the use of these drugs, it is hoped that they are not prescribed unless it is fairly certain that other drugs, with fewer or less severe side effects, will not be just as efficacious. Vestibulotoxic drugs (those that are known to affect the vestibular organs) include streptomycin and gentamycin.

Tuberculosis, which only a short time ago was declining in frequency, is experiencing resurgence. This disease can cause cochlear hearing loss, especially when the prolonged use of **ototoxic** drugs is mandatory, such as in tuberculosis sanitaria, and the patient's hearing should be monitored frequently so that any loss of hearing, or its progression, may be noted. In such cases, decisions regarding continued use of the medication must be made on the basis of the specific needs of the patient. Although the final decision on drug use is always made by a physician, it is within the purview of audiologists to make their concerns over hearing loss known.

Quinine is a drug that has long been used to combat malaria and to fight fever and reduce the pain of the common cold. Many patients who have taken this drug have complained of annoying tinnitus and hearing loss. Quinine is still prescribed (although with less frequency) for certain disorders and continues to be marketed as an over-the-counter medication.

Other drugs that have been associated with hearing loss include aspirin, certain diuretics, nicotine, and alcohol. It is usually expected that these drugs will not affect hearing unless they are taken in large amounts and over prolonged periods of time. Certainly, there are many individuals who appear to consume these substances in what might be considered excess with no side effects. The individual's own constitutional predispositions must surely be a factor here.

It has been recognized for some time that hearing loss from ototoxic drugs initially occurs, in most cases, in the high-frequency range (Jacobson, Downs, & Fletcher, 1969). Thus, physicians prescribing potentially ototoxic drugs often have time to consider alternate medications before the hearing loss encroaches on the frequencies that are more essential to discriminating speech. One of the difficulties in testing ultra-audiometric frequencies (above 8,000 Hz) has been the interference patterns that are set up when pure tones with short wavelengths are presented to the external auditory canal. Even slight differences in placement of the earphone may cause difficulty. That problem has been lessened with the use of insert earphones (Valente, Valente, & Goebel, 1992). Using extended high-frequency audiometry can assist in detecting early hearing loss from noise, chemotherapy, kidney disease, and otitis media, as well as ototoxicity, and can be helpful in understanding some causes of tinnitus in patients who have normal hearing through the usual audiometric frequency range.

The American Speech-Language-Hearing Association (1994) has published guidelines for monitoring patients who receive cochleotoxic drugs. Elements of these guidelines include the following:

1. Specific criteria for identification of toxicity.
2. Timely identification of at-risk patients.
3. Pretreatment counseling regarding potential cochleotoxic effects.
4. Valid baseline measures (hearing tests) performed before treatment or shortly after treatment begins.
5. Periodic monitoring evaluations at intervals timed to document progression of hearing loss.
6. Follow-up evaluations to determine post-treatment effects.

In addition to prescribed medications that can be ototoxic, some so-called recreational drugs can create irreversible hearing loss. Bilateral sensory/neural hearing loss arising from both cochlear and neural pathology can result from cocaine or heroine use in isolation and in combination, as in "speedballing" (Fowler & King, 2008).

Otosclerosis

As mentioned in Chapter 10, otosclerosis is a disease of the bony labyrinth that causes a conductive hearing loss when the new bone growth affects either the oval window or the round window. Although it is uncommon, if otosclerosis involves the cochlea, sensory or mixed hearing loss results, and the hearing loss may be either bilateral or unilateral. Although there are no binding rules, the audiometric configuration is generally flat, and speech recognition is not severely affected. There is a characteristic appearance of this condition that can be seen on CT scans but not MRIs. Attempts have been made to arrest the progression of cochlear otosclerosis with sodium fluoride, but the effectiveness of this treatment has not been proved.

Barotrauma

Barotrauma was mentioned as a cause of conductive hearing loss. In addition, sudden changes in middle-ear pressure, as from diving, flying, or even violent sneezing, may cause a rupture of the round window or a tearing of the annulus of the oval window. The resulting fistula (perilymph leak) can often be surgically repaired and may reverse a permanent or fluctuating cochlear hearing loss and/or vertigo. Barotrauma can produce a mild to profound hearing loss.

Noise-Induced Hearing Loss

The industrial revolution's introduction of high levels of noise brought a greater threat to the human auditory system than evolution had prepared for. Documented cases of noise-induced hearing loss go back more than 200 years. Hearing losses from intense noise may be the result of exposure to high-level sounds, with subsequent partial or complete hearing recovery, or of repeated exposure to high-level sounds, with permanent impairment. Cases in which hearing thresholds improve after an initial impairment following noise are said to be the result of **temporary threshold shift (TTS)**; irreversible losses are called **permanent threshold shift (PTS)**.

A number of agents may interact with noise to increase the danger to hearing sensitivity. Research has shown that aspirin, which has been known to produce reversible hearing loss after ingestion, synergizes with noise to produce a greater temporary threshold shift than would otherwise be observed (McFadden & Plattsmier, 1983). Although the effects of aspirin on permanent hearing loss have not been demonstrated, it certainly seems prudent for audiologists to advise that people who must be exposed to high levels of noise should refrain from taking this drug, at least at times closely related to exposure.

Men appear to have a higher incidence of hearing loss from noise than do women (Ewertson, 1973), perhaps because as a group they have greater noise exposure, both on the job and during leisure activities. This tendency may indeed have an earlier origin, as the prevalence of noise-induced threshold shift among U.S. children age 6 to 19 years is greater than 14 percent among boys, while the prevalence stands at a lower 10 percent among girls (Niskar et al., 2001). There is evidence that children are suffering increased amounts of hearing loss from items such as toy phones, musical instruments, firecrackers, stereo systems, and toy guns, some of which produce noise levels up to 155 dBA (Nadler, 1997). The fact that children's arms are shorter than adults' results in anything noisy held in the hand being closer to the ear. Although there are recommended guidelines for childhood hearing screening (see Chapter 7), there are no U.S. federal mandates for screening within this population. Clearly, hearing awareness should be presented to school-age children as part of any activities that may be considered by the school speech-language pathologist or educational audiologist for May, Better Hearing and Speech Month or October, Audiology Awareness Month.

Postmortem electron microscope studies (see Figure 11.10) have shown loss of hair cells and their supporting structures in the basal end of the cochlea and nerve degeneration in the osseous lamina (Johnson & Hawkins, 1976) in patients with noise-induced hearing loss. The hearing loss may be due to biological changes in the sensory cells, physical dislodging of hair cells during high sound-level stimulation, changes in the cochlear blood supply with consequent alterations in the function of the stria vascularis, loss of the outer hair cells, rupture of Reissner's membrane, detachment of the organ of Corti from the basilar membrane, or a variety of other causes.

FIGURE 11.10 These electron microscopic images show intact hair cells (A) and a section of the basilar membrane (B) with significant missing hair cells in the basal end of the cochlea. (*Source:* The National Institute for Occupational Safety and Health.)

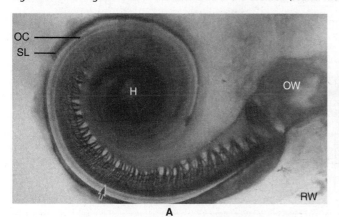

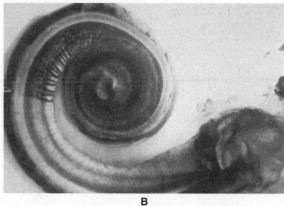

Acoustic trauma is the term often used to describe noise-induced hearing loss from impulsive sounds such as explosions and gunfire. A common audiometric configuration, shown in Figure 11.11, depicts what has been called the **acoustic trauma notch.** Characteristically, the hearing is poorest in the range between 3000 and 6000 Hz, with recovery at 8000 Hz, suggesting damage to the portion of the basal turn of the cochlea related to that frequency range. As a rule, the amounts of hearing loss are similar in both ears when individuals acquire noise-induced hearing losses in the workplace. Rifle shooters generally show more hearing loss in the ear

FIGURE 11.11 Audiogram showing a typical acoustic trauma notch at 4000 Hz. SRTs and WRSs are normal, showing little difficulty in quiet because the hearing loss is primarily above the critical frequency range for hearing and understanding speech. It can be expected that the patient experiences considerable difficulty in understanding speech in the presence of background noise, and additional speech audiometrics to objectively demonstrate this should be considered. Note that the two- and three-frequency pure-tone averages fail to reflect any loss of hearing sensitivity, while the variable pure tone average does.

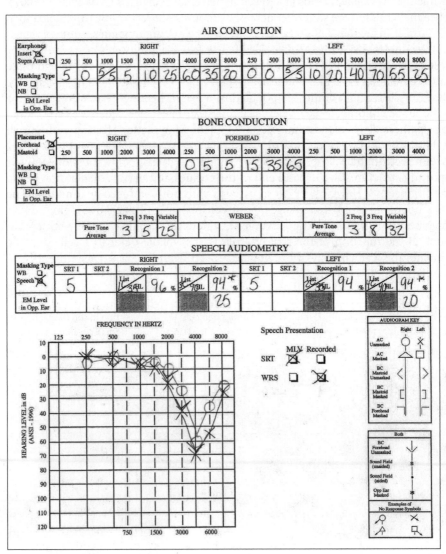

opposite the shoulder to which the rifle stock is held; that is, right-handed s[...] hearing loss in their left ears. A survey in Canada on noise-induced hearin[...] revealed greater loss in the left ear, probably produced by the rush of air [...] on the driver's side (Dufresne, Alleyne, & Reesal, 1988).

The acoustic trauma notch is not found in all cases of noise-induced hear[...] restricted to this cause. It is strongly suggestive of noise, however, and should be co[...] with supporting evidence, such as the clinical history. To help ensure that a noise notch [...] missed on routine evaluations, hearing should always be tested at 3000 and 6000 Hz, even if sensitivity at adjacent octave and mid-octave frequencies is normal. Some audiometers are designed to test frequencies higher than conventional audiometers: up to 16,000 Hz. The use of high-frequency audiometry can yeild earlier detection of cochlear noise damage (Mehrpavar, Mirmohammadi, Ghoreyshi, Mollasadeghi, & Loukzadeh, 2011) as well as damage from oto-toxic medications (Abujamra et al., 2013).

Industrial noise is a factor long recognized as a cause of hearing loss. The term *boilermaker's disease* was coined many years ago to describe the hearing losses sustained by men working in the noisy environs of that industry. Although boilermakers may be fewer in number today, modern technology has produced new and even noisier industries. Exposure to jet engines, drop forges, pneumatic hammers, subways, loud music, and even computers has been documented as causing hearing loss. Fifty years ago, a study of the effects of noise on hearing revealed that older populations in societies that have lower noise-exposure levels exhibit better hearing sensitivity than do those populations in other societies (Rosen, Bergman, Plester, El-Mofty, & Hammed, 1962). Of course, differences in diet, lifestyle, and so on, may also account for the better hearing sensitivity of the older members of more primitive societies.

Noise in society is an ever-increasing problem. Millions of dollars are paid to military veterans in compensation for hearing loss, which is the largest compensable disability among veterans: a disability likely to increase given the increase in global hostilities. Insurance companies, whose coverage includes noisy industries, have been forced to become increasingly concerned with the effects of noise on hearing. Aside from the psychological, social, and vocational handicaps imposed on patients with noise-induced hearing loss, the financial figures have led to concern on the part of government and industry alike.

After a number of proposals, lawsuits, and reversals, the Occupational Safety and Health Administration (OSHA; 1983) has recommended a scale on which the time that a worker may be safely exposed to intense sounds is decreased as the intensity of the noise is increased. Under this rule, the maximum exposure level before hearing-conservation measures must be implemented is 85 dBA for an eight-hour workday. For every 5 dB increase in noise above 90 dBA, the allowable exposure time is cut in half. OSHA's standards for hearing conservation have the legal backing of a federal regulation, but the National Institute for Occupational Safety and Health (NIOSH) has promulgated guidelines that, for many audiologists, are becoming the benchmark for standard of care (National Institute for Occupational Safety and Health, 1998). The NIOSH guidelines are more stringent than those set by OSHA in several areas, including noise monitoring, noise exposure limits, hearing monitoring practices, and the training of audiometric technicians. For example, NIOSH endorses a more protective 3 dB time-intensity tradeoff rather than OSHA's 5 dB exchange rate. Table 11.1 contrasts the OSHA recommended noise standard with the more stringent NIOSH recommendations.

Sound-level meters, or individually worn noise dosimeters, are used to measure the intensity of sound in noisy areas, such as in factories and around aircraft, to determine whether the noise levels fall within or exceed the **damage-risk criteria** set up by OSHA or recommended by NIOSH. The use of any damage-risk criteria is oversimplified, in part because the specified intensities listed do not take into consideration the concentration of sound energy in different

TABLE 11.1 Maximum Sound Exposure Levels as a Function of Duration of Exposure Set to Protect Workers' Hearing*

dB SPL	85	88	90	92	94	95	97	100	105	110	115
NIOSH (hour limit)	8	4			1	¾	½	¼			
OSHA (hour limit)			8			4		2	1	½	¼

Lawnmowers, subways, and truck traffic can measure above 90 dBA. Rock concerts, band practices, and car stereos with aftermarket subwoofers are frequently measured in excess of 110 dBA.

Sources: National Institute for Occupational Safety and Health, 1998; Occupational Safety and Health Administration, 2010. Modified from Niquette and Eply, 2010.

frequency bands. In addition, the impulsive characteristics of offending sounds have also not been considered because most of the sound-level meters used have an averaging time of about 125 milliseconds, while the peaks of many sounds occur within 25 to 50 microseconds. Because it takes some time for the brain to average the sounds, they may be more intense than their psychological interpretations appear and therefore more dangerous than thought.

Lipscomb (1992) points out that readings from noise dosimeters can be misleading and can appear substantially different, depending on how the instrument is set. Hearing conservation is really not an area in which audiologists should merely dabble without the proper background and knowledge.

Because of the increasing interest in noise-induced hearing loss in industry, a number of hearing-conservation programs have been developed in the United States and around the world. Lipscomb (1992) defines a comprehensive hearing-conservation program (HCP) as one that (1) identifies people who are at risk for noise-induced hearing loss, (2) abates dangerous noise levels as economically as possible, and (3) protects employees who are at risk for noise-induced hearing loss.

Workers are being advised about the dangers of noise and are encouraged to wear hearing protectors such as those shown in Figures 11.12 and 11.13. It is likely that hearing protectors may provide a false sense of security, assuring wearers that they are "safe" from noise damage. However, many problems are associated with fitting and wearing hearing protectors, and the amount of sound attenuation found in the laboratory may be considerably more than that actually obtained on the job (Berger & Casali, 2000). The more experience individuals have in fitting earplugs in their own ears, the greater the sound attenuation provided. Davis, Richards, and Martin (2007) reported no significant difference in the attenuation provided by muff-style hearing protection for untrained users and those trained in the use of muffs. However, four other styles of hearing protectors were found to provide either significantly greater attenuation or less variability in the attenuation provided when users were given direct instruction in their use, speaking to the importance of the audiologist's direct involvement in the selection and initial use of hearing protectors. Audiologists should warn hearing aid users that the hollow shell of a turned-off hearing aid provides little effective protection. A demonstration of the proper use of earplugs and earmuffs as hearing protection devices may be seen in the video titled Hearing Protection.

Many preemployment physical examinations now include pure-tone audiometry, but OSHA (1983) requires the first test to be carried out within six months of employment. After that, annual tests (defined as no further apart than 15 months) must be made. Routine tests may be contaminated by recent noise exposure, and the amount of temporary threshold shift and time to recovery is determined, in large part, by the intensity of the previous exposure. According to Melnick (1984), some TTS does not recover for a week or even longer.

FIGURE 11.12 Commercial earplugs designed to attenuate high noise levels. (*Source:* Oaktree Products, Inc.)

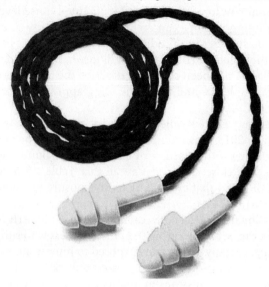

FIGURE 11.13 Commercial earmuffs designed to be worn in areas of intense noise. (*Source:* Oaktree Products, Inc.)

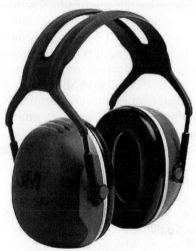

The amount of hearing loss shown by a person exposed to high noise levels in the workplace can vary for many reasons. Genetic factors are always a consideration, as are disease, aging, and noise exposure off the job site. The insidious nature of noise-induced hearing loss often results in long delays before the onset of hearing problems and consultation with a hearing specialist.

A surprising amount of the noise-induced hearing loss seen today is caused by other than work-related activities. It has been known, almost since their innovation, that airbag deployment can cause hearing loss, tinnitus, hyperacusis, and balance disorders (Price & Kalb, 1999). This is not surprising, given that an airbag impulse can generate a noise from 160 to 170 dB SPL. Many millions of people are engaged in hobbies involving motorboats, snowmobiles, motorbikes, and racecars, in addition to the use of guns. What may be viewed as quieter recreation may even pose potential risk to participants. Documented noise levels when using some styles of thin-faced titanium golf clubs can create an impact noise at ear level approaching 130 dB SPL, which may be sufficient to produce either temporary or permanent hearing threshold shifts for susceptible golfers (Buchanan, Wilkinson, Fitzgerald, & Prinsley, 2008). The term *recreational audiology* has been coined to describe the activities of professionals involved in finding these hearing losses and recommending appropriate precautionary steps.

Testament to growing noise levels in society is exemplified by the exuberant outbursts of excited sports fans around the world. In October 2013, fans at the Kansas City Chiefs' Arrowhead Stadium set a new record for loudest sports venue with measures of 137.5 decibels sound pressure level (Guinness World Records, 2013). The close reader may recall that Table 3.3 noted pain from intense sounds begins at 125 dB SPL and that even short-term exposure to sounds exceeding 140 dB SPL can cause permanent hearing loss.

Exposure to intense sounds by professional musicians has caused a special concern for this group. Musicians generally rely more on the sense of hearing than many others who suffer from noise-induced hearing loss and may spend many hours a day exposed to intense sounds. Research suggests that attendance at a single rock/pop concert can create significant postconcert shifts in hearing and reduction in otoacoustic emissions amplitude, indicating a negative impact on outer hair cell function (Derebery, Vermiglio, Berliner, Potthoff, & Holquin, 2012). The long-term cumulative effect on young concert attendees clearly raises public health concerns.

Aerobic instructors and their students may be at particular risk from intense music exposure; studies have suggested that physical exercise plus noise results in greater threshold shifts than exposure to noise alone (Vittitow, Windmill, Yates, & Cunningham, 1994), possibly due to the effects on the cochlea of changes in metabolic activity during exercise. It is not just musicians and music lovers who can put themselves at risk of the adverse effects of intense sound. A coincidental finding for beluga whales reveals that music played above 95 dBA SPL for more than two hours in the festivities ballroom of the Georgia Aquarium not only can be harmful to human hearing but is transferred through the viewing window of the adjacent marine mammal aquarium at levels that may potentially generate stress in the captive whales (converted to dB relative to 1 micropascal [μPa] for underwater measures) (Scheifele, Clark, Miller, Gaglione, & Starke, 2009).

The original impetus for the birth of the audiology profession was acquired hearing loss following military service in World War II, and modern weaponry continues as a major contributor to noise-induced hearing loss (see Figure 11.14). The Department of Veterans Affairs has ranked tinnitus and hearing loss as the two most frequent disabilities in the "war on terror" (U.S. Department of Veterans Affairs, 2008). Nearly 100,000 troops who have served in Iraq and Afghanistan collect disability for tinnitus, with the numbers on disability for permanent hearing loss not far behind.

A patient with apparent noise-induced hearing loss should be advised to limit further exposure to loud noise and to use protective earplugs or earmuffs whenever exposure is necessary. Periodic hearing examinations to monitor progression should also be encouraged. Hunters, target shooters, and snowmobile drivers are often a particularly difficult group to work with because of their reluctance both to wear hearing protectors and to limit their sport. Music enthusiasts who use stereo headphones or portable stereo systems are often at risk for hearing loss because of the high levels of sound delivered directly to their ears. Special hearing protection that does not distort sound quality is available for musicians. Some audiologists have found a new market in the area of recreational audiology as they work toward addressing the hearing protection needs of those whose hobbies endanger their hearing.

FIGURE 11.14 Military personnel are regularly exposed to damaging noise levels. Unexpected roadside bombs, ambushes, and sudden firefights do not afford time for soldiers to insert military-issued hearing protection. (*Source:* U.S. Department of Defense.)

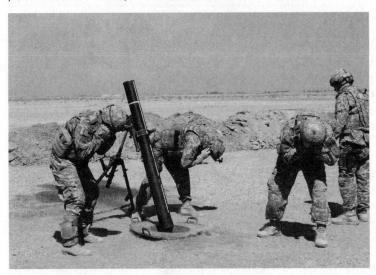

Often, initial examination of hearing is made on the basis of a complaint of tinnitus alone. In patients with an acoustic trauma notch, the tinnitus is often described as a pure tone and can be matched to frequencies in the 3,000 to 6,000 Hz range. Many such patients are unaware of the existence of hearing loss and may even deny it. By the time progression of the impairment has been demonstrated to patients, their communicative difficulties have worsened considerably. The persuasiveness and tact of the audiologist in counseling such patients is of paramount importance.

Shargorodsky, Curhan, and Farwell (2010) examined complaints of tinnitus among over 14,000 subjects in the 1999–2004 National Health and Nutrition Examination Surveys and calculated the frequency of tinnitus in the overall U.S. population. They concluded that approximately 50 million U.S. adults reported having at least occasional tinnitus, and 16 million adults reported having frequent tinnitus. Not surprisingly, the prevalence of frequent tinnitus increased with increasing age. Non-Hispanic whites had higher incidences of frequent tinnitus compared with other racial/ethnic groups. Hypertension and former smoking were associated with an increase in odds of frequent tinnitus. Loud leisure-time, firearm, and occupational noise exposure also were associated with increased odds of frequent tinnitus. Among those who had an audiogram, increased incidence of tinnitus was associated with low- to mid-frequency and high-frequency hearing impairment. Frequent tinnitus was associated with generalized anxiety but not major depression. Refer to Chapter 15 for additional discussion of tinnitus management.

Lovers of loud music are enthralled by the introduction of the earbuds that are used with iPods and MP3 players. Their improved comfort and sound quality encourage the wearers to increase the sound output of the devices to enhance the personal enjoyment of music. Not only are preferred listening levels higher when earbuds are used, levels of background noise interfere with music reception through earbuds more than through over-the-ear headphones, consequently causing users to seek even higher volume levels (Hodgetts, Rieger, & Szarko, 2007). They are often used by joggers or those working out on gym equipment whose physical stress helps to mask the danger of the increased sound intensity. The fact that the earbuds are pressed into the external auditory canal, thereby decreasing the air volume between them and the tympanic membrane, can increase the SPL of the signal as much as 9 dB over more traditional receivers. The ensuing hearing losses often resemble the audiometric features seen in patients whose losses are attributed to aging. The increased damage risk from these devices mandates greater cautionary efforts by hearing healthcare professionals regarding the use of these devices. While research suggests that MP3 listening levels may not be as great a concern for an adult-professional population, routine, long-term use levels are not clearly documented among younger listeners (Hodgetts et al., 2007).

With continued funding through the U.S. Department of Defense, research on a "hearing pill" containing antioxidants may be shown to positively affect the cochlea following noise exposure. Progress continues to be made on this patented pharmaceutical agent as a post-exposure treatment for military personnel as well as those who voluntarily subject their ears to excess levels of recreational noise or music.

There is increasing evidence that noise has other adverse effects besides hearing loss. Noise may play a role in increased anxiety levels, loss of the ability to concentrate, higher divorce rates, greater incidence of illness, and loss of sleep. The ongoing search for U.S. energy independence has led to the development of wind farms across the country (see Figure 11.15). While insufficient to damage hearing, the wind turbine noise has been found to be more disturbing than comparably loud transportation noise or industrial noise, possibly due to the rhythmic swishing noise and the fact that it continues unabated through the night (Pedersen, van den Berg, Bakker, & Bouma, 2009). These ongoing sounds can result in sleep deprivation and subsequent health problems for nearby residents. Additional research has looked at the possible acoustic effects of land-based and off-shore wind farms on wildlife on land and in the sea and air. According to Hempton and Grossman (2009), there is no place left on earth that is free of human-generated noise 100 percent of the time. Clearly humans' noise imprint on the world around them is pervasive.

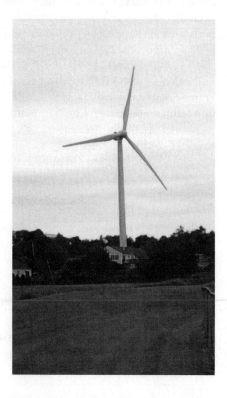

FIGURE 11.15 Low-frequency noise accompanied by a perceived swishing sound generated by wind turbines may result in sleep deprivation and accompanying health problems for nearby residents. (*Source:* Lisa A. Miller.)

Tobacco Smoke and Sensory/Neural Hearing Loss

It has long been accepted that tobacco smoke is linked to a wide variety of serious illnesses and cancers. The effects of cigarette smoke, both primary and secondary, were discussed in Chapter 10 as contributors to otitis media and therefore to conductive hearing loss. It is now becoming increasingly clear that these substances may be a major contributory element in permanent sensory/neural hearing loss.

Although the link between cigarette smoking and sensory/neural hearing loss has been known for more than four decades, recent work on a number of tests, including otoacoustic emissions (Negley et al., 2007) indicates that not only the outer hair cells may be involved, but also symptoms of central auditory processing disorders. Particularly at risk are children of mothers who smoked during pregnancy as well as those exposed to secondhand smoke. As a matter of fact, it is likely that the growing number of hearing losses in preteens, teenagers, and young adults previously ascribed to exposure to intense sounds (such as loud music) may, in fact, be caused by direct or secondhand smoke or that the two factors may synergize (Wild, Brewster, & Banerjee, 2005). A likely cause, at least in part, is the reduction in oxygen in the cochlea caused by cigarette smoke.

Radiation-Induced Hearing Loss

The use of radiotherapy for the treatment of brain tumors and head and neck cancers can adversely affect any of the auditory structures, from the external auditory meatus through the more central auditory pathways. The majority of radiation-induced conductive hearing losses arising from acute complications to the middle-ear system and occurring in up to 40 percent of patients (Jereczek-Fossa, Zarowski, Milani, & Orecchia, 2003) are not permanent. However, nearly one-third of patients whose radiotherapy extends to the cochlea experience permanent sensory hearing loss. The combined use of radiation and chemotherapy places a patient at higher risk for hearing loss. Patients scheduled to undergo radiation should have a preradiation baseline auditory assessment, with a repeat evaluation at the conclusion of radiotherapy. Given the delayed onset of radiation-induced hearing loss and its documented progression, regular monitoring of hearing status is essential. Audiological management of radiation-induced hearing loss is complicated by the fact that speech recognition can be significantly poorer than would be predicted by the pure-tone hearing loss (Bass & White, 2008).

Cochlear Hearing Loss Following Surgical Complications

Sometimes even the best middle-ear surgeon not only fails to improve hearing with corrective surgery but, in fact, makes it worse. Many otologists estimate that a cochlear hearing loss following stapedectomy is probable in 1 or 2 percent of those operated on. The odds appear very good, except, of course, for the unfortunate few.

An early practice to ensure mobility during stapedectomy was to palpate the ossicular chain to check for a light reflex on the round window. This is no longer done because it has been found to generate traveling waves of amplitude greater than most environmental sounds that can cause cochlear damage.

Excessive bleeding, or other surgical complications, may account for some cases of cochlear hearing loss following middle-ear surgery, but some cases of even total hearing loss in the operated ear cannot be related to any specific cause. Some technically perfect operations are also followed by total deafness. Evidently, for specific physiological reasons, some patients do not tolerate the surgery well. The term *fragile ears* has been assigned to this group, and it is unfortunate that these cases cannot be predicted preoperatively. Common complications of middle-ear surgery include transitory vertigo and alterations in the sense of taste.

Sudden Idiopathic Sensory/Neural Hearing Loss

Sudden idiopathic sensory/neural hearing loss (SISNHL) refers to a hearing loss, usually unilateral, that may develop over the course of a few days or occur seemingly instantaneously, with many patients claiming that they awoke from sleep in the morning to find that their hearing had changed. Generally, a SISNHL is defined as a decrease of at least 30 dB over at least three octaves within a period no greater than three days (Zadeh, Storper, & Spitzer, 2003). Although a number of etiologies have been suggested, they break down into broad categories that include autoimmune diseases, viral or other infections, rupture of the basilar membrane, vascular disorders, tumors, or other neurological disorders. A viral origin may be more suspect if respiratory infection has preceded the loss. While such hearing losses may occur among patients of any age, they are most frequent by far in the adult population.

The nutrition of the cochlea is supplied by the stria vascularis, which is fed by the internal auditory artery, with no collateral blood supply. If a spasm occurs in that artery, total unilateral deafness may result, although the sustained loss may be substantially less for some individuals. A sudden loss of hearing should always be treated as a medical emergency, with diagnosis including a number of blood tests, magnetic resonance imaging, and neurological testing. Therapy is often directed at vasodilation. The sooner therapy is instituted following the onset of symptoms, the better is the prognosis for complete recovery.

A relatively new procedure has shown to be beneficial in many cases. A myringostomy is performed and a cylindrical wick is threaded through the PE tube with one end of the wick positioned against the round window membrane. The patient applies steroid drops to the external ear canal, which are drawn through the wick by capillary action and delivered to the inner ear via absorption through the round window. This approach to the administration of steroids for the treatment of sudden idiopathic hearing loss permits the delivery of relatively high concentrations of the medicine, simultaneously minimizing the systemic side effects often observed when these medications are taken orally (Silverstein, Thompson, Rosenberg, Brown, & Light, 2004). The self-administration of the drops significantly reduces the number of physician visits required if medication is administered through transtympanic injections.

If **vasospasm** is suspected as an underlying cause of the hearing loss, treatment often includes immediate hospitalization, with intravenous administration of the appropriate medications. At times, hearing recovery is complete. Vestibular symptoms, such as vertigo and nausea, as well as the often accompanying tinnitus, may also abate. In some patients, symptoms disappear spontaneously, whereas in others they persist in the form of severe or total unilateral hearing loss.

Ménière's Disease

Another cause of sudden unilateral hearing loss is **Ménière's disease.**[5] The seat of the difficulty lies within the labyrinth of the inner ear. In a normal inner ear, the endolymph is maintained at a constant volume and contains specific concentrations of chloride, sodium, potassium, and other electrolytes, which allows the structures to function normally.

The disorder is characterized by sudden attacks of vertigo, tinnitus, vomiting, and unilateral hearing loss. Although usually unilateral, bilateral Ménière's disease has been observed in 5 to 10 percent of the studied cases of aural vertigo. Many patients describe the onset of symptoms in the same way. The difficulty may begin with a sensation of fullness in one ear, followed by a low-frequency roaring tinnitus, hearing loss with great difficulty in speech recognition, the sensation of violent turning or whirling in space, and vomiting. Although these may be considered the classic symptoms associated with Ménière's disease, not all symptoms are present in each case. Indeed, some may have what has come to be known as cochlear Ménière's disease, which may be characterized solely by fluctuating and progressive sensory hearing loss and possible aural fullness accompanying a sudden drop in hearing. Similarly, a second subcategory known as vestibular Ménière's disease may present solely with spells of vertigo with no change in hearing. The symptom of aural fullness helps differentiate this condition from vestibular **neuritis** (Pulec, 1996), or inflammation of the auditory nerve. The qualifiers of *cochlear* or *vestibular* are dropped if more inclusive symptoms of Ménière's disease develop subsequently.

Ménière's disease may occur as a result of a blow to the head, infection, degeneration of the inner ear, allergy, or (in rare circumstances) a tumor. In many cases the cause is entirely undetermined. Many authorities believe that it is caused by endolymphatic hydrops, the oversecretion or underabsorption of endolymph. As the fluid pressure builds in the cochlear duct, the pressure on the hair cells produces the tinnitus and hearing loss. If the pressure builds sufficiently, the vestibular apparatus becomes overstimulated, and vertigo ensues. According to Lawrence (1969), excessive endolymphatic pressure alone could not alter the function of the inner ear unless the metabolic or ionic balances were disturbed, as by a rupture of Reissner's membrane. In earlier times treatment was designed to limit fluid intake and retention through diuretic drugs, but the opposite approach is taken today, assuring that the patient has adequate fluid ingestion. Alcohol, smoking, and caffeine (in the forms of chocolate, cola drinks, coffee, and tea) all tend to increase symptoms.

It is likely that a change in the elasticity of the basilar membrane, combined with the loading of the cochlear duct produced by the increased endolymphatic pressure, cause the hearing loss to be in the low frequencies. This may also account for the harmonic distortion and the diplacusis. The displacement of the basilar membrane probably affects the shearing action between the tectorial membrane and the organ of Corti. The displacement of the basilar membrane probably decouples the tips of the hair cells from the tectorial membrane, which can explain the tinnitus, loudness recruitment, and the distortion that results in decreased speech recognition scores.

Sedatives, tranquilizers, and vestibular suppressants have all been used. Reports on the success rates of different therapies vary in the medical literature; some have even been described as placebo effects. More recently, wicks placed through a PE tube, as described earlier for treatment of sudden idiopathic sensory/neural hearing loss, have been used to reduce symptoms of vertigo related to Ménière's disease. Anxiety and allergic factors have been considered as causes of Ménière's disease, which affects more men than women and rarely affects children. Other causes may be trauma, surgery, syphilis, hypothyroidism, and low blood sugar.

Ménière's disease may be extremely handicapping. The paroxysmal (sudden, without warning) attacks of vertigo may interfere with driving an automobile, or even with performing one's job. The disease has been called the "labyrinthine storm" because of the sudden and dramatic appearance of symptoms; it is characterized by remissions and exacerbations. Cases of bilateral hearing loss due to Ménière's disease are helped best with multimemory hearing aids, which offer more than one pattern of amplification to address fluctuating hearing loss.

Surgical approaches to Ménière's disease are often aimed at decompressing the endolymphatic sac or draining the excessive endolymph by inserting a shunt into spaces in the skull so that the fluid can be excreted along with cerebrospinal fluid. Ultrasonic and freezing procedures

FIGURE 11.16 (A) Worksheet illustrating sensory/neural hearing loss in the right ear. Masking was required for bone conduction but not for air conduction due to the increased interaural attenuation provided by insert receivers. (B) Audiogram showing a unilateral (right) sensory/neural hearing loss observed in a patient with Ménière's disease. Word recognition is impaired in the right ear. Even with the larger interaural attenuation provided by insert receivers, masking for WRS is required for speech audiometrics at lower sensation levels.

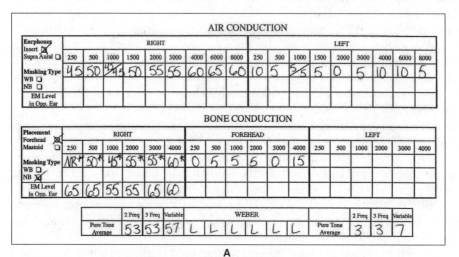

AIR CONDUCTION

Earphones Insert ☒ Supra Aural ☐	RIGHT									LEFT								
	250	500	1000	1500	2000	3000	4000	6000	8000	250	500	1000	1500	2000	3000	4000	6000	8000
Masking Type WB ☐ NB ☐	45	50	45/55	50	55	55	60	65	60	10	5	5/5	5	0	5	10	10	5
EM Level in Opp. Ear																		

BONE CONDUCTION

Placement Forehead ☒ Mastoid ☐	RIGHT						FOREHEAD						LEFT					
	250	500	1000	2000	3000	4000	250	500	1000	2000	3000	4000	250	500	1000	2000	3000	4000
Masking Type WB ☐ NB ☒	NR*	50*	45*	55*	55*	60*	0	5	5	5	0	15						
EM Level in Opp. Ear	65	65	55	55	65	60												

	2 Freq	3 Freq	Variable	WEBER							2 Freq	3 Freq	Variable
Pure Tone Average	53	53	57	L	L	L	L	L	L	Pure Tone Average	3	3	7

A

SPEECH AUDIOMETRY

Masking Type WB ☐ Speech ☒	RIGHT					LEFT			
	SRT 1	SRT 2	Recognition 1	Recognition 2		SRT 1	SRT 2	Recognition 1	Recognition 2
	50		List 60% HL	List 56% HL		5		List 100% HL	List 100% HL
EM Level in Opp. Ear			15	25					

Speech Presentation

	MLV	Recorded
SRT	☒	☐
WRS	☐	☒

B

have also been used. In extreme cases, the entire labyrinth has been surgically destroyed or the auditory nerve severed to alleviate the vertigo and tinnitus. Even such dramatic steps as these are not always entirely successful. Audiological findings in Ménière's disease are shown in Figures 11.16 through 11.19. Specific diagnosis of this condition can often be accomplished with electrocochleography (Ferraro, 1992).

FIGURE 11.17 Results on immittance for the patient with Ménière's disease illustrated in Figure 11.16B. The tympanogram is normal for both ears but shows a lower point of maximum compliance on the left ear because of increased pressure in the inner ear. Static compliance is normal for both ears, but it is lower in the left ear than in the right ear. Tympanometric width is normal for both ears. The sensation level of the acoustic reflex is reduced in the right ear, suggesting a lesion of the cochlea.

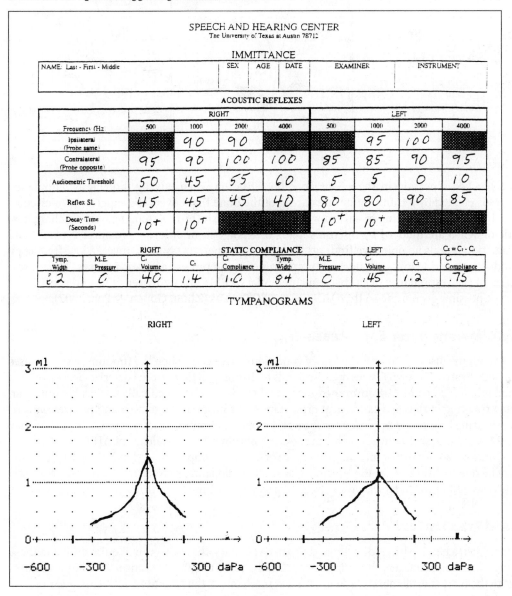

Semicircular Canal Dehiscence Syndrome

Also known as superior canal dehiscence syndrome because the superior semicircular canal is much more frequently affected than the posterior canal, **semicircular canal dehiscence syndrome (SCDS)** can mimic the symptoms of other otologic pathologies and be easily misdiagnosed. Due to its symptoms of dizziness, vertigo, and disequilibrium, SCDS has frequently been misdiagnosed as a peripheral vestibular disorder. In addition to vestibular symptoms, patients with SCDS may present with complaints often associated with a patulous eustachian tube such

FIGURE 11.18 Results of auditory brain-stem response testing on the patient with a cochlear hearing loss (Ménière's disease) in the right ear (see Figure 11.16). Absolute latencies are shown in Figure 11.19.

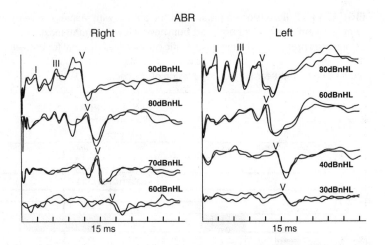

as a blocked sensation in the ear or an echo sensation when talking, known as autophony. SCDS is created by a thinning or weakening of the bone that covers the superior semicircular canal, essentially resulting in a third window in the labyrinthine system. Symptoms characteristic of SCDS are induced by intense sounds or change in middle-ear pressure. Typical ENG evaluation reveals no objective findings. Routine audiometrics typically reveal a low-frequency conductive hearing loss with normal tympanometry and present acoustic reflexes. The muscle reflex of the vestibular-evoked myogenic potential (VEMP) is highly sensitive and specific for SCDS, possibly even more so than the results of CT scans (Zhou, Gopen, & Poe, 2007).

Autoimmune Inner-Ear Disease

Autoimmune diseases are inflammatory conditions that occur when the immune system causes the body to attack its own tissues because it fails to distinguish them from bacteria, viruses, or cells from other organisms. **Autoimmune inner-ear disease (AIED)** specifically attacks the inner ear, often resulting in the classical clinical presentation of a bilateral fluctuating and progressive sensory hearing loss, which may occur over several months. Tinnitus, aural fullness, and vertigo may accompany this potentially reversible inner-ear syndrome. The prevalence of AIED is believed to be quite low; however, a significant percentage of bilateral symptoms in Ménière's disease patients may be due to AIED. As in the treatment of sudden idiopathic sensory/neural hearing loss, steroids can be administered via a wick for absorption into the inner ear through the round window.

Head Trauma

Often when a hearing loss is directly related to a head injury, the audiogram is quite similar to those typical of acoustic trauma, showing a "notch" in the 3,000 to 6,000 Hz range. In addition to damage to the tympanic membrane and middle-ear mechanism, the structures of the inner ear may be torn, stretched, or deteriorated from the loss of oxygen following hemorrhage. If a fracture line runs through the cochlea, the resulting hearing loss is severe to profound and may be total. External and/or internal hair cells may be lost, and the organ of Corti may be flattened or destroyed. Trauma to the skull may also result in complications such as otitis media or meningitis, which may themselves be the cause of a hearing loss. Hearing loss may result from head trauma, even without fracture, if there is a contusion of the cochlea, or if a strong pressure wave is conducted through the skull to the cochlea (Schuknecht, 1993). This may be ipsilateral or contralateral to the skull insult.

FIGURE 11.19 Latency-intensity functions for Wave V derived from the auditory brain-stem response tracings shown in Figure 11.18 on the patient with a unilateral (right) cochlear hearing loss (see Figure 11.16B). The latencies are normal for the left ear and increased for the right ear, primarily at lower intensities. Otoacoustic emissions are absent in the affected ear.

SPEECH AND HEARING CENTER
The University of Texas at Austin 78712

NAME: Last - First - Middle	SEX	AGE	DATE	EXAMINER	RELIABILITY	INSTRUMENT

OTOACOUSTIC EMISSIONS
(Present or Absent)

☑ TEOAE Level **80** dB Peak SPL
☐ DPOAE Level F₁____ F₂____

Right | | | | | Left
500	1000	2000	4000	6000	500	1000	2000	4000	6000
A	A	A	A	A	P	P	P	P	P

AUDITORY BRAINSTEM RESPONSE
ABR WAVE V LATENCY-INTENSITY FUNCTION

RIGHT O - O
LEFT X - X

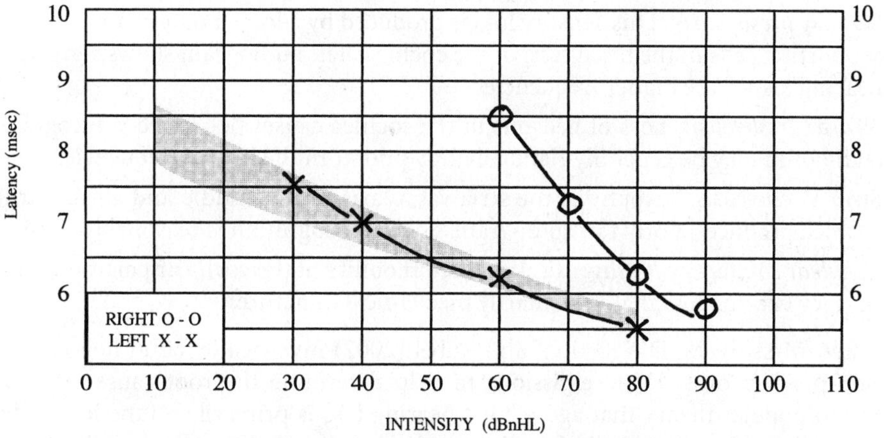

SHADED AREA REPRESENTS Normal Wave V Range for patients older than 16 mos. for 30 clicks per second

EAR	nHL		Absolute Latency (ms)			Interpeak Latency (ms)			Latency Change w/ Increased Rate	
	dB HL	Click Rate	I	III	V	I-III	III-V	I-V	V	Click Rate
RIGHT	90	33.1	1.6	3.75	5.8	2.15	2.05	4.2		
LEFT	80	33.1	1.52	3.7	5.6	2.18	1.9	4.08		
Interaural Differences										

Amplitude Ratio (V same or > I)   R NL L NL
Estimated Air Conduction Threshold   R ≤60 L ≤30
Estimated Bone Conduction Threshold   R ____ L ____

Head injuries, acoustic trauma, diving accidents, or overexertion may cause rupture of the round window membrane, or a fistula of the oval window with a perilymph leak into the middle ear. When there is the possibility of a fluid leak, the fistula test, using an immittance meter as described in Chapter 6, can be of great assistance in medical diagnosis.

Presbycusis

The caseload of any audiology clinic includes a large number of patients who have no contributing etiological factors to hearing loss except advancing age. It would be inaccurate to assume that lesions in **presbycusis** (hearing loss due to aging) are restricted to the cochlea, regardless of the relationship to noise exposure mentioned earlier. The aging process produces alterations in many areas of the auditory system, including the tympanic membrane, ossicular chain, cochlear windows, and central auditory nervous system. There is probably some relationship to general oxygen deficiency caused by arteriosclerosis. A precise definition of the age at which presbycusis begins is lacking in the literature, but it should be expected in men by the early 60s and women by the late 60s, all other factors being equal. It is possible that the hearing mechanism begins to deteriorate slowly at birth.

A common characteristic of presbycusis is significant difficulty in speech recognition, which Gaeth (1948) has called **phonemic regression.** Many older people report that they often understand speech better when people speak slowly than when they speak loudly. A number of "typical" presbycusic audiometric contours have been suggested.

The classical work on presbycusis is by Schuknecht (1993), who defined four different, but overlapping, causes of this hearing loss:

1. *Sensory presbycusis.* This sensory loss is produced by a loss of outer hair cells and supporting cells in the basal turn of the cochlea. The audiogram shows a greater hearing loss in the higher frequencies.

2. *Neural presbycusis.* Loss of neurons in the cochlea causes poor speech recognition. The audiogram may be generally flat or slightly poorer in the higher frequencies.

3. *Strial presbycusis.* Atrophy of the stria vascularis in the middle and apical turns of the cochlea produce a fairly flat audiogram. Speech recognition is reasonably good.

4. *Cochlear conductive presbycusis.* Impaired mobility of the cochlear partitions produces a sensory hearing loss that is primarily mechanical in nature.

Gates, Mills, Nam, D'Agostino, and Rubel (2002) investigated adult hearing loss using distortion-product otoacoustic emissions to help determine the root cause of presbycusis. Contrary to popular theory that age-related hearing loss is primarily a function of decreased outer hair cell activity, their findings indicate strial degeneration may be the primary contributor to presbycusis.

Some gender effects have been noted regarding the audiometric configuration of presbycusic patients. Jerger, Chmiel, Stach, and Spretnjak (1993) surveyed a large number of audiograms over a 50-year period and found that elderly males tend to show greater hearing loss above 1,000 Hz, whereas elderly females have poorer sensitivity below 1,000 Hz, even when accounting for environmental factors such as noise exposure. This same finding of a greater prevalence of sloping audiometric configurations for males than females has been reported within a non-elderly population as well (Ciletti & Flamme, 2009). Possible explanations for this gender difference are the greater presence of cardiovascular disease in elderly females and the increase in variety and amounts of noise exposures among men.

Approximately 25 percent of adults between the ages 45 and 64 years and 40 percent of those over age 65 have some degree of hearing loss (Glass, 1990). Hearing loss in this context is defined as a handicap in social, emotional, vocational, and psychological areas (American

CHECK YOUR UNDERSTANDING

Speech-Language-Hearing Association, 1992). Efforts are being made to screen elderly citizens for hearing loss, in ways similar to screening infants and school children, in order to identify problems and seek solutions as early as possible. Such screening tests must be effective, high in sensitivity and specificity, and yield a high predictive value.

ACTIVITIES

EVOLVING CASE STUDIES

Chapter 11 is on the subject of the inner ear, so you are asked here to look at Case Study 3. The term *sensory/neural* is actually a broad one because it suggests that a given hearing loss is either sensory (in the inner ear) or neural (on the auditory nerve), although it may, of course, be both. The former is the more usual lesion site and is demonstrated here. Discussion below briefly reviews what we know about this case. Before reading the following entry, remember that following Chapter 7 you were asked to predict the results for acoustic immittance, acoustic reflex thresholds (ARTs), otoacoustic emissions (OAEs), and auditory brain-stem response (ABR) measures. In addition, based on what you know so far about this case and the tests you have studied, you can predict that the area causing the hearing loss is cochlear. Some of the other site-of-lesion tests described in Chapter 7 are not discussed here, but you may feel free to conjecture about the possible outcomes of those tests.

Case Study 3: Sensory/Neural Hearing Loss—Inner-Ear Disorder

As presented in Chapter 4, this 76-year-old male patient has a moderate loss similar to Figure 4.14. Given no air-bone gaps greater than 10 dB in this audiogram (and presumably in the audiogram you had predicted following reading of Chapter 4), this patient clearly has a sensory/neural hearing loss. As was stated in Chapter 5 (and as you may have predicted at that time), speech-recognition scores would be somewhat reduced with this loss. The probability is that the tympanograms are normal (Type A) with acoustic reflex thresholds, ipsilateral and contralateral, occurring at low sensation levels. OAEs are probably absent, and if ABR testing were completed, the latency-intensity functions for Wave V in both ears would resemble those shown for the right ear in Figure 11.17. All test results up to this point are consistent with a cochlear site of lesion or sensory hearing loss.

Summary

The inner ear is a fluid-filled space, interfaced between the middle ear and the auditory nerve. It acts as a device to convert sound into a form of electrochemical energy that transmits information to the brain about the frequency, intensity, and phase of sound waves. The vestibular portion of the inner ear provides the brain with data concerning the position and movement of the body.

When the cochlear portion of the inner ear becomes abnormal, the result is a combination of sensory hearing loss and dysacusis. Bone-conduction and air-conduction results essentially interweave on the audiogram, and word recognition generally becomes poorer in direct relation to the amount of hearing loss. Results on tympanometry and static immittance in the plane of the tympanic membrane are usually within normal limits, unless the sensory loss has a superimposed conductive component, resulting in a mixed hearing loss. Acoustic reflex thresholds are expected at low sensation levels. In pure cochlear hearing losses, the latency-intensity functions obtained from ABR testing are rather steep, showing longer latencies close to threshold. If the outer hair cells are damaged, causing more than a mild hearing loss, otoacoustic emissions are absent.

If any of the behavioral site-of-lesion tests discussed in Chapter 7 are performed, patients with cochlear hearing loss are expected to show high SISI scores and moderate amounts of tone decay (especially in the higher frequencies). Recruitment of loudness can usually be found, which often complicates auditory rehabilitation.

Habilitation or rehabilitation of patients with sensory hearing losses of cochlear origin is considerably more difficult than for patients with conductive lesions. Medical or surgical correction is usually obviated by the very nature of the disorder; however, there are several important exceptions. Combinations of harmonic and frequency distortion and loudness recruitment often make the use of hearing aids difficult but not impossible. Auditory rehabilitation of patients with cochlear disorders is of special concern to audiologists.

REVIEW TABLE 11.1 Common Causes of Cochlear Hearing Loss According to Age at Onset

Prenatal	Childhood	Adulthood (All of Column 2, Plus . . .)
Anoxia	Birth trauma	Autoimmune inner-ear disease
Heredity	Drugs	Labyrinthitis
Rh factor	Head trauma	Ménière's disease
Toxemia of pregnancy	High fever	Otosclerosis
Trauma	Kidney infection	Presbycusis
Viral infection (maternal)	Noise	Vasospasm
	Otitis media	
	Prematurity	
	Surgery (middle ear)	
	Systemic illness	
	Venereal disease	
	Viral infection	

Frequently Asked Questions

Q How does otitis media cause a sensory/neural hearing loss?

A *Otitis media is a major cause of cochlear hearing loss. Enzymes produced by the infected fluids in the middle ear may diffuse through the round window and damage the inner-ear structures.*

Q Does tinnitus have a treatment or cure?

A *A host of treatments has been used, including medication, surgery, hypnosis, and biofeedback. Some treatments such as tinnitus retraining therapy have high success rates in reducing the annoyance of tinnitus, but even these are not a cure.*

Q If a patient suffers from mild tinnitus, does caffeine worsen the effects of the tinnitus? If so, what amount of caffeine is safe to drink without worsening the effects of the tinnitus?

A *Caffeine has been implicated as an aggravator of tinnitus, but individual tolerances vary widely.*

Q Can Ménière's disease cause permanent hearing loss in the low frequencies?

A *The audiometric contour in Ménière's disease is usually flat and often shows a greater loss in the low frequencies.*

Q What can be done to treat autoimmune inner-ear disease?

A *Numbers of drugs have been tried, including steroids.*

Q What is the function of the organ of Corti?

A *The organ of Corti is the end organ for hearing and transduces the mechanical energy in the middle ear to an electrochemical code to be transmitted to the brain.*

Q If a person has vertigo that never goes away, is there some sort of medicine or treatment to help him or her live a normal life?

A *There are both medical and surgical treatments for vertigo, but some patients fail to respond to either.*

Q What is the function of the ampullae?

A *The ampullae contain the cristae, which are the end organs of the semicircular canals.*

Q Is the Rh factor in blood genetic? Are some people born with the factor and some without?

A *Yes, those born with the factor are termed Rh positive and those without it are Rh negative. It is a heterozygous condition, so if even one gene is received from a parent who is Rh positive, the baby's blood will be Rh positive.*

Q Is presbycusis only a loss in the cochlea, or can it occur in any part of the ear?

A *Almost any part of the auditory system can be affected by aging.*

Q If endolymphatic hydrops causes Reissner's membrane to rupture, as in Ménière's disease, can the membrane heal, or will there always be an ionic imbalance and resulting symptoms?

A *In many cases, the membrane does indeed heal. However, symptoms may return.*

Q How does cardiovascular disease affect the hearing of elderly people?

A *Anything that interferes with normal blood supply can cause anoxia, resulting in cell damage. Structures most susceptible to anoxia are found in the brain and the inner ear.*

Q Why do some viruses, like mumps, cause unilateral hearing loss most often, while most others cause bilateral hearing loss?

A *This is unknown.*

Q Why do rifle shooters experience more hearing loss in the ear opposite their shooting side?

A *The loud sound of a rifle discharging comes from the end of the barrel as the bullet breaks the sound barrier. With the stock held to the right shoulder, and the head cocked, the end of the barrel is closer to the left ear.*

Q Does OSHA have standards for concert halls, amphitheaters, and so on? Why can people stand so close to speakers if it is known that this is so dangerous to their hearing?

A *OSHA supplies damage-risk criteria for noise exposure. Why people expose their hearing to such intense music is a matter of preference and is not understood by most people concerned with hearing conservation (like audiologists). OSHA does not govern these venues.*

Q Do acoustic trauma and head injury patients all show a notch in the 3,000–6,000 Hz range because this is the area with frequencies around the promontory, leaving them most susceptible to trauma?

A *This is generally but not always correct.*

Q Are the numbers (percentages) of individuals with presbycusis increasing over time?

A *Yes because people in general are living longer.*

Q What characterizes Ménière's disease?

A *This question has many answers, including sudden onset of unilateral hearing loss, roaring tinnitus, vertigo, very poor speech recognition in the affected ear, a sensation of aural fullness, and remissions and exacerbations.*

Q What is the ultrasonic procedure used to treat Ménière's disease?

A *The ultrasonic procedure destroys the inner ear, leaving the patient with no hearing in the operated ear but hopefully relieved of vertigo.*

Q Is sudden idiopathic sensory/neural hearing loss unilateral or bilateral?

A *It can be either.*

Q Should sudden idiopathic hearing loss be treated as an emergency?

A *Any sudden hearing loss should be considered an emergency. In many cases, prompt and appropriate treatment can result in restoration of hearing.*

Q Under the OSHA standards, what is the maximum level of exposure for an eight-hour workday?

A *The maximum level of noise exposure for an eight-hour workday is 85 dBA SPL before a hearing conservation program must be in place. For every 5 dB above 90 dBA SPL, the time of exposure must be halved.*

Q Do men or women have a higher incidence of hearing loss?

A *As they age, men tend to lose their hearing earlier, but by the late eighties both sexes show about the same amount of loss. There are some data to suggest that by the nineties women actually have poorer hearing than men.*

Q What is the characteristic of an acoustic trauma notch on an audiogram?

A *The characteristic of an acoustic trauma notch on an audiogram usually shows increased hearing loss with increased frequency, with the greatest loss between 3,000 and 6,000 Hz and recovery at 8,000 Hz. There are always exceptions to this generalization.*

Q What are improvements in hearing thresholds after an initial impairment following noise called?

A *Temporary threshold shifts (TTSs).*

Q Phonemic regression is a common characteristic of what disorder?

A *Phonemic regression is not uncommon in presbycusis and is construed to mean the word-recognition difficulties experienced by elderly patients. In addition to generalized problems in discriminating speech, many elderly individuals are found to understand better when speech is slowed down.*

Q How do drugs that address the Rh factor work?

A *When women are found to have elevated levels of antibodies related to the Rh factor, some drugs can reduce the production of more antibodies during pregnancy.*

Q Why is the cochlea not responsive to frequencies above 20,000 Hz?

A *There is evidence that responses to sounds by bone conduction or under water go to much higher frequencies than the normally expected 20,000 Hz by air conduction. Apparently the middle ear acts as a low-pass filter, not allowing the higher frequencies to reach the cochlea.*

Q Is it possible for cerumen to carry HIV and then infect another person?

A *This has been debated, but so far HIV has not been isolated in human cerumen.*

Q How long does it take to recover from a noise-induced temporary threshold shift (NITTS)?

A *This varies considerably from patient to patient.*

Q How do physicians decide whether it is worth it to give a patient a cochleotoxic drug?

A *Such decisions are made based on whether the risks to the patient's life and health from an antibiotic outweigh the likelihood of hearing loss.*

Q Can Reissner's membrane and the basilar membrane ever be ruptured or dislodged? If they can, how does it occur?

A *It is believed that such ruptures are precisely what happens when the pressure from the endolymph increases abnormally during attacks of Ménière's disease. There are also risks of such ruptures from barotrauma.*

Q Why are otoacoustic emissions more prevalent in women than in men, and why are they more common in the right ear than the left ear?

A *We do not know the answer to this question.*

Q What part of the brain is affected by athetotic cerebral palsy?

A *It is thought to be the globus palidus in the extrapyramidal tract. Although concomitant damage may arise in the brain stem, the cochlea is thought to be the primary site for loss of hearing sensitivity.*

Q During the caloric test, how does the water or air (warm or cold) get through the tympanic membrane and to the inner ear if there is no perforation in the tympanic membrane?

A *The temperature of the heated or cooled water or air alters the temperature first of the intact tympanic membrane, then the air in the middle ear, which generates eddies in the endolymph, which in turn produces the vertigo and nystagmus.*

Q Can smoking cigarettes cause a hearing loss due to anoxia of the hair cells in the cochlea? If so, are heavy smokers more susceptible to hair cell death than light smokers?

A *In addition to causing anoxia caused by constriction of blood vessels, cigarette smoke contains a number of other substances, like carbon monoxide, which are cochleotoxic.*

Q If a mother smokes while she is pregnant, does the fetus have a higher risk of hearing damage?

A *Yes. For some time, pregnant women have been advised not to smoke and to keep secondhand smoke away from babies and children.*

Q What is the most common form of cerebral palsy with a hearing loss as a symptom?

A *Athetosis.*

Q What is the etiology of an idiopathic sensory/neural hearing loss?

A *The word* idiopathic *suggests a disorder of unknown cause.*

Q What does the acronym COWS stand for?

A *Cold—opposite, warm—same. This is the direction of the fast component of nystagmus during caloric testing for ENG.*

Suggested Reading

Feuerstein, J. F., & Chasin, M. (2009). Noise exposure and issues in hearing conservation. In J. Katz, L. Medwetsky, R. Burkard, & L. Hood (Eds.), *Handbook of clinical audiology* (pp. 678–698). Baltimore: Lippincott Williams & Wilkins.

Gelfand, S. A. (2004). *Hearing: An introduction to psychological and physiological acoustics.* New York: Marcel Dekker.

Musiek, F. E., & Baran, J. A. (2007). *The auditory system: Anatomy, physiology, and clinical correlates.* Boston: Allyn & Bacon.

Toriello, H. V., Reardan, W., & Gorlin, R. J. (2004). *Hereditary hearing loss and its syndromes* (2nd ed.). New York: Oxford University Press.

Endnotes

1. For Ernst Reissner, German anatomist, 1824–1878.
2. For Alfonso Corti, Italian anatomist, 1822–1888.
3. For Hermann Ludwig Ferdinand Helmholtz, German physicist and physiologist, 1821–1894.
4. For Georg von Békésy, Hungarian physicist and Nobel Prize winner, 1899–1972.
5. Named for Prosper Ménière, French physician, 1799–1862, who first described this syndrome.

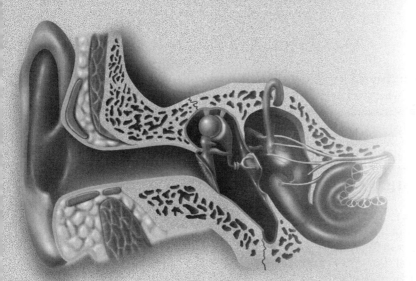

CHAPTER 12

The Auditory Nerve and Central Auditory Pathways

LEARNING OBJECTIVES

The tests described in this chapter for site-of-lesion diagnosis in the brain have met with varying degrees of clinical acceptance and are offered to the new student in diagnostic audiology because they seem to be the most appropriate ones at the time of this writing. At the completion of this chapter, the reader should be able to

- Provide a general description of the complexities of the central auditory system and the difficulties of diagnosing disorders in the brain.
- Initiate and interpret test procedures for proper diagnosis of auditory disorders beyond the cochlea.
- Discuss management considerations for retrocochlear pathology.

THE PREVIOUS THREE CHAPTERS have been concerned with the propagation and conduction of sound waves through the outer and middle ears, and the transduction in the cochlea of these pressure waves into neural activity to be processed by the central auditory system. Because sound is meaningful only if it is perceived, an understanding of its transmission to, and perception by, the brain is essential to the audiologist. Much remains to be learned about how the nervous system transmits, receives, and processes information related to sound.

Diagnosis of disorders of the auditory system from the outer ear through the auditory nerve (also called the acoustic nerve and the vestibulocochlear nerve) is best made through the test battery. This battery includes pure-tone and speech audiometry, measurements of acoustic immittance at the tympanic membrane, and measures of auditory brain-stem response (ABR) and otoacoustic emissions (OAEs). This chapter's treatment of the anatomy and physiology of the central auditory system is designed mainly to introduce the reader to these processes; therefore, the chapter is far from complete. As in the previous chapter, this presentation relies heavily on what has been learned in the foregoing sections of this text. For a deeper understanding of these issues, the reader is encouraged to pursue the suggested readings listed at the end of this chapter.

From Cochlea to Auditory Cortex and Back Again

Almost without exception, every anatomical structure on one side of the brain has an identical structure on the opposite side of the brain. For clarity, a block diagram (see Figure 12.1), rather than a realistic drawing, is shown to illustrate the auditory pathways. This diagram represents the anatomical arrangement in the system and illustrates the directions of neural impulses and the primary waystations from cochlea to auditory cortex. A comprehensive review of the anatomy and physiology of the auditory nerve and its waystations is provided by Muziek and Baran (2007).

Nerve fibers pass from the cochlea through the **internal auditory canal,** which begins at the cochlear modiolus and terminates at the base of the brain. The internal auditory canal also carries the vestibular portion of the VIIIth nerve, whose fibers are innervated by the utricle, saccule, and semicircular canals. There are approximately 30,000 nerve fibers in the cochlear

FIGURE 12.1 Ascending auditory pathways. As illustrated, several decussations, or crossover points, beginning at the level of the cochlear nucleus, provide bilateral representation to signals presented to just one ear. (*Source:* Dr. Chris Matyear as a modification of the figure by Yost & Nielsen, 2000.)

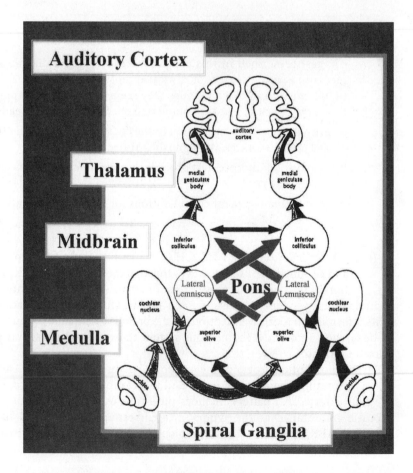

portion and 20,000 in the vestibular portion. The auditory portion of the VIIIth nerve actually spirals through the internal auditory canal. The nerve fibers form a cylindrically arranged bundle, or cable, with fibers that arise from the basal (high frequencies) turn of the cochlea, forming the outer portion, and fibers that arise from the apical (low frequencies) areas, forming the center, together creating the nerve trunk. In addition to the VIIIth nerve, the internal auditory canal, which runs a distance of approximately 10 mm in adults, also carries the internal auditory artery and fibers of the VIIth (facial) nerve.

The **auditory nerve** extends 17 to 19 mm beyond the internal auditory canal, where it attaches to the brain stem, at which the **cerebellum, medulla oblongata,** and **pons** join to form the **cerebellopontine angle (CPA).** At this level, the auditory and vestibular portions of the VIIIth nerve separate. One part of the cochlear bundle descends to the **dorsal cochlear nucleus,** and the other ascends to the **ventral cochlear nucleus.**

As mentioned in Chapter 11, neurons from the cochlea are arranged in an orderly fashion according to frequency. The arrangement of fibers in the cochlea is repeated in the auditory nerve and central auditory structures, and is said to represent **tonotopic** organization. Tonotopicity is the spatial representation of the frequency layout of the cochlea in retrocochlear structures. The auditory nerve fibers terminate in the cochlear nuclei—basal turn fibers in one area, apical turn fibers in other areas, and so on. The different cell types of the cochlear nucleus react differently to the incoming auditory nerve impulses, thus modifying input to the brain.

The brain is characterized by many **decussations,** or crossover points, that unite symmetrical portions of its two halves. Specialized nerve-fiber bundles called **commissures** unite similar structures on both sides of the brain. The first decussation in the auditory pathways occurs after the cochlear nucleus at the level of the **trapezoid body** of the pons, representing the beginning of bilateral representation of a signal presented to just one ear.

The **superior olivary complex (SOC)** receives input from both the ipsilateral and contralateral cochlear nuclei. The large number of neural inputs allows the superior olivary complex to sense the direction of a sound source by analyzing small differences in the time or intensity of a sound arriving at the two ears. In addition to its major function as a relay station for neural activity on the way to the cerebral cortex, the superior olivary complex also mediates the reflex activity of the tensor tympani and stapedius muscles of the middle ear. Some of the cells of the superior olive interact with some neurons of the facial nerve. Intense sounds produce activation of certain motor fibers of the facial (VIIth cranial) nerve, which innervate the stapedial branch of this nerve. The decussations at this anatomical point explain the contraction of the stapedius muscles in both middle ears when sound is presented to just one ear. A diagram of the ascending pathways through the superior olivary complex was shown in Figure 7.6, with the discussion of the acoustic reflex pathways.

The **lateral lemniscus** provides a major pathway for the transmission of impulses from the ipsilateral lower brain stem. Some fibers terminate in the nucleus of the lateral lemniscus, others course to the contralateral lemniscus, and still others continue to the **inferior colliculus.** The inferior colliculus receives afferent stimulation from both superior olivary complexes. Neurons that connect the inferior colliculus with the next relay station, the **medial geniculate body,** represent the third or fourth link in the ascending auditory system. A few fibers bypass the inferior colliculus to reach the medial geniculate body directly from the lateral lemniscus.

The medial geniculate body, located in the **thalamus,** is the last subcortical relay station for auditory impulses. Of its three main areas, the ventral division is responsible primarily for auditory information. After this point, nerve fibers fan out as the **auditory radiations** and then ascend to the auditory cortex. Because there are no commissural neurons at the level of the medial geniculate body, no decussations exist there.

The areas of auditory reception are in the **temporal lobes** on both sides of the cerebral cortex in an area called the **superior temporal gyrus** or **Heschl's gyrus.** There is evidence that the selective representation of frequency, observed at specific places in the cochlea, is repeated in the auditory cortex, although to a lesser degree. Apparently, the temporal area is concerned primarily with the frequency characteristics of sound, the **insular** area with the temporal aspects of sound, the **parietal lobe** with association of sound with past experiences (and because this area has inputs from all sensory modalities, the auditory stimulus is compared or matched with input from other senses), and the frontal area with the memory of sounds.

It was once believed that the auditory cortex was the only center for auditory discrimination. It is now known that many discriminations may be mediated subcortically. Perceptions of pitch and loudness can be maintained in animals whose cortices have been surgically removed. Although discrimination of some simple sounds may be retained, the understanding of speech requires at least minimal integrity of the auditory cortex.

The auditory system is generally considered to be a sensory system (like the skin or the eyes). It provides the brain with information transmitted to the cochlea in the form of pressure waves and transduced by the cochlea into neural activity to be sent to the brain. In addition to the **afferent** pathways, the auditory system contains a complex **efferent** system of descending fibers. These descending fibers correspond closely with the ascending fibers and connect the auditory cortex with lower brain centers and with the cochlea. One presumed purpose of this descending system is to provide inhibitory feedback by elevating the thresholds of neurons at lower stations in the auditory tract. It is true, however, that some descending connections have an excitatory function, but their purpose is not clearly understood.

Development of the Auditory Nerve and Central Auditory Nervous System

Relatively little information is available on the prenatal development of the VIIIth nerve and central auditory nervous system. Development of the nervous system (neurogenesis) in general is still poorly understood. In humans, the VIIIth nerve begins to form at about the 25th gestational day and appears almost complete at about 45 days. It is probable that the efferent fibers develop later than the afferent fibers. The cochlear and vestibular ganglia appear by the 5th week.

Improved understanding of the embryogenesis and fetogenesis of the central auditory pathways will undoubtedly provide insights into the causes of some types of lesions of the auditory nervous system. It is generally agreed that the entire nervous system forms from the ectoderm.

Summary of the Auditory Pathways

The auditory nerve and central pathways are tremendously complex. The ascending (afferent) system provides stimulation from one ear to both sides of the brain, including the temporal cortex. Descending efferent fibers from each side of the brain provide inhibition to both cochleas.

The waystations in the auditory system perform the complex processing of the incoming nerve impulses. The series of cochlear nucleus, superior olivary complex, lateral lemniscus, inferior colliculus, and medial geniculate body are not simply parts of an elaborate transmission line whereby the coded information of the VIIIth nerve is relayed to the cortex. Recoding and processing of information take place all the way up through the system.

Hearing Loss and the Auditory Nerve and Central Auditory Pathways

Because there are many collateral nerve fibers and so much analysis and re-analysis of an acoustic message as it travels to the higher brain centers, it is said that the auditory pathways provide considerable *intrinsic redundancy.* There are also many forms of *extrinsic redundancy* in speech messages themselves, such as the usual inclusion of more words than necessary to round out acceptable grammar and syntax. Also, the acoustics of speech offer more frequency information than is absolutely essential for understanding. For example, the average telephone only transmits frequencies between about 300 and 3000 Hz, far less than the frequency range for normal hearers, and yet voices can be clearly understood. People with normal auditory systems rarely appreciate the ease these factors provide in understanding spoken language. Those who are deprived of some intrinsic redundancy may not show much difficulty in discrimination until the speech message has been degraded by noise, distortion, or distraction, limiting the extrinsic redundancy.

Lesions in the conductive portions of the outer and middle ears and the sensory cells of the cochlea result in the loss of hearing sensitivity. The extent of the hearing loss is in direct proportion to the degree of damage. Loss of hearing sensitivity, such as for pure tones, becomes less obvious as disorders occur in the higher centers of the brain. For these reasons, even though site-of-lesion tests may be extremely useful in diagnosing disorders in the more peripheral areas of the central auditory pathways, such as the auditory nerve and cochlear nuclei, these tests frequently fail to identify disease in the higher centers.

Disorders of the Auditory Nerve

Lesions of the auditory nerve result in hearing losses that are classified as neural. Bone conduction and air conduction interweave on the audiogram, and there is usually little or nothing in the general audiometric configuration that differentiates cochlear from VIIIth nerve disorders. Johnson (1977) points out that in more than 50 percent of a series of patients with acoustic tumors, consistent audiometric configurations appeared but could not be differentiated from cochlear lesions according to audiometric patterns. In fact, a small percentage of patients with acoustic neuromas have normal pure-tone audiograms and normal ABR findings (Telian, Kileny, Niparko, Kemink, & Graham, 1989). Two common early symptoms of auditory nerve disorders are tinnitus and high-frequency sensory/neural hearing loss. Whenever cases of unilateral or bilateral sensory/neural hearing loss with different degrees of impairment in each ear occur, alert audiologists suspect the possibility of neural lesions. The philosophy that *all unilateral sensory/neural hearing losses are neural in origin until proved otherwise* is a good one to adopt.

A second symptom of auditory nerve disorders is apparent when there is a discrepancy between the amount of hearing loss and the scores on speech-recognition tests. In most cochlear disorders, as the hearing loss increases, the amount of dysacusis also increases. When difficulties in speech recognition are excessive for the amount of hearing loss for pure tones, a neural lesion is suggested. In some cases of VIIIth nerve disorder, hearing for pure tones is normal in the presence of speech-recognition difficulty. Despite these statements, it must be remembered that, even in cases of neural lesions, patients' speech-recognition scores may be perfectly normal.

Lesions of the VIIIth nerve may occur as a result of disease, irritation, or pressure on the nerve trunk. Etiologies for these include tumor, meningitis, hemorrhage, and trauma. Because the cochlear nerve extends into the brain for a short distance beyond the end of the internal auditory canal, some lesions of this nerve may occur in the canal and some in the cerebellopontine angle.

Tumor of the Auditory Nerve

Most tumors of the auditory nerve are benign and vary in size depending on the age of the patient and the growth characteristics of the **neoplasm.** Usually these tumors arise from sheaths that cover the vestibular branch of the VIIIth nerve. The term usually applied to these tumors is **acoustic neuroma,** although some neuro-otologists believe that the term *acoustic neurinoma* is more descriptive of some growths that arise from the peripheral cells of the nerve. Because most acoustic neuromas arise from the Schwann cells[1] that form the sheath of the vestibular branch of the VIIIth nerve, it has been suggested that the term *vestibular schwannoma* would be most descriptive.

An acoustic neuroma is considered small if it is contained within the internal auditory canal, medium-sized if it extends up to 1 centimeter into the cerebellopontine angle, and large if it extends any farther (Pool, Pava, & Greenfield, 1970). The larger the tumor within the canal, the greater the probability that pressure will cause alterations in the function of the cochlear, vestibular, and facial nerves, as well as the internal auditory artery. The larger the tumor extending into the cerebellopontine angle, the greater the likelihood that the pressure will involve other cranial nerves and the cerebellum, which is the seat of balance and equilibrium in the brain. It is difficult to predict the growth rate of acoustic neuromas, but most increase slowly in size, on the average of 0.11 cm per year (Strasnick, Glasscock, Haynes, McMenomey, & Minor, 1994).

Acoustic neuromas occur in the United States at the rate of about 1 per 100,000 each year. Most cases occur in adults over the age of 30, although naturally there are exceptions. These tumors comprise about 6 percent of all intracranial tumors, 30 percent of brain-stem tumors, and far and away the majority of tumors in the cerebellopontine angle (Kim, Klopfenstein, Porter, & Syms, 2004). About 95 percent of these tumors are unilateral, and all are thought to be the result of the absence of a tumor-suppresser gene (National Institutes of Health [NIH] Consensus Statement, 1991). Acoustic neuromas have been known to occur in both ears, either simultaneously or successively. One disease, **neurofibromatosis (NF),** or von Recklinghausen disease,[2] may cause dozens or even hundreds of neuromas in different parts of the body, including the internal auditory canal.

The earlier in their development acoustic neuromas are discovered, the better the chance for successful surgical removal. Audiological examination is very helpful in making an early diagnosis. Most hearing clinics do not see patients with early acoustic neuromas, however, because hearing loss is not a primary concern in the initial stages. As the tumor increases in size, VIIIth nerve symptoms, such as tinnitus, dizziness, hearing loss, and speech-recognition difficulties, become apparent. While the increase in the size of an acoustic neuroma usually shows progressive unilateral hearing loss as the first symptom, it is often accompanied by facial weakness or numbness and alterations in the senses of taste and vision. If the tumor grows very large, it can cause speech and swallowing difficulties and eventually hydrocephalus and death.

Because acoustic neuromas are usually benign, they do their damage by pressing on the brain or other cranial nerves. When these tumors occur within the internal auditory canal, they are called intracanicular; when they are outside the canal, they are called extracanicular. Decisions on whether to operate depend on a number of variables, including the age of the patient and the age at onset of the tumor; the tumor's size and precise location; the patient's preference; and, of course, the symptomatology.

Modern approaches to removal of acoustic neuromas carry with them lower rates of mortality and morbidity (a fatal outcome versus the appearance of complications such as facial weakness and hearing loss) than do many neurosurgical approaches. Any surgery carries the risk of infection and, in the case of brain surgery, leaks of cerebrospinal fluid, and occasional strokes and death. Neurosurgery is the treatment of choice for large tumors (greater than 4 to 5 cm) but other options are available for smaller lesions.

In the 1990s, the use of the **gamma knife** first appeared. which involves the application of focused beams of gamma radiation. These rays usually do not destroy the tumor but rather arrest its growth. The rays can be precisely aimed at specific abnormalities and, by not requiring surgical incision, practically eliminate the common risks of infection and complications from general anesthesia and blood transfusion. Usually performed as an outpatient procedure, it allows for treatment of otherwise inaccessible lesions, minimizes damage to surrounding tissue, and is painless, which frees most patients from post-treatment medication.

Emerging today is a preference for the **cyberknife,** which allows for staged, or fractionated treatments, usually numbering three to five, and is more comfortable for the patient. This noninvasive radiosurgery allows time between treatments for healthy tissues, including the VIIIth and VIIth nerves, to recover from the radiation. At this time, the cyberknife appears to be the safest approach for acoustic neuroma treatment, but much more in the way of research and clinical trials is needed.

Although acoustic neuromas usually result in gradually progressive hearing loss, pressure on the internal auditory artery may result in interference with the blood supply to the cochlea and cause sudden hearing loss and/or progressive sensory hearing loss as a result of anoxia in the cochlea. Changes in blood supply to the cochlea may cause cochlear symptoms to appear, such as misleading ABR patterns and complaints of loudness recruitment, possibly resulting in the misdiagnosis of cochlear disease as the primary disorder.

Cranial nerves other than number VIII may be affected as an acoustic tumor increases in size. Symptoms of Vth (trigeminal) nerve involvement include pain and numbness in the face. Occasionally, nerve VI (abducens) becomes compressed, causing double vision (diplopia). VIIth (facial) nerve symptoms include the formation of tears in the eyes; alterations in the sense of taste; and development of facial weakness, spasm, or paralysis. Abnormalities of the facial nerve often result in the loss of the corneal reflex; that is, the patient's eyes may not show the expected reflexive blink when a wisp of cotton is touched to the cornea. Dizziness and blurred vision may also occur. The loss of both ipsilateral and contralateral acoustic reflexes may result when measurement is taken with the probe in the ear on the same side as an impaired facial nerve (see Table 7.2H). As the IXth (glossopharyngeal), Xth (vagus), or XIIth (hypoglossal) cranial nerves become involved, difficulty in swallowing (dysphagia) and speaking (dysarthria) may ensue. When the brain stem is compressed as a tumor increases in size, symptoms include coma and eventually death. Audiologists should always consider the possibility of an intracranial tumor when patients present symptoms that include headache, vomiting, lethargy, respiratory distress, and unilateral hearing loss. Figure 12.2A and B show test results illustrating a high-frequency sensory/neural hearing loss. The findings of tests for the patient illustrated are typical of an acoustic neuroma, but in any given case one or more of these results may differ from what is expected. Auditory nerve lesions cannot be diagnosed on the bases of a "typical" audiometric configuration.

Proper audiological diagnosis consists of utilizing information from a battery of tests. As shown in Figure 12.2, speech-recognition scores are poor in the impaired ear. Acoustic reflexes are absent in many cases (see Figure 12.3), even at very high stimulus levels (Anderson, Barr, & Wedenberg, 1969). If an acoustic reflex can be obtained, the time required for its amplitude to decay

FIGURE 12.2 (A) Test results for a patient with a slight high-frequency sensory/neural hearing loss in the left ear and normal hearing in the right ear. Masking is required for bone conduction at only three frequencies when testing the left ear. (B) Audiogram exemplifying a left acoustic neuroma. Although speech-recognition testing was performed in quiet, word recognition is much poorer than expected even when repeated at a higher intensity. Naturally, proper masking is essential in this case, especially for bone-conduction and speech-recognition testing at high intensities.

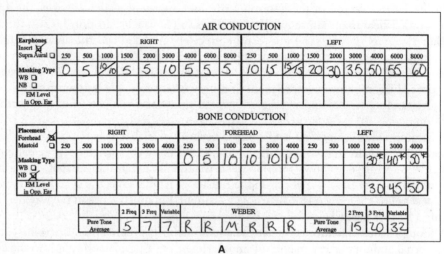

A

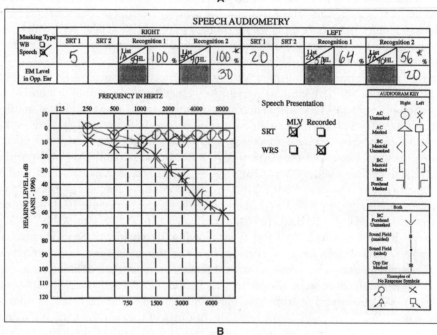

B

by 50 percent is markedly reduced in the low frequencies (less than 10 seconds). In 10 cases of acoustic neuroma described by Anderson and colleagues, the acoustic reflex half life was less than 3 seconds for frequencies at and below 1,000 Hz. Jerger, Oliver, and Jenkins (1987) reported on several cases of acoustic tumors in which the most dramatic finding was the decrease in acoustic reflex amplitude when the eliciting stimulus was presented to the ear on the affected side. ABR

FIGURE 12.3 Results on immittance measures for the theoretical patient illustrated in Figure 12.2. Tympanograms and static compliance are normal for both ears. The acoustic reflexes are normal when the tone is presented to the right (normal) ear. Reflex thresholds are elevated when tones are presented to the left ear (acoustic neuroma) in the low frequencies and absent for the higher frequencies. Reflex decay time is very rapid in the left ear in the low frequencies, with no decay in the right ear.

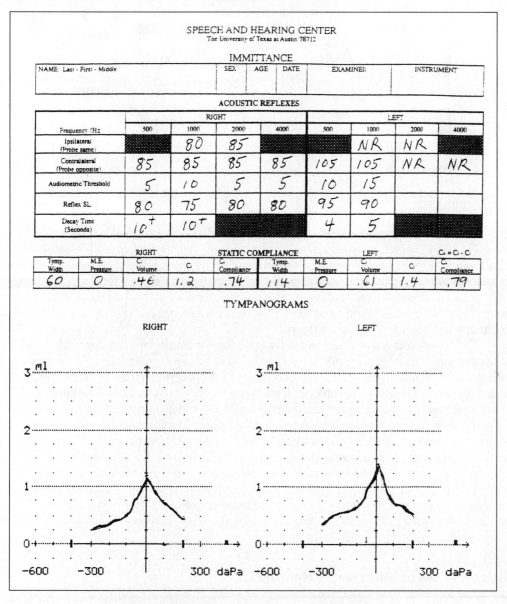

latencies in the affected ear are markedly increased (see Figures 12.4 and 12.5), and otoacoustic emissions are present because there is apparently no damage to the cochlea (Figure 12.5). Valente, Peterein, Goebel, and Neely (1995) find that elevated or absent acoustic reflexes and abnormal findings on ABR testing were the best tests of correct diagnosis of acoustic neuromas. Josey (1987) reports the ABR has heightened test sensitivity to surgically confirmed lesions, to 97 percent. The audiological test battery approach for acoustic neuromas is now often streamlined to pure-tone and speech audiometry, acoustic reflex assessment, OAEs, and ABR. A limitation of ABR testing

FIGURE 12.4 Results of auditory brain-stem response testing on the patient with an VIIIth nerve hearing loss (acoustic neuroma) in the left ear (see Figure 12.2). See the latency-intensity functions for Wave V in Figure 12.5.

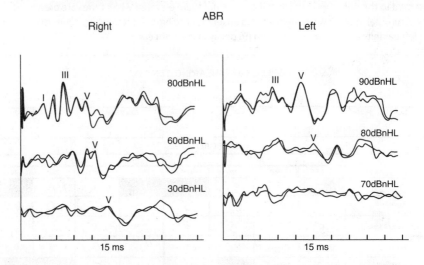

presents itself in the presence of hearing poorer than 75 dB HL at 1,000 to 4,000 Hz (Josey, 1987). As discussed in Chapter 7, more recent use of the stacked ABR has resulted in the identification of smaller acoustic neuromas than previously identified through standard ABR measures. When the magnitude of hearing loss precludes ABR testing, the physician's referral for diagnostic imaging may be based on audiometric and immittance results coupled with the patient's reported symptoms. The absence of OAEs in some cases may be the result of a concomitant, often unrelated, cochlear lesion and may confuse diagnosis.

Confirmation of acoustic neuroma is made through an interdisciplinary approach. Vestibular tests often show a number of abnormal signs, including spontaneous nystagmus with the eyes closed and generally decreased vestibular function on the affected side. An increase in the amount of protein in the cerebrospinal fluid is helpful in determining the presence of tumors. New advances in the specialty of medical imaging have vastly improved acoustic neuroma verification.

While it is important to consider the medical needs first for patients with acoustic neuroma, audiological regards should not be ignored. In postoperative patients and those electing to delay surgery, the hearing needs should be considered. Naturally, an ear with profound neural deafness does not respond favorably with the use of a conventional hearing aid. However, some patients with profound or total deafness in one ear, and normal or near normal hearing in the other ear, have found that using an osseointegrated auditory implant can be of assistance. As discussed in Chapter 14, the aid is worn at the bad ear, and sound is conducted via bone conduction to the cochlea of the better ear.

Other Causes of VIIIth Nerve Hearing Loss

Because of their dramatic symptoms and the danger they pose to the life of the patient, acoustic neuromas come to the audiologist's mind first when VIIIth nerve signs appear. This is a safe and prudent attitude, but other conditions of the auditory nerve can produce identical audiological symptoms. These conditions include **acoustic neuritis** (inflammation of the vestibular or cochlear nerve) and **multiple sclerosis (MS).** A safe and prudent philosophy would be to assume that all unilateral sensory/neural hearing losses should be suspected of being acoustic tumors until proven otherwise.

FIGURE 12.5 Results of otoacoustic emissions testing showing the presence of these emissions in both ears at all frequencies. Latency-intensity functions for Wave V derived from the auditory brain-stem response tracings shown in Figure 12.4, based on the patient with a unilateral retrocochlear hearing loss caused by an acoustic neuroma in the left ear (Figure 12.2). Wave V latencies are normal for the right ear and markedly increased for the left ear at all the sensation levels tested.

SPEECH AND HEARING CENTER
The University of Texas at Austin 78712

NAME: Last - First - Middle	SEX	AGE	DATE	EXAMINER	RELIABILITY	INSTRUMENT

OTOACOUSTIC EMISSIONS
(Present or Absent)

☑ TEOAE Level **20** dB Peak SPL
☐ DPOAE Level F₁ ____ F₂ ____

	Right						Left		
500	1000	2000	4000	6000	500	1000	2000	4000	6000
P	P	P	P	P	P	P	P	P	P

AUDITORY BRAINSTEM RESPONSE
ABR WAVE V LATENCY-INTENSITY FUNCTION

RIGHT O - O
LEFT X - X

INTENSITY (dBnHL)

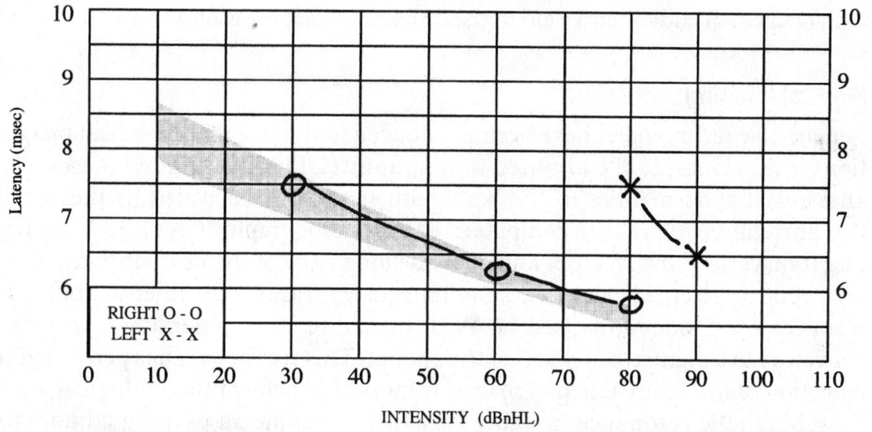

SHADED AREA REPRESENTS Normal Wave V Range for patients older than 16 mos. for 30 clicks per second

EAR	nHL		Absolute Latency (ms)			Interpeak Latency (ms)			Latency Change w/ Increased Rate	
	dB HL	Click Rate	I	III	V	I-III	III-V	I-V	V	Click Rate
RIGHT	80	13.1	1.9	3.8	5.8	1.9	2.0	3.9	6.0	89.1
LEFT	90	13.1	1.68	4.0	6.6	2.32	2.6	4.92	Absent	89.1
Interaural Differences										

Amplitude Ratio (V same or > I)   R **NL** L **NL**
Estimated Air Conduction Threshold   R ____ L ____
Estimated Bone Conduction Threshold   R ____ L ____

Auditory Neuropathy Spectrum Disorder

Auditory neuropathy spectrum disorder (ANSD) occurs when patients have normal outer-hair-cell function in the cochlea, but the responses on the VIIIth nerve that carries electrical signals to the brain fail to occur in synchrony; that is, they are dys-synchronous. The result is that, instead of a smooth transition of information from the cochlea to the brain stem, the information is not relayed in a consistent manner. The degree of this dys-synchrony usually varies from individual to individual, and it often fluctuates in the same person (Hood, 2007).

Patients with ANSD often exhibit a mild to moderate sensory/neural hearing loss with speech-recognition difficulties disproportionate to the degree of the measured loss. These patients may also present with other peripheral neuropathies. In contrast, patients with acoustic neuroma exhibit preservation of ABR Wave I with an attenuation or delay of subsequent waves, unless a profound loss exists that results in the absence of all waveforms. These patients' tumors are usually evidenced on **magnetic resonance imaging (MRI).** In comparison, patients with suspected ANSD may show an absence of all ABR waves when hearing thresholds may be only moderately impaired and there is no evidence of lesions of the VIIIth nerve or the brain stem on MRI. In addition, normal cochlear outer-hair-cell function is evidenced by the presence of evoked oto-acoustic emissions (Starr, Picton, Sininger, Hood, & Berlin, 1996). The type of VIIIth nerve lesion present in these patients is not clear. Rapin and Gravel (2006) lament that ANSD is too frequently diagnosed based soley on audiological criteria rather than when behavioral, electrophysiologic, and pathologic testing indicate pathology of the spiral ganglion cells and their VIIIth nerve axons. The hearing loss seen in ANSD appears slowly progressive and does not demonstrate much benefit from hearing aids; however, other rehabilitative efforts including speechreading, **cued speech,** and cochlear implantation (see Chapter 14) may be helpful. Physiological tests in conjunction with behavioral audiometrics aid in the differential diagnosis of ANSD.

Medical Imaging

Remarkable technologies have been introduced to the science of medical imaging. The revolutionary development of **computed tomography (CT)** has permitted the viewing of numerous anatomical abnormalities in the body with sensitivity unrivaled by previous techniques. In this procedure, often called computerized axial tomography (CAT), an X-ray transmitter scans in a transverse plane (at right angles to the long axis) of the head or body, along a 180-degree arc, while an electronic detector simultaneously measures the intensity of the beam emerging from the other side of the patient. With the aid of a computer, the detector's information is converted to a picture, or "slice," of the patient. This technology has permitted the noninvasive detection of intracranial hemorrhages, tumors, and deformities with great sensitivity.

Magnetic resonance imaging (MRI) has become an exciting adjunct to CT scanning. Using ionizing radiation to obtain images, MRI employs magnetic fields and radio waves to produce images in the different planes of the body. One of the most satisfying aspects of this technology is that the waves are believed to be harmless. Furthermore, the technique is excellent for seeing many soft-tissue masses, such as acoustic neuromas, even when they are as small as just a few millimeters in diameter. An MRI scan of an acoustic neuroma is shown in Figure 12.6.

During head scans with both CT and MRI, the patient remains motionless while the head is scanned from within a large machine in the shape of a doughnut that surrounds the head. Patients often find lying still on their backs difficult, and some who suffer from different degrees of claustrophobia become quite upset, even though the procedure is considered harmless. Often a chemical, such as gadolinium, is injected into the arm so that it can flow into the brain and serve as a contrast medium, allowing a mass to be seen more clearly. The noise

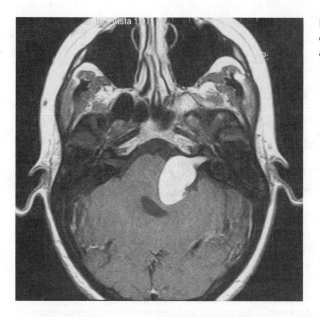

FIGURE 12.6 MRI scan showing a clinical orientation of a tumor in the left internal auditory canal. (*Source:* Robert W. Keith, Ph.D.)

emitted by many imagers is so loud that many radiologists provide foam hearing protectors for their patients.

In a series of 100 patients with acoustic neuromas reported by Josey, Glasscock, and Musiek (1988), 93 had sufficient hearing to allow ABR testing, and 97 percent of that group showed abnormal ABR results, reflecting the lesion. By contrast, 69 percent of the lesions were correctly identified by medical imaging alone. This result dramatizes the need to use both procedures in diagnosis.

Telian and Kileny (1988) reported three case histories in which ABR, ENG, CT, and MRI at times suggested different problems. In other words, some of the tests resulted in both false positive and false negative results. Telian and Kileny also concluded that false negative ABR responses are more likely to occur when an acoustic tumor is in the cerebellopontine angle than when it is in the internal auditory canal.

Abnormal ABR findings have been demonstrated in some cases of acoustic neuroma where no hearing loss exists. Despite this great sensitivity, the rate of false negative findings is, not surprisingly, slightly higher for ABR than for MRI, especially in cases of very small tumors that produce only slight pressure on the auditory nerve. The fact that ABR is so much less expensive than MRI ensures its continued use as a screening procedure for these tumors (Turner, Robinette, & Bauch, 1999).

Positron emission tomography (PET) is a procedure that utilizes radioactive materials emitted from the body after injection. This procedure is considered safe because the radioactivity levels decay very rapidly. PET is designed more to detect biochemical than anatomical changes in the patient, and it can be useful in the diagnosis of conditions like multiple sclerosis, Parkinson disease, stroke, schizophrenia, and even depression.

Disorders of the Cochlear Nuclei

The cochlear nuclei represent the first of the relay stations in the central auditory nervous system and the last point at which entirely ipsilateral representation is maintained. Because the tonotopic layout of these nuclei allows for frequency analysis, lesions in these areas may produce clinical loss of hearing sensitivity. Beyond the cochlear nuclei, a stimulus presented to one ear is processed and transmitted along fibers on both sides of the brain.

Audiologists work under the assumption that lesions central to the cochlea produce results specific to retrocochlear disorders on special diagnostic tests. Such results are usually observed with VIIIth nerve lesions, but they are not always observed in the cochlear nuclei.

Causes of Cochlear Nuclei Disorders

Damage to the cochlear nuclei is difficult to diagnose with certainty without postmortem study. Lesions in the nuclei, like those on the auditory nerve, may result from disease, toxicity, irritation, pressure, or trauma.

Rh incompatibility was discussed briefly in Chapter 10 as a prenatal cause of cochlear hearing loss. Postmortem studies have shown deposits of bilirubin in the cochlea, as well as in different areas of the brain, including the cochlear nuclei. Goodhill (1950) coined the term *nuclear deafness* to describe the site of lesion in children with hearing loss who have cerebral palsy secondary to Rh incompatibility.

The term **kernicterus** has been used for some time to describe the condition characterized by bile deposits in the central nervous system. Kernicterus often results in degeneration of the nerve cells that come into contact with liver bile.

Conditions that interfere with or alter the blood supply to the cochlear nuclei may result in hearing loss. Such disorders, called *vascular accidents,* include the rupturing of blood vessels as well as clots that obstruct the arterial space. These clots may be either *thromboses,* which form and remain in a specific area of the vessel, or *embolisms,* which are formed by bits of debris that circulate through the system until they reach a narrow passageway through which they cannot pass. Either one may obstruct the blood vessel or cause it to burst. Arteries have also been known to rupture where aneurysms (dilations in the blood vessels) form, because aneurysms usually cause the walls to become stretched and thin. Cases of obstruction or rupture of blood vessels within the brain are called **cerebrovascular accidents (CVAs)** or *strokes.*

An increasingly common condition today is arteriosclerosis, or hardening of the arteries. In addition, the narrowing of the lumen within an artery may be associated with accumulations of fatty debris due to improper diet, insufficient exercise, or metabolic problems. When blood supply to critical nerve cells is diminished, the result is **anoxia,** which alters cell metabolism and may cause destruction of nerve tissue.

A number of congenital defects of the brain including the central auditory pathways have been described in the literature. These defects may be the result of birth trauma or agenesis of parts of the brain.

Pressure within the brain stem may also produce hearing loss. This pressure may be caused by tumors (either benign or malignant), by increased cerebrospinal fluid pressure produced secondary to trauma, or by direct insult to the head. Hemorrhage produced by vascular or other accidents may also cause pressure and damage.

Syphilis (lues) can produce damage anywhere in the auditory system, from the outer ear to the cortex. Cells are damaged or destroyed either by direct degeneration of the nerve units or, secondarily, by CVAs associated with the infection.

Degeneration of nerve fibers in the brain is expected with advancing age. Although presbycusis was listed as one of the causes of cochlear hearing loss, it has become accepted that, with aging, changes occur nearly everywhere in the auditory system, including the brain stem. Diseases such as multiple sclerosis can produce degeneration of nerve fibers in younger people as well.

Disorders of the Higher Auditory Pathways

The types of disorders that affect the cochlear nuclei may also affect higher neural structures. Tumors, for example, are not limited to specific sites. Head injury, the major cause of death or serious brain damage among young people in the United States, can produce lesions in a variety of sites. Lesions may encompass large portions of the brain or be localized to small areas.

Factors influencing audiometric results include not only the sizes of the lesions but also their locations. Lesions of the temporal cortex, such as from CVA or epilepsy, usually lead to abnormal results on special tests in the ear contralateral to the lesion. Lesions in the brain stem are not so predictable.

Jerger and Jerger (1975) point out that when a lesion is **extra-axial** (on the outside of the brain stem), audiometric symptoms appear on the same side of the head. Such patients often show considerable loss of sensitivity for pure tones, especially in the high frequencies. When the lesion is **intra-axial** (within the brain stem), central auditory tests may show either contralateral or bilateral effects. Often, hearing sensitivity for pure tones is normal or near normal at all frequencies.

Auditory Processing Disorders

The principal function of the central auditory system is to organize concurrent or sequential auditory input into definite patterns. The subsequent ability to comprehend and develop spoken language depends primarily on the success of the entire auditory system to process speech signals. In an attempt to avoid implicating an individual anatomical site by recognizing the interplay between peripheral and central pathologies, participants of a consensus conference recommended the clinical entity previously referred to as **central auditory processing disorder (CAPD)** be more operationally defined as **auditory processing disorder (APD)** (Jerger & Musiek, 2000). Although the conference addressed APD in children, it seems logical to extend this operationally inclined definition to auditory processing disorders of adults as well. Many with APD have difficulty in the interpretation of auditory information in the absence of a concomitant loss of peripheral hearing sensitivity. These processing difficulties are further compounded in the presence of surrounding auditory, or sometimes even visual, distractions. Discussion of the management of auditory processing disorders is presented in Chapter 15.

On occasion, patients present with complaints of decreased hearing abilities, although subsequent routine hearing tests reveal normal peripheral hearing. These patients may be distressed over their difficulties in auditory functioning within social contexts and concerned with potential deterioration in their hearing. In the absence of identifiable peripheral pathology or disconcerting unilateral symptoms, most of these patients are discharged with simple reassurance, leaving unanswered questions regarding the underlying problem. Patients following this scenario have been classified as having **obscure auditory dysfunction (OAD)** (Saunders & Haggard, 1989, 1993). It is probable that given testing directed specifically at auditory processing, many of these patients would be found to have an auditory processing disorder, resulting in the elimination of the obscurity of the diagnosis.

APDs occurring later in life, secondary to disorders such as CVAs, head trauma, brain tumor, or multiple sclerosis, have less chance of recovery than do APDs in the pediatric population. Because of the adaptive properties of the younger central nervous system, children have the advantage of compensatory development of other areas within the system. Auditory processing deficiencies may result in lack of attention to auditory stimuli. This increases distractibility, decreases auditory discrimination and localization abilities, and makes comprehension of speech more difficult. Difficulty with auditory figure–ground differentiation results in a decreased ability for selective attention. One cause for these deficiencies in children appears to be the decrease and fluctuation in the intensity of auditory input secondary to recurrent otitis media.

Minimal Auditory Deficiency Syndrome

The animal brain is characterized by an extremely well-organized system of representation for response to incoming signals. When there is deprivation of sensory input, such as to visual or auditory signals, marked changes may take place in the brain (Schwaber, 1992). The tendency of cells to become altered in order to conform to their environments is called **plasticity.** Changes in structures in the brain may take place as a result of the sensory deprivation caused by either cochlear or conductive hearing losses.

The slight or mild hearing loss that is often associated with otitis media may go undetected in very young children. Even when it is correctly diagnosed, parents and physicians alike are relieved when symptoms abate and the child appears normal in all respects. Experts have recognized that even these transient and very mild conductive hearing losses may affect the development of skills essential to the learning of language. The term ascribed to this set of circumstances is the **minimal auditory deficiency syndrome (MADS).**

What may be happening in the young human brain has been demonstrated in the laboratory on experimental animals (e.g., Webster & Webster, 1977). Within 45 days, mice with conductive hearing loss surgically induced shortly after birth showed smaller neurons in the cochlear nuclei, superior olivary complex, and trapezoid body than did mice in the control group. Katz (1978) reported that the attenuation of sound may produce similar effects in children and contribute to the development of learning disabilities.

Concern over the relationship between language disorders and otitis media was demonstrated by Rentschler and Rupp (1984). These researchers found that 70 percent of a group of speech- and language-impaired children also had histories of hearing problems, and they suggested persistent monitoring of children with middle-ear disorders through tympanometric measures.

Although the population they studied was small, Gunnarson and Finitzo (1991) looked at a group of children with conductive hearing loss and the later effects on the electrophysiology of the brain stem. They concluded that there do appear to be effects of early transient hearing loss on auditory brain-stem responses and that adequate sensory input to the central auditory nervous system is important to the brain during critical developmental periods.

The American Academy of Audiology (2000) issued a position paper on the guidelines for diagnosing and treating otitis media in children. Although some controversy continues to exist, many are now convinced of a cause-and-effect relationship between early and recurrent otitis media and later learning and communication disorders. It is not the extent of the hearing loss that is the precipitating factor, but rather the fluctuating nature of the disorder and the fact that differences in hearing sensitivity between the two ears of a child may result in abnormal development of auditory processing skills, which depend on binaural interactions in the brain. There is no disagreement that the primary responsibility for treating otitis media lies within the medical domain; however, the diagnosis and management of subsequent hearing loss is the responsibility of the audiologist.

The American Academy of Audiology (2000) recommends the following:

1. *Identification.* This includes screening at-risk children such as those who develop otitis media at or before the age of six months, those who attend daycare centers, those with cleft lip or palate or Down syndrome, and Native Americans. Screening should include

the functions of the middle ear, hearing, and language development. Children who fail the screening should be referred for in-depth testing and possible remediation. Those failing communication screenings may need referral for further evaluation and communication therapy from a speech-language pathologist.

2. *Assessment.* Air- and bone-conduction audiometry for both ears should be carried out to determine the degree of hearing loss and the audiometric configuration. Speech audiometry, along with acoustic immittance tests and a battery of tests for auditory processing disorders, should be administered when practicable. Referral to speech-language pathologists should be made on the basis of the outcome of these tests.

3. *Audiometric monitoring.* Periodic audiometric follow-up should be completed, even when the child is asymptomatic. Hearing tests should be carried out at the beginning of every school year and at least once during the winter. Parents or caregivers should be kept apprised of hearing test results, and their concerns over their children's hearing status should be carefully heeded. Parents or caregivers and teachers should also be taught skills for dealing with their children during exacerbations of hearing loss, ways of recognizing the possible development of hearing loss, and systems for minimizing the disruption of classroom learning by attention to the learning environments of at-risk children.

Although it is recognized that not all children who suffer repeated bouts of otitis media develop conditions that cause them to fall short of their genetic potential for learning, prudence demands that all persons who interact with these children should be alerted to the potential dangers.

Central Deafness

Cases of central deafness are extremely rare, occurring when both hemispheres of the brain are severely compromised. Although responses to behavioral audiometric tests may be absent, these patients typically have normal acoustic reflexes and ABRs. Such findings are usually secondary to vascular lesions of the middle cerebral artery or its branches.

Tests for Auditory Processing Disorders

Lesions in the auditory nerve and cochlear nuclei produce obvious and dramatic hearing symptoms in the ear ipsilateral to the lesion. As stated earlier in this chapter, once the level of the olivary complex is reached, both sides of the brain are involved in the transmission of auditory information. Even large lesions in the brain may produce either no audiological symptoms or symptoms that are very subtle. For this reason, emphasis must be placed on developing tests that are specifically sensitive to lesions in the central auditory system, many of which are reviewed in this chapter.

For the most part, tests using pure tones have been unsuccessful in identifying central auditory lesions. Because pure-tone tests have been disappointing, much of the past and current emphasis in diagnosing auditory processing disorders has been placed on speech tests, many of which are available commercially.[3] As Keith (1981) points out, tests to evaluate these disorders in children share certain characteristics, including language-dependent administration and scoring. Clearly tests that rely on speech stimuli must be used with caution if the patient exhibits speech-recognition difficulties. Given this caveat, one can expect more nonverbal tests for auditory processing disorder in the future.

Gaps-in-Noise Test

The Gaps-in-Noise (GIN) test (Musiek et al., 2005) represents a measure to assess temporal-processing abilities with a nonverbal task. During this test, the individual identifies the presence of gaps between 2 and 20 ms in duration within a 6-second broadband noise signal. The effect of any existing frequency-specific hearing loss is minimized through the use of a broadband test signal, and the relatively simple nature of the task limits the effects of patient language and cognitive skills. The test can be performed with any clinical audiometer connected to a CD or other type of player. Another commercially available temporal-processing test, the Random Gap Detection Test (RGDT), similarly limits the effects of patient language skills and has established normative data for children, adults, and older adults (Keith, 2000).

Masking-Level Difference

The phenomenon of binaural release from masking, or **masking-level difference (MLD),** has been known for some time (Hirsh, 1948). To determine the MLD, the binaural threshold is determined for a low-frequency tone presented in phase to the two ears in the presence of a binaural noise, also in phase. When the threshold is remeasured with the tones 180 degrees out of phase with the noise, a threshold improvement is found on the order of 10 to 15 dB. Abnormal MLDs in normal-hearing subjects strongly suggest a brain-stem lesion (Noffsinger, Martinez, & Schaefer, 1985), but positive findings have also been observed in cases of acoustic neuroma, presbycusis, Ménière's disease, and particularly multiple sclerosis (Mueller, 1987a). MLDs have also been measured using speech signals.

Although the effects of cochlear and cortical lesions on MLD are somewhat unpredictable, there is general agreement among researchers (e.g., Olsen & Noffsinger, 1976) that the release from masking is either absent or significantly less than normal in patients with lesions in the brain stem. If the clinician has access to a device capable of shifting the phase of the pure tone without affecting the phase of the noise, simply measuring several binaural pure-tone thresholds may provide additional insight into site of lesion.

While the advantages of including MLD testing in the assessment of auditory processing disorders have been documented for some time, including the fact that this test represents another non-language-based assessment, the lack of practical administration of this assessment tool has frequently relegated it to the realm of research investigations. A simplified protocol for the administration of MLD testing using a standard audio player (Wilson, Moncrieff, Townsend, & Pillion, 2003) holds promise for increasing clinical use of this measure of auditory perceptual abilities. Unlike the Gaps-in-Noise test, approaches to measuring MLD through any approach may be complicated by any degree of peripheral hearing loss.

The Dichotic Digits Test

Musiek (1983) describes a version of the **dichotic digits test** as being useful for diagnosing both brain-stem and cortical disorders, although it may not be possible to tell one lesion site from the other on the basis of this test alone. Twenty sets of two-digit pairs are presented at 50 or 60 dB above the SRT. The digit *7* is omitted because it is the only one that has two syllables. The patient hears two successive pairs of two digits and is asked to repeat all four digits. The test can also be done with three-digit pairs but may result in low scores for some individuals because of short-term memory difficulties. For this reason, Mueller (1987a) believes that the two-digit pair test is probably better for detection of lesions in the central auditory nervous system.

Performance-Intensity Function Testing

Jerger and Jerger (1971) described the use of the **performance-intensity function for PB words (PI-PB)** as a method of screening for central auditory disorders. As discussed in Chapter 5, it is unlikely that word-recognition test lists are truly phonetically balanced, and research suggests that attempts at such balancing may not even be necessary (Martin, Champlin, & Perez, 2000). In addition to testing with words, performance-intensity functions have been assessed with sentence-length speech-recognition tests as well. Patients with normal hearing sensitivity who show differences in the scores and shapes of the PI curves may be suspected of central disorders. Speech-recognition tests are presented to the patient at a number of levels—for example, 60, 70, 80, and 90 dB HL. The tests are scored, and a graph may be drawn for each ear; the graphs show the speech-recognition scores as a function of presentation level.

If a significant difference in scores occurs between ears (20 to 30 percent), it may be suspected that a central lesion is present on the side of the brain opposite the poorer score. Sometimes rollover of the curve occurs; that is, at some point, scores begin to decrease as intensity increases (see Figure 12.7). Rollover suggests a lesion on the side of the brain opposite the ear with the rollover or a lesion of the VIIIth nerve on the same side (Figure 12.2). PI functions may not be helpful in detecting central lesions if a loss of hearing sensitivity is also present. A rollover ratio is derived by the following formula:

$$\text{Rollover ratio (\%)} = \frac{\text{Max} - \text{Min}}{\text{Max}}$$

"Max" is the highest score and "Min" the lowest score obtained at an intensity above that required for the "Max" (Jerger & Jerger, 1971). Rollover ratios of .40 suggest cochlear lesions, whereas ratios of .45 or greater indicate an VIIIth nerve site. High rollover ratios are also seen in some elderly patients (Gang, 1976), which probably reflects some degree of central presbycusis.

Two factors must be considered when determining rollover ratios. First, the procedure is not helpful if all speech-recognition scores are low. Second, for the greatest accuracy, a number of levels must be tested. Establishing complete performance-intensity functions can be very time-consuming. When a central pathology is suspected, however, a comparison of performance of a high-intensity speech-recognition measure (90 dB HL, tolerance permitting) with that of an estimate of maximum performance (closely estimated by testing at 5 to 10 dB above

FIGURE 12.7 Typical performance-intensity functions for words showing the normal increase in word-recognition scores with increased intensity and the rollover (decreased discrimination beyond a certain level) evident in some ears contralateral to a central auditory disorder.

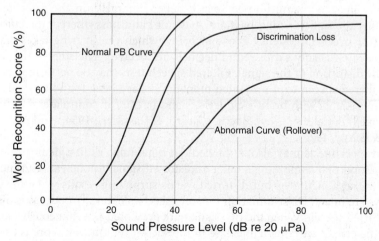

the most comfortable level) may be revealing. A decrease of 20 percent or more at the higher level can be considered an indication of central involvement. Because this is a measure significantly above threshold, masking of the contralateral ear must usually be employed.

Listening in Spacialized Noise Test

Capitalizing on the central auditory system's need to utilize binaural cues adequately to differentiate the location of competing signals from the message that one is listening to, the Listening in Spacialized Noise test (Cameron, Dillon, & Newall, 2006) creates a virtual (under earphones) three-dimensional listening environment to detect auditory figure–ground discrimination deficits. This test, which can be administered with standard audiometric equipment and a personal computer, may have a higher specificity in identifying children with problems in binaural processing. It uses special distribution of sound sources for suppression of auditory distractions: a common difficulty reported for children suspected of having auditory processing difficulty.

Filtered Speech Tests

Although standard tests for speech recognition do not usually identify central lesions, it has been known for many years that distortion of the speech signal presented monaurally often results in reduced speech-recognition scores in the ear contralateral to a central lesion (Bocca & Calearo, 1963; Goetzinger & Angell, 1965). This statement is true if the lesion does not impair the symbolization and memorization processes of the brain, which may result in much more demonstrable symptoms. Subsequent studies of distorted speech testing with suspected central lesions has used speech signals that have been periodically interrupted, masked, compressed in time, presented at low sensation levels, and filtered. Filtering some frequencies from the speech spectrum has become the most popular of these methods. These test methods often follow Bocca's (1967) early suggestion that distorted sentence materials are superior to isolated words because they put greater stress on the brain's capacity for pattern recognition.

A speech signal may be passed through a filter that rejects the low frequencies and passes the highs (high-pass filter) or one that rejects the high frequencies and passes the lows (low-pass filter). A signal may also be processed through a filter that rejects both high and low frequencies above and below a prescribed range, so that only a band of frequencies is allowed through. This is called band-pass filtering and is usually described in terms of the range from the lowest to the highest frequencies passed.

Difficulty in recognizing filtered speech depends largely on the filter characteristics, such as whether the signal is high-pass, low-pass, or band-pass filtered; the cutoff frequency of the filter (the precise frequency above or below which the filtering takes place); and the filter rejection rate (usually expressed in decibels per octave). The steeper the rejection rate, the greater the distortion of the signal. Filtered speech tests may be performed monaurally or binaurally. Filtered speech tests presented monaurally have been found to yield scores markedly poorer in patients with brain-stem lesions and in the ear contralateral to temporal lobe lesions (Antonelli & Calearo, 1968; Bocca, Calearo, & Cassinari, 1954; Hodgson, 1967; Jerger, 1960; Lynn & Gilroy, 1977).

Filtered speech tests may also be carried out binaurally, as first demonstrated by Bocca (1955), who found that combining a quiet undistorted signal to one ear with the same signal to the other ear, at a high level but distorted, yields surprising results when the central auditory pathways are intact. Discrimination for soft speech is naturally poor, as is discrimination for loud, distorted speech. When the two signals are presented simultaneously (soft to one ear, distorted to the other), a dramatic increase in the speech recognition score is observed as the two signals are fused in the brain. No such summation of scores was observed by Jerger (1960) or Calearo (1957) in patients with temporal lobe disorders.

Band-Pass Binaural Speech Audiometry

Matzker (1959) was first to develop a test wherein different filtered portions of a speech signal are presented to each ear. Discrimination for either a low-frequency band-passed signal alone or a high-frequency band-passed signal alone yields very poor speech intelligibility. If the brain stem is normal, the two signals are fused when presented simultaneously. Inability to demonstrate this binaural fusion suggests a lesion in the brain stem.

One method for this test has been described by Smith and Resnick (1972). The low-frequency band of words is presented at 30 dB SL through one channel of a two-channel speech audiometer. The high-frequency band, controlled by the hearing-level dial of the second channel, is presented 10 dB above the level set for the low band. Three test conditions exist:

1. Low band to the right ear, high band to the left ear (**dichotic**).
2. Low band to the left ear, high band to the right ear (dichotic).
3. Both bands to both ears (**diotic**).

The Smith and Resnick (1972) procedure with CNC words, which they call dichotic binaural fusion, has gained some clinical prominence. There appear to be no differences in the three scores in patients with normal hearing, cochlear lesions, or lesions of the temporal lobe. Patients with brain-stem disorders show significant diotic-score enhancement over one or both of the dichotic scores.

In a similar test, Palva and Jokinen (1975) found that patients with disorders of the auditory cortex show poor scores when both bands are presented to the ear contralateral to the lesion, although their dichotic scores are good. Patients with brain-stem lesions show especially poor scores for binaural fusion.

Martin and Clark (1977) employed a comparison of diotic and dichotic presentations of the **Word Intelligibility by Picture Identification (WIPI) test** to young children so that a picture-pointing procedure could be used as a screening test for children with auditory-processing disorders. They found that diotic presentation improved discrimination scores by 10 percent and that a control group did about as well on the more difficult dichotic task as on the diotic one. As with any screening test for children who show normal hearing on standard audiometric procedures but whose histories suggest the possibility of central deficits, those who fail the test should be referred for in-depth testing of auditory processing abilities (see Table 12.1).

Synthetic Sentence Identification Tests

The synthetic sentence identification (SSI) test, described in Chapter 5, may be used to identify lesions of the central auditory system. The sentences are made more difficult to identify by using a competing message, a recording of continuous discourse. This may be an *ipsilateral competing*

TABLE 12.1 Band-Pass Filter Settings Used in Five Studies of Binaural Fusion

Study	*Low-Frequency Band (Hertz)*	*High-Frequency Band (Hertz)*
Matzker (1959)	500–800	1815–2500
Hayashi, Ohta, and Morimoto (1966)	300–600	1200–2400
Franklin (1966)	240–480	1020–2040
Smith and Resnick (1972)	360–890	1750–2200
Palva and Jokinen (1975)	420–720	1800–2400

message (ICM), which is presented to the test ear along with the synthetic sentences, or it may be a *contralateral competing message (CCM),* which is presented to the opposite ear. With the test materials (SSI) fixed at a given sensation level, the competing message may be varied in intensity so that a number of message-to-competition ratios (MCRs) are obtained (Jerger, 1973).

According to Jerger (1973), normal-hearing persons perform at the 100 percent level on the SSI-ICM test with an MCR of 0 dB, 80 percent with an MCR of –10 dB, 55 percent with an MCR of –20 dB, and 20 percent with an MCR of –30 dB (competing message 30 dB above the sentences). Patients with lesions of the brain stem show large differences in scores between the right and left ears on this test. With an increase in the level of the competing message, scores deteriorate more rapidly than normal when the test is performed in the ear contralateral to the lesion. For example, for a patient with a lesion of the left brain stem, SSI-ICM scores will be poorer in the right ear than in the left ear.

The SSI-CCM test is performed in precisely the same manner as the SSI-ICM, the only difference being that the competing message is presented to one ear and the sentences are presented to the opposite ear. The MCR is varied up to –40 dB.

Persons with normal hearing and normal central auditory function perform very well on the SSI-CCM test, even at MCRs of –40 dB. The competition of the other ear seems to have little effect on the ability to understand the synthetic sentences. Patients with lesions of the temporal lobe perform well when the sentences are presented to the ear on the same side as the lesion while the competing message is presented to the other ear. When the sentences are presented to the ear on the unimpaired side and the competition is presented to the ear on the same side as the cortical lesion, deterioration of scores ensues. For example, in a left cortical lesion, SSI scores will be good with sentences in the left ear and competition in the right ear, but scores will be poor with sentences in the right ear and competition in the left ear. Jerger (1973) therefore believes that the use of ipsilateral and contralateral competing messages with the SSI not only reveals central disorders but actually separates lesions of the brain stem from those in the cortex.

Competing Sentence Test

Building on work begun a decade earlier, Williford (1977) reported on the use of natural sentences in diagnosing central auditory disorders. The Competing Sentence Test (CST) is made up of natural sentences and, unlike the SSI procedure, uses an open-message set. To make the procedure useful, of course, a competing message is presented to the opposite ear.

The primary message is presented at a level 35 dB above the pure-tone average (PTA), while the competing message is presented at 50 dB above the PTA. Both sentences are the same length and on the same subject (e.g., time, food, weather, family). Fifteen sentences are used. The patient is told to repeat only the primary (softer) sentence. Because many brain-injured patients have difficulty in attending to soft stimuli or those under conditions of adverse message-to-competition ratios, modifications of the original method have been developed (Bergman, Hirsch, Solzi, & Mankowitz, 1987).

Patients with lesions of the temporal lobe show the greatest difficulty when the primary sentence is presented to the ear contralateral to the lesion. Simple versions of the procedure have been used successfully to identify children with learning disabilities. Children tend to improve on this test as they get older, which is not surprising because the central auditory nervous system probably continues to mature until about 9 years of age.

Rapidly Alternating Speech Perception

A test has been designed that rapidly alternates six- or seven-word sentences between the ears (Williford, 1977). The 20 sentences, presented at 50 dB above the SRT, are switched back and forth every 300 milliseconds. The procedure is called the **Rapidly Alternating Speech**

Perception (RASP) test. For the patient to understand and repeat the sentences, brain-stem function must be normal because any segment presented to one ear alone is presumably too short to allow discrimination.

The Staggered Spondaic Word Test

Katz (1962, 1968) developed a test of dichotic listening that has undergone more standardization on English-speaking adults than most of the other tests for central auditory disorders and has been shown to differentiate between normal children and those with learning disabilities (Berrick et al., 1984). The **Staggered Spondaic Word (SSW) test** is a measure of dichotic listening that utilizes spondees in a suprathreshold manner. Pairs of different spondaic words are presented to each ear, with some timing overlap for both ears. The first syllable of one spondee is presented to one ear, and while the second syllable is presented, the first syllable of the other spondee is presented to the other ear. Then the second syllable of the second spondee is presented alone. This procedure is diagrammed as shown:

	Time ---------->		
	1	2	3
Right ear	OUT	SIDE	
Left ear		IN	LAW

Naturally, the very nature of this test precludes the use of masking, but insert receivers are useful in increasing the interaural attenuation. Poor scores on the SSW test suggest a lesion in the higher brain centers on the side contralateral to the low-scoring ear. Although the SSW test is very popular, one lasting complaint concerns the amount of time needed to follow the complex scoring system. At least one computer program is now available for this purpose. Mueller (1987b) has suggested that diagnosis with the SSW test may be carried out simply by computing the score for each ear on the basis of the percentage of words identified correctly.

Time-Compressed Speech

With special recording devices, it is possible to speed up the playback of speech stimuli without significantly creating the perception of higher vocal pitch. This **time-compressed speech** has been studied by using the words from the NU-6 lists. Central auditory lesions are best identified at 60 percent time compression (Kurdziel, Noffsinger, & Olsen, 1976). Kurdziel and colleagues found that, in some brain lesions, time-compressed word-recognition scores were poor in the ear contralateral to the lesion, whereas in other cases scores remained normal in both ears. There has not been much information in the recent literature on the use of time-compressed speech in cases of central auditory nervous system damage.

Screening Test for Auditory Processing Disorders

The **Screening Test for Auditory Processing Disorders (SCAN)**[4] was devised as a rapid procedure to detect auditory processing difficulties in children ages 3 to 11 so that their risk factors may be determined and specific management strategies applied. Its standardization (Keith, 1986) appears to be more extensive than some of the other tests for central auditory disorders. The SCAN comprises three subtests. The filtered-word subtest contains two lists of 20 monosyllabic words that are low-pass filtered at 1,000 Hz (with a rejection rate of 32 dB per octave) and are presented by recording to one ear at a time. The auditory figure-ground subtest likewise contains two monosyllabic 20-word lists, presented to each ear in the presence of a background noise made up of a multitalker babble. A signal-to-noise ratio of +8 dB is used. The competing-word subtest comprises two lists of 25 monosyllabic words presented dichotically (one word introduced to each ear simultaneously). The child is instructed to repeat the word heard in the right ear followed by the word heard in the left ear. Comparisons to other tests for central auditory disorders suggest that the SCAN may be a useful procedure (Keith, Rudy, Donahue, & Katfamma, 1989).

In response to a need for well-standardized central auditory tests for persons over 11 years of age, Keith (1994, 1995) modified the SCAN for use with older subjects. The SCAN-A is an upward extension of the SCAN designed for use with adolescents and adults with neurological disorders and learning disabilities. A caution was raised by Woods, Pena, and Martin (2004) about the possible contamination of results on the SCAN based on ethnic differences so these should be considered carefully in interpretation.

Acoustic Reflex Test

Comparison of ipsilateral and contralateral acoustic reflexes can be of great value in determining the integrity of the crossover pathways in the trapezoid body of the brain stem. For example, if a patient has normal hearing and normal ipsilateral acoustic reflexes in both ears, it is highly probable that the cochleas, the VIIth and VIIIth cranial nerves, and the middle-ear mechanisms are intact on both sides. If the contralateral reflexes are absent in the same individual, the most likely explanation is that damage exists within those crossover pathways (see Table 7.2I and J).

Auditory Evoked Potentials

Auditory brain-stem response audiometry has been useful in diagnosing central auditory disorders as long as any hearing loss in the two ears is essentially symmetrical and no more than a mild loss exists in either ear (Musiek, 1983). The presence of concomitant peripheral lesions may confound interpretation of ABR results if lesions are present in both the cochlea and the brain stem. Central lesions generally slow the conduction velocity of electrical impulses sent through the nerve fibers. Musiek suggests the following general observations:

Wave I (all waves) delay	Lesion in outer, middle, or inner ear
Wave I–III delay	Lesion in auditory nerve or lower brain stem
Wave III–V delay	Lesion in higher brain stem

In testing for lesions of the brain stem, it is useful to compare the latencies and intervals of Waves I, III, and V as a function of increased click rates. Although the ABR results may provide important diagnostic information in testing for central auditory lesions, interpretation can be difficult when it is complicated by the absence of some waves, the influence of unusual audiometric configurations, and the patient's age and body temperature. The ABR is generally the most sensitive and specific test currently available for diagnosis of auditory brain-stem lesions, although the use of the complete central test battery remains important (Chermak & Musiek, 1997).

The P300, or cognitive potential of the late auditory evoked response, is elicited by an "oddball" paradigm whereby the subject tries to discriminate between a frequently occurring stimulus and a rarely occurring stimulus. For example, a 1,000 Hz tone burst is presented

80 percent of the time, and a 2,000 Hz tone burst is presented randomly 20 percent of the time. The subject is asked to count only the higher-pitched tones. The waveform elicited by the rare (2,000 Hz) stimulus shows a large positive peak with a latency of approximately 300 milliseconds. Reduction in amplitude, or increase in the latencies of the P300, has been found in elderly individuals, those suffering from dementia, and head trauma patients. This procedure is thought to hold future promise as a diagnostic procedure for other disorders of the central auditory nervous system. Indeed, Hall (2007) reports an abnormal P300 response in a large number of children being assessed for auditory processing disorder.

Otoacoustic Emissions

It has been emphasized in this text that otoacoustic emissions (OAEs) have come into their own as a powerful clinical tool with a variety of applications (see Chapter 7). For example, Jerger, Ali, Fong, and Tseng (1992) report on a patient with multiple sclerosis in whom it was possible to identify the source of the speech-recognition difficulty she experienced in one ear as retrocochlear. The presence of distortion product OAEs in this case suggested that at least the outer hair cells of the cochlea were functioning normally. The diagnosis of a more central lesion was confirmed by MRI of the brain. Cevette, Robinette, Carter, and Knops (1995) also reported on the important contribution OAEs can make to the diagnosis of multiple sclerosis.

Although the role of OAEs in the diagnosis of acoustic neuroma is limited, OAEs have been used in intraoperative monitoring and as a preoperative and postoperative measure of cochlear function. In the operating room, distortion-product OAEs have been demonstrated to reveal earlier evidence of cochlear compromise than monitoring with ABR (Telischi, Widick, Lonsbury-Martin, & McCoy, 1995).

Cases of auditory neuropathy/auditory dys-synchrony are relatively uncommon. However, the ability of OAEs to assess cochlear function objectively helped to identify this clinical entity when absent ABRs were seen in the presence of only mild to moderate hearing loss. It may be anticipated that further reports of the increasing clinical utility of OAEs will be forthcoming.

Approaching APD Through a Battery of Tests

While administration of electrophysiological tests is more costly than that of behavioral measures, behavioral tests are not always feasible, for example, with patients with aphasia or central deafness. The sensitivity of testing for lesions of the auditory nerve and central auditory pathways increases when behavioral and electrophysiological measures are combined. In addition, the audiologist's confidence in making a diagnosis of auditory processing disorder is heightened when abnormalities are found in both the behavioral and electrophysiological domains (Chermak & Musiek, 1997).

The Bruton Conference on auditory processing disorders recommended a battery of tests including behavioral and electroacoustical/electrophysiological measures (Jerger & Musiek, 2000). On the behavioral side, participants advocated a combination of pure-tone audiometry to assess for peripheral hearing loss, performance intensity function testing to compare performance between the ears, dichotic tasks, and measures of auditory temporal processing. Recommended electroacoustic/electrophysiologic measures included immittance measures to rule out middle-ear disorder and to identify acoustic reflex abnormalities, OAEs to rule out inner-ear disorders, and ABR and middle latency response as measures of auditory structures at brain-stem and cortical levels. The diagnosis of APD is best carried out through a team approach, capitalizing on the backgrounds of audiologists, speech-language pathologists, and educational psychologists.

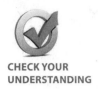

CHECK YOUR UNDERSTANDING

ACTIVITIES

Clinical COMMENTARY

The aim of behavioral measures of central function has changed over the years. While these tests were originally designed to help identify the site of lesion of neuropathology, this role has largely been supplanted by the more objective electrophysiological and electroacoustical measures and the advances in medical imaging. Today, behavioral measures of central auditory function are more frequently employed as screening measures for potential disorders rather than as diagnostic indices. Their true value to the audiologist has evolved in their ability to describe the communication impact of auditory processing disorders. Therapeutic intervention can be designed and implemented more successfully if it is based on the study of communication impact. For discussion of management of auditory processing disorders, see Chapter 15.

EVOLVING CASE STUDIES

As mentioned in Chapter 11, the term *sensory/neural* can be an ambiguous one. In the context of this chapter, it refers to the neural element of the word. Although relatively rare, retrocochlear lesions, those beyond the cochlea, often have serious medical considerations. One of the more common of these considerations is a tumor on or beyond the auditory nerve (VIII). Because these problems usually present, at least initially, in one ear, a sensible approach in audiological diagnosis is to suspect the possibility of such lesions in all cases of unilateral sensory/neural hearing loss until proven otherwise. In such instances, a medical referal, to a neuro-otologist if possible, is mandatory if special audiological tests are positive, or even suggestive, of such a lesion.

Case Study 4: Sensory/Neural Hearing Loss—Auditory Nerve Disorder

As described earlier, this 36-year-old female presented with a gradually progressive sensory/neural hearing loss in her left ear. An alerting find was a relatively poor score during word-recognition testing, with some rollover in the left ear, while the findings in the right were normal. Immittance measures, which are often significantly helpful in such cases, showed normal typanograms, further eliminating conductive disorders. However, she showed elevated or absent acoustic reflex thresholds, both ipsilaterally and contalaterally, and significant acoustic-reflex decay in her impaired ear at 500 Hz. These findings suggest the performance of additional audiological tests, such as otoacoustic emissions, which would predictably be normal; auditory brain-stem response testing, which would be expected to reveal abnormal Wave V latencies; and other auditory evoked potentials. Medical diagnoses would probably include magnetic resonance imaging.

Summary

This chapter dealt with the function and audiological diagnosis of lesions of the auditory nerve and central auditory nervous system. Although considerable mystery continues to surround the central nervous system, nowhere is this mystery greater than in the higher auditory pathways. Impulses that pass from the cochlea are transmitted by the auditory nerve to the cochlear nuclei, which are waystations for transmission to higher centers and areas for complex frequency and temporal analysis. The cochlear nuclei also represent the highest centers at which the processing of neural stimuli corresponds to auditory information obtained from just one ear. From the cochlear nuclei, auditory information is processed by the superior olivary complexes, the lateral lemnisci, the inferior colliculi, and the medial geniculate bodies. Impulses are finally transmitted to the cortex by the auditory radiations. Because of the numerous decussations at higher centers, there is representation of each ear on both sides of the brain, with greater representation on the opposite side.

Caution should always be exercised when an audiologist attempts to determine the site of a lesion affecting the auditory system. For example, a patient may have both a cochlear and a central disorder. Most auditory tests give results that reflect primarily the first lesion reached by the stimulus (the most peripheral lesion) but can be further complicated by the more central lesion. Ruling out one anatomical area of the auditory system should not result in a diagnosis of a lesion in a specific region elsewhere.

Both behavioral and electroacoustical/electrophysiological procedures have been devised for testing central disorders, but none has been demonstrated to be infallible. Much research is needed to improve techniques for detecting disorders in the central pathways and pinpointing the area of damage. There is little doubt that this is one of the most challenging areas for research in diagnostic audiology. Thirty-five years ago, Williford (1977) lamented that audiology had only scratched the surface in its efforts to diagnose APD and that practical treatment programs were even less developed. Despite considerable progress to date, these are areas that still need much additional exploration.

REVIEW TABLE 12.1 Audiological Symptoms of Retrocochlear Lesions

VIIIth Nerve and Cochlear Nucleus	Central Pathways
Decruitment; no recruitment	Poor binaural fusion
Marked tone decay at all frequencies	Low SSI-ICM scores
Rapid acoustic reflex decay	Low SSI-CCM scores
Elevated or absent acoustic reflexes	Increased Wave III–V interval
Marked increase in ABR Wave V latencies	SRS for distorted speech poor in ear contralateral to lesion
Present otoacoustic emissions	
SRS for distorted speech poor in ear ipsilateral to lesion	

Frequently Asked Questions

Q What is the usual inclusion of more words than necessary to round out acceptable grammar and syntax called?

A *Extrinsic redundancy.*

Q In what way does multiple sclerosis cause damage to the VIIIth cranial nerve and thus create hearing loss?

A *MS strips away the protective myelin sheath from cranial nerves. When the auditory nerve becomes demyelinated, it ceases to function normally.*

Q Can minimal auditory deficiency syndrome be a result of a lack of language input?

A *Yes.*

Q Is the difference between a central and peripheral hearing loss the same as the difference between a conductive and sensory/neural hearing loss?

A *In contemporary parlance, we no longer speak of central disorders as hearing loss. The old term,* central deafness, *is no longer in use.*

Q What is the last subcortical relay station for auditory impulses?

A *The medial geniculate body in the thalamus.*

Q Where do tumors usually arise in the auditory nerve?

A *Most of these intracanicular (within the internal auditory canal) tumors arise from the Schwann cells on the vestibular branch of cranial nerve VIII. For this reason, they are sometimes called "Schwannomas."*

Q Are the tumors found on the auditory nerve usually malignant or benign?

A *They are usually benign.*

Suggested Reading

Chermak, G. D. & Musiek, F. E. (2014). Handbook of central auditory processing disorder: Comprehensive intervention (2nd ed.). San Diego: Plural Publishing.

Musiek, F. E., & Baran, J. A. (2007). *The auditory system: Anatomy, physiology, and clinical correlates.* Boston: Allyn & Bacon.

Tillery, K. L. (2009). Central auditory processing evaluation: A test battery approach. In J. Katz, L. Medwetsky, R. Burkard, & L. Hood (Eds.), *Handbook of clinical audiology* (pp. 627–641). Philadelphia: Lippincott Williams and Wilkins.

Endnotes

1. For Theodore Schwann, German anatomist and physiologist, 1810–1882.
2. For Friedrich Daniel von Recklinghausen, German pathologist, 1833–1910.
3. Auditec of St. Louis (800-669-9065).
4. SCAN and SCAN-A available from The Psychological Corporation, Harcourt Brace Jovanovich (800-228-0752).

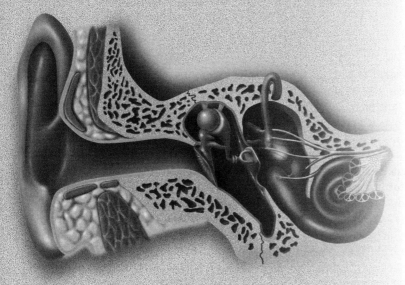

CHAPTER 13

Nonorganic Hearing Loss

LEARNING OBJECTIVES

This chapter should alert the reader to the problem of nonorganic hearing loss and some of the symptoms that make its presence known. At the completion of this chapter, the reader should be able to

- List several terms that have been used to describe nonorganic hearing loss and recognize the implications behind these terms and why some may not be appropriate.

- Describe how some of the objective measures of hearing described in Chapter 7 may be applied to the evaluation of those with nonorganic hearing loss, which tests may provide qualitative evidence (evidence of existence), and which provide a more quantitative measure of nonorganic hearing loss.

- Outline tests using a standard two-channel clinical audiometer that can provide qualitative or quantitative evidence of nonorganic hearing loss.

PATIENTS WHO CLAIM TO HAVE HEARING LOSS, but actually have normal hearing or a lesser hearing loss than portrayed, are more than infrequently seen in audiology clinics. It is paramount that audiologists recognize these patients when they present themselves so that their cases may be properly managed. This chapter is dedicated to a discussion of this problem.

There are several reasons why an individual might decide to fabricate or exaggerate a disability, and there are many forms of expression for this decision. Lawsuits have been filed for compensation for whiplash, back pain, memory loss, cognitive deficits, spinal-cord injury, weakness, dizziness, tinnitus, and, of course, hearing loss. In addition, there is a host of litigious actions, many of which are related to claims for workers' compensation. Some children may express nonorganic hearing loss as a means of acquiring peer acceptance, parental affection, decreased academic pressures, and so on.

The past four chapters have discussed anatomical areas in the auditory system and hearing losses associated with lesions in each of these areas. The term **nonorganic hearing loss** is used in this text to describe an apparent loss of hearing without any organic disorder or with insufficient pathological evidence to explain the extent of the loss.

The source of patient referral, medical history, symptoms, and behavior both during and outside formal hearing tests are factors to be considered before making a diagnosis of nonorganic hearing loss. Patients may exaggerate a hearing loss because they are incapable of more reliable behavior, because they are willfully fabricating or exaggerating a hearing disorder, or, perhaps because they have some psychological disorder. There may, of course, be an interaction among these factors. Observation of the patient and special tests for nonorganic hearing loss often lead the audiologist to the proper resolution of the problem. Above all, audiologists must be alert to patients who present spurious responses during routine audiometric procedures.

Terminology

There have been ongoing problems with the terms that audiologists and other specialists concerned with hearing disorders use to describe what is referred to in this text as *nonorganic hearing loss*. Some other common terms that have been used are listed below:

- *Nonorganic hearing loss.* The term nonorganic hearing loss has been popular for some time and is common in the literature. The problem with this label is that it may convey the notion that the entire hearing loss, as presented by the patient, contains no organic explanation. Because many nonorganic hearing losses have at least some physical basis, with added embellishment, the term leaves something to be desired. Nevertheless, it appears to be the most useful term available and is widely accepted.

- *Erroneous hearing loss.* The term erroneous hearing loss (Martin & Clark, 2012) was suggested as an alternative because it does not imply an all-or-none entity. While there are advantages to this term, other terms are much more clinically ingrained. As such, this term has not become popular.

- *Pseudohypacusis.* Some clinicians prefer **pseudohypacusis** (Carhart, 1961), which literally means "false hearing loss." Originally spelled *pseudohypoacusis,* this term suffers from the same limitations as *nonorganic hearing loss.* The objection comes from the notion that the patient has no organic pathology whatsoever (Mendel, Danhauer, & Singh, 1999; Stach, 2003; Ventry & Chaiklin, 1962). The correct medical parlance implies that there is either no underlying pathology or that any present disorder does not explain the extent of a hearing loss (Roeser, Buckley, & Stickney, 2000). This meaning is not always conveyed in reports by audiologists.

- *Functional hearing loss.* Another common term for nonorganic hearing loss is **functional hearing loss** (Ventry & Chaiklin, 1962). Physicians and psychologists often use the term functional to describe the symptoms of conditions that are not organic in nature. One of the many problems with the use of the word functional in a hearing loss context is that the term may be viewed from its other definition, which relates to some kind of function or malfunction.

- *Psychogenic hearing loss.* Some audiologists have used **psychogenic hearing loss** to describe a fabricated or exaggerated problem of unconscious origin, as opposed to one that is consciously feigned (*psychogenic* means "beginning in the mind"). More recently this has been replaced by **conversion disorder** because the underlying process is one of psychological stresses being converted to overt physical symptoms (Shahrokh & Hales, 2003). Both *psychogenic hearing loss* and *conversion disorder* speak to the etiology of the problem and should be eschewed by audiologists for a number of reasons.

- *Hysterical deafness.* An older term, **hysterical deafness,** is a carryover from the Freudian era and is overly simplistic. This is in part true because of the all-or-none implications and the suggestion that the behavior is entirely on an unconscious level. Martin (2009) has stated, "Since the word 'hysterical' derives from the Greek 'hystera' (womb) the term is actually pejorative and its disuse is appropriate for this reason as well."

- *False or exaggerated hearing loss.* Peck (2011) suggests that **false or exaggerated hearing loss** be used when the audiologist observes inconsistencies in test results or in patient behavior. This is a new term, so only time will determine whether it will be widely adopted.

- *Factitious disorder.* The human psyche is far too complex for a simple contrast between intentional and unintentional motivations. Austen and Lynch (2004) discuss the use of a number of paradigms as alternatives to the dichotomy that exists in the traditional attempts to separate behavior into that which is deliberate versus that which is not. They advocate for another term, **factitious disorder,** and recommend a new nomenclature in dealing with the categorization of nonorganic hearing losses. It is recognized that persons who deliberately pretend to have a disorder that they do not have, such as hearing loss, are not necessarily free of psychological influences. While complex, many of these recommendations appear valid.

- *Malingering.* One term probably used far too often is **malingering.** A malingerer is a deliberate falsifier of physical or psychological symptoms for some desired gain. Malingering is also frequently suspected (often unjustly) in association with automobile and industrial accidents, when payment may be involved to compensate patients for damages. Many patients who are called auditory malingerers actually have some degree of hearing loss. In addition to the potential for psychological damage to the patient and the risk of inaccuracy in diagnosis, calling someone a "malingerer" is tantamount to calling him or her a liar, which brings with it potentially serious litigious implications.

Although *nonorganic hearing loss* is the term used in this text, the reader should be aware of other terminology and should know that this label does not suggest cause, as do terms like *malingering* or *psychogenic*. There is no way to know for certain whether a patient with a feigned or embellished disorder is malingering, has a psychological disorder, or exhibits a combination of the two. Unless the patient admits to lying, or the confirmed diagnosis of an emotionally induced disorder is made by a qualified psychologist or psychiatrist, audiologists should settle for more general terms. In any event, terminology should be chosen carefully when communicating with patients, their families, and referral sources (Snyder, 2001).

Patients with Nonorganic Hearing Loss

Patients manifesting symptoms of nonorganic hearing loss may be of any age, sex, or socioeconomic background. It is probable that more adult males have been suspected of this disorder because emphasis has been placed on eliminating its possibility among men applying to the Department of Veterans Affairs for compensation for hearing loss.

Most of the studies performed on patients with nonorganic hearing loss have been carried out on adult males because they have been "captive audiences," as in military studies. This leads one to wonder whether there are any age or gender differences in this respect, and the paucity of data along these lines regarding nonorganic hearing loss is not helpful. Some generalizations to nonorganic hearing loss may be made, however, from the literature on interpersonal communication.

Some nonorganic hearing losses may be looked on as one form of deception, which can be defined as an intentional, conscious act. According to Burgoon, Buller, and Woodall (1989), in general, men find deceit more permissible than do women. They further claim that when women lie, it is usually to protect significant others, whereas men who lie tend to do so for more self-serving reasons. Because children's abilities to plan and execute deception successfully improve with age (as they develop strategies for this purpose), we may assume that young children are less likely to feign a hearing loss successfully than are adults or older children. However, there are reasons to believe that nonorganic hearing loss may be more common in children than has previously been thought and that the dynamics that result in such behaviors may be much more deeply seated than has been supposed (Johnson, Weissman, & Klerman, 1992). Nonorganic hearing loss in children may signal long-term emotional problems (Brooks & Goeghegan, 1992) or serious distress (Riedner & Efros, 1995).

The only true way to discover the kinds of strategies patients with nonorganic hearing loss use in attempts to deceive their examiners is to ask them. This is obviously impossible, so Martin, Champlin, and McCreery (2001) studied 30 adults with normal hearing and paid them according to how diligently they tried to malinger a hearing loss on the usual routine tests. Based on their findings, malingerers may incorporate a combination of strategies to feign a hearing loss. For example, they may initially not respond to stimuli at all or randomly respond but then switch to a loudness judgment, responding to a predetermined reference level of loudness. According to this study, the majority of subjects who use more than one strategy use a combination of loudness judgment and a counting method. Specifically, malingerers may use the *loudness judgment* strategy for the evaluation of the first ear and then switch to the *counting with a loudness reference* strategy. For the evaluation of the first ear, the malingerer may simulate a hearing loss by responding to a predetermined reference level of loudness. Once the patients figure out the standard presentation procedure, they may switch to the counting strategy for the evaluation of the other ear. That is, they may simulate a hearing loss in the second ear tested by responding to every third presentation following the predetermined loudness reference. This type of combination exemplifies the importance of not adhering to standard procedures when nonorganic hearing loss is suspected.

Ross (1964) has described the development of nonorganic hearing loss in children under some circumstances. Very often, children with normal hearing inadvertently fail screening tests performed in public schools. There are many reasons for failure to respond during a hearing test besides hearing loss: Equipment may malfunction, ambient room noise may produce threshold shifts, students may have difficulty in following instructions, and so on. Children may find that as soon as school and parental attention focus on a possible hearing problem, they begin to enjoy a degree of gain in the form of favors, excuses for poor grades, and special attention. By the time some children are seen by hearing specialists, they may be committed to perpetuating the notion that they have hearing losses. Ross believes that public school referrals to audiologists or physicians should be made only after the individual responsible for the screening is fairly certain that a hearing loss exists.

There are probably myriads of reasons why individuals might show nonorganic hearing loss. If a patient is, in fact, malingering or deliberately exaggerating an existing hearing loss, the motivation may be financial gain. Other reasons may simply be to win attention or to avoid performing some undesirable task. Because the underlying reasons are more difficult to understand, this avoidance has been considered a form of **conversion neurosis.** Whatever the dynamics of nonorganic hearing loss, they may be deeply enmeshed in the personality of the patient, and a cursory look at these dynamics in any single chapter must be recognized for its superficiality.

Indications of Nonorganic Hearing Loss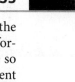

There are many signs that alert the audiologist to nonorganic hearing loss. These include the source of referral, the patient's history, his or her behavior during the interview, and performance on routine hearing tests. Sometimes the symptoms of nonorganic hearing loss are so overt that they are easily recognized, even by nonprofessional personnel. At times, the patient with nonorganic hearing loss is the comic caricature of a hard-of-hearing person, appearing to have no peripheral vision when approached in the waiting room, and so on. The audiologist should be alert for exaggerated hearing postures or extremely heavy and obvious reliance on lipreading. Many patients with problems related to nonorganic hearing loss show no such easily recognized signs.

When a patient is referred to an audiologist with the specification that there is compensation involved, nonorganic hearing loss immediately becomes a prime consideration. Such referrals may be made by the Department of Veterans Affairs, insurance companies, attorneys, or physicians. To be sure, only a small number of such patients show behavior consistent with nonorganic hearing loss. The incidence of nonorganic hearing loss in this group, however, is bound to be higher than in the general population.

Clinical COMMENTARY

It is difficult to estimate what percentage of a clinical population may exhibit nonorganic hearing loss, but surely its occurrence varies depending on the patients served by a particular audiology clinic. It has been estimated that nearly 25 percent of patients seen for evaluation in conjunction with applications for compensation for work-related hearing loss have some involvement with nonorganic hearing loss. As patients of any age can find reason to exhibit a nonorganic hearing loss, astute clinicians are always on the alert for this possibility.

Performance on Routine Hearing Tests

One of the first clues to nonorganic hearing loss is inconsistency on hearing tests. The test-retest reliability of most patients with organic hearing loss is usually quite good, with threshold differences rarely exceeding 5 dB. When audiologists find differences in pure-tone or speech thresholds that exceed this amount, they must conclude that one or both of these measures is incorrect. Sometimes, of course, the cause of such inconsistency is wandering attentiveness, and bringing the matter to the patient's awareness solves the problem. In any case, the patient should be advised of the difficulty, and increased cooperation should be solicited.

One of the most common symptoms of nonorganic hearing loss is incompatibility between the pure-tone average and the speech-recognition threshold (SRT). In audiograms that are generally flat, the agreement should be within 5 to 10 dB. If the audiometric configuration becomes irregular, as in sharply falling high-frequency hearing losses, the SRT may be closer to the two-frequency average, or even at or better than the best of the three speech frequencies. In older patients, or those suffering from abnormalities of the central auditory nervous system, the SRT is sometimes poorer than the pure-tone average. When the SRT is better than the pure-tone average without an explanation such as audiometric configuration, nonorganic hearing loss is a strong possibility.

That the patient with nonorganic hearing loss often shows inconsistencies between thresholds for speech and pure tones is understandable. If, for example, a person were malingering, the objective would be to respond consistently to sounds above threshold, as if they were at threshold. Patients must therefore remember how loud a signal was the last time they heard it so that they can respond when the sound reaches that same loudness again. This is why test-retest differences are often so revealing. Some patients with nonorganic hearing loss have an uncanny ability to replicate their previous responses to speech or pure tones, but they fail in equating the loudness of the two. When spondees and pure tones are presented at the same intensities, the spondees may appear louder, probably because the energy is spread over a range of frequencies.

Performance on other than threshold tests is sometimes helpful in detecting nonorganic hearing loss. Sometimes a patient with nonorganic hearing loss, due to his or her lack of sophistication about audiology, will yield excellent word-recognition scores at 30 dB SL. Patients who choose to pretend to have poor speech recognition may merely count the number of words and remember how many were deliberately missed in order to be consistent.

Determination of acoustic reflex thresholds is discussed in Chapter 7, and the results of this test produced by different kinds of auditory lesions are described in Chapters 9, 10, 11, and 12. Except in cases of cochlear damage, the acoustic reflex threshold is expected to be at least 65 dB above the behavioral threshold. When the reflex threshold is less than 10 dB above the voluntary threshold, nonorganic hearing loss is a probability (Lamb & Peterson, 1967).

Acoustic reflex testing will often turn up evidence of nonorganic hearing loss even when it might not otherwise be suspected. Consider the case shown in Figure 13.1. This patient claims to have no hearing in his left ear and yet he presents with normal acoustic reflex thresholds whenever the reflex-activating signal is presented to his left ear, with either ipsilateral or contralateral stimulation. This, of course, is impossible if the hearing loss shown is genuine.

Another suggestion of nonorganic hearing loss comes from the apparent lack of cross hearing in unilateral cases. Considerable attention is paid in Chapters 4 and 5 to contralateralization of pure tones and speech. When individuals feign a loss of hearing in one ear,

FIGURE 13.1 Theoretical results on immittance tests performed on a patient simulating a total loss of hearing in the left ear with normal hearing in the right ear. The tympanograms are normal for both ears, as are the acoustic reflex thresholds, whether the reflex-activating signal is presented ipsilaterally or contralaterally, an impossible finding.

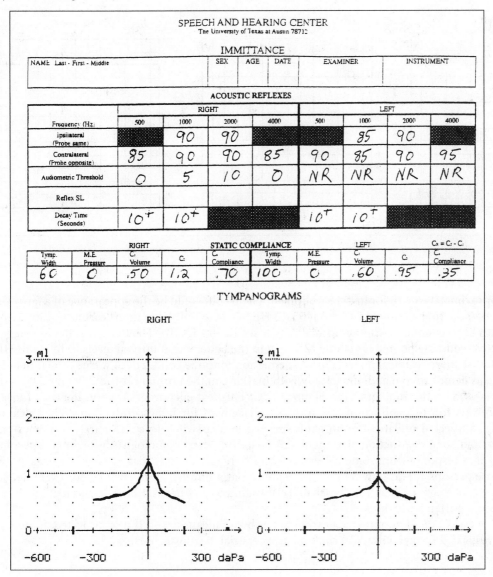

without the knowledge of the phenomenon of cross hearing, they often give responses showing normal hearing in one ear and a profound (or total) loss in the other ear, exceeding the most extreme values of interaural attenuation (see Figure 13.2A). A lack of cross hearing is especially noticeable for mastoid bone-conduction tests, where any interaural attenuation is negligible. In fact, a truly profound loss of hearing in one ear would appear as a unilateral conductive hearing loss. The air-conduction thresholds would be obtained from the non-test ear with about 55 dB lost to interaural attenuation (assuming supra-aural earphones;

FIGURE 13.2 Theoretical test results showing normal hearing in the right ear and (A) a false total loss of hearing in the left ear (no evidence of cross hearing by air conduction or bone conduction); (B) a true total loss of hearing in the left ear showing tones cross-heard in the right ear, giving the appearance of a conductive hearing loss; and (C) a total loss of hearing in the left ear with proper masking in the right ear.

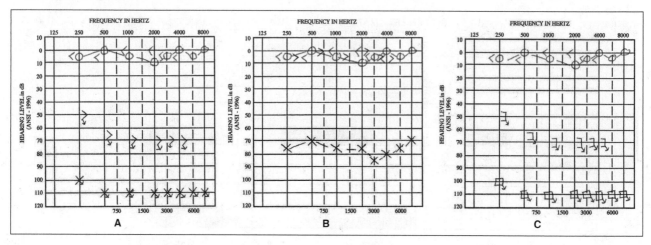

approximately 85 dB for insert earphones). The result would be the appearance of a fairly flat air-conduction audiogram of about 55 dB HL (again, 85 dB HL if insert earphones are used), with bone conduction in the normal range (see Figure 13.2B). The bone-conduction signals delivered to the poorer ear would be heard in the better ear at normal levels (0 to 10 dB HL) because there is almost no interaural attenuation for bone conduction. A true total unilateral loss is demonstrated audiometrically with masking in the normal ear (note the masked symbols used on the audiogram) in Figure 13.2C. This text encourages the routine use of insert receivers for air conduction and forehead placement for bone conduction. When dealing with suspected unilateral nonorganic hearing loss, a switch to supra-aural earphones and mastoid bone-conduction placement may be useful. Many audiologists have noted a peculiar form of response from some patients with nonorganic hearing loss during SRT tests. Often these persons repeat only half of each spondee at a number of intensities; for example, *hot* (for "hot dog") or *ball* (for "baseball"). Why this occurs has not been explained, but it has been reported fairly often.

Suspicion of nonorganic hearing loss is by no means proof. If it is suspected, it must be investigated further with great caution, using special diagnostic tests.

Tests for Nonorganic Hearing Loss

The primary purpose of special tests for nonorganic hearing loss is to provide information about the patient's hearing, even though cooperation may be lacking. Behavioral tests for nonorganic hearing loss may be performed with pure tones or with speech. Some tests may be carried out with the usual diagnostic audiometer, and other tests require special equipment. Unfortunately, many of the tests are merely qualitative; that is, they produce evidence of nonorganic hearing loss, but they do not reveal the patient's true thresholds of hearing. Other tests are quantitative and reveal information about the patient's actual thresholds.

Objective Tests

Nothing could be better suited to the testing of patients with nonorganic hearing loss than procedures that require no voluntary responses. By determining auditory thresholds in such a manner, the very lack of required cooperation would tend to discourage some patients from attempting to malinger. Some tests are available that can be administered with this objective in mind.

Acoustic Reflex Tests

An addition to the many uses already described for acoustic immittance meters in Chapter 7 is a method of estimating hearing sensitivity for patients who are unwilling or unable to cooperate. Following up on some earlier work on differential loudness summation, Jerger, Burney, Mauldin, and Crump (1974) developed what has come to be known as the **sensitivity prediction from the acoustic reflex (SPAR)** test. Margolis (1993) has shown that, with this procedure, hearing losses in excess of 30 dB can be detected with sensitivity and specificity greater than 90 percent.

The SPAR test is based on the fact that acoustic reflex thresholds become lower as the signal bandwidth gets wider. Stated differently, to elicit the reflex, a normal-hearing person requires greater intensity for a pure-tone than for a wide-band noise. The usual difference is about 25 dB. Patients with sensory/neural hearing losses of mild to moderate degree show only a 10 to 20 dB difference, whereas patients with moderately severe losses show less than a 10 dB difference. Of course, patients with severe losses show no acoustic reflex for either stimulus. To estimate the degree of hearing loss, the acoustic reflex thresholds (in dB SPL) at 500, 1,000, and 2,000 Hz are averaged and compared to the threshold for the broadband noise.

Auditory Evoked Potentials

The use of auditory evoked potential (AEP) audiometry, described in Chapter 7, lends itself nicely to examining many difficult-to-test patients, especially those with suspected nonorganic hearing loss. Predicted thresholds obtained through some of these objective procedures have a close correlation with behavioral thresholds, allowing clinicians to discern both the hearing levels as well as the configuration of any existing hearing loss. For a demonstration of patient preparation and recording of the ABR, see the video entitled Auditory Brain Stem Response.

Otoacoustic Emissions

Transient-evoked otoacoustic emissions (TEOAEs), also described in Chapter 7, may be of great value in the detection of nonorganic hearing loss (Musiek, Bornstein, & Rintelmann, 1995). Gollegly, Bornstein, and Musiek (1992) presented six cases in which voluntary thresholds were elevated but TEOAEs were normal. Gollegly (1994) concludes that TEOAEs can serve as a screening test for persons suspected of falsifying audiometric data, although if there is a possibility of a retrocochlear disorder, ABR testing should also be done. OAEs can be used to separate patients with hearing sensitivity better than 20 to 25 dB HL from those with hearing poorer than 30 dB HL. In such testing, TEOAEs are more sensitive for testing at 1000 Hz, while distortion-product OAEs are more sensitive from 4,000 to 6,000 Hz. The two appear equally sensitive for assessment of 2,000 and 3,000 Hz (Gorga et al., 1997; Prieve et al., 1993).

When otoacoustic emissions are normal and retrocochlear pathology is ruled out, a reasonable conclusion to draw is that patients with elevated voluntary thresholds are manifesting behaviors suggesting nonorganic hearing loss. Absence of OAEs does not mean that some exaggeration of auditory threshold is not taking place. OAEs, like some other hearing tests that do not require behavioral responses, have been referred to as **objective audiometry.** These tests may be objective in the sense that patients do not play a voluntary role in stating when they hear a stimulus. Interpretation of responses, however, is at times a very subjective matter. For a demonstration of performance of otoacoustic emissions, see the video entitled Otoacoustic Emissions.

Many behavioral tests for determining nonorganic hearing loss have been developed over the years. Much like a lot of the behavioral site-of-lesion tests discussed in the historical note within Chapter 7, many of these tests have been replaced by the more objective measures just presented. Of the behavioral tests, the **Stenger test** is still widely used clinically because it is highly reliable and easily performed using most clinical audiometers.

The Stenger Test

The Stenger test was designed for use with unilateral hearing losses. This test is based on the Stenger principle; that is, when two tones of the same frequency are introduced simultaneously into both ears, only the louder tone is perceived. The test works best when there is a large difference (at least 25 dB) between the admitted thresholds of the two ears. Using a two-channel audiometer, a single pure-tone source may be split and controlled by two separate attenuators, or tones may be generated by two separate oscillators. If two oscillators are used, the tones must be locked in phase to avoid beats.

The thresholds of each ear for the desired frequencies are obtained first. Then, using one channel of the audiometer, a tone is introduced 10 dB above the threshold of the "better" ear. A response should always be obtained. A tone is then presented 10 dB below the admitted threshold of the "poorer" ear. A response will be absent for one of two possible reasons. The first, obviously, is that the patient does not hear it because it is below threshold. The second is that the patient may be unwilling to respond to a tone that he or she does in fact hear. At this point, both tones are introduced simultaneously, 10 dB above the better-ear threshold reading and 10 dB below the poorer-ear threshold reading.

If patients fail to respond, it is because they hear the tone in the poorer ear, which they do not wish to admit. They will be unaware of the tone in the better ear, owing to the Stenger effect, and so will not respond at all. This is called a positive Stenger. If the patient responds when both ears are stimulated, this is called a negative Stenger and suggests the absence of nonorganic behavior, at least at the frequencies tested.

When positive results are found on the Stenger test, more quantitative information may be obtained. This is done by presenting the tone at 10 dB above the threshold for the better ear and at 0 dB HL in the poorer ear. With successive introductions, the level of the tone in the poorer ear is raised in 5 or 10 dB steps. The patient should always respond because the 10 dB SL tone in the better ear provides clear audibility. If responses cease, the level of the tone in the poorer ear should be noted.

The lowest intensity that produces the Stenger effect is called the **minimum contralateral interference level.** This level may be within 20 dB of the actual threshold of patients with nonorganic hearing loss. Although some clinicians always perform the Stenger test by finding the minimum contralateral interference level, use of the screening procedure described first in this section often saves considerable time when Stenger results are negative.

A negative result on the Stenger test is fairly conclusive evidence that there is no significant nonorganic component in the "poorer" ear. A positive Stenger tells the audiologist that the threshold results obtained in the poorer ear are inaccurate, but it does not reveal the true organic thresholds (although they may be approximated by noting the minimum contralateral interference levels).

The Speech Stenger Test

Sometimes called the modified Stenger, the speech Stenger test may be carried out, using spondaic words, in exactly the same fashion as with pure tones. The principle is unchanged and requires that spondees be presented by a two-channel audiometer. The SRTs are obtained for each ear, using channel 1 for one ear and channel 2 for the other ear. Spondees are then presented 10 dB above the better-ear SRT, 10 dB below the level recorded as SRT of the poorer ear, and finally at these levels simultaneously. Criteria for positive and negative on the speech and pure-tone Stenger tests are identical.

Like the pure-tone Stenger test, the modified version for speech signals often helps to identify the presence of nonorganic hearing loss but may not reveal the precise organic threshold of hearing. The speech Stenger test has the advantage over the pure-tone version in that there is no need for concern over the two tones beating. Determination of the minimum contralateral interference level for spondees may be made to help in estimating the SRT.

The Doerfler-Stewart Test

Historically, one of the first tests for nonorganic hearing loss, the **Doerfler-Stewart test,** capitalized on known test inconsistencies for threshold measures by testing with spondees in the presence of noise, thereby exaggerating patient inconsistencies (Doerfler & Stewart, 1946). This is a confusion test and is rarely used today.

The Lombard Test

The **Lombard test** is based on the familiar phenomenon that people increase their vocal levels when they speak in a background of noise. If a noise is presented to the ears of persons who do not hear the noise, they will, of course, not change the loudness of their voices. If, however, the level of a person's voice goes up as noise is added, it is obvious that the noise is audible to that person. The Lombard test is not a strong test for nonorganic hearing loss and attempts at finding normal values—that is, how many decibels above threshold a noise must be to cause the reflex—have failed.

The Delayed-Speech Feedback Test

People monitor the rate and loudness of their speech through a variety of feedback mechanisms, for example, tactile, proprioceptive, and primarily auditory feedback. After a phoneme is uttered, it is processed through the auditory system, and the next phoneme is cued. Simultaneous feedback is essential for smooth articulation of speech sounds.

If a person's voice is recorded, delayed 0.1 to 0.2 seconds, and played back, this **delayed auditory feedback (DAF)** causes subjects to alter their speech patterns, in some ways creating an effect similar to stuttering. Speakers may slow down, prolong some syllables, increase their loudness, or find it very difficult to speak at all. The creation of delayed feedback audiometry was inevitable as a test for nonorganic hearing loss. Surely a speaker's voice played back with a short delay can have no effect on speech production unless it is heard.

For some, speech changes have been observed as low as 10 dB above the SRT, while others can tolerate delayed-speech feedback at very high sensation levels with no apparent breakdowns in their speech or voice patterns. Possibly due to this variability, these tests have never gained wide popularity among audiologists.

The Pure-Tone Delayed Auditory Feedback (DAF) Test

The principle of delayed auditory feedback has also been applied to pure tones by presenting a brief tone (50 milliseconds) through the patient's earphone 200 milliseconds after the subject taps a silent switch with his or her index finger. The short delay from the tap on the key to the audibility of the tone causes subjects to modify the tapping pattern they are instructed to follow. If the tone is inaudible, tapping behavior continues uninterrupted. Ruhm and Cooper (1962) found that positive results on pure-tone DAF tests occur at sensation levels as low as 5 dB; thus, the examiner may infer that the patient's hearing threshold is no poorer than 10 dB below the DAF threshold. Occasionally patients are seen who cannot or will not tap consistent patterns. In such cases the test cannot be performed.

Of all the tests described so far in this section, pure-tone DAF comes closest to doing what is necessary: identifying the patient's true organic thresholds. However, like delayed auditory feedback with speech, this test, too, has never gained popularity among audiologists.

Variations on Békésy Audiometry Using a Conventional Audiometer

At this time very few clinics perform Békésy audiometry (described briefly in Chapter 7) as a routine procedure (Martin, Champlin, & Chambers, 1998). It was used to identify nonorganic hearing loss when the pulsed-tone thresholds showed poorer hearing than the continuous-tone thresholds (called the Type V pattern) (Jerger & Herer, 1961), a phenomenon that is accentuated when the off-time of the signal is made longer (Hattler, 1970), when the intensity of the signal is decreased rather than increased (Chaiklin, 1990), or when some of these approaches are combined into a Békésy Ascending Descending Gap Evaluation (BADGE) (Hood, Campbell, & Hutton, 1964). This comparison of ascending- (using a continuous tone until audibility is signaled) and descending- (using a pulsed tone until inaudibility is signaled) threshold searches has also been described using a conventional audiometer and works quite well as a qualitative measure of nonorganic hearing loss (Cherry & Ventry, 1976; Harris, 1958; Thelin, 1997; Woodford, Harris, Marquette, Perry, & Barnhart, 1997). Schlauch, Arnce, Lindsay, Sanchez, and Doyle (1998) recommend an ascending procedure for SRT and a descending procedure for pure tones to identify nonorganic hearing loss.

Martin, Martin, and Champlin (2000) developed a procedure called **CON-SOT-LOT,** which stands for "continuous tone, pulsed tone with a standard off-time (50 percent), and a lengthened off-time (80 percent)." The procedure is carried out with an audiometer manually, depressing the interrupter every other pulse to create the lengthened off-time. It is also used in a descending format (beginning well above the patient's admitted threshold) and an ascending format (beginning at a level well below the patient's admitted threshold). All this totals six tests per frequency, but the test runs very quickly and has been found to be very difficult for patients exhibiting nonorganic hearing loss to "beat." There clearly is evidence (Martin & Monro, 1975; Martin & Shipp, 1982; Monro & Martin, 1977) that knowledge about the principles underlying some audiometric measures may assist the patient in "beating" some tests. Some procedures are more resistant to practice or sophistication than are others. Audiologists must consider these factors in working with patients demonstrating nonorganic hearing loss.

The Varying Intensity Story Test

Another way of confusing a patient who may have a nonorganic hearing loss is to administer the **Varying Intensity Story Test (VIST)** (Martin, Champlin, & Marchbanks, 1998). The patient is asked to listen to a story in one ear, parts of which are presented above the admitted threshold (+10 dB SL) and parts below this level (–30 to –50 dB SL). The story is delivered so rapidly that it is difficult for listeners feigning a hearing loss to be certain what information was obtained that should and should not be admitted to. This test requires the use of a two-channel audiometer and a stereo recording of the story.

At the completion of the test, the patient is given a short test. The story in Figure 13.3 has the advantage that the theme changes from a discussion of china (the dishes) to China (the country), when information presented at the softer level is included.

If the patient correctly answers any questions based on information presented below the admitted threshold, the conclusion must be drawn that hearing is no worse than the level at which that information was presented. This test can demonstrate graphically to

FIGURE 13.3 Sample of a Varying Intensity Story Test.

CHINA	
PART I	PART II
PRESENTED ABOVE THRESHOLD	PRESENTED BELOW THRESHOLD
China,	despite overpopulation.
is well known for its delicate beauty	and its rugged terrain.
Many popular styles of	cooking originating in
china exist today.	
Patterns	of beautiful gardens
of flowers and geometric	landscaping
designs are equally common	in many modern Chinese cities.
Hand-painted scenes	of the natural beauty of China
can be found	in many museums
if one knows where to look.	Books about
China owned by your grandmother probably	contain much misinformation, because early 20th century China
is quite different from modern china. The computer age	has arrived and
changed the way complex designs are printed	on all types of textiles.
on modern china.	A new age has dawned.

patients that, if they are deliberately feigning or exaggerating a hearing loss, the examiner is aware of it.

Other Confusion Tests

Often tests are administered that are designed to confuse patients suspected of nonorganic hearing loss in hopes they will abandon this behavior. A series of tones may be introduced above and below the voluntary threshold, and the patient may be asked to count the tones and report the number that was heard (Ross, 1964). This becomes a problem for patients with non-organic hearing loss because they have to remember which tones they are willing to admit to hearing. The same procedure may be used to pulse the tones rapidly from one ear to the other in a unilateral case. The tones should be above the threshold of the "better" ear and below the admitted threshold of the "poorer" ear (Nagel, 1964).

The yes-no method, described by Frank (1976), is often useful in finding pure-tone thresholds for children. The child is instructed to say yes when a tone is heard and no when a tone is not heard. An ascending method is used. Many children falsifying test results will say no coincidentally with tonal presentation below their admitted thresholds. This method is easy and fast and makes life simpler for the audiologist when it works. Naturally, the more sophisticated children are, the less likely they are to be tripped up by such an obvious subterfuge.

Nonorganic hearing loss may be identified by a standardized test for lipreading ability (Utley, 1946). The patient may be seated facing the examiner through the observation window separating the patient room from the control room. Lights in the patient room should be dimmed to minimize glare. The patient wears the audiometer earphones and is given one form of the test, with the intensity set well below admitted threshold but above the level estimated as threshold by the audiologist. A different form of the test is given in identical fashion, but with the microphone switched off. Patients often do considerably better on the test when they hear, possibly because they are eager to prove they are good lipreaders.

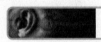

Tinnitus

Tinnitus is a common clinical concern, affecting an estimated 50 million U.S. adults. This topic is covered in detail in other chapters of this text, but it warrants discussion here because it is the Department of Veteran Affairs' most commonly claimed disability, which may at times be reported fictitiously for financial gain.

The process of evaluating tinnitus as a disability is complicated by the fact that its cause is usually, but not necessarily, associated with hearing loss. Additionally, the functional impairment created by tinnitus is difficult to assess. Because no direct tests are known to exist that can objectively substantiate complaints of "ringing" or other head noises, the entire assessment of disability is based on subjective appraisal.

According to a ruling made several years ago, a veteran with a plausible history of military noise exposure who reports "recurrent" tinnitus will most likely receive 10 percent service connection rating for life. The frequency and duration of each episode is not necessarily a factor, and medical causation need not be established. The determining interview with the veteran is usually, but not necessarily, carried out by an audiologist. Because there is no way to truly substantiate the complaint, the veteran usually receives a pension regardless of how often, loud, or distracting the tinnitus is.

When there is an application to the Department of Veterans Affairs for compensation for tinnitus without concurrent hearing loss, detailed service and medical histories are obtained and the complaint is evaluated based on those sources. Compensation has been granted to those veterans without hearing loss, but it is naturally more difficult to obtain. There are no truly useful data on such applications in the private sector.

Further research into the evaluation and compensation for tinnitus is more than warranted. It seems likely that the disability and annoyance factors may frequently exceed the amount of reparation offered. Denial of compensation for those who may be fabricating or exaggerating the complaint must also be investigated.

Management of Patients with Nonorganic Hearing Loss

Openly confronting either an adult or pediatric patient demonstrating nonorganic hearing loss rarely results in improved test validity. After all, cooperation is hardly forthcoming in the presence of hostility. Clinicians may advise the patient that test inconsistencies exist, but they may try to shift the "blame" for this to their own shoulders, using such explanations as "Perhaps I didn't make it clear to you that you are to raise your hand even if the tone is very soft. You've been waiting until the tone is relatively loud before you've signaled. I'm sorry that I didn't make this clearer before, but let's try again." This provides patients with an honorable way out, which they often take.

Silver (1996) provides guidelines for the management of a number of nonorganic conditions, including nonorganic hearing loss. Silver also urges the avoidance of confrontation and labeling but rather the supplying of benign explanations for the behavior. Veniar and Salston (1983) advise that the patient may be told that the inconsistency of test results may be more a matter of poor listening than poor hearing, which may have a better outcome in rehabilitation.

As may be seen from the preceding sections of this chapter, a number of tests for nonorganic hearing loss are at the disposal of the audiologist. In most cases, it is not difficult to uncover nonorganic hearing loss. Many tricks have been used. For example, audiologists may cover their mouths when speaking to patients who profess heavy reliance on lipreading. Patients may be given instructions through the audiometer below their admitted SRTs, such as "Remove the earphones; the test is over." Any movement of the hands toward the receivers tells the audiologist that the patient has heard the instruction and reacted before realizing that it was below his or her admitted threshold.

The greatest problem in dealing with patients with nonorganic hearing loss concerns the determination of the true threshold and how to manage these patients. If all patients with nonorganic hearing loss were liars whose dishonesty is motivated by greed or laziness, perhaps the job would be easier. It is possible, however, that many patients with nonorganic hearing loss may be deeply troubled. As stated earlier, some hearing losses may be entirely feigned, others merely exaggerated, and still others produced because of some emotional difficulty. Peck (2011) notes that the exhibited hearing loss should be viewed as a possible symptom of an underlying psychosocial problem. If the audiologist is able to get the patient to admit true organic thresholds, the underlying causal problem may persist. While adults more often feign hearing loss for financial gain, this is unlikely the motivation for children.

Children who maintain that a physical disorder exists often have a psychological need for the favorable attention that they perceive may attend the disorder, and this need may require investigation before behavioral measures yield success. It is certainly within the audiologist's purview to "screen" for possible psychosocial disturbances in a child's life that may underly nonorganic hearing loss. Often something is disturbing these children at home (e.g., a pending divorce or abuse), at school (e.g., a school bully or pressure for improved academic performance), or in the neighborhood. Directly questioning the child and/or the parent on potential difficulties or disturbances may raise concerns that should be investigated further through referral to the school psychologist. It should be explained to the parent that consultation with the school counselor can help identify the issues that led to the hearing test failure, so the child and the family can address these concerns together. The supportive therapy that can be provided through this referral is often the most efficacious treatment for the child with nonorganic hearing loss (Andaz, Heyworth, & Rowe, 1995). Parents should be encouraged to see their children in these circumstances as resourceful, not deceitful. It is indeed the clever child who can create circumstances that provide some psychological support when confronting significant life stressors (Clark & English, 2004).

Certainly an accurate test of a child's demonstrated hearing loss is the goal of every audiologist. However, accurate results may be more readily attained through conventional means after the potential underlying motivators for the exhibited nonorganic behavior have been addressed. If, in the audiologist's best judgment, hearing is normal, it may be unwise to suggest that hearing loss is viewed as a true possibilty and futher testing should be postponed. The audiologist's referral report to the school counselor should request a "return referral" for additional testing, when the counselor deems appropriate, to document accurate hearing test results (Clark, 2002).

One of the temptations that all professional persons must avoid in working with patients with disabilities is that of making value judgments. Although we may be curious about the psychodynamics of a given situation, we cannot assume the role of psychiatrist with a patient suspected of having a psychogenic hearing loss. We also cannot play prosecutor, no matter how convinced we are that a patient is malingering. Malingering can be proved without question only if the patient admits to it, and that is rarely, if ever, seen.

CHECK YOUR UNDERSTANDING

When nonorganic hearing loss is demonstrated, it may be an unwise practice to draw the audiogram. Too many persons are prone to glancing at the red and blue symbols, with no study of the actual results and what they mean. When suspicious results are observed, it may be better to write "suspected nonorganic hearing loss" across the audiogram, to force anyone reading it to look more carefully at the report that should accompany the results of any hearing evaluation. In writing reports, audiologists should avoid the word *malingering,* but they should not hesitate to use the term *nonorganic hearing loss* if they believe this to be the case. Referral to psychiatrists or psychologists of adult patients exhibiting nonorganic hearng loss are sometimes indicated, but they should be made very carefully. Exactly how a patient should be advised of test results is an individual matter and must be dictated by the experience and philosophies of the audiologist.

ACTIVITIES

EVOLVING CASE STUDY

This chapter concerns special tests for nonorganic hearing loss, a diagnosis that appears to fit Case Study 5. All that is present so far is a history and set of symptoms that appear to indicate that this patient, for whatever reason, is not reporting his ability to hear in an accurate fashion. The very first test tip-off was the lack of a shadow curve for all the threshold tests. If, in fact, the patient truly had no hearing in his left ear, his audiogram would not have appeared like the one in Figure 13.2A; rather, it would have looked like Figure 13.2B, which indicates cross hearing for both air conduction and bone conduction and appears like a conductive hearing loss in the left ear. Because of the possibility of cross hearing, masking would have been carried out, and the results would appear like those shown in Figure 13.2C. Therefore, results like those shown in Figure 13.2A are almost impossible on an organic basis.

Because audiologists cannot read the minds of their patients, the true motivation in this instance cannot be known. An exception would be the highly unlikely possibility that the patient admits that he is malingering, that is, deliberately falsifying test results for external gain (in this case, money). Many of the tests described in this chapter assist in nailing down the diagnosis of nonorganic hearing loss and possibly predicting the patient's true organic hearing thresholds. Before reading the comments below for Case Study 5, try to determine which tests you would use, in their logical order, and what the findings might be, assuming that this is, in fact, a nonorganic hearing loss.

Case Study 5: Nonorganic Hearing Loss

The most popular test for unilateral nonorganic hearing loss is the Stenger test (both the pure-tone and speech versions). These tests would be expected to be positive in this case, and, if the minimum contralateral interference levels were as low as 30 or 40 dB HL, it could be predicted that the patient has normal hearing in his left ear. For the pure-tone test, a number of frequencies should be tested.

A variety of tests are described in Chapter 7 that can be applied to this patient if additional evidence of nonorganic hearing loss is required. Otoacoustic emissions (OAEs) would take a short amount of time and could be carried out during the period allocated for a complete audiometric evaluation. In the presence of a positive Stenger test, if OAEs are normal in both ears, the hearing could be expected to be normal as well. Absent OAEs in the left ear might suggest that the patient is exaggerating a true hearing loss rather than fabricating it. Auditory brain-stem response (ABR) testing is much more time consuming and would probably require rescheduling. If the results are similar for both ears on ABR, normal hearing might be concluded. A mild loss in the left ear is still a possibility.

Counseling patients with nonorganic hearing loss can be difficult and must be approached carefully. This delicate topic will be addressed in the case studies reviewed in Chapter 15.

Summary

Some patients seen in audiology clinics show symptoms of nonorganic hearing loss. They may be malingering, exaggerating hearing losses, or suffering from emotional disorders. There may also be other reasons for test results to be inaccurate. The responsibility of the audiologist is to determine the true organic thresholds of hearing, even if this must be done with less than the full cooperation of the patient.

A number of tests can be performed when nonorganic hearing loss is suspected. Some of them merely confuse patients and provide evidence of nonorganic hearing loss; they might also convince the patients that they must be more cooperative. Other tests actually help determine auditory thresholds.

Audiologists have an obligation to serve patients even when they are uncooperative. The problems of writing reports and counseling are much greater with patients with nonorganic hearing loss than with those showing no evidence of this condition.

REVIEW TABLE 13.1 Summary of Tests for Nonorganic Hearing Loss

Name of Test	Pure-Tone Signal	Speech Signal	Special Equipment Required	Tests for Unilateral Loss	Tests for Bilateral Loss	Estimates Threshold
ABR	X		X	X	X	X
Békésy Audiometry	X		X	X	X	
Confusion tests	X	X		X	X	
CON-SOT-LOT	X			X	X	
DAF—pure tone	X		X	X	X	X
DAF—speech		X	X	X	X	
Doerfler-Stewart		X			X	
Lombard		X			X	
OAE	X		X	X	X	X
SPAR	X		X	X	X	X
Stenger	X	X		X		
TEOAE	X		X	X	X	
VIST		X		X		

Frequently Asked Questions

Q How is the Lombard test performed and why is it given to a patient?

A *The patient is asked to read a short, simple passage several times, and then a noise is presented via earphones. If the patient speaks more loudly, it is assumed that he or she has heard the noise. If the level of the noise is below, at, or only slightly above the patient's admitted threshold, a positive Lombard is implied. One of the many problems with this test is that it fails to quantify the amount, if any, of nonorganic hearing loss.*

Q When should you perform the speech delayed auditory feedback test?

A *This is an older test that is rarely performed today. You must have the capability to perform this test on your audiometer, and many audiometers today are not capable of performing this test. There are many newer, better tests to perform.*

Q What are the strategies patients with nonorganic hearing loss use in attempting to trick an audiologist?

A *They may try to remember the loudness of a signal at which they have responded and wait for this loudness to be repeated before responding. In some cases, they figure out the system that the audiologist is using, like the ASHA method that begins at 30 dB HL and then increases in 10 dB steps. When they realize what the system is, they may simply count the number of presentations before responding to maintain consistency. The obvious solution to this, of course, is to vary the intensities randomly at which stimuli are presented.*

Q What is usually the first clue in recognizing a nonorganic hearing loss?

A *The big tip-off is inconsistency. This may be within the same test or between different tests, such as the relationship between the PTA and the SRT.*

Q What is the lowest intensity that produces the Stenger effect?

A *The minimum contralateral interference level may be as low as 20 dB.*

Suggested Reading

Martin, F. N. (2009). Nonorganic hearing loss. In J. Katz, L. Medwetsky, R. Burkhard, & L. Hood (Eds.), *Handbook of clinical audiology* (6th ed., pp. 699–711). Baltimore, MD: Lippincott Williams and Wilkins.

Peck, J. E. (2011). Pseudohypacusis: False and exaggerated hearing loss. San Diego, CA: Plural Publishing.

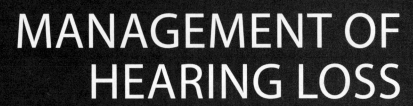

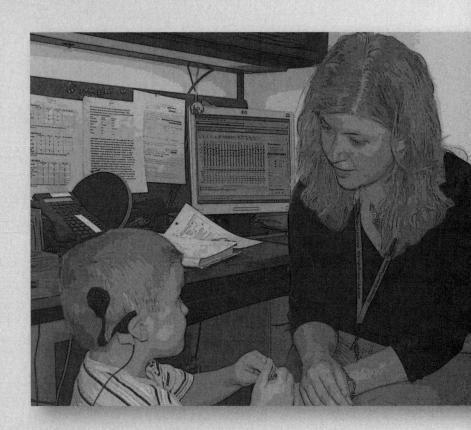

The final part of this book is devoted to audiological management. All previous chapters on hearing disorders and their identification and quantification are of paramount importance to an audiologist's educational preparation and professional responsibilities because the subsequent management of hearing loss rests on the information and skills obtained. However, it is within the realm of the treatment that audiologists provide to their patients where true autonomy can be found. These final two chapters present the thrust of what creates the independent audiology professional. Chapter 14 covers the subject of amplification/sensory systems and how they may be used to improve the communication of people with hearing loss. The closing chapter involves general patient treatment and is concerned with improving the lives of individuals with auditory disorders through specialized training and patient and family counseling.

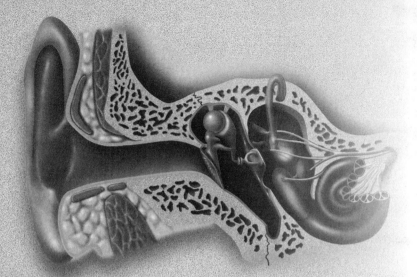

Amplification/Sensory Systems

LEARNING OBJECTIVES

This chapter provides an overview of the evolution of amplification systems and the hearing aid styles and circuit options, including implantable options that are available at the opening of the 21st century. At the completion of this chapter, the reader should be able to

- Describe the differences between analog and digital hearing aids.

- Define the electroacoustic properties of hearing aids.

- Delineate the different styles of hearing aids.

- List the factors to consider in hearing aid selection and verification procedures for both children and adults.

- Recognize when assistive listening and alerting devices designed to augment the benefit derived through traditional amplification or to bring greater awareness of auditory signals may be useful and describe a variety of these devices.

- Describe the types of implantable hearing aids and who might be considered a candidate for implants.

AMPLIFICATION AND SENSORY SYSTEMS, either personal (in the form of hearing aids or implants) or supplemental (in the form of assistive devices such as television amplifiers), comprise a major component of management endeavors for the patient with hearing loss. When audiological treatment is indicated, consideration should be given to amplification in the form of hearing aids. Although it is true that some patients cannot use or do not desire hearing aids, amplification should be considered for all patients with hearing impairment as part of a total rehabilitation program.

The task of the audiologist is to find the amplification/sensory system(s) most appropriate to the patient's needs and capabilities that will provide the greatest possible enhancement of speech understanding. This task becomes more challenging when working with very young children or individuals with multiple handicaps who cannot fully participate in the treatment process, those adult patients who deny the family's perceived need for treatment, or the elderly whose declining mental and/or physical capabilities impede the treatment process.

Hearing Aid Development

Documentation of the historical development of devices to aid human hearing has been most fully chronicled by Berger (1988). The use of devices to collect and amplify sound for those with hearing loss may well be nearly as old as the human race. The earliest reference to sound collectors indicates that animal horns and seashells were employed to gather sound waves and direct them into the external auditory canal. While many other devices were contrived through the years to collect and direct sound energy (see Figure 14.1), it was not until the late 19th century that the first electronic hearing aid was produced. Because of size and weight, early electronic hearing aids often limited their users to the proximity of a table that could support the devices. Although some early carbon hearing aids could be body-worn (see Figure 14.2), it was nearly 40 years after the development of electronic hearing aids before the **vacuum tube** allowed for any significant miniaturization. The vacuum tube also brought a significant increase in power and frequency bandwidth so that electronic amplification became feasible for a larger range of hearing losses than could be reached with the earlier carbon instruments.

The first **transistor,** developed by Bell Telephone Laboratories in 1947, was not initially useful in hearing aid design. However, an early refinement, the germanium junction transistor, found its first commercial use in hearing aids. Because of the junction transistor's smaller size and lower battery voltage requirements, significant miniaturization of hearing aids rapidly followed. Hearing aids have continued to evolve and improve through the use of **integrated circuits,** computer technology, and increased miniaturization. For years, audiologists have found hearing instrumentation to be the most rapidly developing and changing aspect of their clinical practice. The profession can look for this trend to continue.

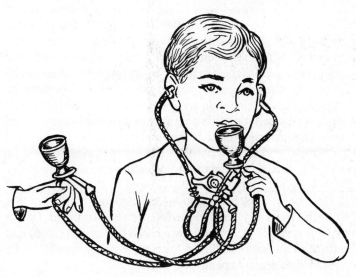

FIGURE 14.1 The Sexton Conversation Tube, an example of a sound collector for hearing enhancement. Presented by Samuel Sexton at the American Otological Society in July 1885. (*Source:* Reproduced with permission from the International Hearing Society.)

FIGURE 14.2 A complete carbon hearing aid consisting of a double carbon microphone for increased power, an earphone-style receiver with headband, and battery, circa 1910. (*Source:* John Hawks, Curator of the Kenneth W. Berger Hearing Aid Museum and Archives, Kent State University.)

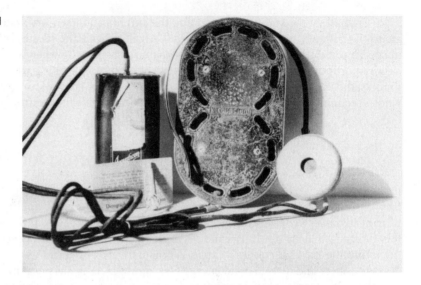

Hearing Aid Circuit Overview

Hearing aids may be thought of as miniature, personalized public-address systems. Sounds that strike the microphone (input transducer) are amplified, transmitted electrically to a miniature loudspeaker (output transducer), and then into the patient's external ear canal. Some hearing aids utilize a bone-conduction vibrator for the output transducer, and others are partially or fully implanted.

Hearing aids are signal processors; that is, they alter the signal input to improve it for the wearer. **Analog hearing aids,** so called because the electrical signals generated are analogous to the sound that comes into the instrument, have involved technology much like the grooves of a phonograph record resemble the sound waves that were used when the record was cut (Pascoe, 1991). Analog technology involves modifying a continuous electrical signal. In today's hearing aid market, analog hearing aids are seldom seen, having been replaced by more sophisticated circuitry capable of providing greater benefits to those with hearing loss.

Completely **digital hearing aids** convert sound waves into numbers that are stored as binary digits (0s and 1s referred to as "bits"), the way a computer stores data. A digital instrument changes the continuous electrical signal by means of an analog-to-digital (A/D) converter into a series of many separate bits, which represent the frequency, intensity, and time patterns of the signal. When a signal is in digital form, advanced processing operations can be carried out with lightning-fast speed. The altered signals are changed back to analog form by a digital-to-analog (D/A) converter. Digital hearing aids are capable of providing improved clarity of signals and enhanced signal-to-noise ratios that are superior to those obtained with more traditional analog instruments. Digital technology has the potential to allow hearing aids to store sounds that enter the instrument and to separate wanted signals (those that will be used) from those that are unwanted (e.g., noise). Digital technologies allow separate amplifier characteristics to be stored in the hearing aid's memory, to be accessed by the wearer during different listening conditions (e.g., hearing in quiet, hearing in noise, listening to music) or that are activated automatically based on the types of sounds in the listener's environment. Digital hearing aid fittings comprise over 90 percent of hearing aids purchased (Kirkwood, 2004) and now approach 100 percent. Despite the superiority of digital instruments, they should not be perceived by clinicians, or represented to patients, as panaceas.

A "hybrid" hearing instrument allows for the digital shaping of the sound response of the hearing instrument, while the actual processing of the signal is through analog technology. Referred to as "programmable" hearing aids, like their digital counterparts, these precursors to digital hearing aids could be coupled to computers and programmed more precisely to an individual's hearing loss configuration and loudness tolerance levels than analog hearing aids. While these instruments once were less expensive than fully digital instruments, they no longer carry this advantage and consequently have been replaced by the newer digital instruments.

In addition to the usual on-off switches and volume controls, even early-style analog hearing aids have internal and external adjustments to modify the amplification obtained in different frequency ranges, albeit not as precisely as their digital counterparts. All hearing aids can be manufactured with **compression** circuitry to reduce loud sounds and keep them within the patient's dynamic range. Because patient loudness discomfort levels are not increased by the amount of sensory/neural hearing loss, this circuitry is a valuable addition for those with loudness recruitment.

Another valuable addition to hearing aid circuitry is the directional microphone, which helps suppress sounds from behind a listener, thereby increasing the signal-to-noise ratio of the desired signal. The advantages of directional microphones for listening to speech in noise is well documented (Amlani, 2001), and this feature is standard on most of today's digital hearing aids.

Some hearing aids also contain electromagnetic coils that, when switched into the circuit, bypass the microphone so that the user can hear more clearly over the telephone. These so-called telecoils have been used for improved telephone communication systems for many years, and today all corded telephones must be compatible with hearing aids, and many cordless phones are as well. Given the early integration of telephone use into the lives of children today, parents should be fully instructed on the use of telecoils. In addition to telephone use, telecoils allow access to a variety of assistive listening devices. As such, Ross (2002) has recommended that this useful circuit be renamed "**audiocoil**."

One of the more revolutionary additions to hearing aid circuit options is the incorporation of Bluetooth technology to allow a wireless interface not only to computer programming software, allowing easier adjustment of amplification characteristics in the clinic, but also connectivity to other Bluetooth-compatible devices such as personal music players, televisions, land-line phones, and cell phones.

Depending on the desires of the patient, or the needs dictated by his or her physical limitations, many of the circuits in some of today's more advanced hearing aids can be set to function automatically. Automatic audiocoils can switch themselves on when they sense a telephone is approaching the ear, and then switch back to the microphone circuit when the phone is removed from the ear. Hearing aids can "listen" to the level of sounds in the environment and automatically activate directional microphones as needed. Many of today's hearing aids are dispensed without a volume control but with compression circuitry that will automatically compensate for changes in the levels of incoming signals. The continued advancements in hearing aid technology may make hearing aids more complicated technically, but they are becoming easier for the consumer to use.

Electroacoustic Characteristics of Hearing Aids

Hearing aids are usually described in terms of their electroacoustic properties, which include **output sound-pressure level (OSPL), acoustic gain, frequency response,** and **distortion.** Until the **Hearing Aid Industry Conference (HAIC)** (1961, 1975), these characteristics were loosely defined, which led to a number of misconceptions. The most recent specifications for hearing aids are published by the American National Standards Institute (ANSI, 2003). Measurements are made on an artificial ear with a 2 cm^3 coupler to accommodate the external receiver of the hearing aid, or to hold the plastic tubing that comes from the receiver. Although the 2 cm^3 coupler measurement does not represent the hearing aid's function in a real ear, it does provide a standardized system for comparing different hearing aids. Most modern audiology clinics utilize a special hearing aid test system (see Figure 14.3) that contains a sound-treated enclosure for the hearing aid, a sweep-frequency audio oscillator and loudspeaker, and a microphone that picks up the signal after amplification by the hearing aid so that a curve can be printed out showing the characteristics of the signal after amplification. With these test boxes, important electroacoustic properties of the hearing aid are measured and a graph is automatically drawn that shows the response of the hearing aid over a frequency range of 125 to 10,000 Hz. For a demonstration of the use of a hearing aid test box, see the video entitled Hearing Aid Test Box Measurements.

Output Sound-Pressure Level

It is obvious that some control must be exercised by the manufacturer over the maximum sound pressure emitted from a hearing aid. If this pressure were unlimited, it could damage the wearer's hearing. The output sound-pressure level (OSPL), previously called the saturation sound-pressure level (SSPL), is the greatest sound pressure that can be produced by a hearing aid. The OSPL is considered one of the most important measurements and is usually made by using an input signal of 90 dB SPL with the hearing aid turned to full volume (OSPL90).

Acoustic Gain

The acoustic gain of a hearing aid is the difference, in decibels, between an input signal and an output signal. The gain (volume) control of the hearing aid is adjusted to its desired position, and a signal of 50 or 60 dB SPL is presented to the microphone. If the output SPL is 100 dB with an input of 60 dB SPL, the acoustic gain is 40 dB. **High-frequency average (HFA)** full-on gain is the average gain at 1000, 1600, and 2500 Hz when the volume control is turned as high as it can go. Although these measurements reflect maximum gain, they do not represent a true

FIGURE 14.3 Hearing aid test system including sound chamber for 2 cm^3 electroacoustic analysis of hearing instruments and probe-microphone measurements. (*Source:* Audioscan.)

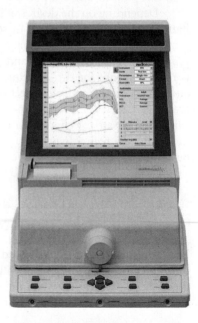

picture of the gain of the instrument for the patient because hearing aids are rarely worn at full-volume settings. The American National Standards Institute (2003) standard is used for measuring acoustic gain below the aid's full-on position. This **reference test gain** allows for a more realistic appraisal of the way hearing aids might perform for a patient, although anatomical differences among users can alter performance. The most accurate means to measure the gain an individual receives is through measures of increased sound-pressure level delivered by the hearing aid as measured at the tympanic membrane with a **probe-tube microphone.**

Frequency Response

The range of frequencies that any sound system can amplify and transmit is limited. In the case of hearing aids, this range is restricted primarily by the transducers (microphone and receiver) and by the earmold configuration. Modern ear-level aids can provide wider frequency response ranges than their predecessors because of advances in technology. The frequency response of a hearing aid is determined by first measuring the reference test gain over a wide frequency range. Figure 14.4 shows a tracing from an in-the-ear hearing aid that provides maximum amplification in the 1500 to 6000 Hz range. To determine the frequency response, a line is drawn parallel with the baseline, which is 20 dB below a level showing the average gain at 1000, 1600, and 2500 Hz. The points of intersection of this line with the response curve may be considered the frequency range of the instrument.

Distortion

When a sound leaving a hearing aid differs in its frequency spectrum from the input signal, **frequency distortion** has taken place. **Amplitude distortion** refers to the differences in the relationships of the amplitudes of the input and output signals.

When sounds of one frequency are increased in amplitude, they may cause the electronic or mechanical portions of an amplifying system to be overstressed. This **harmonic distortion** can be expressed as the percentage of distortion of the input signal. The greater the distortion of a hearing aid, the poorer the quality of the amplified sounds of speech.

Other Hearing Aid Parameters

Modern hearing aid test equipment allows for a number of other checks to be made on the characteristics of hearing aids. Some of these checks include **equivalent input noise level,** battery drain, the performance of telephone induction coils, and the dynamic characteristics of circuitry, which alter the gain of the hearing aid as a function of the input signal (**automatic gain control**). Although definitions and descriptions are not presented here, the interested reader is encouraged to check the suggested reading list at the end of this chapter.

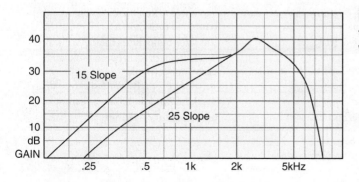

FIGURE 14.4 Frequency response characteristics of a typical in-the-ear hearing aid. Measurements were made with a 2 cm^3 coupler and 60 dB SPL input level.

Clinical COMMENTARY

Children with hearing loss need a high-quality input of oral communication if they are to develop the essential phonological, morphological, lexical, and semantic features of spoken language. Yet for more than three decades, research has consistently demonstrated that more than half of all children with hearing loss attend their classes wearing ineffective hearing aids. Too often no one in the child's educational environment takes the initiative to ensure that a program of daily hearing aid monitoring is completed. Certainly a child should not begin a speech-language therapy session without a brief check of hearing aid function (see Table 14.1). A daily visual and listening inspection of a child's hearing aids can be completed in less than 90 seconds by parents, teachers, or a child's speech-language pathologist (see Figure 14.5). While vitally important, this check should not, however, be construed as a replacement for thorough periodic electroacoustic evaluations and hearing-performance checks.

TABLE 14.1 Common Hearing Aid Problems and Their Solutions

Complaint	Explanation	Solution
Weak sound	Partial obstruction in earmold[†]	Clean earmold.
	Partial obstruction in tubing[†]	Clean/replace tubing.
	Weak battery[*]	Replace with new battery.
Intermittent sound	Broken cord[‡]	Replace cord.
	Weak battery[*]	Replace with new battery.
	Dirty battery contacts	Clean contacts with cotton swab and alcohol.
	Dirty controls	Move switches and controls through all positions to dislodge dirt; roll volume control several times through entire range; spray with contact cleaner.
	Internal	Return aid for servicing.
No sound	Dead battery[*]	Replace with new battery.
	Incorrect battery	Replace with proper battery.
	Battery improperly inserted	Remove battery and replace correctly.
	Obstruction in earmold[†]	Clean earmold.
	Obstruction in tubing[†]	Clean/replace tubing.
	Twisted tubing[†]	Untwist or replace tubing.
	Broken cord[‡]	Replace cord.
	Broken receiver[‡]	Replace receiver.
	Set for telephone coil	Move to microphone position.
	No explanation	Return aid for servicing.
Aid works but is noisy	Acoustic feedback	Check for tight-fitting mold.
		Check connection between mold and receiver or earhook.
		Check for properly inserted earmold.
		Check for crack in tubing or earhook.
	Internal feedback	Return aid for servicing.

[*] *Use a battery tester that places a load on the battery.*

[†] *Body type or CROS (contralateral routing of offside signals) aid only.*

[‡] *Body type or bone-conduction aid only.*

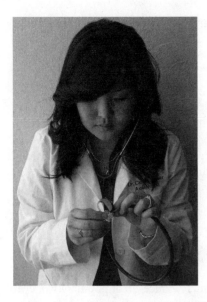

FIGURE 14.5 Visual and listening checks of hearing aids should be routinely conducted before hearing, speech, and language therapy. Together with electroacoustic analysis of a hearing aid's performance, they are integral components of the audiologist's hearing-check procedures. (*Source:* Carissa Weiser, AuD.)

Surprisingly, research has revealed that many elderly adults' hearing aids are also operating at less than peak performance. Clearly speech-language pathologists providing services to adults who wear hearing aids should begin therapy sessions only after a check of hearing aid function. Those with malfunctioning hearing aids should be referred to their audiologists.

Bilateral/Binaural Amplification

A primary goal of any hearing aid fitting is to restore audition to as near normal a state as possible. As such, every attempt should be made to provide binaural hearing, assuming sufficient residual hearing and no contraindications presented by anatomical abnormalities. It should be noted that a bilateral hearing aid fitting does not ensure binaural hearing, especially if significant asymmetries exist between the two ears. However, when aided binaural hearing is achieved, research has documented patient comments that speech is clearer, louder, and less contaminated by background noise. In addition, localization of a sound source is usually enhanced with binaural hearing aids. Evidence suggests that a unilateral hearing aid fitting may result in auditory deprivation effects to the unaided ear (Gelfand & Silman, 1993; Silverman, Silman, Emmer, Schoepflin, & Lutolf, 2006), which lends further credence to bilateral hearing aid fittings. Surveyed audiologists fit nearly 80 percent of their patients with two hearing aids (Strom, 2004). Carter, Noe, and Wilson (2001) report, however, that some people with a preference for monaural fittings that cannot be explained by peripheral auditory findings demonstrated a left-ear deficit on dichotic digit tasks, suggesting a physiologic basis for this preference. In addition, in a small percentage of cases, speech recognition is so poor in one ear that bilateral aids decrease, rather than increase, the intelligibility of speech.

Types of Hearing Aids

Hearing aids come in a variety of shapes, sizes, colors, and types. Among the hearing aids available today are the body-type, eyeglass, behind-the-ear, in-the-ear, in-the-canal, and completely in-the-canal instruments. Fully digital circuitry is available in even the smallest size hearing instruments. For a video illustration of the various types of hearing instruments, their components, and battery insertion, see the video titled Hearing Aids.

Body-Type Hearing Aids

Body-type hearing aids are rarely used today. These instruments contain the microphone, amplifier, circuit modifiers, and battery compartment within a case that may be clipped to the wearer's clothing or worn in a pocket or a special pouch. A cord carries the electrical signals to a receiver, which is coupled to the patient's ear through a custom-fitted earmold (see Figure 14.7). Because instruments are now available that can be worn on the ear and still provide the power previously found only in body-type instruments, the use of body aids has dropped sharply.

Eyeglass Hearing Aids

Hearing aids built into the temple bars of eyeglasses were among the first attempts at head-worn amplification following development of the transistor. The once-great popularity of eyeglass aids has diminished considerably in recent years, largely because of increased interest in in-the-ear (ITE) hearing aids and the dissatisfaction of having to wear two prostheses in one, which creates practical problems when one needs repair or replacement. Today, few manufacturers make or service this style of hearing aid.

Behind-the-Ear Hearing Aids

Hearing aids worn behind the ear (see Figure 14.6A and B) and coupled via a hollow plastic elbow, or ear hook, to a molded plastic insert can be used by patients with mild to profound hearing losses. For some patients and for some degrees of hearing loss, behind-the-ear (BTE) instruments are preferred, but for many years they comprised only approximately 20 percent of hearing aids dispensed. Almost all BTE hearing aids and some receiver-in-canal hearing aids are fit with custom earmolds. BTE hearing aids are used routinely with children because their ears grow rapidly, necessitating frequent replacement of earmolds (see Figure 14.8), which are less costly to fabricate than recasing custom hearing instruments such as in-the-ear and in-the-canal hearing aids. For a demonstration of one procedure for taking custom earmold impressions for hearing aids, see the video titled Earmold Impressions.

Open-Fit Hearing Aids

In recent years, BTE hearing aids have surged to over 70 percent of the hearing aid market. This jump is almost entirely due to the recent emergence of open fit and receiver-in-canal BTE instruments. Open-fit hearing aids are often significantly smaller than traditional BTE instruments and are coupled to the ear with a very thin tubing, which adds to their cosmetic advantage. The open-designed ear tip provides a comfortable fit largely free of what has become known as the occlusion effect, the booming sound many hearing aid wearers complain about when listening to their own voices.

Because the ear canal is left largely open, increasing the likelihood of acoustic feedback, the open-fit style hearing aid's fitting range is limited to mild to moderate hearing losses. Problems with **acoustic feedback** generally become greater as hearing aids decrease in size or as the fitting becomes more open. Acoustic feedback is a whistling sound that is the result of a cycle caused by the amplified sounds leaving the receiver (speaker), reaching the microphone,

FIGURE 14.6 Types of air-conduction hearing aids: (A) BTE hearing aid and (B) as seen on the ear with a thin-tube open fitting; (C) small receiver-in-the-canal hearing aid and (D) as worn; (E) full-shell in-the-ear hearing aid and (F) as worn; (G) in-the-canal hearing aid and (H) as worn; (I) completely-in-the-canal hearing aid and (J) as worn; (K) invisible-in-canal hearing aid and (L) as worn. (*Source:* Starkey Hearing Technologies.)

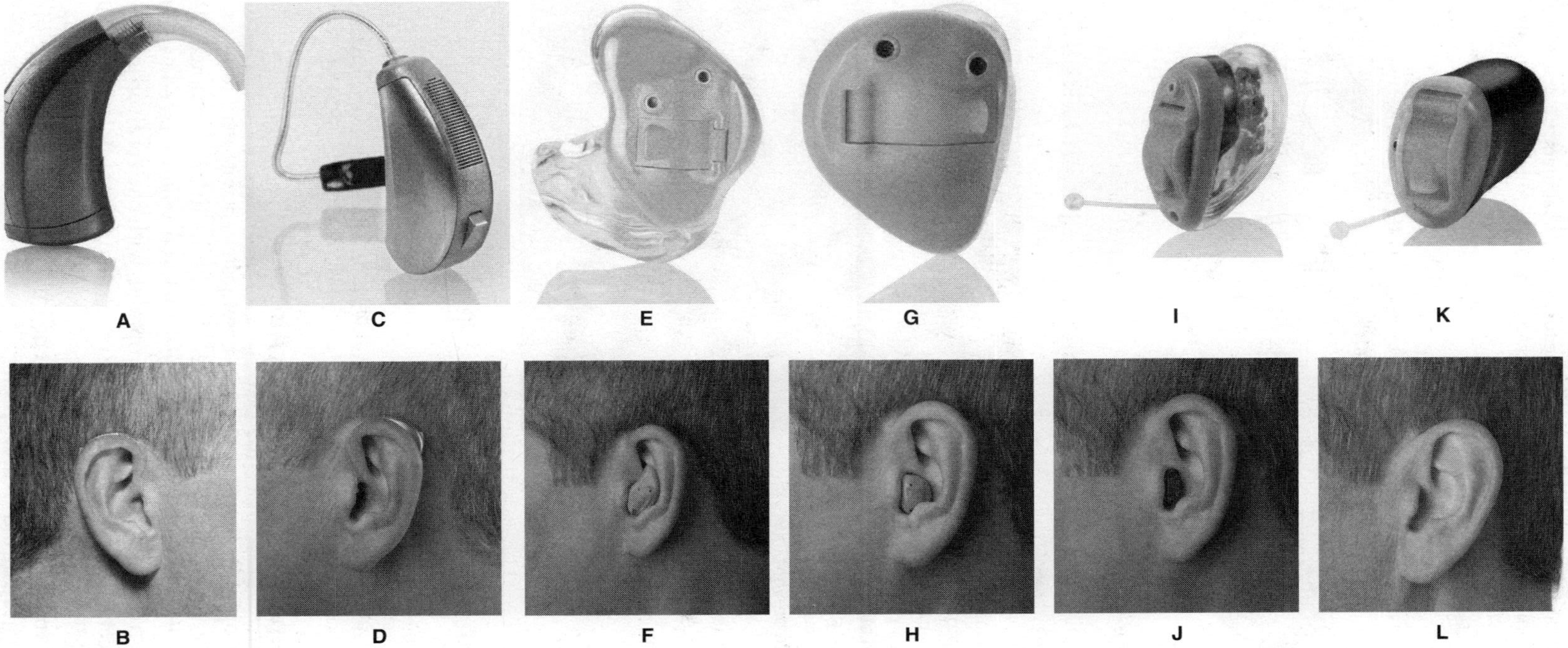

FIGURE 14.7 Five types of earmolds, showing (A) shell type for severe impairment; (B) skeleton; (C) open-bore canal for enhanced high frequencies; (D) minimum contact mold for reduced occlusion effect; (E) micro mold that fits in the canal with a retrieval line attached for removal. (*Source:* Westone Laboratories, Inc.)

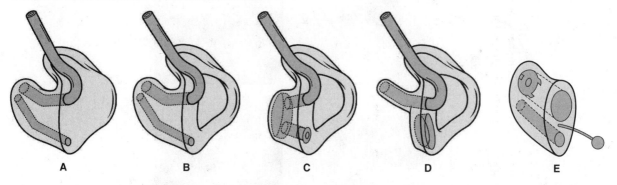

A   B   C   D   E

FIGURE 14.8 Because of the rapid growth of their ears, young children may need new earmolds every three to six months. When making ear impressions for laboratory fabrication of earmolds, the audiologist must place a small cotton or foam block deep into the ear canal to ensure the impression material does not run down to the tympanic membrane. Careful bracing is required to prevent injury if a child unexpectedly moves his or her head. (*Source:* Clark Audiology, LLC.)

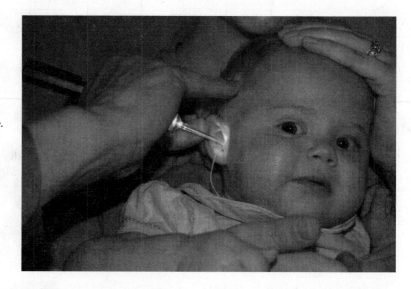

and receiving repeated amplification. Feedback can be substantially managed in many hearing aids with digital circuitry designed with feedback suppression capability.

Receiver in Canal Hearing Aids

Most open-fit hearing aids are now designed with the receiver placed in the ear canal (see Figure 14.6C and D). This placement results in greater fidelity than when sound must travel through a tube. The chance for feedback is further reduced when the receiver is moved further away from the hearing aid microphone with the receiver in canal (RIC) design (also known as receiver-in-the-ear [RITE] hearing aids). When fit with a tightly sealed earpiece in the ear canal (Figure 14.7E), rather than with an open tip, these hearing aids can be fit without feedback and can be used with most degrees of hearing loss, providing a cosmetic advantage that many hearing aid wearers prefer.

In-the-Ear Hearing Aids

First developed in the late 1950s, instruments that are worn entirely in the concha and external auditory canal (see Figure 14.6E and F) with the circuitry built into the earmold itself are still the most prevalent of the hearing aid styles worn within the ear. Originally useful only for mild hearing losses, they can now be used for hearing losses that range from mild to moderately severe because of improved technology.

In-the-Canal Hearing Aids

A major breakthrough in hearing aid design was the development of hearing instruments that fit entirely into the external auditory canal (see Figure 14.6G and H), with only a slight protrusion into the concha. In-the-canal (ITC) aids are somewhat limited in power by their size, but with today's feedback suppression circuits they can be used by some patients with losses in the moderately severe and severe range. This design takes advantage of the natural acoustic properties of the pinna, which are largely ignored by body, eyeglass, ITE, and BTE instruments. The smaller size of the canal hearing aids makes them less useful than the ITE aids for some elderly patients.

Completely-in-the-Canal Hearing Aids

The completely-in-the-canal (CIC) aid (see Figure 14.6I and J) is barely noticeable in many ears when it is inserted deep in the external auditory canal. Ideally designed for mild or moderate hearing losses, the benefits of this instrument go beyond the obvious cosmetic appeal and include relatively easier use with telephones, lessening of wind-noise problems, increase of the usable gain of the instrument (because the amplified sound is closer to the tympanic membrane), and maximization of the contributions to hearing made by the pinna and the concha. Despite its small size and deep fitting within the ear canal, frequently the cosmetic advantage for the CIC instrument is not as great as that for the open-fit style and RIC hearing aids. The smaller size of these instruments requires smaller batteries, which must be considered when working with a patient with reduced manual dexterity. In addition, as with some of the canal hearing aids, coupling to assistive listening devices is not possible. These limitations may explain why these cosmetically advantageous hearing instruments are not as popular as one would expect.

Invisible-in-the-Canal Hearing Aids

The smallest style instrument available is the invisible-in-the-canal (IIC) aid (see Figure 14.6K and L) cannot be fit unless the size of the patient's ear canal will accommodate the electronics of the instrument. However, when size permits this hearing aid cannot be seen without a very close and purposeful inspection of the ear. All of the advantages and disadvantages of the CIC hearing aid would hold true for the IIC as well.

Single-Day-Fit Hearing Aids

Nearly 80 percent of those with hearing loss have yet to seek the treatment they need to improve their hearing. In an attempt to make hearing aids more appealing to this large, underserved population, inexpensive disposable hearing instruments were brought to the market in the 1990s. These instruments have a 40-day use-life (generally the life of the battery) and a price under $100 for a binaural set. These products come with a variety of circuit options for the audiologist to select from and three sizes purported to fit a majority of adult ears.

It was hoped by those who produce these hearing aids, as well as those who dispense them, that they would appeal to the younger demographic of people with hearing loss who often have only mild to moderate hearing loss and an active lifestyle and to those who are looking for an introduction to amplification because they may not be fully convinced that they have a significant hearing problem. While disposable hearing aids have experienced some success in Europe, they were not widely accepted in the United States. The more recently developed receiver-in-the-canal hearing aids (Figure 14.6 C and D) offer the same single-day fitting of the disposable hearing instruments given that they require no impression of the ear and can be dispensed in one office visit, potentially granting it significant market appeal to the baby boomer generation.

CROS Hearing Aids

A patient with an unaidable unilateral hearing loss has a particular kind of listening difficulty, which can include trouble hearing soft speech from the "bad side." Little had been done in the way of amplification for such problems until Harford and Barry (1965) described a specially built instrument called **CROS (contralateral routing of offside signals)**. In this configuration, the microphone is mounted on the side of the impaired ear, and the signal is sent to the amplifier and receiver fitted at the side of the normal-hearing ear. The signal may be routed electrically through wires that are draped behind the head for BTE and ITE aids. The most popular method today is by way of FM transmitters and receivers, eliminating the need for wired connections. The signal presented to the canal of the "good" ear, either through a plastic tube or through a custom earmold, may contain an additional opening to allow unamplified sounds to enter the external ear canal normally. In this way patients hear from the "good" side in the usual fashion, but they also hear sounds from the "bad" side as they are amplified and led to the better ear.

The use of the CROS hearing instrument has expanded beyond its original intended use for unilateral hearing loss. It has been used both monaurally and binaurally (CRIS-CROS) for high-frequency losses and in other difficult cases in which traditional fitting results in acoustic feedback. A **BiCROS hearing aid** configuration allows for implementation of the traditional CROS principle, with the addition of amplification delivered directly to the better-hearing ear when this ear also has some degree of hearing loss. Variations of the CROS system are available for different types of hearing losses (Dillon, 2012).

While the CROS feature can be valuable in eliminating the difficulties of hearing from only one side, difficulties with understanding speech in noise may continue because all sounds are still received unilaterally. Indeed, Kenworthy, Klee, and Tharpe (1990) indicated that the introduction of additional noise into a normal, or near normal, ear might be a detriment to children in a classroom setting. Today, increasing numbers of patients with unilateral deafness consider use of bone-conduction implants, which are discussed later in this chapter.

Bone-Conduction Hearing Aids

Bone-conduction hearing aids are selected for those patients with conductive hearing loss and otological conditions that preclude the use of air-conduction amplification (see Figure 14.9). These conditions may include persistent or recurrent ear drainage or hearing loss resulting from congenital ear canal anomalies. The transducer is a vibrating receiver that is pressed firmly against the mastoid process. As vibration of the skull stimulates both cochleas from a single bone-conduction instrument, true binaural hearing, arising from timing and intensity differences of sounds reaching the two ears, is not attainable. Less than half a percent of all hearing aids prescribed are bone-conduction hearing aids.

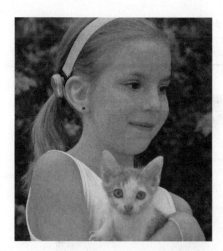

FIGURE 14.9 The vibrating receiver of a soft-band bone-conduction hearing aid sends sound waves to the cochlea through the bone-conduction auditory pathways of the skull. (*Source:* Oticon Medical.)

Implantable Bone-Conduction Devices

There are many people who suffer from conductive hearing losses for whom surgery either has failed to improve their hearing or is not an option. A number of these people have been helped in the past by bone-conduction hearing aids, but these devices are often found to be uncomfortable and/or unsightly. Some patients have shown preference for a device that can be surgically implanted under the skin in the mastoid area. The procedure may be performed as outpatient surgery, using either local or general anesthesia. Several designs of such devices are now available (see Figure 14.10) (Miller & Sammeth, 2008).

For one design, a screw hole is prepared following a surgical incision in the mastoid, which is closed after the instrument is firmly screwed into place. After the incision has healed (about eight weeks), the patient is fitted with the induction device (which fits directly over the implant) and either an at-the-ear or body-worn battery-powered processor. Bone-conduction hearing implants statistically provide better performance than traditional bone-conduction hearing aids (Christensen, Smith-Olinde, Kimberlain, Richter, & Dornhoffer, 2010). In addition, patients report good sound quality, elimination of the acoustic feedback found with traditional hearing aids, and preference for this device over their previously worn hearing aids (Ghossaini, Spitzer, & Borik, 2010; Johnson, Meikle, Vernon, & Schleuning, 1988).

Referring to implantable bone-conduction devices as hearing aids created confusion for patients in the past given that many private insurance carriers and Medicare do not provide coverage for hearing aids but do reimburse for the surgically implanted device known as either an osseointegrated auditory prosthesis, an osseointegrated cochlear stimulator, or simply a bone-anchored hearing implant.

Naturally, because hearing stimulation is by bone conduction, patients must have significant air-bone gaps and reasonably good bone-conduction thresholds in at least one ear. They are often used successfully with bone-conduction pure-tone averages as poor as 45 dB. Due to the successes demonstrated with early bone-anchored hearing implants, the Food and Drug Adminstration (FDA) has approved its use for children as young as 5 years of age, for bilateral implantation, and for unilateral hearing loss (Spitzer, Ghossaini, & Wazen, 2002). In the case of congenital or sudden-onset unilateral deafness following autoimmune inner-ear disease or acoustic neuroma removal, a bone-anchored hearing implant can be placed on the deaf side, where it receives sound and delivers it through the bones of the scull (transcranial routing of signals [TROS]) to the opposite ear's normal-functioning cochlea (Wazen et al., 2003).

There are some caveats for users of bone-anchored hearing implants. For example, the sound processors of these devices are more sensitive to damage from extreme weather conditions than are

FIGURE 14.10 The Cochlear™ BAHA®, an osseointegrated auditory implant (Coclear™ BAHA® BP 100 Bone Conduction System): (A) Bilateral routing of bone-conducted sound; (B) the BAHA attaches to an abutment connected to a titanium screw threaded directly into the mastoid bone, allowing transmission of sound directly via the titanium screw. (*Source:* BAHA® provided courtesy of Cochlear™ Americas, © 2010 Cochlear Americas.)

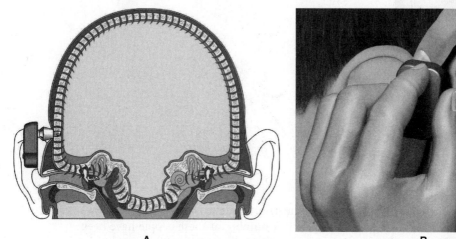
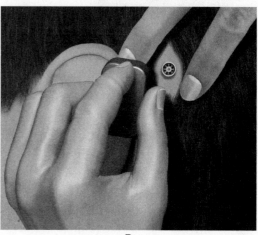

A　　　　　　　　　　　　B

traditional hearing devices, or they can be extracted due to trauma. While the implant itself, and the abutment, can remain in place, patients must have the processor removed before a magnetic-resonance scan can be performed. And just as with any amplification device, users of these instruments must take care around young children to prevent accidental ingestion of batteries.

Middle-Ear Implants

The impetus behind the development of middle-ear implants has been improved fidelity by driving the ossicles and/or cochlea directly without occlusion of the outer ear and reduction of acoustic feedback (because the energy is not transduced back to an acoustic signal). Designed primarily for moderate to severe sensory/neural hearing loss, these devices are increasingly being used with mixed hearing loss as well.

In August 2000, the first middle-ear hearing prosthetic received clearance from the FDA for commercial implantation in the United States for individuals 18 years and older (Food and Drug Adminstration, 2000). These partially implanted devices consist of three components: (1) an external audio processor that transmits sound across the skin to (2) an implanted receiver, which in turn transmits the converted electrical signal to (3) a transducer mounted onto the ossicular chain (see Figure 14.11A and B). Later-developed fully implantable middle-ear hearing prosthetics (Bassim & Fayed, 2010), like partially implanted devices, appeal to some patients because of their reported advantages of improved sound clarity, reduced feedback, and the elimination of the occlusion effect. However, given the cosmetic advantages of some of the newer more conventional hearing aids, the high cost of surgical implantation and the potential surgical side effects, it is unlikely that middle-ear implants would be considered by most patients who have a viable nonsurgical alternative.

Cochlear Implants

Early attempts to stimulate the cortex of the brain electrically to reproduce auditory sensations in people with profound sensory/neural hearing loss were abandoned for a variety of technical reasons, but they led to the development of several systems for electrical stimulation of the

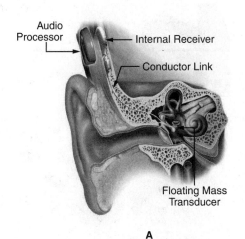

Audio Processor
Internal Receiver
Conductor Link
Floating Mass Transducer

A

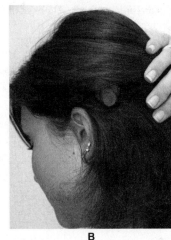

B

FIGURE 14.11 Partial middle-ear implant showing (A) anatomical cross-sectional view of device components and (B) physical appearance of the audio processor as worn. (*Source:* MED-EL Corporation.)

cochlea. Prior to cochlear implants, **vibrotactile aids,** designed on the principle that vibratory patterns can be generated on the skin that are directly related to the acoustic wave that strikes the microphone of the device, met with moderate success for those who could not use conventional amplification.

Studies demonstrate improved sound detection, enhanced perception of intonation, and greater speechreading performance through the use of vibrotactile stimulation (Auer, Bernstein, & Coulter, 1998; Galvin et al., 1991; Plant, 1998). Although less invasive a solution than cochlear implantation, vibrotactile aids fall significantly short of the positive results of cochlear implants and have never enjoyed a wide acceptance and use except when cochlear implantation is not a viable option.

In the absence of viable hair-cell function, the **cochlear implant** (House, 1982) allows for direct stimulation of the auditory nerves (see Figure 14.12). The internal receiver, which is implanted under the skin behind the pinna, consists of wire electrodes and a tiny coil. Up to 22 active electrodes are placed 22 to 24 mm into the scala tympani within the cochlea (see Figure 14.13A). Ground electrodes are placed outside the bony labyrinth, often in the temporalis muscle. A small microphone attached to an earhook feeds electrical impulses to a speech processor housed in a behind-the-ear casing, as in Figure 14.12B, or a body-worn unit similar to a body-style hearing aid. The processor codes the speech information, which is subsequently delivered to a transmitter, which in turn converts it to magnetic impulses that are transmitted to the electrode array (see Figure 14.12). An electrical signal is induced from the magnetic field in the cochlea and flows on to stimulate the auditory nerve.

The external components of the device are not actually fitted to the cochlear implant recipient until four to six weeks after the surgery, when healing is complete. After the external components are in place, the audiologist adjusts the stimulus parameters of the speech processor to transfer the temporal, frequency, and intensity cues of speech signals most effectively to the implanted electrode array. The subsequent program set for the speech processor is called a map. A fully implanted cochlear implant, with no external components, is anticipated to be available within a few years.

Only a small number of adverse effects from cochlear implant surgery have been reported, and many of these have been corrected with revisions in the instruments and surgical procedures. As the cochlear implant device was improved and diagnostic tests were expanded, candidacy for implantation grew to include children with profound congenital hearing losses. Today, the same number of children receive cochlear implants as do adults, often with success

FIGURE 14.12 Example of an ear-level cochlear implant device showing its internal components (Cochlear™ Nucleus® CP512 cochlear implant) and external components (CP810 Sound Processor and CR110 Remote Assistant). (*Source:* Nucleus® 5 photo provided courtesy of Cochlear™ Americas, © 2010 Cochlear Americas.)

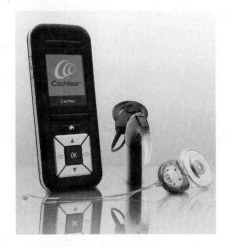

FIGURE 14.13 (A) Implantation of a multielectrode array of a cochlear implant device. (*Source:* Cochlear Americas.) (B) Physical appearance of the cochlear implant processor as worn.

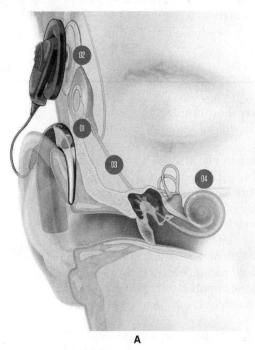

A

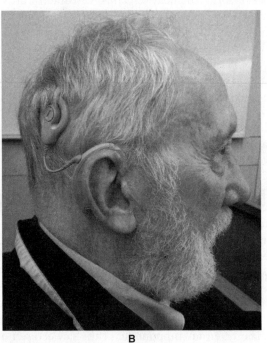

B

that far exceeds that which could have been attained with even the best in traditional amplification. Regardless of how candidacy for cochlear implantation may change as future technology develops, several key questions, which are outlined in Table 14.2, must be addressed.

The degree of success with implantation hinges on a variety of personal and support factors, but generally adults with postlinguistic deafness of shorter duration and children implanted before 2 years of age attain the highest levels of success. A cochlear implant is not a quick fix for any candidate. Adult cochlear implant candidates, as well as parents of children to be implanted, must be guided toward realistic expectations before the surgery itself and must be fully committed to the time and effort that are required for success.

TABLE 14.2 Is a Cochlear Implant the Answer? Questions to Be Addressed

- Is implantation consistent with the patient's medical/health status?
- Is implantation physically feasible (e.g., a viable auditory nerve and a patent internal auditory canal)?
- Will implantation yield greater communication benefit than traditional hearing aids?
- Will patients' psychological status, family dynamics, and educational and rehabilitation settings support successful implantation and the ongoing use of the device?

With the expansion of universal newborn hearing screening, increasing numbers of children at younger ages will be identified as potential implant candidates. Successful cochlear implantation with children depends on coordinated interaction with a team of professionals working in concert with dedicated parents. A cochlear implant team may include an otologic surgeon, the child's pediatrician, a psychologist, an audiologist, a speech-language pathologist, and/or an auditory rehabilitation therapist. The audiologist determines the audiological candidacy of potential implant recipients and is instrumental in the programming ("mapping") of the sound processor. The audiologist and the speech-language pathologist and/or auditory rehabilitation therapist serve as liaisons to the child's educational setting to help ensure that the child's teachers are familiar with the cochlear implant device and to provide needed educational recommendations.

Svirsky, Robbins, Kirk, Pisoni, and Miyamoto (2000) found that children deafened before 3 years of age who receive a cochlear implant and appropriate habilitation maximize their chances of interacting within the hearing world. Indeed, Connor, Craig, Raudenbush, Heavner, and Zwolan (2006) found children implanted before 2.5 years of age had significantly stronger outcomes in consonant-production accuracy and vocabulary compared with age-matched peers who received implants later. Nicholas and Geers (2003) reported much improved personal and social adjustment levels of young cochlear-implant recipients compared with previously reported adjustment problems among deaf children. The only remaining obstacle to pediatric implantation is the ethical considerations presented by those who question if others should make implantation decisions for children who are too young to choose whether they wish to try to live in a hearing world or reside within the Deaf community (Chute & Nevins, 2000; Lane & Bahan, 1998).

Adult implant recipients, as well as parents of pediatric recipients, are usually advised that they may not be able to discriminate among many of the sounds of speech. In spite of this, both objective and subjective outcome measures document the successes of cochlear implantation (Simons-McCandless & Parkin, 1997; Zwolan, Kileny, & Telian, 1997). Although frequency discrimination is far from perfect, voices may be heard at normal conversational levels, providing sound awareness and cues such as rate and rhythm that can assist the listener in speechreading. Many patients have reported that hearing their own voices allows them to monitor their vocal pitch and loudness much more effectively than was possible prior to implantation. A surprising number of patients demonstrate a marked ability to discriminate speech, even over the telephone. A growing number of cochlear implant recipients are also receiving the known benefits of binaural hearing through the appropriate fitting of traditional hearing aid amplification to the nonimplanted ear (Ching, Hill, Dillon, & van Wanrooy, 2004).

The American Board of Audiology has instituted a specialty certification for audiologists working with cochlear implant recipients. It is unfortunate that surveys indicate that large numbers of speech-language pathologists (in some surveys approaching 80 percent) receive no training in their education programs on the evaluation and treatment of children with cochlear implants yet may be required to provide services to these children who are on their caseload (Cosby, Culbertson, Hudson, Bengala, & Joyner, 2009). Clearly this area, just as so many areas in hearing-loss management, requires a commitment from audiologists and speech-language pathologists toward life-long learning through continuing education.

Ongoing audiological management for those with cochlear implants includes programming the implant device parameters and monitoring its performance. For children too young to respond overtly to behavioral measures, performance evaluation can be attained through the electroacoustic measures discussed in Chapter 7, with stimuli delivered to the cochlear implant. In addition to assessment of improved hearing levels, periodic audiological evaluations assess improvement in sound and speech detection and the auditory reception of speech.

As experience with cochlear implants has increased and the design of the instruments has improved, the number of physicians doing implant surgery and the number and variety of recipients have increased. Because of reports in the news media, there is presently considerable interest in cochlear implants, and audiologists may be asked for information about them. It should always be pointed out that the cochlear implant is intended for those patients with hearing impairments so severe that they cannot be helped with other less invasive devices.

Auditory Brain-Stem Implants

Patients with bilateral acoustic neuromas that threaten either life or neurologic function are usually left with a loss of auditory function upon tumor removal. As they have no remaining cochlear nerve to stimulate, cochlear implantation provides no benefit. Advances in neuro-otology permit the cochlea and first-order neurons to be bypassed, permitting direct stimulation of the cochlear nuclei.

Only patients with **neurofibromatosis type 2,** 90 percent of whom exhibit bilateral acoustic neuromas, are eligible for auditory brain-stem implantation (ABI) under protocols set by the U.S. Food and Drug Administration (Hitselberger & Telischi, 1994). However, future applications of ABI may include patients with bilateral temporal bone fractures or bilateral agenesis of the cochlea (Weber, 2002). As with cochlear implantation, the implanted electrode is coupled through a transcutaneous magnetic connector to an external sound processor. While ABI creates an enhanced auditory awareness and improved speechreading performance, communication improvement is not as great as that obtained for cochlear implant recipients, regardless of the extent of auditory rehabilitation received following implantation.

Vibrotactile Instruments

Despite all attempts to take advantage of residual hearing, some patients simply cannot be helped by any of the devices just described. There is clear benefit to the use of instruments that amplify sound, not to augment hearing per se, but to provide tactile stimulation on the surface of the skin. An interest in such stimulation continues because, unlike cochlear implantation, vibrotactile aids are noninvasive and thereby pose less risk to young children than surgery and because some cochleas are congenitally ossified and cannot be implanted.

 # Selecting Hearing Aids for Adults

The selection of appropriate hearing aids and the subsequent acceptance of their use depend on a number of factors, not the least of which is the patient's motivation to follow the audiologist's recommendations. Clearly a comprehensive case history, assessment of the patient's perception of the impact of the loss, and a full diagnostic hearing evaluation are prerequisites to the selection of amplification, but none of these possess a clear predictive value of hearing aid use. A measure of the level of noise that patients are willing to accept when listening to speech may provide a greater indication of hearing aid use than any other of the audiologist's tests (Nabelek, Freyaldenhoven, Tampas, Burchfield, & Muenchen, 2006). This "acceptable noise level" is expressed as the decibel difference between the most comfortable listening level for cold running speech and the maximum background noise level the listener will accept.

In the past, general guidelines were used for determining whether a given patient should try hearing aids. Today audiologists often find such rules confining and lacking in usefulness. An old common rule was to recommend a hearing aid if the average hearing loss at 500, 1,000, and 2,000 Hz exceeded 30 dB in the better-hearing ear. Restriction to this kind of guideline ignores a number of critical factors, such as age, duration of hearing loss, speech-recognition ability, audiometric contour, intelligence, vocation, education, financial resources, physical limitations, and (perhaps most important of all) motivation to use hearing aids.

Before the era of modern middle-ear surgery, most patients wearing hearing aids had conductive hearing losses. Because these patients usually had good word-recognition ability and tolerance for loud sounds, many physicians encouraged them to try hearing aids. However, patients with sensory/neural hearing losses were discouraged from wearing hearing instruments because of their greater difficulties with speech recognition and loudness tolerance. Complaints that the instruments merely amplified the distortion they heard, as well as problems with loudness recruitment, led many clinicians to conclude that patients with sensory/neural hearing loss were often poor risks for amplification. It is unfortunate that this misperception lingers among many physicians, despite the numerous improvements in hearing aid electronics.

With advances in middle-ear surgery, the number of people with conductive hearing loss wearing hearing instruments has decreased, while the number with sensory/neural losses has increased. This latter fact is partly a result of improvements in the instruments and partly because of the influence of rehabilitative audiology. Selecting hearing aids for persons with sensory/neural loss involves much more than simply scrutinizing the audiogram and making a recommendation. In many cases, an adjustment period of several weeks with new hearing instruments can be a determining factor.

Carhart (1946) described a procedure for hearing aid evaluation that was used for many years. This procedure included making measurements in the sound field using a number of different tests, performed both unaided and with a variety of different hearing aids. In addition to doubts about how replicable results with sound-field speech audiometry with hearing aids can be, other problems presented themselves, casting doubt on the validity of the traditional comparative methods. However, the goals for hearing aid selection stated nearly four decades ago by Carhart (1975) still hold true today. These goals dictate that the ideal hearing aid fitting should (1) provide a restoration of adequate sensitivity for speech and environmental sounds too faint to hear without hearing aids; (2) provide a restoration, retention, or acquisition of the clarity (including intelligibility and recognition) of speech and other sounds within ordinary, relatively quiet environments; (3) achieve the same when these sounds occur in noisier environments; and (4) ensure that higher intensity sounds are not amplified to an intolerable level. Today's electronics address these goals more effectively than at any time in the past.

To meet these goals, today's approach to hearing aid fittings is by prescription, followed by some means of verifying the performance of the chosen circuit. A variety of prescription methods are currently employed by audiologists to match, as closely as possible, the acoustic characteristics of the earmold and hearing aid to the acoustic needs of the patient. In addition to more sophisticated electroacoustic circuit modifications than previously available, through venting and special earmold designs low-frequency energy can be de-emphasized for patients with hearing losses that are primarily in the higher frequencies. Mid-frequency energy can be modified with acoustic dampers or filters in the tubing of the earmolds or ear hooks of the aids, and high-frequency energy can be enhanced with bell-shaped tubing or belled receiver openings. Many of the prescriptive calculations done today are completed by computer algorithms that select frequency/gain response characteristics, compression needs, and output limits based on entered threshold information and frequency-specific uncomfortable loudness levels.

Verification and Validation of Hearing Aid Performance for Adults

Audiologists have come to realize that, despite the important measurements made in hard-walled 2 cm^3 couplers, the real ear behaves quite differently. Amplified sound-pressure levels in the human ear are not accurately represented by the artificial cavity. Astute audiologists also recognize that reliance on hearing aid laboratory fitting software calculations, which are based on the dimensions of the average adult human ear, can falsely represent the accuracy of a hearing aid fitting. In fact, more than half of the hearing aids fit in a clinic may vary significantly from prescribed settings when fitting accuracy is based on software calculations with no subsequent verification (Azah & Moore, 2007). These realizations have encouraged the measurement of hearing aid characteristics within the external auditory canal of the patient with tiny probe microphones (see Figure 14.14). Such verification measurements reflect not only the acoustic characteristics of the hearing aid, but also the natural individual resonance of the ear itself and the interactions among these effects (Mueller, Hawkins, & Northern, 1992). Verification with probe-microphone measures are unfortunately not attained by many audiologists, a practice that Palmer (2009) notes is not in keeping with established professional protocols.

When the earmold of a hearing aid is placed into the external ear canal, its first effect is to act like a plug, creating an additional hearing loss and altering the natural resonance of the ear. This is known as the **insertion loss.** Therefore, the first job of the hearing aid is to overcome the hearing loss it has created and the way the natural ear properties have been altered. For these reasons, *in situ* (in position) measurements are extremely valuable in determining important considerations such as the real-ear unaided gain, the real-ear aided gain, and the **insertion gain.** With the programming capabilities of digital hearing aids, it is possible to use probe-tube measurements to tailor the response of the hearing instrument more closely to the sound-pressure needs of the individual. For a demonstration of a probe-tube real-ear measurement system for hearing aids, see the video titled Hearing Aid Real Ear Measurements.

FIGURE 14.14 A soft silicone tube is placed in the external ear canal near the tympanic membrane to obtain probe-microphone (real-ear) measures of the acoustic characteristics of the hearing aid as worn.

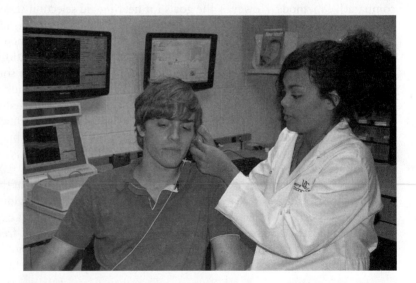

The suitability of amplification cannot be judged solely on the basis of how closely aided thresholds approximate normal threshold levels. It is often impossible to reach normal threshold levels or even a full audibility of the **speech spectrum** with some severe or profound hearing losses because of the constraints of acoustic feedback and loudness tolerance levels associated with some hearing losses (see Table 14.3). Probe-microphone measures of hearing aid gain to assess audibility and hearing aid maximum output to prevent overamplification should be combined with aided sound-field speech-recognition measures as the recommended verification protocol because probe-microphone measures alone do not assess an individual's cognitive processing abilities.

It should be noted that verifying a hearing aid's ability to meet prescribed goals of amplification does not ensure a patient's favorable perception of benefit. Some formal means of validation that the patient's perceived amplification needs have been addressed should be included within any hearing aid fitting process. This may take the form of a pre- and post-fitting administration of a hearing-loss-impact questionnaire or other self-assessment measure. It is unfortunate that many audiologists continue to fail to attain formal verification or validation of their hearing aid fittings.

Clinical COMMENTARY

Before the widespread clinical availability of probe-microphone measures of hearing aid performance, sound-field threshold tests with hearing instruments were common and are still used in some clinics today. Thresholds measured both with and without hearing aids at a number of different frequencies show the **functional gain** at different frequencies. This procedure is fraught with a variety of weaknesses when practiced with adults, weaknesses that are only magnified when attempted with children. Such testing in 5 dB increments at sound levels that do not activate a hearing instrument's compression can give misleading information about the degree of amplification for conversational speech. In lieu of functional gain measures, measured gain values attained through probe-microphone testing may be extrapolated onto the audiogram for a visual representation of hearing aid gain.

TABLE 14.3 Aided Threshold Goals

*Average Hearing Threshold** *(dB HL)* +	*Average Aided Real Ear Gain* =	*Aided Threshold Goal[†] (dB HL)*
Hearing Loss Descriptor[‡]		
–10 to 15	NA	NA
16 to 25	4 to 10	12 to 15
26 to 40	10 to 20	16 to 20
41 to 55	20 to 30	21 to 25
56 to 70	30 to 40	26 to 30
71 to 90	40 to 50	31 to 45
91+	46+	45 to 55

*Average 0.5, 1, and 2 kHz re: ANSI-1989.
[†]Goal based on sensory/neural hearing impairment. Conductive and mixed hearing losses tolerate more gain, resulting in a goal for lower thresholds.
[‡]From Goodman (1965) as modified by Clark (1981).
NA = not applicable.
Source: Clark, 1996.

Selecting Hearing Aids for Children

The general goal of any hearing aid fitting is to provide for reception of soft, moderate, and loud sounds within a variety of environments while maintaining comfortable listening. Attaining this goal with children, especially those who may have a variety of coexisting conditions, presents a true challenge to the pediatric audiologist who must consider the hearing aid fitting within the context of each child's circumstances.

A child who is mature enough to perform behavioral hearing tests and is found to be in need of amplification may be tested by modifying certain adult selection procedures. The absence of receptive language skills, of course, usually precludes the use of speech audiometry in pediatric testing. Sometimes it is realized that a small child needs amplification even though no behavioral audiometric results have been obtained. Digital hearing instruments provide the electroacoustic flexibility so that modifications can be made as further information is obtained about the child's hearing sensitivity.

Clinical COMMENTARY

It is neither necessary nor ethically appropriate to delay a child's hearing aid fitting until full audiometric data have been determined. The earlier the age at which amplification through properly adjusted hearing aids can be provided, along with auditory training and speech-language therapy, the better the chances for development of normal language and intelligible speech and voice. At a minimum, prior to hearing aid fitting, low- and high-frequency, ear-specific hearing threshold data should be attained through auditory-evoked potentials, as discussed in Chapter 7. Behavioral measures may be obtained for older infants and young children through visual reinforcement audiometry and condition play audiometry as discussed in Chapter 7. Those children for whom a full hearing profile has not been determined should spend some time during each communication therapy session being conditioned to play audiometry. No hearing assessment is considered fully complete until behavioral thresholds have been determined.

Verification and Validation of Hearing Aid Performance for Children

Using probe-microphone-assessment procedures commonly employed with adults to verify hearing aid performance fails to verify hearing aid fittings adequately with children. One reason for this is the significant variation in the resonance properties of a child's smaller external ear compared to the average adult's ear, upon which targets are based. If a single aided probe-microphone measure can be attained from a child, the difference between this measure and one obtained through a 2 cm^3 hearing aid analyzer can be determined at discrete frequencies. Knowing the real ear–coupler difference in hearing aid performance can allow all further hearing aid adjustments and measures to be completed through the analyzer without the child's active cooperation. Expected aided performance can then be extrapolated from the measured data.

As with adults, verifying that hearing instruments are performing as desired in a clinical setting is not the same as demonstrating the benefits and limitations of hearing aid use. Toward this end, aided speech-perception measures should be attained at the earliest date. Speech audiometrics that may be used with children are discussed in Chapters 5 and 8. In addition, functional assessment questionnaires can be completed by parents and educators to assess the validity of pediatric fittings and to aid in further remedial planning for children (Anderson, 1989, 2002; Anderson & Smaldino, 2000).

Hearing Aid Acceptance and Orientation

One of the obvious requirements in deriving maximum benefit from pediatric amplification is to get children to wear their hearing instruments. There are several reasons why some children are resistant. They may find their hearing aids physically uncomfortable, acoustically unpleasant, or cosmetically unappealing. Whereas vanity forces many adults to select the least conspicuous instrument, children are often attracted by those that are brightly colored and appealing. Allowing children to participate in the choice of the color of the instrument and earmold, whenever possible, makes them partners, rather than passive participants, in the selection process.

There is no way to stress the importance of providing amplification to children, when indicated, at the earliest possible time. The notion that such action might be "too soon" is simply untrue. Children's acceptance of amplification is critical to the success of rehabilitation, and their enthusiasm toward acceptance varies considerably. The sudden presentation of loud, distorted, and unfamiliar sounds can be frightening to children. They may be confused and annoyed by the earmolds or the hearing aids themselves. For the small child, there is no way for explanations to precede the wearing of hearing aids. The attitudes portrayed by the audiologist, speech-language pathologist, family, and others can make a great and lasting difference in children's attitudes toward amplification. It is important that children not learn to use their hearing aids as instruments of punishment against their elders. Children have been known to pull hearing aids from their ears and throw them to the floor when they become angry with their parents.

Much of the stigma thwarting adult acceptance of wearing hearing aids was reduced by President Ronald Reagan's hearing aid fitting in the early 1980s and President Bill Clinton's hearing aid fitting in 1997. Because of this, along with the continued growth of the older segment of the population and the fact that more people than ever before can now be helped to hear better through corrective amplification, the number of hearing aids dispensed each year is well positioned for future growth. Clearly, hearing aid dispensing is a role for which audiologists in training should be prepared.

Acceptance of amplification is highly dependent on the provision of clear and complete instructions in the proper use and care of the instruments and the expected benefits and limitations of the selected hearing system. Table 14.4 outlines the primary considerations in orienting new users of hearing aids, be they adults or children and their caregivers.

The dynamic nature of hearing instruments and the devices used to adjust them and measure their performance is such that the technology will probably be changed and updated on an almost constant basis in the foreseeable future. Science has truly come to the assistance of the hearing aid user. Nevertheless, it is essential that patients themselves play active roles in the selection and maintenance of their hearing instruments (see Figure 14.15).

TABLE 14.4 Hearing Instrument Orientation Topics for Adult and Pediatric Hearing Aid Users, Family Members, and Educators

- Cleaning hearing aids and guarding against moisture
- Insertion and removal of hearing instruments
- Overnight storage of hearing aids
- Insertion and removal of batteries
- Battery life, toxicity, and storage
- Recommended wearing schedule
- Basic troubleshooting
- Telephone and other HAT (hearing assistance technology) coupling
- Basic hearing aid maintenance
- Hearing aid insurance, loss and damage policies, and loaner hearing aid programs
- Recommended follow-up and monitoring

FIGURE 14.15 A hearing aid vacuum designed for home use to suction cerumen accumulation routinely from the receiver port of a hearing aid. Routine maintenance of hearing aids is integral to their successful use and long-term function. (*Source:* JodiVac, LLC.)

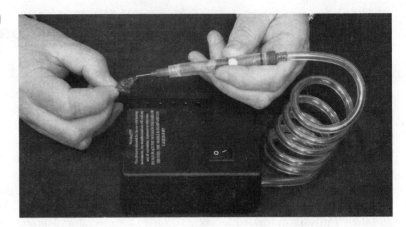

Dispensing Hearing Aids

Until the late 1970s, the bylaws of the American Speech-Language-Hearing Association (ASHA) did not allow its members to dispense hearing aids directly. Such sales were considered unethical because it was felt that the audiologist's objectivity might be compromised if any profit motive were injected into the selection process. The tide of this entire subject has turned. Not only are audiologists in many practice settings dispensing hearing aids directly to patients, but university training programs have been preparing students for this practice for many years.

Under proper conditions, direct dispensing of hearing aids appears to be an ideal procedure. The audiologist must be (1) aware of the characteristics and adjustments of the aids to be dispensed, (2) able to provide simple repairs, (3) capable of taking earmold impressions and modifying earmolds (see Figure 14.16), and (4) able to provide a total audiological treatment program suited to each individual's needs. In addition, direct dispensing provides the unique opportunity for a patient to receive an entire rehabilitation program from one highly trained professional. Before embarking on a hearing aid dispensing program, however, the audiologist must be aware of any pertinent state licensing laws. Many states now permit audiologists to dispense hearing aids without obtaining a second license through the hearing aid dispensers' licensing board.

Two separate professional groups dispense hearing aids in the United States. While some nonaudiologist hearing aid dispensers provide their services admirably, as a group they lack the professional training and expertise of the audiologist. The most efficient and successful means for a patient to procure hearing aids is through a qualified professional, who can:

- Take a comprehensive case history and provide a full diagnostic hearing evaluation to determine the type and degree of any existing hearing loss and the existence of any possible otologic pathology necessitating medical attention.
- Select instrumentation based on an individual's hearing loss, lifestyle, and listening needs.
- Modify the selected instruments' electroacoustic parameters to the most advantageous settings.
- Verify that the final settings address the acoustic needs presented by the hearing loss and determine that the benefit obtained is perceived as a true improvement by the patient.

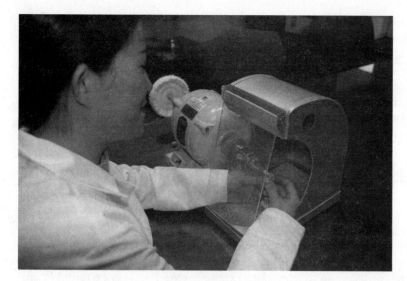

FIGURE 14.16 Earmolds and hearing aids can be ground and buffed when needed for greater physical comfort. The sound opening of the mold or hearing aid can be "belled" or scooped out to enhance high-frequency amplification, and vent openings can be enlarged to decrease the amount of low-frequency amplification.

- Orient the patient fully to the needed care and maintenance of the instruments and the requisite steps toward the adjustment to amplified sound.
- Determine, with the individual and family, what supplemental devices may augment the benefit derived through amplification.
- Provide communication instruction to offset the residual hearing difficulties that are always present even with the most effective hearing aids.

It is unfortunate that consumers can purchase hearing aids through the Internet, bypassing the professional service component of the dispensing process. This approach to hearing healthcare, while appearing more cost effective, deprives many of the full hearing potential they might otherwise have received and runs the risk of failing to obtain treatment for a condition that may require medical attention.

Hearing Assistance Technologies

The inherent limitations of hearing aids often necessitate the use of a variety of technologies, including various **assistive listening devices (ALDs)** and vibratory or visual alerting systems. One of the major disadvantages of wearable hearing aids is the environmental noise between the microphones of the hearing aids and the talker, which creates adverse signal-to-noise ratios and decreased speech intelligibility. The closer the talker is to the listener's hearing aids, the fewer the effects of intervening room noise. In addition, reverberation and other acoustic characteristics of any room may affect important parameters of sound waves as they travel through air. Getting talker and listener close together in space is often difficult in classrooms, as well as in a variety of other listening situations.

Older auditory training units were hard-wired, meaning that the microphone and amplifier were physically connected to receivers worn by the listener. This configuration severely restricted the person speaking to proximity to the microphone and limited the person listening to a fixed location at the receivers. Three types of assistive listening systems commonly used today interface in a variety of ways with personal hearing aids or small earphone receivers for use in classrooms, theaters, hospitals, houses of worship, auditoriums, retirement facilities, libraries, and personal offices and homes. These systems utilize transmitters and receivers that allow freedom of movement for the talker and the listener.

In a frequency modulated (FM) system, the talker wears a small microphone, and signals are transmitted along a radio frequency (RF) carrier wave. Receivers worn by the listener allow the signal to be demodulated and delivered to the user in a variety of ways, including an **induction loop** that is worn around the neck. With a neck-worn induction-loop fitting, the signal is then amplified for the user via the telecoils/audiocoils within the hearing aids. In lieu of the induction neck loop, a wire from the FM receiver unit permits coupling directly to the hearing aids or through earbud inserts or earphones (see Figure 14.17C). Both of these means of coupling the FM receiver to the hearing aids are rapidly being replaced by technological advances that have permitted the miniaturization of the FM receiver, allowing the receivers themselves to be directly coupled to the hearing aids.

Speech may also be delivered directly to hearing aids through infrared systems (IR) that utilize light frequencies invisible to the human eye to carry speech signals to a receiving unit worn by the listener (see Figure 14.17A). The receiving unit transduces the light signal into an auditory signal that may then be amplified to the desired level. Smaller infrared light systems may be used in the home for listening to television. Large-area systems may be found in cinemas, theaters, and houses of worship.

FIGURE 14.17 Examples of a few hearing assistance technologies for use by individuals with hearing impairment: (A) an infrared system for transmission and reception of auditory signals through invisible light frequencies, useful for watching television and attending events in many live theaters and cinemas; (B) amplified cordless phone with caller ID; (C) FM system with microphones in both the transmitter and receiver for increased auditory signals, shown with earphones but also available with a neck loop that interfaces with hearing aid telecoils; (D) captioned telephone with text display used with the relay service; (E) smoke detector system that activates a bed vibrator for vibrotactile alerting; (F) amplified neck loop that picks up a Bluetooth signal from a cell phone and creates an induction signal for the hearing aid telecoil. (*Source:* beyondhearingaids.com.)

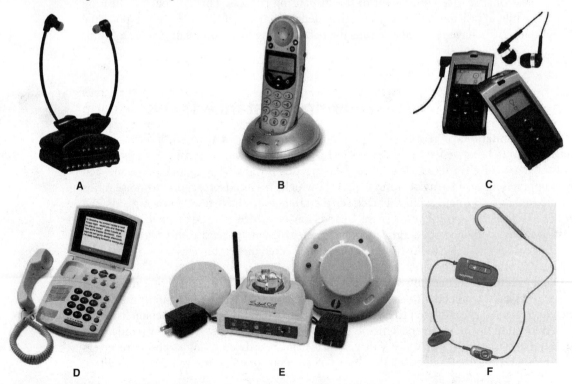

A   B   C

D   E   F

A third system employs the same induction-loop principle used with the neck loop described earlier. In this system, an electromagnetic field is created by a loop of wire around the room. As with the neck loop, the user receives the signal via the telecoils/audiocoils within the hearing aids. Parts of Europe are far ahead of the United States in utilization of induction-loop technology. Overseas it is not uncommon to find banks, groceries, information kiosks, and other venues wired for sound reception through hearing aids' telecoils/audiocoils (Meyers, 2002, 2010). With this technology, hearing aid users standing on an electromagnetic induction pad can switch to their audiocoils to hear speech through their hearing aids while eliminating or greatly reducing all background interference. In 2006, the Gerald R. Ford International Airport in Grand Rapids, Michigan, became the first airport in the United States to utilize this technology. Induction-loop systems are less expensive than either FM or IR systems, although some signal purity is sacrificed through electromagnetic coupling. A joint initiative started in 2010 between the Hearing Loss Association of America and the American Academy of Audiology to "loop America" should bring an increase in the use of induction loops in public places, with a concomitant increase in hearing aid utility. Certainly, different systems may be more appropriate for different purposes (Ross, 2002; Tyler & Schum, 1995), but it clearly is time that audiologists proactively recommend telecoil/audiocoil circuitry for all of their patients.

In classrooms, either FM or IR technology can be coupled to sound-field speakers (see Figure 14.18), providing greater acoustic accessibility of the teacher's instruction for all students in the room. Sound-field amplification must not be construed to be a replacement for a personal FM system. The former typically improves the classroom signal-to-noise ratio by 10 to 20 dB, the latter by as much as 20 to 30 dB. While some children's hearing losses require the greater signal-to-noise ratio provided through a personal FM unit, sound-field technology has proven beneficial for children with fluctuating conductive hearing loss, unilateral hearing impairment, and slight permanent hearing loss (10 to 25 dB HL), as well as those with language, learning, attention, processing, or behavioral problems (Flexer, 1999).

A valuable addition to the array of assistive listening devices is the personal listening system. Many people with hearing impairment may benefit from these less expensive, basic amplification devices that are not custom fit yet are fairly compact in size with large, easy-to-use controls. These devices are especially valuable in nursing homes, where looking after small hearing instruments can be a great inconvenience and where patients often lack the fine motor control required of smaller units. An increasing number of physicians are learning the value of personal-listening systems through audiologists. Confidential patient/physician dialogue is easily restored through these units for patients who have not yet been fitted with appropriate hearing aids (see Figure 14.19).

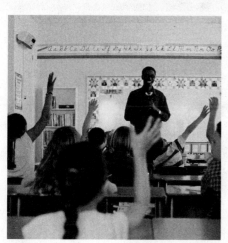

FIGURE 14.18 Classroom signal-to-noise ratios are enhanced as a teacher's voice is picked up by an infrared pendant microphone and transmitted to an IR speaker mounted on the wall to the left. (*Source:* FrontRow.)

FIGURE 14.19 In the absence of hearing aids, a Pocketalker® or similar amplifier to enhance communication may be used to maintain more private conversations between healthcare providers and their patients in compliance with privacy legislation. These devices may also be plugged directly into the television set or other audio-output jacks to provide direct sound to the user's ears, thereby improving the signal-to-noise ratio. (*Source:* Clark Audiology, LLC.)

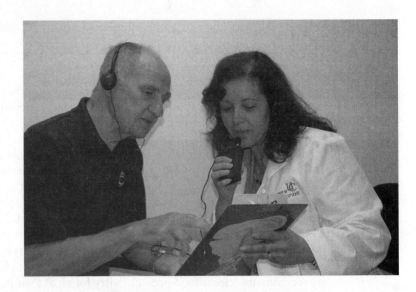

CHECK YOUR UNDERSTANDING

ACTIVITIES

Also included in the general category of hearing assistance technology are signaling or alerting units, which have been called environmental adaptations (Vaugn, Lightfoot, & Teter, 1988) (see, e.g., Figure 14.17E). The first of these devices amplified ringers of telephones and the talker's transmitted voice. More recently developed devices alert individuals through flashing lights or vibrations to the presence of emergency signals such as smoke or fire alarms; crying babies; or mundane but important signals such as timers, doorbells, and alarm clocks. Additional instruments to improve communication on the telephone include telecommunication devices for the deaf (TDDs), also known as text telephones (TTs) or captioned telephones (see Figure 14.17D). All television sets larger than 13 inches sold after 1992 are equipped with telecaptioning decoders to allow printed text to be viewed on the screen. Modern technology and microcircuitry have created instruments that can markedly improve the quality of life for those with a hearing loss.

EVOLVING CASE STUDIES

Chapter 14 is the first of two chapters in this book that deal directly with the audiologist's treatment of hearing loss. The diagnostic evaluations performed by audiologists are designed to afford insight into the etiology of a given hearing loss as well as the consequences of hearing loss on patients' interactions with family and the educational, vocational, and social aspects of life. When a hearing loss is identified that cannot be corrected using medicine or surgery, it becomes the audiologist's mission to restore auditory function as fully as possible.

Chapter 14 has discussed considerations about the selection and use of a variety of amplification options. Several of the six case studies you have been following throughout this text might benefit from amplification. Before reading the case study entries below, ask yourself for each what type and style of amplification would be appropriate, which ear(s) you would fit, the types of circuit options you might consider, and whether any hearing assistance technologies beyond hearing aids would be appropriate.

Case Study 1: Conductive Hearing Loss—Outer-Ear Disorder

Just as this young boy has presented unique challenges within the assessment process, so too, does he present challenges for remediation. Clearly air-conduction hearing aids would be inappropriate for this child given the absence of external ear canals. Given his good bone-conduction hearing levels, the bone-conduction hearing aid he has should work well. The FDA requires a child be at least 5 years old before considering a bone-anchored hearing implant. Before proceeding with a bone-anchored implant, a fairly invasive procedure, one might begin with a noninvasive soft-band bone-conduction device to demonstrate to the child and parents the benefits derived through hearing by bone conduction (see Figure 14.9). This is not necessary for this child as he currently wears a bone-conduction hearing aid. Given that both cochleas are stimulated from a single bone-conduction device, the detriments of auditory deprivation to an unaided ear are not a concern here. However, bilateral hearing restoration is possible for this child through a bilateral implantation and should be considered. Given the lack of cochlear distortion common with sensory/neural hearing loss, this child should do well with amplification. Full orientation stressing safety concerns with bone implants, especially during sports activities, will need to be provided to both the parent and the child.

Given the degree of hearing loss by air conduction (see Figure 9.10), it can be expected that hearing levels with any amplification device will not fully restore hearing to normal levels. As such, some of the classroom instructional modifications would be appropriate, as would exploration of hearing limitations that may be addressed through other hearing assistance technologies.

Case Study 2: Conductive Hearing Loss—Middle-Ear Disorder

One would hope that the conductive loss this patient experiences could be managed successfully through medical intervention. However, if medical intervention is not a possibility or if a significant hearing loss remained following such intervention, the audiologist would need to address the use of amplification with this patient. Air-conduction hearing aids are always superior to bone-conduction hearing aids when their use is possible. However, if the unresolved conductive hearing loss is accompanied by drainage from the ear, or if the pathology is exacerbated when the canal is closed with a hearing aid, special considerations would need to be made. This is unlikely to be the case here because the otologist reported, and your testing confirms, intact tympanic membranes.

Given the mild to moderate nature of this loss (see Figure 4.13), it may be possible to proceed with air-conduction hearing aids using a receiver-in-the canal, over-the-ear style. An open-canal fitting most likely would not be needed because the sensation of occlusion is less likely with a conductive hearing loss and may preclude adequate boost of the signal for the lower frequencies. A less sophisticated digital circuit would probably be appropriate because the more advanced circuits are designed to contend with the reduced sound-processing capabilities of cochlear hearing loss, a difficulty this patient does not have. Conductive hearing losses do not cause the same tolerance problems common to sensory/neural hearing losses, frequently resulting in a patient's desire for higher levels of gain and output. If the canal must remain open, and acoustic feedback cannot be avoided with an open-fit instrument, a bone-conduction hearing aid may be required for this patient. Many patients with a permanent need for bone-conduction amplification report better hearing with an implanted bone-conduction hearing aid. As stated above, given the intact tympanic membranes, these considerations should not be an issue as air-conduction hearing aids should work well.

The use of select hearing assistance technologies (HATs) should be discussed with this patient for times when the hearing aids are not worn or do not fully address the listening limitations. In particular, these technologies may include a vibratory alarm clock, TV amplifier, and an amplified smoke alarm. Additional HATs and the use of further management suggestions, which will be discussed in Chapter 15, are typically not as necessary with patients like the one in this case study, given the degree of loss and the lack of cochlear involvement.

Case Study 3: Sensory/Neural Hearing Loss—Inner-Ear Disorder

You may recall that this 76-year-old male patient has a moderate sensory/neural loss similar to that shown in Figure 4.14 with somewhat reduced speech-recognition abilities that were further compromised when tested at conversational intensities (45 dB HL). The improvement at intensities above conversational levels was a first indication that amplification would benefit this patient. While research suggests that a small number of older adults may do better with monaural amplification, the advantages of a bilateral hearing aid fitting are generally great enough so that two hearing aids would be recommended for this patient.

The needs of a mild to moderate hearing loss can often be met with any style hearing aid. An instrument placed wholly in the ear or canal is often easier to insert than a behind-the-ear instrument if significant arthritis is a complicating factor. Otherwise a discreet receiver-in-the-ear, over-the-ear hearing aid can be a good option because it allows for inclusion of an audiocoil (also known as a telecoil), which will prevent feedback when using the phone and allow connection to the increasing looping options that are becoming available. Because manual dexterity was not found to be a compromising factor, this patient might express a preference for canal-style hearing aids, which should do well. This size hearing aid also allows for an audiocoil. Today's digital hearing aids allow for considerable adjustment to tailor the frequency response to the configuration of the hearing loss. The circuit will provide the compression circuitry requisite for the reduction in the dynamic range expected with a sensory hearing loss.

The sophistication level of the selected circuit depends on an exploration of this patient's listening needs and communication environments, but may include directional microphones to enhance signal-to-noise ratios. Probe-microphone measures to verify the aids' performance while in the ear are a must to ensure a proper fit, as is a measure to assess perceived benefit derived from amplification. Hearing aid acceptance depends directly on this patient's motivation to use hearing aids and the audiologist's ability to convey the expected benefits appropriately.

Given that hearing aids cannot fully restore hearing to normal levels, the audiologist should explore whether any hearing assistance technologies would be beneficial following an initial adjustment with hearing aids. One might expect a significant reduction in difficulties in hearing conversations, the television, and the telephone, but the devices that may have been recommended for the patient with conductive loss in Case Study 1, such as an amplified smoke alarm and a vibratory alarm clock, may be beneficial. In addition, a companion microphone may be beneficial for listening in areas of considerable background noise, as is frequently the case when dining out. This patient should be informed of the availability of large-area hearing assistance technologies in locations such as cinemas and theaters, which is required by the Americans with Disabilities Act. Additional management suggestions to further improve communication will be considered when this case study continues at the end of Chapter 15.

Case Study 4: Sensory/Neural Hearing Loss—Auditory Nerve Disorder

As stated in Chapter 12, patients with test results consistent with a disorder of the auditory nerve must be further evaluated medically. Removal of an acoustic neuroma frequently results in a total loss of hearing, although outcomes can be more favorable but still leave varying degrees of hearing loss, both better and worse than presurgery hearing levels. These tumors are generally slow growing and, depending on the age of the patient, the physician may choose to monitor the hearing instead of proceeding to surgical removal. However, given that this patient is only 36 years old, recommendation for treatment is likely. If the tumor is surgically removed and hearing is lost, and depending on motivation and expressed hearing difficulties, this patient would be a candidate for either a CROS hearing aid, with sound routed from the left side to the right ear, or an osseointegrated auditory implant (see Figure 14.10). If there was a degree of residual hearing remaining that could benefit from direct amplification to the left ear, an air-conduction hearing aid would be an appropriate consideration. The audiologist, in consult with the patient, would select the style and circuit type for the hearing aid. It is possible that further hearing assistance technologies could be beneficial and this should be explored. In adverse listening environments, communication strategies for the patient or the communication partner may be helpful as well.

Case Study 5: Nonorganic Hearing Loss

There is always a possibility that a nonorganic hearing loss has an underlying organic component; that is, an existing hearing loss is being exaggerated. Until the patient is forthcoming with accurate hearing test results, it would be inappropriate to discuss amplification.

Case Study 6: Pediatric Patient

As mentioned when this case study was introduced in Chapter 2, this 3-year-old girl passed her neonatal screening. As with all screening measures, some with a hearing disorder will pass the screening (false negative), just as some with no disorder will be incorrectly identified (false positive). While it is possible that the hospital's neonatal screening failed to identify this child's hearing loss, it is also possible that the loss was of delayed onset. In either event, we can expect that the revelation of the diagnostic findings in Chapters 8 and 11 may have been devastating to the parents. As presented in Chapter 15, an emotional impact of the audiologist's test findings is frequently present whether working with children or adults, but is especially evident when talking with parents.

The counseling skills of audiologists are never so tested as they are when talking with the parents of a newly diagnosed child with a hearing loss. This includes discussions of the loss itself and the rehabilitative measures that need to be pursued if the child is to reach the highest possible potential. Certainly, the topic of hearing aids must be broached as soon as the emotional impact of the news delivered has subsided enough so that information of this nature can be adequately processed. This most probably will not be at the same office visit in which diagnostic findings are presented, although discussion of hearing aids and management in general terms may be touched on briefly.

Given the power levels currently available in ear-level hearing aids, body-level hearing aids are rarely recommended, usually being reserved only for those cases in which delays in neuromuscular development preclude a child from holding his or her head upright. In-the-ear style hearing aids for this young girl would not be appropriate given the degree of loss and the fact that her ears are still growing rapidly, which would require frequent refabrication of the hearing aid shell. The programmability of digital hearing aids allows for circuit modifications as further details of her hearing levels become available. Research has never definitively revealed an advantage to frequency response shape or gain levels that are different from those that would be prescribed for an adult with a similar degree of hearing loss. However, research has demonstrated that children who are actively acquiring speech and language skills should have a greater signal-to-noise ratio than adults. As such, hearing aids with direct audio input capabilities for the use of a personal FM system would be important for this child.

This child was referred by a speech-language pathologist, who would need to ensure the child's enrollment in both individual and group speech and language therapy along with active involvement by the parents. Progress should be closely monitored with an eye toward consideration of cochlear implantation for this child. Additional management considerations will be addressed when we visit this case study for the last time at the end of Chapter 15.

Summary

Devices designed to augment sound transmission to aid human hearing have evolved from simple sound collectors to instruments that employ some of today's most sophisticated miniature electronics. The styles and circuit options available are designed for both the hearing needs and cosmetic concerns of an ever-growing population of persons with hearing loss.

The audiologist's selection of appropriate amplification must always be followed by some means to verify that the performance received closely approximates the performance expected. The electroacoustic parameters of all hearing aids must meet certain standard specifications, and their performance should be monitored to ensure that adherence to standards is maintained.

As discussed further in the next chapter, the recommendation and fitting of appropriately selected hearing instruments are only the first steps within the complete hearing (re) habilitation services provided to patients. When the audiologist's treatment efforts with patients reveal the need for greater sound augmentation than hearing aids alone can provide, the appropriate recommendation and instruction for assistive listening/alerting devices should be given. To offer less than the full array of options available to those with hearing loss falls short of optimum patient care.

Frequently Asked Questions

Q Is a hearing aid available that attenuates random noise from the background and amplifies speech only?

A *Research has been devoted for many years to noise-suppression circuitry in hearing aids. While these devices are more useful than they have been in the past, it is unreasonable to hope that all background noise will vanish while wearing hearing aids.*

Q Why does sound through hearing aids seem different?

A *The range of frequencies amplified by hearing aids is limited, cutting off the higher and lower ranges. In addition, even the best hearing aids have some distortion, which leads to loss of the naturalness of speech.*

Q What are the known side effects of cochlear implants?

A *We assume that you are referring to the surgery itself. As in any surgery there is the risk of infection. There have also been reports of meningitis following this surgery.*

Q Are there many organizations that help families that cannot afford hearing aids?

A *There are many such private organizations like the SERTOMA Club. In addition, assistance can be found in many state departments of health.*

Q Are all current hearing aids digital?

A *Some of the less sophisticated digital hearing aids have come down considerably in cost. Today most hearing aids are digital, with many manufacturers eliminating their analog line of products.*

Q What is the best way to reduce acoustic feedback?

A *Tightly fitting earmolds are the first step. When the most commonly used instruments were of the body type, moving the receiver as far as possible from the microphone was usually recommended when feedback was a problem. Some behind-the-ear instruments follow this logic by placing the receiver of the hearing aid into the ear canal. Many digital hearing aids also have feedback suppression circuitry.*

Q Can audiologists dispense hearing aids?

A *More clinical audiologists are now dispensing hearing aids than those individuals who are not so licensed. Many states have eliminated the need for audiologists to hold two licenses, one as an audiologist and one as a hearing-aid dispenser, with the audiology license covering all the professional activities of the audiologist. This has been a trend that will doubtless continue.*

Q What is an FM system used for?

A *FM systems are used primarily in theaters, auditoriums, and classrooms to improve the signal-to-noise ratio for the listener.*

Q What are the most common reasons for people not wanting to wear hearing aids?

A *Although hearing aids have improved, some people have such difficulty with the tolerance of loudness and have so much distortion in their ears that they believe hearing aids simply do not help enough to justify their use. Many of these individuals could be helped with proper motivation and treatment by an audiologist. There will always be problems for people who shun what they believe to be a stigma attached to wearing hearing aids and, while public education may help with this, vanity is something that will never completely disappear.*

Q What is the difference between analog and digital hearing aids?

A *Digital hearing aids allow for an analysis of the input signal prior to amplification to help decrease the intensity of unwanted sounds. Digital hearing aids also allow for greater manipulation of the signal to match the amplification requirements of a hearing loss more closely.*

Q What are the advantages and disadvantages of middle-ear implanted hearing aids?

A *Any surgery has the potential for complications. This and the cost of a surgical procedure are the disadvantages of middle-ear implants. The advantages are the reduction of acoustic feedback and the elimination of the occlusion effect.*

Q Who is eligible for an auditory brain-stem implantation?

A *Following acoustic neuroma removal, the patient does not have a cochlear nerve for stimulation with a cochlear implant. This patient can benefit from auditory brain-stem implantation.*

Q What are vibrotactile aids?

A *Vibrotactile aids can provide vibratory tactile stimulation of the patterns of speech through small vibrators worn on the chest, neck, wrist, or back of the hand.*

Q What are the different types of assistive listening devices?

A *Assistive listening devices can be divided into those that improve signal-to-noise ratio (such as infrared, FM, and induction loop) and those that alert persons to auditory stimuli through either vibration or light.*

Q Who are the best candidates for cochlear implants?

A *Those persons who cannot receive adequate auditory stimulation for speech reception through acoustic hearing aids are candidates for cochlear implantation. Children younger than 18 to 24 months typically are not implanted. Adults with prelinguistic hearing loss are rarely good candidates for cochlear implantation. Advocates of Deaf culture believe cochlear implants deprive an individual of her or his birthright to a place within the Deaf community.*

Q Has the increase in contact lenses and eye surgery contributed to the shift away from eyeglass hearing aids?

A *Not really. When electronic hearing aids were first developed, the goal was always to make them head worn. It was the miniaturization of hearing-aid design following development of the transistor that allowed this to be accomplished in housing separate from the glasses. In addition, the disadvantages encountered when repair needs arise in a device that is shared with another sensory aid such as eyeglasses led to the shift away from eyeglass hearing aids.*

Suggested Reading

Dillon, H. (2012). *Hearing aids (2nd ed.)* Turramurra, Australia: Boomerang Press.

Thibodeau, L. M. (2014). Hearing assistance technology systems as part of a comprehensive audiologic rehabilitation program. In J. J. Monatano & J. B. Spitzer (eds.), *Adult audiologic rehabilitation (2nd ed.)* (pp. 349–374. San Diego: Plural Publishing.

Zwolan, T. A. (2010). Cochlear implants. In J. Katz, L. Medwetsky, R. Burkard, & L. Hood (Eds.), *Handbook of clinical audiology* (pp. 912–933). Philadelphia, PA: Lippincott Williams and Wilkins.

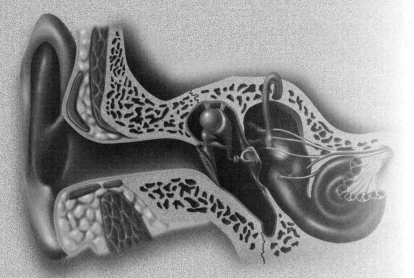

CHAPTER **15**

Audiological
Treatment

LEARNING OBJECTIVES

This chapter is designed to introduce the reader to various aspects of patient management, such as taking histories, counseling, writing reports, cooperating with other professionals, and providing audiological treatment. Less emphasis is placed on precise methodologies here than in previous chapters; the intention is to give the reader a brief overview of several different aspects of audiology not previously detailed in this text. At the competition of this chapter, the reader should be able to

- Obtain a proper case history, attending to both the possible pathology underpinnings of hearing loss and the communication impact of the loss.

- Determine when referral to other specialists is necessary to ensure proper hearing loss management.

- Recognize the different styles for writing reports to address the concerns pertinent to a variety of professionals who may work with a patient who has hearing loss.

- Recognize some of the factors that can affect, positively and negatively, the counseling given to patients and their families.

- Discuss the principles of hearing-loss management for both children and adults.

- Describe educational options for children with hearing loss.

- Demonstrate an understanding of multicultural issues and their impact on patient care.

C LINICAL AUDIOLOGISTS have responsibilities that transcend diagnosis. When a medical condition causes or contributes to a patient's hearing problem, proper otologic consultation must be sought. In the absence of medical treatment, or after its completion, the audiologist is the logical person to take charge of the patient's total audiological management program. If it is decided that hearing aids are indicated for a patient, the audiologist should select and fit the appropriate instruments and provide the needed orientation and follow-up care to ensure optimum efficiency in their use.

The American Speech-Language-Hearing Association (ASHA) scope of practice has long recognized that both speech-language pathologists and audiologists provide aural rehabilitation to children and adults. Frequently, and especially with children, rehabilitation efforts achieve their highest levels of success when audiologists and speech-language pathologists work in concert for the communication enhancement of those with hearing loss.

All preceding materials in this text have led to what must be summarized briefly in the following pages. An understanding of normal and abnormal auditory functioning, together with diagnostic procedures, is without merit unless it culminates in activities that improve the lives of persons with hearing impairment.

Patient Histories

Proper documentation of a patient's history may be as important as the audiometric examination. The manner in which the history is recorded may follow one of several formats, ranging from informality to close adherence to a printed form. Some audiologists prefer to ask only questions that appear to relate to the patient's particular complaints and jot their remarks down informally. This approach requires much skill and experience and allows for possible omission of essential questions.

Some case history forms are lengthy and contain more items than are essential for gathering data pertinent to a particular hearing problem. Short forms like those in Figures 15.1 and 15.2 have proven useful in the majority of cases. Although in some busy audiology centers case histories are recorded by ancillary personnel (technicians or clerks) or are mailed to patients for completion before evaluation, it is best for the audiologist to ask the questions or at least to review the questionnaire with the respondent or caregiver.

Any case history form must provide space for a statement of the problem, including why the services of the audiologist are sought. It is helpful to know the patient's own attitude about the appointment. Knowing the reason for the visit to the clinic can provide powerful insights before the rest of the history has been completed or the first test has been administered. Information about the duration and degree of hearing loss should be gleaned, along with family history of ear disease or hearing impairment, noise exposure, or trauma to the ear or head. Reports of vertigo, tinnitus, past surgery related to the ear, previous hearing tests, and so on, are most important. History of experience with hearing aids is valuable. Developmental histories of children should be obtained along with any childhood illnesses or accidents and any regressions in development associated with them.

The manner in which questions are answered may be revealing. Often a patient or caregiver hesitates in answering some questions, which may suggest that not too much credence should be given to the answers. This hesitancy sometimes reflects disagreement among family members. However, the fact that questions are answered rapidly, and with apparent self-assurance, does not, in itself, ensure validity. People who have repeatedly answered the same types of questions, perhaps posed by different specialists, become practiced at responding

FIGURE 15.1 Sample of a form for recording a pediatric history of hearing loss and related conditions.

PEDIATRIC CASE HISTORY

File # _____ Date: _____

Last Name_____ First Name_____ Date of Birth _____
Sex ( )M ( )F   Parent / Guardian_____

How did you hear of us? _____

GENERAL MEDICAL INFORMATION
What is the name of your child's pediatrician? _____
Were there any pregnancy complications (Illness, accident, medications)? _____
_____
Were there any birth complications (Low birth weight, jaundice, anoxia, other) ? _____
_____
Has your child had a vision evaluation? (and where)_____
Has your child had any serious illness (Mumps, rubella, cytomegalovirus, other)?_____
Is there a history of ear infection? _____
Has your child had ear surgery or injury to the ear ?_____
Does your child have any allergies? _____
Is your child currently taking any medications? _____
Other relevant medical information:_____

HEARING LOSS AND DEVELOPMENTAL INFORMATION
Is there a previously documented hearing loss (where tested and what age)? _____
_____
Is there a family history of childhood hearing loss? _____
Is your child aware of environmental sounds and other's speech? _____
Is your child's speech and language age appropriate? _____
Is your child currently in speech therapy (and where) ?_____
Is your child's motor development age appropriate? _____
Does your child have any known behavioral disorders or coexisting handicaps ? _____
_____

OTHER INFORMATION
What is the sex and ages of siblings?_____
What is your child's school, grade, and teacher? _____
How would you rate performance in school? _____
Does your child currently wear hearing aids?_____
How does your child generally communicate (sign language, speech, gestures)? _____
_____

RELEASE OF INFORMATION

I give permission for release of reports, test results, and recommendations to or from the pediatrician, the referral source, or others as specified.

_____   _____
Signature (Relation to child)   Date

FIGURE 15.2 Sample of a form for recording an adult history of hearing loss and related conditions.

ADULT CASE HISTORY

File No. _____ Date: _____

Last Name: _____ First: _____ Sex ( )M ( )F Date of Birth _____

How did you hear of us? _____

GENERAL MEDICAL INFORMATION

Who is your primary care physician? _____
Do you take any of the following types of medication (circle)? : blood pressure / heart disease / arthritis / daily aspirin / blood thinning / other _____
Do you have any vision disorders? _____
Do you have a chronic or serious illness? _____
Do you have any allergies? _____
Other relevant medical information: _____

HEARING HISTORY

Y N   Do you have a known hearing loss? (Rt ear) (Lt ear) (Both) _____
Y N   Is your hearing loss stable? _____
Y N   Is there a family history of hearing loss? _____
Y N   Have you had a previous hearing evaluation and where? _____
Y N   Do you now, or have you ever, worn hearing aids? _____
Y N   Do you have noises in your ears (Rt ear) (Lt ear) (Both)? _____
Y N   Do you have vertigo or dizziness? _____
Y N   Have you ever had recreational, military, or employment noise exposure ? _____
Y N   Do you have pain, discomfort, or drainage in the ear ? _____
Y N   Do you have a history of ear infection? _____
Y N   Have you had ear surgery ? _____
Y N   Have you had an injury to your ears? _____
Other _____

LISTENING SITUATIONS

Please rank the top 4 listening situations in which it is important for you to hear well:

___ conversation with 1 person	___ telephone	___ television	___ in the car
___ in small groups	___ in large groups	___ restaurants	___ movie / theatre
___ at religious services	___ in meetings	___ work places	___ outdoors
___ listening to music			

RELEASE OF INFORMATION

I give permission for release of reports, test results, and recommendations to or from my family physician, the referral source, or others as specified.

_____   _____
Signature   Date

and may find themselves answering questions incorrectly with aplomb. The clinician should try to elicit objective responses as much as possible. Statements of a diagnostic nature, such as "I have Ménière's disease," or "My child has a conductive hearing loss," should be investigated thoroughly because they may represent the respondent's incorrect reflection of a previous diagnosis.

A variety of questionnaires exist to provide information on patients' own perceptions of the impact of their hearing loss within various areas of their lives (Alpiner & McCarthy, 2000; Geier, 1997). These questionnaires frequently have companion forms for the spouse or significant other to complete so that comparisons of perceptions are revealed. These self-assessment measures can be an invaluable adjunct to case histories, serving to clarify the impact of a given hearing loss and aiding in the subsequent recommendations for audiological treatment.

 # Referral to Other Specialists

Audiologists may refer their patients to other specialists for a variety of reasons. They may feel that additional help is needed for either diagnosis or treatment and may require the talents of professionals such as otologists, speech-language pathologists, psychologists, genetic counselors, and educators. When referring, a proper report should be sent to provide as much pertinent information as possible. In accordance with the Health Insurance Portability and Accountability Act (HIPAA) (1996), it is mandatory that the patient or guardian signs a release form authorizing the audiologist to provide such information to interested parties. The form, properly filed, may prevent possible legal difficulties.

An audiogram or other data obtained on hearing tests should not be forwarded without qualifying remarks. The audiologist should not suppose that the recipient of test results will totally understand and interpret them correctly. At the other extreme, the audiologist should not include long, verbose reports conveying details of each and every test. Professional time is valuable and should not be occupied in reading unnecessary verbiage. In fact, it is probable that long reports are either not read at all or are only scanned for the pertinent facts.

Each report must be written specifically for the type of specialist to whom it is sent. Audiologists should realize that reports sent about the same patient to an otologist and to a speech-language pathologist might differ greatly in the type of information included and in the manner in which statements are made. In addition, two otologists may differ in the type of information or degree of interpretation they desire. As audiologists get to know particular referral sources, they develop an awareness of how reports should be written for each one. Some may require very formal documents, whereas others prefer informal synopses. A commonly used format for report writing provides an easy outline for comprehensive reports as well as more cursory notes (see Table 15.1).

TABLE 15.1 The SOAP Format for Report Writing

S	(subjective): Relevant complaints/reason for visit; subjective observations and family, medical, and otologic history.
O	(objective): Tests or procedures completed; findings and test conditions.
A	(assessment: A summary of the "S" and "O" to provide a diagnostic statement and the implications of the findings.
P	(plan): Appropriate recommendations; follow-up.

Briefly, the organization of a report sent to a professional person might be as follows:

- *First paragraph.* Identification of the patient (name, age, sex, short statement of history); the reason for referral.
- *Second paragraph.* Statement of the type and degree of hearing loss; reference to results that require special attention from the audiometric worksheets and tympanograms; interpretation of test results where needed; implications for communication difficulties.
- *Third paragraph.* Specific treatment plans or recommendations, such as hearing aids; speech, language, or hearing therapy; return for follow-up; avoidance of noise exposure; and so on.

Audiology clinics and audiologists are often judged by the reports they send to other professional workers. Messy forms and poorly written or carelessly proofread reports may cause the recipient to deduce that the audiological examination was also poorly done. Reports should be sent as quickly as possible after evaluations. Audiologists represent their clinics and their profession, and good public relations may be as important to the proper management of the patient as good and accurate testing because one reflects the other.

Clinical COMMENTARY

Reports to speech-language pathologists should include information on the limitations to speech understanding presented by hearing loss. Familiarity with hearing-test procedures discussed in Chapters 4 and 5 can be invaluable to the speech-language pathologist who works with patients with hearing loss. Speech-language pathologists should develop a close working relationship with audiologists in their community to facilitate dialogue on behalf of their patients.

Liaisons with Otolaryngologists

It is obvious that the audiologist is not the person to recommend or perform surgery or medical treatment. This is the duty of the physician, preferably an otologist in the case of ear disease. However, most otologists are neither trained nor interested in the intricacies of diagnostic audiology or the nonmedical aspects of audiological treatment. Many cases of hearing loss have no medical underpinnings, thereby obviating medical intervention. In other important, difficult, or contradictory cases, however, consultation between the otologist and the audiologist is of great advantage to the patient. It is a mistake to think of the relationship between audiology and otology as one in which the audiologist merely provides audiometric services for the use of the physician in a diagnosis. In such situations, the role of the audiologist may deteriorate to that of technician. The association between medicine and audiology should be a symbiotic one, a professional relationship that leads to improved patient management.

In referring patients to a physician, audiologists should state in their reports the areas of concern and the reasons for referral. Recommendations for specific treatment should, of course, not be made. If the patient has a disorder that appears partially or fully reversible (e.g., containing a conductive component caused by otitis media), the audiologist should reschedule the patient for testing following medical attention to ascertain the degree of hearing improvement derived. After an air-bone gap is closed, the sensory/neural portion of a mixed loss may appear different from the pretreatment bone-conduction audiogram. A reevaluation of audiological treatment needs may be required in such cases.

Liaisons with Clinical Psychologists

Sometimes psychological consultation is required because the patient's problem is, at least partially, complicated by an emotional disorder. The training of most audiologists provides a sufficient vocabulary of psychological terms and association with psychological tests to permit interpretation of a psychologist's report. As in referrals to physicians, when referring a patient to a psychologist, audiologists should state their particular concerns about the patient and their reasons for referral. In addition to assistance with emotional disorders, the psychologist can provide information about the patient's performance versus potential—for example, whether a child is reaching academic capabilities or needs some special help. At times, it is not until after consultation that a decision is made about whether the audiologist or the psychologist will become the central figure in the rehabilitation of the patient.

Liaisons with Genetic Counselors

One aspect of audiologist–caregiver interaction that must not be overlooked is the possible need for genetic counseling. Smith (1994) points out that this counseling should not merely provide medical and genetic information, but should also provide support for family members as they learn to deal with their child's hearing loss. The need to direct families to genetic counselors may be more than ethical: Failure to make such recommendations, when they are indicated, may place the clinician in legal jeopardy.

According to Smith (1994), families seek genetic counseling for a variety of reasons once they realize that such services are available. They may be interested in the etiology or prognosis of their own or their children's hearing loss, or they may wish to learn the probability that a later child will have a similar condition. In some cases, if the parents have impaired hearing, they may look at the probability of having an offspring with a hearing loss as a positive outcome.

The year 2003 brought the first use of embryonic genetic screenings for deafness (Robeznieks, 2003). As discussed later in this chapter, a full culture has evolved among the deaf, which embraces its own language and beliefs. This minority group has seen its numbers decrease for years. First, its future members were mainstreamed into public schools and away from the schools for the deaf in which its culture is primarily transmitted, then numbers have further eroded as cochlear implantation has become an increasingly common treatment for pediatric deafness. The use of genetic technologies for the potential business of "designing babies" is seen by some as one more threat to those who live within the Deaf culture.

It is not for the audiologist to judge what decisions should be made on the basis of genetic counseling or the findings of embryonic genetic screenings. Rather, it is the audiologist's responsibility to ensure that families are aware of available genetic counseling services and to know the team to whom referrals should be made. Such a team usually includes a geneticist (a medical doctor), a genetics counselor (usually holding a master's or doctoral degree), and others as needed.

Liaisons with Speech-Language Pathologists

Although many audiologists have reasonably good academic backgrounds in speech-language pathology, most have limited clinical experience. Historically, the similarities in the backgrounds and early training of audiologists and speech-language pathologists have been parallel, and so audiologists probably identify more closely with speech-language pathologists than with other specialists.

An audiologist often sees patients because the speech-language pathologist wishes to know if some aspect of a communication disorder is related to a hearing problem, as well as the extent of this relationship. In the case of young, language-delayed children, the identification of a hearing disorder may play a large role in (re)habilitation. In such cases, collaboration among specialists can result in the proper planning of remediation. Some voice or articulation disorders are directly related to the inability to discriminate sounds or to hear in some frequency ranges.

Reports sent from audiologists to speech-language pathologists should be frank and direct. Audiologists should state their opinions regarding the type and extent of hearing impairment, and they should recommend referral to other specialists, such as otolaryngologists or psychologists, if indicated. The audiologist may state an opinion regarding the effects of hearing loss on a patient's speech but should refrain from specific recommendations regarding therapy.

In working with some pediatric patients, an audiologist may have little more than a clinical hunch about the child's hearing. Phrases such as "hearing is adequate for speech" appear frequently in reports. In such cases, strong recommendations should be made so that follow-up testing is conducted at intervals until bilateral hearing sensitivity can be ascertained. Honest errors made by audiologists may not be caught until valuable time has been lost unless there is routine follow-up. The speech-language pathologist who may be working with a child for speech and language delay is in a prime position to ensure that follow-up hearing tests are scheduled.

Liaisons with Teachers of Children with Hearing Impairments

Reports sent to teachers of children with hearing impairment are, in many respects, the same as those sent to speech-language pathologists. Events and developments of recent years have brought clinical audiologists and teachers closer together for the betterment of children with hearing disorders, largely because of the trend toward removing children from the self-contained environment of traditional schools for the deaf into the mainstream of education.

To permit children with hearing loss to compete with their hearing contemporaries, the combined efforts of the two specialties of clinical audiology and education of the deaf have come into closer harmony than ever before. This is largely true because of the emphasis now being placed by many educators on the use of residual hearing. As the barriers between the two groups break down, their formal educations include more overlapping coursework. The harmony achieved can result in teamwork, with the children being the ultimate beneficiaries.

Teachers must learn to understand the implications of audiological management, and audiologists must learn to comprehend the difficulties in the day-to-day management of children in the classroom, especially when those children have impaired hearing. Items of mutual concern include hearing aids, classroom amplification systems, and implications of classroom acoustics. Audiologists' isolation from teachers of children with hearing impairment, and these teachers' reluctance to accept audiological involvement, will disappear as the interactions between these professions continue to increase.

Liaisons with Regular School Classroom Teachers

With the advent of Public Law 94-142, the Education for All Handicapped Children Act of 1975, teachers are educating many children with hearing loss within regular classrooms with no formal preparation in the impact of, and remediation for, hearing impairment. The role of audiology in the delivery of appropriate education for these children, who were mainstreamed into the regular classroom, was a primary impetus for the development of educational audiology as a specialty area within audiology studies (Blair, 1996; Johnson & Benson, 2000).

Educational audiology is still an underrepresented segment of the profession. Regular classroom teachers must usually rely on the information provided by the clinical audiologist in their efforts to meet the educational needs of mainstreamed children with hearing loss. When possible, direct consultation with a child's classroom teacher will go a long way toward helping the teacher and the school address the hearing difficulties a child must endure, even following procurement of appropriate amplification. Reports and/or consultations should go beyond simple documentation of the hearing loss and amplification recommendations and must include specific implications of the hearing loss in concrete and functional terms. These may include factors such as the impact of background classroom noise, resultant fatigue from attempts at visual compensation for the hearing loss, and what high-frequency consonant sounds may still be missed even with amplification (Martin & Clark, 1996). Specific classroom-management suggestions for children with hearing loss (Clark & English, 2004) are welcome additions to any communication with the regular classroom teacher.

Clinical COMMENTARY

Of all the professionals, it is the speech-language pathologist with whom the audiologist may collaborate most frequently when working with children. Given the high number of children with reduced hearing and the general paucity of audiologists employed within educational settings, it is apparent that speech-language pathologists play an integral role in the treatment of and advocacy for children with hearing loss. When a school-age child has been identified as having a hearing loss, the speech-language pathologist may be the only person available to provide the in-service training educators may need. This is not to suggest that audiologists are relieved of their advocacy role for children with hearing loss. No child can have too many advocates for justifiable needs. However, the speech-language pathologist's proximity may consign much of the advocacy responsibility to this professional's shoulders.

Audiological Counseling

For many clinicians in all areas of human healthcare, the word *counseling* means telling patients what is wrong and what must be done about it. Counseling by audiologists must include much more. Audiological counseling is based on the "well-patient model" because the majority of those seen by audiologists are psychologically normal individuals who are trying to cope with the disruption a hearing loss has caused in their lives (Clark, 1994). Those occasional patients who face much deeper psychological difficulty may necessitate referral to mental-health professionals.

The word *care* is one of the primary definitions of counseling, which is usually defined by healthcare providers as a system of information transfer; that is, the counselor (audiologist, physician, hearing aid dispenser) provides directions that the client is expected to follow. This is no surprise because the word *client* comes from the Latin *cliens,* a follower, or one who bows or leans on another (as one's master) for protection. The alternative word *patient,* which is the one used in this text, is not much better because its root is in the Latin *patiens,* to suffer, that is, a person passively receiving care. It is little wonder then that the clinician may expect to operate from the position of power, and the patient from one of subservience. Relationships between patients and their clinicians often come down to the exertion of control (Cassell,

1989), with the clinician exerting authority for what is believed to be in the best interest of the patient. Older, less-educated patients seem to accept a more passive role than their younger, better-educated counterparts (Haug & Lavin, 1983). However, the goal of the audiologist should be to help those they serve to achieve independence and to learn how to solve the problems associated with hearing loss, and the voice of clinical authority must often take a back seat.

Often elderly patients with hearing impairment are not referred to audiologists by other healthcare providers. It is not clear why this is the case, but it may be reasonable to assume that physicians simply expect hearing loss in some patients as a normal consequence of aging, do not realize the extent to which many patients can be helped by counseling and amplification, or do not understand that the impact of the hearing loss is not fully evidenced in a quiet health-care provider's office. In these matters, the audiologist must educate not only the patient and the patient's family, but the medical community as well.

Diagnostic Counseling

It has long been believed that one of the greatest responsibilities of the audiologist is to ensure that test results and diagnostic impressions are imparted adequately to patients and their families. Accurate test results are of paramount importance, but the tests serve merely as instruments to help clinicians give advice and counsel to patients and their families.

To a large degree, the specific approach used and the details included in counseling a patient or family are determined by the audiologist's experience. In the important area of content counseling, it is helpful if the type and degree of loss are explained, and the adult patient, or caregivers of the pediatric patient, acquires a basic understanding of the audiogram. Results of speech audiometry and other diagnostic tests are often not well understood, but if some interest is shown in these tests, the results should be explained in as much detail as the patient desires, using the clearest terms possible with conscious avoidance of audiological jargon. What is surprising to many is that, initially, many people do not appear to show great interest in test results and want to go directly to the "bottom line," with questions about the need for hearing aids, progression of the loss, implications of the loss on general health, and so on. A sensible approach, after testing is completed, is simply to ask what information is desired. If the patient or parent is not prepared to listen, there is not much sense in pouring forth technical information. The counseling role of the audiologist cannot be overstressed because there is evidence that much of what is explained by clinicians is not accurately retained, even by educated and intelligent persons (Martin, Krueger, & Bernstein, 1990).

In some cases, it is necessary to avoid more than a perfunctory explanation of test results, for example, if there is a potentially serious medical condition. On the one hand, an audiologist must not engage in discussions with patients of acoustic tumors and the like; this is the responsibility of the physician. On the other hand, if an audiologist suspects a condition for which a referral is made to an otologist, the patient will surely want to know the reason for the referral, and tact, diplomacy, and counseling skills are often tested under such conditions.

When discussing test results, the audiologist must create an atmosphere of calm professionalism, which is often the basis for patient or caregiver confidence in the clinician. Confidence is not determined by whether the audiologist wears a white coat or shows other outward postures of competence. Ordinarily, clinicians should not be separated from their patients by artificial barriers such as desks and tables. As the physical space between parties is decreased, the opportunities for trust and openness increase. After an explanation of test results has been made, the audiologist should solicit questions from the patient and try to answer them in appropriate detail.

Precisely how to convey to parents or caregivers the nature and extent of their children's hearing loss is not universally agreed upon. Many clinicians use a system of direct information transfer. That is, they present information, insofar as it is known, about a child's hearing loss. Often this includes descriptions of the audiogram, definitions of terms, and options for meeting the child's needs. The intent is to educate the caregivers to the point that they can best handle the child's hearing problems. Clinicians often do not realize that their choice of language, verbal and nonverbal, and even the amount of information provided, may have profound effects, both positive and negative, on the receiver of that information. Care should be taken not to present more information than can be taken in. On the initial confirmation of hearing loss, emotions can be quite raw, often making the cognitive processing of new information limited at best. The wise clinician will pace the delivery of information, possibly withholding details until a subsequent visit, while always questioning the recipient to assess comprehension and emotional reaction to the news being given.

It is natural for clinicians to present diagnostic information to the adults who have accompanied a child to the hearing evaluation. Certainly, when children are young and profoundly hearing impaired, it is their caregivers who must decide how the children are to be educated and what amplification alternatives will be considered. However, when children are old enough and have sufficient communication skills, they should be part of the discussion. This serves to eliminate the resentment that many children feel when they have been excluded from discussions that relate directly to them. Naturally, when children are very young, severely hearing impaired, or with multiple handicaps, it is the adults who should be addressed, but always be attentive to the child's feelings.

It is natural to feel resentment when those discussing our welfare ignore our presence. Yet this happens frequently in health care settings serving elderly people, as well as teenagers. When discussions about the person with the hearing loss are directed solely to others in attendance, that person rapidly begins to feel of marginal importance to the rehabilitative process. Assistive listening devices can be very useful in helping patients through the counseling process if they do not have their own hearing instruments (see Chapter 14).

Emotional Response to Hearing Loss

Parents are often confused and disturbed by new and unusual terminology; thus, even the very words used to describe a child's problems may be critical (Martin, 1994). Martin, George, O'Neal, and Daly (1987) conducted a survey in the United States and learned that parents (or other caregivers) are often not receptive to detailed information immediately after they have learned that their child has an irreversible hearing loss. A qualitative study supports this contention, finding that most caregivers could recall the diagnosis and recommendations that the audiologist had given but had very little recall or understanding of explanations that were given about the actual tests or how the ear worked (Watermeyer, Kanji, & Cohen, 2012).

Initial parental reactions to their child's hearing loss diagnosis include sorrow, shock, denial, fear, anger, helplessness, and blame, although not all of these reactions will necessarily appear and may show up in any order (Martin et al., 1987). It takes varying and sometimes prolonged amounts of time for the diagnosis of hearing loss to be accepted. Acceptance of this diagnosis is often easier for parents and others if they have the opportunity to observe hearing tests as they are performed on their children. By the time an adult patient reaches the audiologist, a greater level of acceptance has often been attained. Yet it is still important that audiologists remain cognizant of the impact their words may carry when relaying diagnostic findings to adults.

The reactions of parents to the realization that their child has a hearing impairment are not always the same. Whether externalized or internalized, it is safe to say that the effect is generally quite intense. As Moses (1979) points out, parents view their children as extensions of themselves, with hopes and dreams of perfection. When an imperfection is uncovered, the dreams become shattered. Because of its "invisibility," hearing impairment often does not appear to be a true disability, which makes the adjustment even more difficult for the parents.

Many people have inferred that adults with acquired hearing loss do not suffer significant shock, disappointment, anger, sadness, or other emotions because they more or less expect the diagnosis they hear. Apparently, however, this is far from true in many cases, and adults may be much more emotionally fragile than had been supposed (Glass & Elliot, 1992; Martin, Krall, & O'Neal, 1989). Assessing the emotional reaction of a patient to the news of a hearing loss often cannot be gauged accurately on the basis of a patient's affect, even by the most sensitive clinician (Martin, Barr, & Bernstein, 1992). As with parents, it is often difficult to distinguish those adults who receive what they perceive to be bad news about irreversible hearing loss in a matter-of-fact way from those for whom the same news is catastrophic.

It is almost always desirable to ask new adult patients to be accompanied to their hearing evaluations by someone significant to them, such as a spouse. The support afforded and the clinical insights gained through such a practice can be immeasurable, yet the involvement of a third party is most often not encouraged as it should be (Stika, Ross, & Cuevas, 2002).When working with children, both parents should be present at the evaluation whenever possible. Observing the tests, as well as the responses given, allows these individuals insights into the nature of the hearing disability that are difficult to comprehend when only explained.

Following the pronouncement that a hearing loss is probably irreversible, the emotional states of parents or adult patients may make it difficult for them to understand and process subsequently presented technical aspects of their hearing disorder and explanations of test results. At the same time, patients complain that they want to have much more information at the time of diagnosis than audiologists, physicians, and hearing aid dispensers usually provide (Martin et al., 1989). A major complaint by those seeking audiological care is that they feel rushed while in the clinician's office. As stated earlier, one solution to this problem is to ask patients or parents what they know about their problems and what they wish to be told. It should be emphasized that further counseling is available, and patients should be encouraged to call for more in-depth discussion of their hearing problems. After people have had a chance to compose themselves, they often think of many pertinent questions or details that they want explained. Opportunities for further consultation with the clinician should be provided at the earliest possible time. Audiological counseling should be viewed as a continuing process, and patients and families should feel that they can come to their audiologist/counselor when they need assistance.

Clark and English (2014) reviewed the states through which many people pass when hearing loss is diagnosed. Parents often go through a period of *denial* as a means of self-defense against what they perceive to be very bad news. The frequently cited seven-year delay between the time adults first suspect that their own hearing has decreased and the time in which assistance is sought speaks volumes on the strength of denial among adults with hearing loss. Often by the time adults get to an audiologist, they have largely worked through their denial. During a state of denial, it is frequently fruitless even to try to provide details of the diagnosis and recommendations for treatment because patients are simply incapable of acceptance at this juncture.

Faced with denial, the audiologist might state, "The idea that your child may have a hearing loss seems difficult for you to accept. Can you tell me what it would mean to you if my diagnosis is correct?" Acknowledging difficulty in accepting the test findings can open a dialogue that may be helpful in moving beyond this aspect of the grieving process. The same approach can be useful when working with adult patients who have not fully reconciled themselves to a newly emerging self-concept as one with hearing loss.

As mourning over the loss of the perfect child continues, parents frequently express *anger* as they relinquish their feelings of denial. This anger may be transferred to loved ones, marital partners, audiologists, physicians, or God, leaving almost no one invulnerable. Adult patients may also be angry at society's lack of understanding of the difficulties they encounter. Unintentionally hurtful statements such as, "He only hears when he wants to hear," only fuel these feelings. Audiologists must be able to function as counselors and accept expressed anger, even if it is directed toward them. Objectivity at this point is crucial.

While traversing through the maze of emotions, parents frequently go through a period of *guilt*. Parents who persist in seeking explanations for the cause of the hearing loss may be looking for a way out of the awful sense that they have somehow done this to their child or are being punished for some past sin. If the guilt is projected toward the other marital partner, the marriage can become shaky; divorce is not uncommon among parents of children with disabilities. Indeed, many parents never pass from the guilt state, with unfortunate consequences for children who may become spoiled or overprotected or may never reach their full potential. Merely telling parents that they need not blame themselves is often fruitless, but the audiologist should try to avoid words or actions that promote guilt. Adult patients, too, may feel guilt over their hearing loss, especially if, as in noise-induced hearing loss, they believe that preventive measures that had been ignored could have circumvented the disorder.

As parents cease reeling from the impact of the "bad news" about their child, they seek ways to maximize the child's potential. Unfortunately, they may become so overloaded with assignments, information, and advice (albeit well meaning) from professionals, family, and friends that they believe they are inadequate for the job at hand. Subsequently, anxiety may increase, which must be dealt with before any form of intervention can become effective for the child. Audiologists must be careful not to overwhelm adults as well. The presentation of too many management options can create confusion and a patient who opts to postpone the purchase of hearing aids and the embarkation of further audiological treatment. What are often presented as "stages" of grief rarely appear in a set order, and persons who seemingly have traversed through a variety of stages can backslide and revisit portions of their grief at later dates.

When presenting diagnostic information that may be painful, audiologists must temper their enthusiasm for launching (re)habilitative efforts with patience and understanding. Reliance on feedback from parents, or adult patients, regarding their anxiety levels during counseling may be misleading. For example, what appears to be a lax or indifferent attitude may be a smokescreen for fear and bewilderment.

Clinical COMMENTARY

Speech-language pathologists and audiologists, like healthcare professionals in other disciplines, frequently must break difficult news to those they serve. As discussed by Clark and English (2014), at these times, clinicians must encourage clients to express their feelings and be prepared to respond with empathy and warmth toward whatever surfaces. Adequate time must be given for both the delivery and receipt of difficult news as well as sufficient temporal space to "regroup" as needed before moving forward into the process of rehabilitation.

Personal Adjustment Counseling

Expanding counseling beyond the mere transfer of information reflects a reconsideration of the counseling roles of audiologists that has been evident in recent years. Counseling should have a supportive base, which helps patients and families to make practical changes in their lives, which, in turn, will help them to develop a more positive approach to their own disabilities, the technological assistance available to them, and the residual communication difficulties that, for many, are inevitable (Clark, 1994; Clark & English, 2004; 2014).

An understanding of the differences between professional and nonprofessional counselors is paramount to the audiologist. Professional counselors are those who are specifically educated and trained in this area and counseling is the primary service they provide. These professionals include psychologists, social workers, and psychiatrists, although modern psychiatry appears to be turning away from a counseling profession to a neurochemical discipline. Nonprofessional counselors include those others who may or may not lack specific and advanced training in counseling but provide their counseling to augment their primary service directly. These may include audiologists, speech-language pathologists, physicians, educators, clergy, attorneys, friends, and family. Psychotherapy is in the domain of professional counselors. Understanding the differences between psychotherapeutic counseling and personal adjustment counseling allows nonprofessional counselors to feel more comfortable within their counseling role. It is the audiologist's role in supportive personal adjustment counseling that is often slighted in patient care, and it must be cultivated for the patient's benefit. Those who perform any counseling at all must know their strengths and limitations and must recognize the critical impact that their words and deeds can have on patients and their families.

Sometimes caregivers opt for a plan of action that is not what the audiologist believes to be in a particular child's best interest. Because of their background and training, many audiologists believe that the first avenue followed should employ the aural/oral approach, maximizing residual hearing with amplification and encouraging communication through speech. A different decision by a parent may appear to be "wrong" to the clinician. The function of the audiologist should be to convey educational and habilitative options to the parents (Clark, 1983). While these alternatives should be explained carefully, objectively, and without bias, it is the parents who make the final decisions regarding hearing-loss management for their children.

Before parents can help their children, they must be helped themselves. They must be taught to cope with the challenge of parenting a child with a hearing impairment. They must learn to continue to give and to accept love, and to include the entire family in normal activities, as well as in activities prescribed for the child with the hearing loss. The audiologist, as a sensitive and empathetic listener, must learn to see beyond the words to acknowledge the feelings of family members. Intervention without personal concern may be useless.

Clinical COMMENTARY

One of the greatest impediments to effective patient counseling is a poor match between the feelings underlying parent or adult patient statements and the response given by the clinician. The parent who states, "Those hearing aids look so big on his tiny ears" is no more commenting on the size of the hearing aids than is the adult who states, "I always thought hearing aids were for old people" is making a comment on hearing loss demographics. Pointing out that hearing aids are much smaller than in the past, or that the audiologist has many patients much younger than the present adult patient, is a clear communication mismatch. A better response in either situation that speaks to the pain underlying the recognized need for hearing aids might be an acknowledgment as simple as, "If it were me, I'm sure I would find it quite difficult accepting the unexpected and unwanted changes that have come into my life." Communication mismatch in patient consultations is all too frequent during encounters with all health professionals, including speech-language pathologists and audiologists.

It is frequently the unasked questions that audiologists must sense and answer. Patients, and their families, are frequently fearful of inquiring about the possible progression of hearing loss. Many older patients fear that it is only a matter of time before they will lose their hearing entirely. Parents of young children may fear further impact on the rehabilitative goals their children are striving to attain. Although progression of hearing loss may or may not have been demonstrated by repeated hearing evaluations, it is possible for the audiologist to play a calming and reassuring role.

All audiologists have seen patients who, for whatever reason, would opt to avoid the treatment offered if they were given the opportunity. These may be adult patients who have not fully recognized the impact of their hearing loss or who have not come to grips with the view of themselves as someone who is no longer a fully functioning, unimpaired adult; teenage students with hearing loss who shun continued use of the visible electroacoustic accoutrements others insist they wear; or very elderly patients who may believe they have outlived their usefulness and see no reason to put forth the efforts others are asking of them. Ultimately, patients act through their own values when making decisions that affect their lives. While it is the responsibility of audiologists to recognize and accept conditions that may affect their patients' decisions, they must also always be prepared to explore with their patients various means that may help them to recognize the value of alternative viewpoints and actions (Clark, 2007; Clark & English, 2014).

In the provision of personal adjustment counseling, the audiologist will be well served by remembering three key points:

1. *Reflect* concerns back to the patient. In so doing, the audiologist ensures that concerns were properly understood while simultaneously conveying an empathic desire to see the problem at hand from the patients' or parents' perspective. Effective reflections come in lead statements such as, "As I understand you, you are saying . . . " or, more simply, "In other words. . . ."

2. *Accept* the patients' or parents' expressed feelings or attitudes as valid views or perceptions of the situation at the moment. It is when we make judgments on feelings and attitudes that sharing stops and assistance wanes. Only after audiologists do these first two can they truly begin the third and next step.

3. *Explore* different avenues that may open opportunities for the future (Clark, 1999, 2000).

What persons with hearing loss, and their families, are asking for is no more than they are entitled to: a concerned and compassionate clinician who is willing to give sufficient time and express appropriate interest in what, to many people, is a profound and disturbing disability. Counseling beyond an information transfer should be an integral component to the services audiologists provide, although it is frequently underdelivered. Further discussion of counseling techniques for audiologists may be found in the suggested reading list at the end of this chapter.

Support Groups

Adult patients and family members of pediatric patients find that support groups are of great assistance in dealing with hearing loss. Participants quickly learn within a group that they are not alone in the difficulties they experience. Support groups addressing the pediatric population may be designed for grandparents or siblings to address their specific issues separate from the traditional parent support groups (Atkins, 1994).

Teens with hearing loss who have been mainstreamed often confront their communication challenges and frustrations unaware that there are others with the same difficulties. Teen support groups not only provide a valuable outlet and learning environment for these children, but also allow parents an opportunity to meet again as a group to address the adolescent issues that were not foreseen in their earlier group experiences when their children were much younger. The consumer support group of the Alexander Graham Bell Association for the Deaf and Hard of Hearing (www.agbell.org) provides online support and regional/state meetings for parents, teens with hearing loss, and others in the family constellation of pediatric hearing loss. For adults with hearing loss, one valuable group, with local chapters around the country, is the Hearing Loss Association of America (www.hearingloss.org), which publishes its own consumer-oriented journal. Audiologists need to make referrals to support groups to supplement the treatment services they are providing their patients of all ages.

Management of Adult Hearing Impairment

The passage of Public Law 101-336, the Americans with Disabilities Act (1991), prohibits discrimination against persons with disabilities in areas such as transportation, state and local government, public accommodations, employment, and telecommunications. The Americans with Disabilities Act was updated for the 21st century with passage of the 21st Century Communications and Video Accessability Act (2010), which provides equal access to a variety of communications technologies. These laws sprang from a grassroots movement and have profound effects for individuals with hearing loss. It should be understood by audiologists that, in addition to obvious technical implications, these laws help to reduce the negative images that are associated with physically and mentally challenged individuals, and they foster renewed sensitivity to the feelings of those with disabilities. Audiologists are urged to consider the words they use in case management, for example, substituting *disability* for *handicap,* because a disabled person is only handicapped when faced with an insurmountable barrier. The person, and not the disability, should be emphasized as part of what has been called the "people first" movement; hence, "person with a hearing loss" should replace "hearing-impaired person."

Adult patients requiring audiological management of their hearing problems are usually adventitiously impaired. Although some of these hearing losses are sudden, for example, as the result of drug therapy or illness, most are gradual, almost insidious. The management of these patients has been termed *aural rehabilitation* and, more recently, **audiological rehabilitation** or *audiological treatment.*

It is important to separate the concepts of **hearing impairment,** an abnormality that is psychological, physiological, or anatomical (defined audiometrically), and **hearing disability,** which relates to an individual's difficulty in performing biologically and socially useful functions, from **hearing handicap,** the ways in which individuals are disadvantaged in fulfilling their desired roles (usually defined on self-assessment scales) (World Health Organization, 1980). While these terms are somewhat ingrained within the practice mindset of many health professionals, audiologists should be aware that the World Health Organization (2001) has moved away from terminology that implies a consequence of disease to a "components of health" classification. Within this newer classification framework, *disability* is replaced by *activity limitations* (e.g., effective communication) and *handicap* is replaced by *participation restriction* (e.g., within social, vocational, and educational arenas).

The degree of participation restriction represented by activity limitations presented by a given hearing impairment can be highly individual and must be taken into account in rehabilitative planning. Indeed, participation restrictions are directly related to the availability of personal amplification, assistive devices, workplace accommodations, societal views toward the disabled, and the presence of supportive legislation.

When labeling activity limitation based on a given level of hearing impairment expressed in terms of the pure-tone average (PTA) (see Table 4.1), it is important to remember that two- and three-frequency PTAs were designed to predict the threshold of speech and, as such, often misrepresent the impact of a given hearing loss. Although these averages are often used in assigning hearing-loss labels, the prediction of speech thresholds and the assignment of hearing-loss labels are two quite different processes. Although the variable pure-tone average (VPTA) discussed in Chapter 4 may serve better for the latter, it should be noted that the accuracy of any labeling system in describing a given individual is contingent on a variety of sometimes unknown factors.

Audiological treatment has changed in recent years for several reasons, including technological breakthroughs and cultural influences. Traditional rehabilitative techniques with adults, such as speechreading and auditory training, continue to be practiced, despite the fact that the data do not consistently prove these approaches alone to be effective. However, there is much that can be done to assist patients and their families in addressing the hearing problems that can become so intrusive in their lives.

While medical science has advanced in the treatment of diseases that cause hearing loss, similar advances have served to prolong life, with the result that, for the first time in history, the population of the United States consists of more older people than younger people. Because hearing loss is one of the almost inevitable results of aging, the number of adults with acquired hearing loss is increasing.

A condition that has been thrust into the public's consciousness in the past several decades is **Alzheimer's disease,**[1] which causes confusion, disorientation, and, what is most commonly associated with this condition, memory loss. The disease begins in late middle life, often results in death within 10 to 20 years, and is said to be the largest single cause of **dementia.** The incidence of Alzheimer's appears to be increasing rapidly, in part because its diagnosis has become much easier with the advent of magnetic resonance imaging (MRI) and positron emission tomography (PET) scans.

It is known that the incidence of Alzheimer's disease increases with age and therefore may be a concomitant occurrence with presbycusis, making hearing-instrument use and other avenues of auditory rehabilitation even more difficult. Because memory loss is an unfortunate companion of aging, and both conditions present their own problems with communication, the challenge to the audiologist is significantly increased in those cases where the conditions coexist (Cacace, 2007). Audiologists must be prepared to meet this challenge.

Before an audiological treatment program can begin, it is essential that the patient's hearing disability be assessed. It has been customary to base this assessment on audiometric data alone. The information provided earlier in this text is essential to patient management, but it does not supersede other information that may also be critical, such as the patient's own view of the disability, individual needs and preferences, socioeconomic status, education, vocation, and a host of other important nonauditory considerations (American Academy of Audiology, 2006).

A number of attempts to assess the degree of activity limitation have been based both on audiometric data and on scales computed with the assistance of the patient. A compilation of scales to assess the impact of hearing loss is provided by Clark and English (2014). Although none of these methods is perfect, they assist the audiologist in compiling data about how the hearing impairment affects the central figure in the treatment process. After all, it does little good to insist that a patient needs wearable amplification when the patient minimizes the effects of the hearing loss and has no intention of using hearing aids.

The goal of adult audiological treatment is always to make maximum use of residual hearing. Residual hearing is useful hearing, and it is not always easily discernible by looking at an audiogram, speech-recognition threshold, or word-recognition score. The patient's residual hearing is the difference, in decibels, between the auditory threshold and the uncomfortable loudness level. The broader this dynamic range of hearing, the better candidate the patient is for hearing aids and audiological rehabilitation.

A number of decisions must be made after the hearing has been assessed. The decision on hearing aids must be made, and proper selection and orientation should be arranged. The nature of the orientation must be selected: that is, whether intervention should be done individually or in groups, who should constitute the specific group, what visual cues should be emphasized, how speech can be conserved, and so on. Treatment efforts must be geared to the individual, whose curiosity and ability to comprehend should not be underestimated. The patient should be educated as fully as possible about hearing loss in general and about the specific disability in particular. How the ear works and what has gone wrong, the effects of the loss on speech communication, implications for progression of the loss, the array of hearing assistance technologies available, and interactions with family and friends must all be discussed openly and honestly with the patient, in the presence of a close friend or family member, whenever possible.

Many audiologists are more comfortable in the role of diagnostician than hearing-loss manager. Modern audiology demands that the clinician be facile in both of these areas; indeed, it is within the latter that audiologists find the greater autonomy. There is an unfortunate tendency in clinical audiology to provide hearing loss treatment largely, if not often solely, through available technology. To fail to provide direct intervention through training in effective communication is a disservice to the patient and to the profession of audiology (Clark, 2009, 2010; Clark, Kricos, & Sweetow, 2010).

Beyond Hearing Aids and Hearing Assistance Technologies

A large-scale study of adults with hearing loss and their family members was conducted by the National Council on Aging (NCOA) (Kochkin & Rogin, 2000). The study documented that untreated hearing loss increases levels of depression, anxiety, anger, and frustration. These findings parallel earlier studies, which have shown a demonstrable increase in functional disability in the elderly for every 10 dB increase in hearing loss (e.g., Bess, Lichtenstein, Logan, Burger, & Nelson, 1989). It is now well documented that the use of hearing aids can improve functional health status in elderly patients with sensory/neural hearing loss due to decreases in the functional, psychosocial, and emotional impacts of reduced communication (Chisolm et al., 2007; Crandell, 1998; Kochkin & Rogin, 2000; Larson et al., 2000) and that the short-term benefits initially reported are sustained into the long term (Bratt, Rosenfeld, & Williams, 2007). In addition, specific communication training has been found to further lessen the negative impacts of hearing loss, and many resources are available that provide useful guidance for audiologists in the provision of both individual and group hearing therapy (e.g., Clark & English, 2014; Wayner & Abrahamson, 1996).

A major task of any dispensing audiologist should be to train the patient with hearing loss in the maximum use of residual hearing. For the greatest effectiveness with hearing aids, this should go beyond the standard mechanics of orientation to the use and care of hearing instruments. In spite of the growing evidence that *auditory training* or, more appropriately with adults, *auditory retraining*, can significantly augment the benefit derived from amplification (Kricos & McCarthy, 2007), this adjunct to the audiologist's services to adults is frequently omitted from the treatment provided. A home-based, interactive, and adaptive computer-based approach to auditory retraining known as LACE (listening and communication enhancement) has been demonstrated to positively impact the communication function of adults (Sweetow & Sabes, 2006) and may prove to be a beneficial adjunct to the general orientation to amplification use the audiologist provides (see Figure 15.3). Not only can auditory retraining improve a patient's communication effectiveness, there is evidence that this improvement can be pharmacologically enhanced (Tobey et al., 2005). These preliminary results may prove to be of considerable benefit to many who strive to attain the highest levels of communicative function possible.

FIGURE 15.3 Many patients augment their hearing rehabilitation at home or in the audiologist's office with computer programs designed to improve listening abilities and speechreading performance.

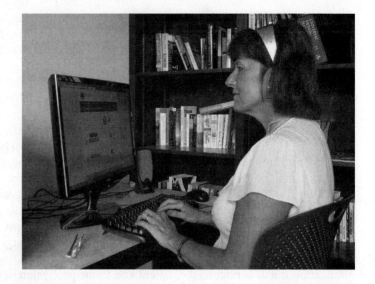

Auditory retraining with adults has evolved to encompass instruction geared to enhance recognition of and intervention for those variables within the environment, or poor speaker or listener habits that impede successful communication (Clark & English, 2004, 2014; Trychin, 1994). Patients should be taught to be more assertive in regard to advising others of their communication needs and to maximize their communicative skills, in part by managing their environments. People should be encouraged to be in the same room with and facing others with whom they speak. Position in the room should be manipulated to take advantage of lighting. Room noise should be minimized during conversation, and hearing assistance technologies should be used when appropriate. The patient's primary communication partners should be actively involved in all training to gain a greater appreciation of realistic communication expectations and to learn ways they can further enhance successful communication. **Hearing therapy,** or communication training, should be integral to a more comprehensive delivery of audiological services and is endorsed by the primary consumer advocacy group for those with hearing loss, the Hearing Loss Association of America, as a recommended adjunct to hearing aid fittings (Self Help for Hard of Hearing People, Inc., 1996). Despite this endorsement, surveys continue to demonstrate that the predominant protocol for hearing aid dispensing has not changed much through the years, with the fitting process reaching completion in most cases within three to five visits (Skafte, 2000).

Clinical COMMENTARY

Unfortunately, for most hearing aid users, maximum benefit with amplification cannot be attained in the traditional three- to five-visit dispensing protocol. Until audiologists begin to provide their patients with more than the mechanics of hearing aid use, it can be expected that general satisfaction levels with amplification, while significantly higher than in the past, will not meet the levels that technological advances are capable of providing.

One of the most effective means of providing communication training is through group classes designed for the individual with hearing loss and a spouse, a close family member, or a friend. The value of group intervention transcends any functional improvement in communication that may be attained. Group work with adults has a psychotherapeutic value that cannot be underestimated. Many adults, particularly older people, become depressed over their hearing losses. They may feel persecuted and alone. Although they may realize, on an intellectual level, that their problems are not unique, emotionally they feel isolated. The mere experience of being with people their own age, and with similar problems, may lift their spirits and aid in their rehabilitation. The opportunity for members of the group to share what has worked for them in their attempts to address their communication difficulties is beneficial to all group members. The educational and emotional values of group intervention can only be approximated. However, even with the strongest attempts at intervention, some adult patients with sensory/neural hearing losses cannot make the adjustment to hearing aids or refuse to attempt to do so.

Group communication training is essential to success for many patients learning to adjust to amplification, but unfortunately, it has yet to be fully embraced by audiologists (Clark, 2001, 2002). Few audiologists provide communication training for adults primarily due to the time investment required for training and the low reimbursement for the provision of these services. It is a misconception that this is time poorly spent because the resultant greater acceptance of hearing aids through such services has its own payoff through fewer hearing aid rejections. Not only is group or individual training rarely provided, many adults with hearing loss may not follow through with recommendations for home study, such as with LACE, believing that today's hearing aid circuitry should fully compensate for their problems or that residual difficulties are a limitation with which they must contend. It is imperative that, at the very least, audiologists discuss communication strategies for persons with hearing loss and those they live with during the hearing aid fitting process (Clark, 2009; Clark & English, 2014).

Speechreading Training with Adults

It is the mistaken concept among many laypersons, and among some professionals as well, that if hearing becomes impaired, it can be replaced by **lipreading,** in which the words of a speaker may be recognized by watching the lips. The term **speechreading** has replaced *lipreading* because it is recognized that the visual perception of speech requires much more than attending to lip movements alone. Recognition of facial expressions, gestures, body movements, and so on, contributes to the perception of speech.

Many speech sounds are produced so that they may be recognized on the lips alone, at least in terms of their general manner and place of production. Some sounds, however, such as /p/, /m/, and /b/, are produced in such a way that they are difficult to differentiate from each other based on visual cues alone. Other sounds, such as /g/, /k/, and /h/, cannot be perceived visually at all.

Although much has been done to investigate the value of speechreading, and numbers of methods are available to teach this skill to people with hearing loss, it is still a considerably misunderstood concept. It is a gross error to believe that speechreading alone can replace hearing in the complete understanding of spoken discourse. It is also an error to believe that more than about 50 percent of the sounds of speech may be perceived through speechreading alone.

For speechreading to be of maximum value to the patient, it should be taught in conjunction with the coping strategies addressed in communication training so that the combined effects of vision and residual hearing may be gained. When the two senses are used simultaneously, they interact synergistically; the combined effect on speech understanding is greater for watching and listening together than for either watching alone or listening alone.

Many people believe that speechreading is an art that requires an innate talent possessed more by some persons than by others. It is probably true that some people are more visually oriented than others. Some people do better on speechreading tests without training than do other people who have had a number of speechreading lessons. Of course, a speaker's poor speaking habits can contribute to the listener's difficulty in speechreading. Direct intervention in developing clear speaking habits has been found to aid in successful speechreading (Caissie et al., 2005).

The methods of teaching speechreading to adults vary considerably in their philosophy and implementation. Some include an analytic approach to the movements of the speaker's lips, whereas others are more synthetic. Computer-assisted training in speechreading that implements CD technology has been used. It is enough to say in this brief discussion that speechreading should be made as natural to the patient as possible, utilizing residual hearing through hearing aids if this is indicated.

Clinical COMMENTARY

The scopes of practice for both speech-language pathologists and audiologists include provision of services in audiological (re)habilitation for adults and children. As the range of audiological rehabilitation services continues to expand, clearly the roles these two professional groups bring to service delivery will differ based on knowledge and skills unique to each profession. Quite frequently, the audiological services provided are a collaborative effort between speech-language pathologists and audiologists. As stated by the American Speech-Language-Hearing Association (ASHA) Board of Ethics, the professional's personal scope of practice in this area is dictated by his or her own education, training, and experience (American Speech-Language-Hearing Association, 2002b).

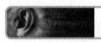

Management of Childhood Hearing Impairment

Although other conditions may contribute to delay the onset of normal language and speech, often hearing loss is the primary problem. Whether a hearing loss is present at birth or develops at some time afterward can make a profound difference in language acquisition. When it exists before the normal development of language, it is referred to as **prelinguistic hearing loss.** A hearing loss that begins after language concepts are formed is called **postlinguistic hearing loss.** Naturally, the later in life a hearing loss begins, the better the chance to conserve the speech and language that a child has already learned through the hearing sense.

One obligation of the audiologist is to pursue medical reversal of a hearing loss as soon as that possibility presents itself. Determination of otologic or surgical treatment is based on medical decisions. Audiologists should make a medical referral immediately when otitis media or other infections are seen, or when there is any indication of a structural deviation that might involve the auditory system. If medical treatment of a hearing loss is impossible, or still leaves the child with some hearing loss, further audiological intervention is needed, including family counseling.

Auditory Training with Children

There are obvious differences in the approaches to patients with prelinguistic and postlinguistic hearing losses. Children who have suffered hearing loss from birth or early childhood cannot call on the memory of speech sounds, and so must begin training in special ways. **Auditory training** programs for children may be quite comprehensive, and specific goals and objectives should be established based on individual needs. Often these programs

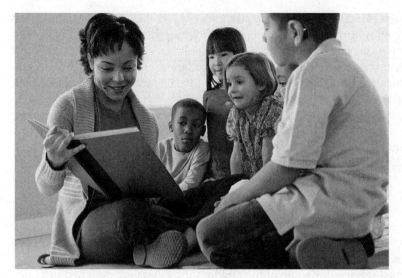

FIGURE 15.4 A major component of any auditory enrichment program is to ensure that a clear signal reaches the ear. Here, the teacher's voice is picked up by a head-worn microphone and sent via FM transmission to the receiver attached to the child's hearing aid. (*Source:* Phonak.)

concentrate on auditory skill development in the areas of sound awareness, sound discrimination, sound identification, and sound/speech comprehension through both formal and informal activities. The more readily the hearing aids are accepted, the sooner training can begin (see Figure 15.4).

Speechreading Training with Children

Speechreading for small children should begin early in life. They should be encouraged to watch the faces of their parents and others. Speech to these children should be slow, simple, and carefully articulated, without exaggeration of the movements of the face and mouth. The error committed by many parents is to mouth speech without voice, in the belief that the exaggerations help the children speechread and that voice is unnecessary because the children are "deaf." Using voice allows the production of the speech sounds to be more natural and, it is hoped, provides some auditory cues if the children's residual hearing has been tapped by amplification.

Educational Options

The Bureau of Education of the Handicapped was established in 1966, which in turn led to implementation of Public Law 94-142 in 1975, the Education for All Handicapped Children Law. This law mandates **mainstreaming** children with disabilities whenever possible and that their education be carried out in the "least restrictive environment." For many children with hearing loss, mainstreaming requires that they spend their entire school day in a regular classroom except for times specifically designed to receive support services related to their disability. Over 25 years ago, more than half of the children with profound hearing losses in the United States were moved away from specialized schools, many of which began to close as a consequence (Lane, 1987). It is unfortunate that the "least restrictive environment" was interpreted as endorsing mainstreaming for *all* children. Restrictive environments may be more appropriately defined as settings that limit a child's classroom potential, and the least restrictive environment is the setting most appropriate for the child (Ross, Brackett, & Maxon, 1991).

The Education of the Handicapped Act Amendments (P.L. 99-457) was enacted in 1986 to provide guidelines for offering assistance from birth to children with hearing loss and other disabilities. The purpose of this law, in addition to offering assistance and guidance to families with younger children, was to develop family-centered programs. Public Law 94-142 mandated the **individual education plan (IEP),** and Public Law 99-457 encouraged the **individual family service plan (IFSP).** The No Child Left Behind (NCLB) Act (2001) mandates high achievement for all students. To meet the spirit of the law for each of these important pieces of legislation, audiologists must not only identify, assess, and plan intervention for children with hearing loss, but must also be familiar with general education curriculum standards, goals, and benchmarks as well as the supports that children with hearing loss may need to attain their highest levels of achievement. Early intervention services include audiometry, speech-language pathology, case management, family training, health services, nutrition, occupational therapy, physical therapy, psychological and social services, transportation, and more. The Individuals with Disabilities Education Act of 1990 (P.L. 101-476) and the Individuals with Disabilities Education Act Amendments of 1997 (P.L. 105-117) added legal clarification. All this legislation places educational audiology on a firm legal footing, although enactment of laws does not always translate into actual services for some of the children these laws are designed to assist. The laws do provide for punitive action, however, against noncompliant schools.

In all states, children who are suspected of having a hearing loss are entitled to free testing. The purpose, of course, is to identify, as early as possible, those children who require special assistance. In many states this is called Child Find. Once the identification is made, audiological services should include appropriate professional referral, habilitative measures (auditory training, language stimulation, speechreading, **speech conservation**), counseling and guidance, and determination of specific amplification needs (Johnson, 1994). The habilitative/rehabilitative components of these services are most frequently provided by speech-language pathologists.

Childhood hearing loss delays the development of receptive and expressive communication skills, creating learning problems that reduce academic performance, create social isolation, lower self-concept, and restrict future vocational options. To help combat the educational implications of childhood hearing loss, the American Speech-Language-Hearing Association (2004b) has detailed the responsibilities of the educational audiologist (see Table 15.2).

A variety of placement options may be available for the formal education of children with hearing loss. These include privately and publicly funded institutions, residential and day schools, and public schools. Of all children in regular classrooms requiring special educational considerations, those with hearing impairment make up the largest groups (Flexer, Wray, & Ireland, 1989). Although classroom teachers have shown an interest in knowing more about their students with hearing loss, they admit that their knowledge base is inadequate for proper management (Martin, Bernstein, Daly, & Cody, 1988). In addition to educational management, teachers must have information about classroom acoustics, individually worn amplification devices, and systems to help improve the signal-to-noise ratios for children.

TABLE 15.2 Responsibilities of the Educational Audiologist

- Creation and administration of hearing-loss identification programs.
- Evaluation of children with identified hearing loss.
- Appropriate referral for medical and professional attention and for further assessment, as needed.
- Creation and administration of programs for the prevention of hearing loss.
- Counseling and guidance of children, parents, and teachers regarding hearing loss.
- Determination of need for and selection and fitting of personal and classroom amplification and hearing assistance technologies, and determination of the effectiveness of such devices.

Source: American Speech-Language-Hearing Association, 2004b.

Clinical COMMENTARY

When children are mainstreamed, direct contact with the classroom teacher is the best way to see that their needs are met. If intervention is handled diplomatically, audiologists and speech-language pathologists will find most teachers are receptive and eager to learn how to help their students. Special help includes assigning preferential seating, providing maximum visual cues, encouraging the use of amplification, providing written supplements to oral instruction whenever possible, and maintaining frequent contact with caregivers. Given the general scarcity of audiologists employed by schools, this important advocacy role for students with hearing loss is often carried out by the speech-language pathologist. It is axiomatic that any system of teaching children with hearing losses, in the classroom or speech and hearing clinic, is most effective if it is complemented by a strong home program. Certainly academic progress must be monitored with the parents on a more frequent basis than with normal-hearing students.

A parental decision to follow a certain course regarding a child's education and training may change, based on the reinforcement received for the efforts made and on new information acquired. The responsibility of the pediatric audiologist is to remain as a source of information and support to families, to follow up the initial diagnosis with regular hearing evaluations, and to assist with hearing aids and other listening devices as needed. Insightful clinicians must develop skills that allow them to facilitate, rather than to direct, families in the series of decisions that are so critical to fulfill the potential of children with hearing impairments.

The reader may have noted that a scrupulous attempt has been made throughout this text to minimize the use of the word *deaf*. Over 40 years ago, Ross and Calvert (1967) pointed out that the "semantics of deafness" might have a profound effect on the ability of a family with a child with a hearing impairment to cope with the problems that arise. The lay public, and to a large extent the professional community, have polarized people into two groups, those who hear and those who do not. When people are labeled "deaf," it means to many that they cannot hear at all and that they will remain mute. This can inhibit the use of residual hearing and the development of spoken language. Ross and Calvert state that ignoring the quantitative nature of hearing loss may affect the child's diagnosis, interaction with parents, educational placement and treatment, and expectations for achievement.

Communication Methodologies

The precise modes of communication by which profoundly hard-of-hearing children should be educated continue to be debated. Increasing numbers of these children are receiving cochlear implants at a young age, thereby circumventing their need for separate instructional communication modalities from their classmates. For children with profound hearing loss who do not have cochlear implants, many people believe that emphasis should be placed on speech, with amplification designed to take advantage of residual hearing. Strict adherents to this philosophy are often called *oralists,* who believe that, because all children live in a world in which communication is accomplished through speech, their adjustment is best made by teaching them to speak so that they will "fit in" with the majority of others.

Other experts believe that manual communication, by signs and fingerspelling, allows nonimplanted children with profound hearing losses to communicate more readily, so that communication skills can be learned more quickly, and specific subjects can be taught. Additionally, the *manualists* often believe that signing serves as a more useful communication system than speech for many of these children given that they will make adjustment to the nonhearing world where they will be accepted more completely.

The debate between manualists and oralists has a history that dates back to the earliest educators of those with hearing loss. While some are purists in their educational approach, others use a combination of signs and spoken messages to deliver their instruction. The following are some of the more familiar teaching methods.

American Sign Language

In American Sign Language (ASL), often called Ameslan, specific and often logical signs are created with the hands. Fingerspelling is used within ASL when no sign exists to represent a given word. (Figure 15.5 shows the manual alphabet.) ASL is often thought to suffer from inaccuracies in English grammar and syntax; however, it is not inaccurate when viewed as a language in its own right. ASL is considered by many educators to be a true language and is accepted by many high schools, colleges, and universities as a means of satisfying foreign-language requirements. For a demonstration of fingerspelling, see the video titled Manual Alphabet.

Auditory-Verbal Approach

Formerly referred to as unisensory or Acoupedics, the auditory-verbal philosophy is based entirely on the use of audition and early amplification with hearing aids. This method stresses the auditory channel as the means for the development of spoken receptive and expressive communication skills.

Aural/Oral Method

Often called the multisensory or auditory-global approach, the aural/oral method attempts to tap the child's residual hearing through amplification and to employ auditory and speechreading training. The child's output is expected to be speech.

FIGURE 15.5 The manual alphabet.

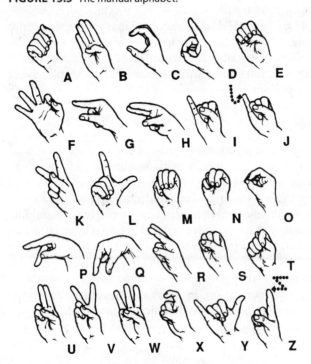

Cued Speech

Cued speech, developed nearly half a century ago by Cornett (1967), was devised to aid speechreading and speech development and employs eight formed handshapes in four positions, which are made close to the face of a speaker so that they may supplement speechreading information. The cues assist in differentiating among sounds that appear to be the same on the lips (for example, /m/, /b/, and /p/). The child must simultaneously attend to both the speechreading and the cues because the cues by themselves are meaningless.

Manually-Coded English

A variety of systems have been devised over the years that can all fall under the more general heading of **Manually-Coded English.** During educational instruction, these systems are usually accompanied by spoken English, which affords a total communication (TC) utilizing signs, residual hearing, and speechreading simultaneously. Proponents of this popular teaching methodology believe that language is learned more quickly and accurately through TC than by other methods, whereas critics maintain that it is unrealistic to expect some children to learn to listen, read lips, and follow signs at the same time.

Examples of Manually-Coded English include Signed English (SE), which follows the rules of English grammar; Signing Essential English (SEE 1), with specific signs for some articles and verbs as well as markers for tense and number; and Signing Exact English (SEE 2), which is a less than normally rigid system of signs that does not necessarily follow precise word order in a sentence. Pidgin Sign English (PSE) is a combination of ASL and some of the elements of systems that use sign markers to delineate plural and tense. An uncommon example of Manually-Coded English is Linguistics of Visual English (LOVE), which follows English word order but employs a slightly different written system. The Rochester Method, known as visible speech, employs the simultaneous use of speech and fingerspelling in a "writing in air" technique superimposed on normal speech. Certainly those systems of Manually-Coded English that do not follow English syntax may leave children at a risk of developing deficits in spoken English.

The Deaf Community

According to Vernon and Mindel (1978), the greatest psychological danger to the child with a profound hearing loss is the inability of the parents, and the professional specialists with whom they deal, to understand the problems involved. Their belief is that the frequent failure of amplification, even with speechreading and auditory training, testifies to the need for the early use of manual communication. They feel that children's psychological and educational needs are not met by forcing them into artificial situations and insisting that they become something they are not—hearing persons. This belief that deafness need not be looked on as a handicap, but rather as a characteristic, is the philosophy of what has come to be called the Deaf community. The term *Deaf* (with a capital D) should be used to denote those who identify themselves with Deaf culture, while the term *deaf* (small *d*) describes the hearing status of the individual (Woodward, 1972). From an audiological standpoint, "deaf" is reserved to describe individuals whose hearing loss is so profound that the auditory channel cannot be used as the primary means for speech reception or speech and language development.

Lane (1992) maintains that the Deaf community should not be regarded as disabled, but should be thought of as a linguistic minority, with its own culture and language: American Sign Language. He speaks of the resentment of this group against the intrusion of the "audists" into the lives and educational decisions of deaf persons. This is a viewpoint that has become increasingly prevalent. Lane (1987) also feels that the community of persons with severe to profound hearing losses is at odds with the professions that were designed to help it: "To achieve intellectual and emotional maturity at full participation in society most deaf children require an education conducted in their primary language, American Sign Language. . . ." Proponents of oral or combined oral and manual approaches to teaching children with hearing impairments may be just as adamant in their beliefs. Educational placement for children with hearing loss is an issue that is not soon to be easily resolved.

 ## Management of Auditory Processing Disorders

Chapter 12 discussed assessment of disorders beyond the cochlea, including auditory processing disorders (APDs). It should be noted that many of today's behavioral measures of central auditory function display their true value in their ability to describe the *communication impact* of auditory processing disorders. APD represents a disturbance or delay in the perception, recall, and organization of auditory information. These difficulties in the perceptual processing of auditory information within the central nervous system may be demonstrated by poor performance in sound localization and lateralization, auditory discrimination, auditory pattern recognition, auditory performance within a background of competing acoustic signals, or with degraded acoustic signals as well as difficulties with a variety of temporal aspects of audition (American Speech-Language-Hearing Association, 2004a). Whether for children or adults who have an auditory processing disorder, therapeutic intervention can be designed and implemented best when it is based on the study of the resultant impact on communication.

Management of APD in Children

Children with APD demonstrate difficulty paying attention or remembering information, require more time to process information, exhibit poor listening skills, and display problems following multistep instructions. In addition, they may have behavior problems and lower academic performance than expected for children with normal hearing and normal intelligence. These children may show a lack of attention to auditory stimuli, thereby increasing distractibility; a decrease in auditory discrimination and localization abilities, making the comprehension of speech more difficult; and difficulty with auditory figure–ground differentiation, resulting in a decreased ability for selective attention. Difficulties in auditory processing may be associated with a variety of conditions, including dyslexia, attention deficit disorder, autism, autism spectrum disorder, specific language impairment, pervasive developmental disorder, or developmental delay. The diagnosis of APD often begins with the child's pediatrician, who will systematically rule out other disorders that may have similar symptoms.

Frequently, APD is not evident until a child enrolls in school and the previous one-on-one home learning environment is replaced by a large classroom with an unfamiliar set of visual and auditory distractions. The child's self-image can deteriorate rapidly as he is repeatedly told he has normal intelligence and hears normally, yet he observes he is not performing as well as his peers.

Therapeutic intervention for APD in children can be best designed and implemented when based on the study of the resultant impact on communication. Often the audiologist and speech-language pathologist work together as a team in the management of APD. Research is ongoing to better understand APD and related childhood disorders and what might comprise the best management approach, with continuous evaluation of the effectiveness of any treatment employed.

Classroom management suggestions (Clark, 1980; Hall & Mueller, 1997) and classroom sound-field amplification or personal FM systems to improve signal-to-noise ratios (see Chapter 14) can be beneficial for children with APD. Classroom modifications to further enhance the signal-to-noise ratio may be as simple as placing tennis balls on the feet of chairs, adding curtains for sound absorption, and providing preferential seating for the student.

Audiological measures may lead to the diagnosis of APD, but the assessment contributions of the speech-language pathologist shed greater light on language ability and the functional deficits of communication that may point to remediation needs. Frequently, speech-language pathologists may work with the child with APD to improve language skills, phonemic recognition, and auditory memory as well as provide auditory training to enhance specific auditory deficits, including sequencing, auditory attention, auditory pattern recognition, auditory discrimination, auditory figure–ground differentiation, and localization.

Some children with auditory processing problems and concomitant language-learning impairment have benefited from speech perception training incorporating recorded speech with speech sound prolongations accompanied by amplification of some of the more salient acoustic features of speech (Cinotti, 1998). This program, known as Fast ForWord, consists of seven games targeting select aspects of language processing. A computer-based program known as Earobics designed for children with literacy problems has also been reported to be useful in the remediation of auditory skills for children with APD.

Auditory integration training (AIT) is another approach purported by some to retrain the auditory system and decrease what proponents refer to as hearing distortions. AIT, a method that has met considerable skepticism over the years, is based on the theory that prolonged listening to loud, frequency-altered music forces the auditory system to respond to a larger than normal frequency and intensity range for sound, resulting in a greater normalization of the auditory system. The American Speech-Language-Hearing Association concluded that AIT has not met scientific standards for efficacy to justify the use of this intervention by either audiologists or speech-language pathologists (American Speech-Language-Hearing Association, 2004e). However, the association did recommend a reexamination of its position should controlled studies that support AIT's effectiveness become available.

It is imperative that either the speech-language pathologist or audiologist advise the teacher of a child with APD of the ramifications of the disorder and the treatment that is being given. Explaining the difference between hearing the sounds of speech and fully comprehending their meaning may be useful in the teacher's understanding of the need for the child to associate the spoken word with its referent to aid comprehension. The greater the teacher's understanding of APD, the greater will be the child's learning success. Similar classroom management suggestions to those given to teachers of children with peripheral hearing deficits are also helpful to the child with APD.

Clinical COMMENTARY

While speech-language pathologists and audiologists may work collaboratively on many fronts within the management of communication disorders, such collaboration may be greatest in the assessment and management of auditory processing disorders in children. Clinical endeavors overlap for these two groups of professionals, with audiologists providing assessment of both the peripheral and central auditory systems and providing management of identified disorders, while speech-language pathologists provide assessment of language skills and provide appropriate intervention in this area.

Management of APD in Adults

Adults with cochlear hearing loss frequently have difficulties in speech sound recognition due to changes in the auditory periphery that attenuate and distort sounds. As some patients age, presbycusis may no longer be simply a cochlear phenomenon but may also affect the central auditory nervous system. This added central presbycusis can make the processing of spoken language even more difficult than it might be with cochlear hearing loss alone, especially when speech is presented rapidly or in the presence of competing acoustic signals. Audiologists frequently see elderly patients whose performance with amplification is significantly poorer than expected based on the audiological evaluation of the peripheral auditory system. Assessment of these patients' speech-recognition performance with auditory competition (as discussed in Chapter 5) can provide significant clinical insights before proceeding to hearing-loss treatment recommendations.

Within rehabilitation, the audiologist's greatest contributions for adults with auditory processing difficulties or central presbycusis often come through the improvement of sound input through signal-to-noise enhancement. This may be accomplished best through instruction on restructuring of the listening environment and the recommendation of personal FM amplification and various other hearing asssistance technologies. (See Chapter 14 for discussion of hearing aissistance technologies.)

The general loss of neurons and brain plasticity that accompanies the aging process may indeed justify a more compensatory approach in the management of auditory processing disorders with adults. In addition, to improve the overall listening environment for adults with central presbycusis, audiologists may provide general communication guidelines that have proven beneficial to patients with more peripheral hearing loss (Clark & English, 2004; Trychin, 1994). The high incidence of some degree of auditory processing difficulties among older adults, and the need to make appropriate recommendations when present, has led many audiologists to routinely incorporate means of screening for the presence of central presbycusis with this population.

While the underlying origins of APD may differ in children and adults, the overall goal of intervention is the same: an improvement in listening skills and spoken-language comprehension. Toward this end, management efforts may be aimed at restructuring listening environments and improving communication strategies coupled with specific auditory processing training. Interested readers may want to consult the suggested reading sections at the end of this chapter for details of a multifactor approach to remediation.

Management of Tinnitus

Tinnitus has been mentioned several times in this text. The term was first coined in the 19th century and comes from the Latin *tinnire,* meaning "to ring or tinkle." Complaints of ear or head noises go back through recorded history and accompany, to some degree, almost every etiology of hearing loss.

Nearly 30 million Americans have tinnitus frequently with no reported accompanying hearing loss (Kochkin, Tyler, & Born, 2011). The prevalence of tinnitus in children may be greater than commonly realized because children are probably less likely to report these sounds unless questioned (Clark, 1984). Graham (1987) reported that more than 60 percent of surveyed children with hearing loss requiring amplification experienced some degree of tinnitus.

While many people with tinnitus do not experience significant deleterious effects, tinnitus can have a negative emotional impact on individuals, affecting concentration, sleep patterns, employment, personal relationships, and social functioning. Indeed, as many as 2.5 million Americans report tinnitus to be so significant as to be considered debilitating (Davis & Refaie, 2000). Early measures of perceived tinnitus loudness suggested levels ranging from 1 to 20 dB SL (Graham & Newby, 1962). However, later measurement methods may be more commensurate with the levels of tinnitus patients' distress, yielding values ranging from 8 to 50 dB SL (Goodwin, 1984). The perceived severity of tinnitus is not solely rated to loudness perception but is influenced by the perceived annoyance and associated disability (Eggermont, 2012). Although the origin of tinnitus has long been a source of debate among clinicians and researchers, investigation of cerebral blood flow suggests that the source of tinnitus may lie within auditory cortical regions of the brain rather than the cochlea itself (Lockwood et al., 1998). This suggests that it may not be damage to the cochlea that gives rise to tinnitus, but rather aberrant changes within the central auditory pathways secondary to more peripheral impairment. However, the origin is not known for certain. It can probably arise from different sites within the auditory system and, if known, would probably not guarantee that an absolute therapeutic intervention could be developed (Sandlin & Olsson, 2000).

Fagelson (2007) describes an association between tinnitus and **posttraumatic stress disorder (PTSD)**. PTSD is a condition that can produce a variety of psychological and physiological symptoms and is seen frequently among combat veterans. The stresses of war and the exposure to dangerously high levels of noise can produce PTSD, with the latter also frequently resulting in noise-induced hearing loss with associated tinnitus. The presence of both these conditions in the same individuals can cause synergistic interactions that can be devastating, a fact that audiologists must constantly take into consideration in dealing with these cases.

Figure 15.6 summarizes many of the contributors to the perception of tinnitus, which has been variously described as "ringing," "crickets," "roaring," "hissing," "clanging," "swishing," and a host of other similar words. Tinnitus of a tonal quality is reported to occur more frequently than "noise-type" tinnitus and is judged by patients to be more annoying (Press & Vernon, 1997). With the formation of the American Tinnitus Association (DeWeese & Vernon, 1975), consciousness has been raised on the subject, and professionals have learned to heed the complaints of tinnitus sufferers. Other than the use of masking sounds to cover up the tinnitus—for example, a radio or white-noise generator at night and hearing aids during the day—little help was available until about 25 years ago. Treatment has included drugs such as vitamins and vasodilators and surgeries such as labyrinthine or vestibular nerve destruction, nerve blocks, and cognitive therapy, all with varying results.

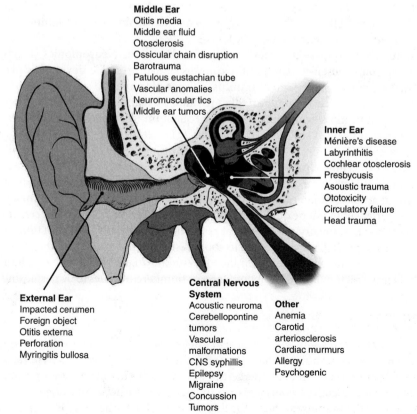

Middle Ear
Otitis media
Middle ear fluid
Otosclerosis
Ossicular chain disruption
Barotrauma
Patulous eustachian tube
Vascular anomalies
Neuromuscular tics
Middle ear tumors

Inner Ear
Ménière's disease
Labyrinthitis
Cochlear otosclerosis
Presbycusis
Asoustic trauma
Ototoxicity
Circulatory failure
Head trauma

External Ear
Impacted cerumen
Foreign object
Otitis externa
Perforation
Myringitis bullosa

Central Nervous System
Acoustic neuroma
Cerebellopontine tumors
Vascular malformations
CNS syphillis
Epilepsy
Migraine
Concussion
Tumors

Other
Anemia
Carotid arteriosclerosis
Cardiac murmurs
Allergy
Psychogenic

FIGURE 15.6 Possible contributors to the perception of tinnitus. (*Source:* Dr. Ross Roeser.)

Audiologists, frequently consulting with a multidisciplinary team, evaluate tinnitus, develop management strategies for combating the effects of tinnitus, and implement treatment and rehabilitation plans for tinnitus sufferers (American Academy of Audiology, 2000). Toward this end, the wearable tinnitus-masking unit has enjoyed some marginal popularity. Most such devices are similar to behind-the-ear and in-the-ear instruments (see Figure 14.6C and E) and are manufactured by some hearing-aid companies. The tinnitus masker produces a band of noise that surrounds the frequency of the tinnitus. When no specific frequency or noise band is reported as characteristic of the tinnitus, a broadband signal may be used as the masker. With patience and gradual adjustments, a close match to a patient's tinnitus can be obtained.

Most patients have given disappointing reports on the effects of tinnitus maskers, but a few are extremely satisfied with the results. Some claim that, not only is the tinnitus relieved by what they observe to be external sounds preferable to their own tinnitus, but also the tinnitus is temporarily absent after the masking device is removed. Although it is not completely understood, this effect may be explained by some residual inhibition in the auditory system. If a hearing loss is present, hearing aids with appropriate gain for the hearing loss often serve as effective tinnitus maskers.

The principles of biofeedback have also been applied for tinnitus relief. Biofeedback allows individuals to monitor their own physiological activity by attaching recording electrodes to special parts of the body; these recording electrodes permit the patient to observe and control the activity. Some patients have learned to monitor and suppress their tinnitus through biofeedback techniques.

Tinnitus retraining therapy (TRT) has been shown to provide patients with a means to habituate to the presence of their tinnitus (Jastreboff & Hazell, 1998). This therapy is based on the observation that the auditory system's contribution to the annoyance of tinnitus may be secondary to that of the limbic (emotional) and the autonomic nervous systems. TRT requires a substantial amount of direct work with patients, but when done properly, it yields a success rate for reducing tinnitus annoyance greater than 80 percent. A comparative investigation between the clinical efficacy of TRT and the use of tinnitus maskers demonstrated significantly greater improvements with TRT (Henry et al., 2006).

One of the more recent tinnitus treatment approaches known as Neuromonics (Davis, 2006) is based on a systematic desensitization of the tinnitus signal through a device that permits an intermittent, momentary perception of tinnitus within a pleasant and relaxing acoustic stimulus. Neuromonics tinnitus treatment reportedly provides rapid and significant reductions in the perceived severity of tinnitus symptoms and a subsequent improvement in the reported quality of life among treated tinnitus sufferers (Davis, Paki, & Hanley, 2007).

Some patients' complaints of tinnitus are much more dire than others with similar amounts of hearing loss in whom one might predict a similar type and degree of tinnitus. Schechter, McDermott, and Fausti (1992) liken the affliction from tinnitus to experiences of pain. They suggest that, given a certain amount of neural activity stimulating the pain centers of the brains of two individuals, the experiences might be quite different, being modified by higher brain centers, and by factors such as mood, personality, and culture. They also suggest that the effects of tinnitus on any given individual's personal life may, at least in some cases, be influenced by that person's psychological state. Given the interactions between the often unknown physiological base of tinnitus and the psychological reaction to it, the phenomenon of tinnitus continues to be perplexing.

Hyperacusis

Some patients with tinnitus report a decreased tolerance to loud sounds known as **hyperacusis**. The majority of sufferers report their hyperacusis to be equally disturbing as, or worse than, their tinnitus (Reich & Griest, 1991). Contrary to the common belief that hyperacusis represents an exceptionally acute sense of hearing, this disorder is more accurately described as a collapse of loudness tolerance. The threshold of loudness discomfort for the patient with hyperacusis has been reported to be inversely related to frequency, with less loudness tolerance as frequency increases. The threshold of discomfort for these patients may be as low as 20 to 25 dB SL for low-frequency sounds (e.g., 250 Hz), declining to as little as 5 dB SL or less for sounds greater than 10,000 Hz (Vernon & Press, 1998). Moorehouse, Waddington, and Adams (2005) report on numbers of individuals complaining primarily of difficult-to-bear loudness of low-frequency sounds. Hyperacusis is a phenomenon separate from loudness recruitment, often considered to result from decreased inhibition within the central auditory system.

Those individuals with hyperacusis may react in a frightened or startled fashion to common sounds such as the telephone ringing or the noise of a vacuum cleaner. These persons may resort to the use of hearing protection to better endure their daily lives, although overprotection of the ears may actually cause a worsening of the condition. In addition to shunning protection of the ears from everyday sounds, audiological rehabilitation has been successful with some patients with hyperacusis through a series of desensitization exercises over a protracted time (Vernon & Press, 1998). Clearly much more is to be learned about the phenomenon of hyperacusis.

Vestibular Rehabilitation

As discussed in Chapters 11 and 12, various lesions of the cochlea and beyond the cochlea related to disease, toxins, trauma, or syndromes can lead to symptoms manifesting as recurrent or constant dizziness, lightheadedness, or vertigo. Indeed, it is estimated that at least half of the U.S. population will be affected by vestibular or balance problems at some time within their lives and that these disturbances can be present within both the pediatric and adult populations (American Academy of Audiology, 2004b). Vestibular problems, which can be acute, chronic, and debilitating for many individuals, can create a blurring of vision, difficulty with balance, dizziness, spatial disorientation, and frequent and sometimes devastating falls.

While some argue that the audiologist's scope of practice should be defined by communicative function, others successfully argue that the anatomical origins of vestibular maladies place their assessment and rehabilitation within the audiologist's purview. Indeed, vestibular assessment and management are within the audiologist's scope of practice (American Academy of Audiology, 2004a; American Speech-Language-Hearing Association, 2004d), and many audiologists have built their careers around vestibular diagnostics and treatment through exercise therapy, habituation, and balance retraining (see Figure 15.7).

Both audiologists and some physical therapists provide services in vestibular rehabilitation or balance retraining with specific goals for their patients (see Table 15.3). These services may take the form of habituation or adaptation exercises, canalith repositioning, and balance retraining exercises. Vestibular habituation or adaptation exercises rely on the brain's ability to retrain its response to sudden movements. Patients are instructed to perform specific movements or assume specific positions that provoke their dizziness and are asked to repeat these movements until the brain habituates the response. Canalith repositioning has been found to be an effective treatment for many who suffer from benign positional vertigo. It involves moving the patient's head in a sequence of positions in order to reposition the otoconia within the semicircular canals. Balance retraining exercises are designed to improve the coordination of muscle responses as well as to enhance the integration of sensory information from the eyes, ears, and muscle receptors governing proprioception. If patients are found to have an impaired ability to maintain their gaze and focus, visual-motor exercises for gaze stabilization and eye-hand coordination may also be provided.

The extent of preparation in vestibular assessment and management that audiology students attain in their professional preparation has increased significantly in most universities with the advent of the professional doctorate in audiology. When training is not sufficient to undertake the responsibilities inherent within vestibular diagnostics and rehabilitation, it is a

FIGURE 15.7 Balance treatment is provided by some audiologists who specialize in vestibular problems. Here, a patient is repositioned from a seated position (A) to a supine position with her head to the right (B) as part of a six-step Eply maneuver to relocate free-floating particles that are inducing vertigo.

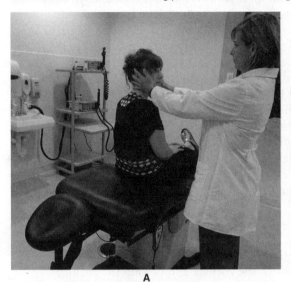

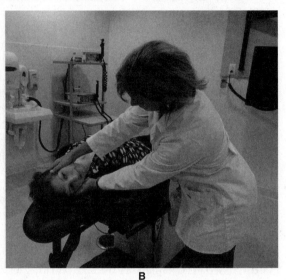

A   B

practitioner's ethical responsibility to ensure the acquisition of requisite knowledge and skills, possibly through postgraduate education.

Clearly, there is a need for the treatment of vestibular disorders because a complaint of dizziness is one of the most common within the primary-care physician's office, with concerns of balance being one of the most frequent reasons for medical consultation and hospital admission for those over 65 years of age (Desmon, 2000). The risk of falling need not be a natural part of the aging process and can be avoided (www.fallpreventiontaskforce.org; see Table 15.4). Given the possible existence of a complicated medical history for the patient with a balance disorder, evaluation and treatment should follow medical evaluation to ascertain if there are any identifiable and medically manageable origins to the stated complaints.

TABLE 15.3 Goals of Vestibular Treatment

- To decrease the frequency, intensity, and duration of dizziness episodes.
- To improve an individual's functional balance.
- To decrease the severity of the related symptoms of nausea, headache, and lightheadedness.
- To improve the individual's performance of daily activities.
- To reduce falls or the risk of falling.
- To develop compensation strategies for coping with disequilibrium and dizziness and the accompanying anxieties.

TABLE 15.4 Fall Prevention Suggestions for the Elderly Patient

- Health conditions and medication history should be assessed for potential contributions to falls.
- Engage in a general exercise program to improve strenth, flexibility, and balance.
- Keep your living space well lit and make generous use of nightlights.
- Clear clutter in the home and secure loose rugs.
- Wear well-fitting, sturdy shoes. Avoid slick soles, high heels, and floppy slippers.
- Install railings and grab bars, and use a cane or walker to ensure stability.

Multicultural Considerations

Ethnic, cultural, and linguistic diversities have been changing throughout the United States for decades. Diversity within our population may arise from a variety of influences, including ethnicity, religion, sexual orientation, geographic region, socioeconomic levels, educational background, mental/physical disability, and age-based peer groups (American Speech-Language-Hearing Association, 2004c). Approximately one out of every three Americans is nonwhite, with Hispanics constituting the most rapidly growing minority group in the United States. The percentages of culturally and linguistically diverse groups among school-age children was nearly twice that of the general population in the latter part of the 20th century (U.S. Bureau of the Census, 1990) and will comprise 22 percent of the school-age population by 2010 (U.S. Bureau of the Census, 2000).

Professionals have an obligation to become familiar with cultures apart from their own and to recognize the diversity existent within a given culture (Atkins, 1994; Ballachanda, 2001; Clark, 1999; Clark & English, 2004; Roseberry-McKibbin, 1997). Certainly, language differences between audiologists and patients can directly influence both the evaluation and the subsequent counseling that is provided (Flores, Martin, & Champlin, 1996). But beyond this, patients from different cultural backgrounds bring to the clinic values and assumptions that may in themselves be foreign to the clinician. Variations within culturally acceptable family dynamics and cultural influences on outward interactions with those perceived to be in positions of authority (like audiologists) can have a direct impact on acceptance and implementation of professional recommendations.

It has been estimated that only about 7 percent of audiologists and speech-language pathologists identify with a racial or ethnic minority background (American Speech-Language-Hearing Association, 2002a). Most Americans are proudly immersed within the dictates of Western culture to an extent that unfortunately breeds considerable ethnocentricity. When an employment setting brings one into repeated contact with persons from a different heritage, it behooves clinicians to become familiar with aspects of the cultures of their patient base. Such familiarity allows us to recognize attitudes and beliefs that need to be acknowledged and accounted for within rehabilitative planning. Roseberry-McKibbin (1997) provides an extensive overview of culturally diverse patients who may seek services from professionals in communicative disorders. As she points out, open and honest discussions, so common to Americans, are not the norm for many cultures. Japanese social norms, for example, dictate that one seeks out harmony and avoids conflict. Such ingrained social patterns do not interface well with some aspects of patient management.

Some Hispanics and Asians believe that only overtly visible physical disabilities merit intervention, a view that may greatly impede attempts at hearing rehabilitation. Individuals from some cultures may feel uncomfortable when professionals ask for family participation in the rehabilitation program because they believe such matters are solely within the province of the professionals. Others may feel attempts at intervention are inappropriate outside the context of family influence.

Certainly, not all people from different linguistic and cultural backgrounds remain steeped within the cultural constructs of their forebears. This is as important for clinicians to hold in mind as is the need for acceptance of differences that may be encountered. When cultural diversities arise, it is paramount that professionals strike a balance between accepting patient and family beliefs and encouraging exploration of available rehabilitative options. For information on how best to interact within a clinical setting with patients from different cultural backgrounds, the reader is referred to www.culturegrams.com and to the Center for Assessment and Demographic Studies, Gallaudet University, Washington, DC.

As described earlier, audiologists must remain cognizant of the views of those who align themselves within the culture of the Deaf community. Regardless of one's views on Deaf cultural issues, the Deaf community can serve as a valuable resource in hearing-loss management for families and professionals alike.

Tele-audiology

The practice of tele-medicine can now provide medical services to populations in remote areas of the world who might otherwise find that their inaccessible locations preclude more traditional medical diagnosis and treatment. The Comprehensive Telehealth Act of 1997 distinguished between tele-medicine provided by physicians and tele-health practices, which might be provided by any healthcare practitioner, including audiologists and speech-language pathologists. These distance-formatted practices may be provided through phone calls, within synchronous sessions using real-time, encrypted videoconferencing, or Internet chats, or within an asynchronous format through the forwarding of documents, electronic records, video clips, audio files, or photo images for review and online comment for subsequent discussion.

The World Health Organization (WHO) reports that hearing loss is now the number one disability, so the development of **tele-audiology** was perhaps inevitable. The vast majority of individuals with hearing loss, perhaps as many as 90 percent of those in need (Nemes, 2010), live away from centers that deliver traditional audiological diagnosis and treatment and can benefit from this approach to care. With tele-audiology, an entire battery of hearing-care services can be delivered to persons in need who do not have the means or opportunity to travel sometimes great distances to receive services traditionally located in urban areas. These regions literally encompass the entire world and can also include low-income areas in the United States.

In audiology, the provision of tele-health services between an audiologist and patient works well, for example, for portions of tinnitus treatment or hearing aid follow-up. Hearing tests can be performed using specially designed devices and can include remote hearing tests as part of the screening process of newborns. Cochlear implant reprograming, hearing aid programming and adjustment, completing probe-microphone measures, and a variety of hearing assessment procedures can be conducted through the assistance of a facilitator on-site with the patient during synchronous consultation with an off-site professional.

Certainly providers of tele-health services must adhere to their profession's ethical guidelines and provide services only within their profession's designated scope of practice. Audiologists and speech-language pathologists must be licensed or registered in their state to provide clinical services. Before engaging in tele-health practices, one must ensure the legalities for clinical treatment are also met for the state in which the recipient of care resides, and this may often necessitate that the clinician have an active license to practice in that state as well. There is little doubt that the desire of the profession of audiology to reach all those in need of hearing healthcare will lead to many changes and improvements in this unique specialty.

 ## Evidence-Based Practice

Practitioners of audiological treatment, like providers of intervention for any human disorder, should provide evidence of benefit derived for the services rendered. This is the underlying principle of **evidence-based practice,** which is most concisely defined as a "conscious, explicit, and judicious use" of the best and current evidence available when making decisions about patient care (Sackett, Rosenberg, Gray, Haynes, & Richardson, 1996). Evidence-based practice utilizes a combination of the practitioner's clinical experience and available research on the interventions provided.

The effective delivery of clinical practice that is based on evidence supporting the best of current procedures and technology is a five-part process entailing a definition of the problem, searching for available evidence to support the contemplated treatment, critically appraising the evidence, detailing recommendations, and assessing the outcome of the treatment delivered (Cox, 2005). Certainly integral to the success of evidence-based practice is the practitioner's ability to allow and encourage the patient's viewpoints and preferences, to elicit the patient's concerns, and to help develop a level of reasonable expectation for success with the rehabilitative intervention. It is the practitioner's responsibility to formulate interventions that offer the best solutions available for each unique individual.

Outcome Measures

Many aspects of healthcare are often delivered with insufficient consideration given to the evidence available that might direct one toward a different approach, or to documentation of the outcomes derived from the approach taken. In audiological treatment, the desired outcome may not necessarily be a resolution of the hearing impairment. Rather, treatment is more directly aimed at compensating for the effects of hearing impairment. The provision of services that do not benefit the patient is a violation of professional ethics and highlights the importance of documenting the positive outcome of audiological treatment.

Given the wide diversity in the patients seen and the auditory and balance problems they may manifest, it is not surprising that there is not a single, best approach to measure outcomes in the practice of audiology. Ideally, the efficacy of treatment provided should be documented through objective measures comparing performance on select tests prior to and following intervention and subjective measures of patients' and families' perceptions of improvement. The latter may be accomplished most easily through a comparative re-administration of the self-assessment questionnaire that may have been given when obtaining case history information. Self-assessment questionnaires to gauge the perceived impact of a disorder on an individual are available for hearing loss, tinnitus, balance difficulties, and other areas or problems treated by audiologists.

CHECK YOUR UNDERSTANDING

ACTIVITIES

EVOLVING CASE STUDIES

Through the course of this text, you have followed six case studies presenting six different types of audiological challenges that you may be called on in the future to address with your patients. Frequently, results obtained on patients necessitate audiological intervention that transcends diagnostic evaluation. It is within the realm of the treatment provided to patients that audiologists reach their highest levels of professional autonomy. There is perhaps no greater responsibility for audiologists than to ensure that their patients' communication function is restored as fully as possible so that they may attain their greatest potential in all areas of their lives. Toward this end, we turn to a final look at our continuing case studies.

Case Study 1: Conductive Hearing Loss—Outer-Ear Disorder

In Chapter 2, this nine-year-old boy arrived at the clinic with bilateral **anotia** and absent ear canals, and wearing a bone-conduction hearing aid (see Figure 14.9). You may recall from Chapter 4 that audiologic evaluation revealed a 50 to 60 dB hearing loss similar to

Figure 9.7. In Chapter 14, it was recommended that he attain bilateral osseointegrated auditory implants (see Figure 14.10). Given the conductive nature of this boy's hearing loss, his auditory performance is not confounded with the cochlear distortions and reduced tolerance for loud sounds so frequently seen in sensory hearing loss. However, devices designed to provide hearing through bone conduction, as with air-conduction hearing aids, rarely restore hearing to normal levels. A school consultation, possibly facilitated through the school speech-language pathologist who had referred the child, would be in order to ensure preferential seating in the classroom as well as exploration of sound-field amplification in the classroom (see Figure 14.18). Depending on his receptive and expressive communication skills, the patient will likely be continuing with speech-language services at his school. Part of these services should include discussions on how to field questions from peers and others regarding his hearing device and how to assert effectively for his own listening needs. Communication training and repair strategies would be also be beneficial to this boy and his family. Hearing treatment is not complete without referral for a genetic consultation.

Case Study 2: Conductive Hearing Loss—Middle-Ear Disorder

In many instances, conductive hearing loss is successfully treated medically and functional hearing is regained following intervention. The audiologist's role lies in the provision of an accurate evaluation prior to treatment and the determination post-treatment that no residual hearing impairment remains. Not only are these losses most amenable to medical intervention, it is these patients who frequently perform most successfully when audiological intervention is required. Due to the absence of active otologic pathology, the 23-year-old woman in this case study was fitted with air-conduction hearing aids, as discussed in Chapter 14. As with any patient who acquires amplification, it is imperative that she be scheduled for routine (annual or semiannual) visits to service her hearing aids and monitor her hearing for any change in sensitivity. Given normal cochlear function, it is unlikely that she will experience the same amplification limitations experienced by the patient in Case Study 3. As such, she may not require the same active spousal involvement in the treatment process nor the same hearing-loss management guidelines.

Case Study 3: Sensory/Neural Hearing Loss—Inner-Ear Disorder

As you may recall from Chapter 14, this 76-year-old patient has a bilaterally symmetrical, mild to moderate sensory/neural hearing loss of cochlear origin, accompanied by reduced speech recognition. It was noted by his wife at the outset of this case study in Chapter 2 that this patient has significantly reduced his interactions with others, particularly avoiding movies, theater events, and religious services. Our goal in the treatment process with the selection and fitting of appropriate amplification that began in Chapter 14 continues here. Even the best hearing aids can restore lost hearing function only partially. While the benefit obtained can be substantial, noted deficits will remain. It is the audiologist's responsibility to ensure that both the patient and any attending significant other, in this case the wife, are fully aware of the expected benefits and limitations of hearing-loss intervention.

To offset the remaining constraints on this patient's hearing, additional hearing assistance technologies that may improve signal-to-noise ratios in public venues should be demonstrated. In addition, it is imperative that the audiologist provides direct instruction in hearing-loss management. As discussed in this chapter, instruction may include identification of sources of communication breakdown (including speaker, listener, and environmental factors) and actions that may be taken to combat each of these in direct attempts to reduce communication stress. Discussions of this sort are always best conducted in a group setting, but when this is not possible, these points should be covered with the patient and spouse, and they should be provided with accompanying handouts.

To ensure long-term satisfaction, this patient should be scheduled to return annually or semiannually for servicing of his hearing instruments and monitoring of his hearing levels, with modification to his hearing aid's circuit settings made as needed. If it has not been completed before, his first six-month checkup would be a good time to repeat any self-assessment measure that was given during his initial evaluation. A comparison of results can quickly document self-perceptions of the benefit received from the intervention given. Such results are becoming increasingly important to audiologists who, like any other healthcare professional, need to justify the efficacy of the services they provide to insurance companies and other third-party payers.

Case Study 4: Sensory/Neural Hearing Loss—Auditory Nerve Disorder

As discussed in Chapter 14, following medical management of an acoustic neuroma, which may be through radiation or surgery or a combination of both, amplification approaches will be dictated to some degree on the level of residual hearing in the left ear. Given the presence of normal hearing for the right ear, speech communication in quiet will be unimpaired, and hearing assistance technologies for signal alerting may not be needed (except possibly when sleeping on the better ear). However, any means to improve signal-to-noise ratios in adverse listening environments should be discussed and demonstrated to this patient. Communication management suggestions for both this patient and her primary communication partners could prove beneficial in select situations (Clark & English, 2014).

Case Study 5: Nonorganic Hearing Loss

You may recall that this patient is a 45-year-old male who has recently sought legal action against his employer because of an alleged hearing loss. Our clinical responsibilities with patients who exhibit nonorganic hearing loss not only includes identification of the behavior, but also determination of true organic hearing levels when possible and referral for professional counseling when indicated. Discussing test findings with a patient whose test results are clearly invalid and without a clear organic basis for the exhibited hearing loss can be one of the more disconcerting and frustrating consultations in which audiologists engage. As discussed in Chapter 13, a direct confrontation with the patient who exhibits nonorganic hearing loss is rarely fruitful. If the clinician assumes responsibility for the inaccurate test results by, for example, blaming poor instructions or equipment difficulties and begins the test again, this may allow the patient to save face and provide more accurate results. It may be helpful to let this patient know that, if difficulties in attaining accurate results on the retest continue, there are other, more objective measures that may be required. If true organic thresholds cannot be voluntarily obtained from this patient and are believed necessary for disposition of the case, ABR testing should be recommended. Short of this, any report to the referral source should speak only to the discrepancies in the test findings and the lack of requisite cooperation to secure accurate results.

It is easy for clinicians to become annoyed with noncooperative patients, especially those who take more than the usually allotted time and interfere with the schedule. It is most important that the audiologist play a nonaccusatory role and avoid any terms that might be considered pejorative. The possibility of legal action has to be carefully avoided. Perhaps even more important is the fact that, especially in the early encounters with patients with nonorganic hearing loss, it is not possible to know the extent of any emotional fragility, and we do not want to contribute to any psychological difficulties the patient may be experiencing. While financial incentives most frequently seem to underly nonorganic hearing loss in adults, the motivators for children most often have a psychosocial underpinnng. As such, approaches with children who exhibit nonorganic hearing loss differ, as discussed in Chapter 13.

Case Study 6: Pediatric Patient

Through several visits with this patient, hearing tests have revealed a severe to profound sensory/neural hearing loss for this 3-year-old girl who possesses no meaningful speech and language. In Chapter 14, it was recommended that this girl be fitted with relatively powerful digital behind-the-ear hearing instruments with direct audio input capabilities to accommodate a personal FM system and thus enhance the signal-to-noise ratio of the speech she hears. It was also expected that she would continue with the referring speech-language pathologist for individual and group speech and language stimulation programs. Monitoring this child's progress in therapy will be one component in any future considerations that may be made toward possible cochlear implantation.

Throughout continued intervention with this patient, the audiologist and the speech-language pathologist must remain cognizant that, nearly universally, families in this situation are undergoing great, prolonged, and painful adjustments. Professional codes of ethics dictate that referrals be made when best practices dictate that this should be done. Certainly, referral to a parent support group would be an excellent step for this child and her family, which may include siblings, grandparents, or other relatives. In addition, constituent-specific support groups should be investigated for grandparents and for any siblings who may be old enough to have their own questions and concerns, expressed and unexpressed, about this new dimension to their home life. The availability of genetic counseling will also need to be broached with the parents, who at some point, often early in the process, will question the origins of this hearing loss and the possibility of its recurrence within their own immediate family or the future families of their children. Privacy legislation dictates that referral to any outside agency or professional person must be accompanied by a signed release from the parents to share pertinent information.

Summary

Diagnosis of the type and degree of a patient's hearing loss is an essential beginning to audiological (re)habilitation. For proper management, the audiologist must become sophisticated in the intricacies of history taking. The importance of a proper professional relationship between the audiologist and the patient (or family) cannot be overstated. Advising and counseling sessions greatly affect the overall management of those with hearing impairment. Audiologists also must maintain good relationships with other professionals who may be involved in the rehabilitation of the patient. Proper relationships are strongly influenced by the exchanges, such as letters and reports, among professionals.

Audiologists should be responsible for the total program of audiological rehabilitation of the adult patient with a hearing loss. They must make the determination of the need for special measures, such as speechreading, communication training, auditory training, the acquisition of hearing aids, tinnitus therapy, or hyperacusis desensitization. If hearing aids are indicated, the audiologist should figure prominently in the selection and fitting procedures.

When working with children, audiologists must muster every resource at their disposal, including interactions with caregivers and other professionals, in designing approaches that will maximize the human potential in every child with a hearing loss. To do less is a disservice to the children, whose futures may be profoundly affected by professional decisions.

Frequently Asked Questions

Q What can be done to improve the signal-to-noise ratio in a classroom?

A *Treatment of the room itself is the first step. Replacing hard surfaces with carpeting, acoustic tile, drapes, and so on, is one way, but it is difficult to find funds for these corrections in the public schools. The use of FM or IR systems can be very helpful for individual students.*

Q Must all audiologists learn American Sign Language?

A *This is not an official requirement, but because many audiologists will on occasion work with patients or families that communicate using American Sign Language, this is a practical thing to do. Individuals with hearing impairment who use this system of communication truly appreciate when hearing individuals make an effort to sign, even if they do so poorly.*

Q How much knowledge about the Deaf culture is an audiologist required to have? Or is there even a requirement?

A *As the Au.D. programs develop, there will be more emphasis in this area. The best answer is "the more, the better."*

Q Who is considered the team manager in hearing loss management?

A *In cases of adult hearing loss management, the audiologist is the primary provider of services, coordinating with others, such as vocational rehabilitation counselors, family physicians, and so on. In pediatric hearing loss, there is frequently more interaction among professionals, with the one in most frequent contact with the child and family assuming the role of team manager.*

Q What is the best means of attaining a case history?

A *The style of attaining case history information varies among clinicians and sometimes within a single clinician, whose style varies according to the type of patient seen. There is no single correct means of obtaining the case history, but the approach taken should ensure that the patient or caregiver is comfortable with the process, the clinician displays*

a level of interested concern, and the time together is free of interruption.

Q When should an audiologist refer a patient for genetic counseling?

A *Any time the etiology of a disorder is unknown, a genetic counseling referral should be made so that parents might better anticipate the likelihood of recurrence in a subsequent pregnancy. In addition, young adults who have a hearing loss should be made aware of genetic counseling services before they plan their own families.*

Q Is emotional or support counseling needed with all the patients an audiologist sees?

A *Information transfer or content counseling is the primary type of counseling audiologists provide to their patients. Personal adjustment, support counseling is certainly within the audiologist's purview and should be effectively infused within clinical practice. Additional counseling is frequently needed to help patients build the motivation they may require to follow through successfully on recommendations. The difficulty many professionals have is recognizing when emotional support counseling is needed. Audiologists should be constantly on the lookout for when more than content information is needed by their patients.*

Q Do most audiologists provide rehabilitation for their patients beyond hearing aid fittings?

A *Most audiologists do not provide rehabilitation beyond the mechanics of hearing aid dispensing and orientation. However, many patients do need more than this minimum. Audiologists should provide information about successful communication strategies, assistive listening devices, and support groups for those with hearing loss to almost all of their patients.*

Q What is auditory training?

A *In its purest sense, auditory training is therapy designed to improve auditory skill development. This is an important* *component of pediatric hearing-loss management; with adults, training usually focuses on the recognition of sources of communication breakdown, the development of better communication strategies and habits, and training to increase assertiveness levels to help others recognize what may be needed to ensure that messages are heard.*

Q Do many audiologists provide treatment for tinnitus or dizziness?

A *Most audiologists do not work in the areas of tinnitus treatment or vestibular rehabilitation. However, these two important areas of audiological management continue to grow.*

Suggested Reading

Brown, A. S. (2009). Intervention, education and therapy for children who are deaf or hard of hearing. In J. Katz, L. Medwetsky, R. Burkard, & L. Hood (Eds.), *Handbook of clinical audiology* (pp. 934–953). Philadelphia, PA: Lippincott Williams and Wilkins.

Clark, J. G., & English, K. M. (2014). *Counseling-infused audiologic care*. Boston, MA: Pearson Education.

Desmond, A. L. (2008). Vestibular rehabilitation. In M. Valente, H. Hosford-Dunn, & R. J. Roeser (Eds.), *Audiology treatment* (pp. 452–470). New York: Thieme.

Medwetsky, L., Riddle, L., & Katz, J. (2009). Management of central auditory processing disorders. In J. Katz, L. Medwetsky, R. Burkard, & L. Hood (Eds.), *Handbook of clinical audiology* (pp. 642–662). Philadelphia, PA: Lippincott Williams and Wilkins.

Montano, J. J., & Spitzer, J. B. (2014). *Adult audiologic rehabilitation (2nd ed.)* San Diego, CA: Plural Publishing.

Newman, C. W. & Sandridge, S. A. (2014). Tinnitus management. In J. J. Montano, & J. B. Spitzer, *Adult audiologic rehabilitation (2nd ed.)* (pp. 467–517). San Diego, CA: Plural Publishing.

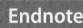

Endnote

1. For Alois Alzheimer, German neurologist, 1864–1915.

Glossary

acoustic admittance (1) The total flow of energy through the middle-ear system expressed in mohms (milliohms). (2) The reciprocal of impedance, which is expressed in ohms.

acoustic feedback The whistling sound that is created when the signal leaving the receiver of a hearing aid leaks back into the microphone and is reamplified.

acoustic gain The difference, in decibels, between the intensity of the input signal and the intensity of the output signal in a hearing aid.

acoustic impedance The total opposition to the flow of acoustic energy (as in the plane of the tympanic membrane). It consists of mass reactance, stiffness reactance, and frictional resistance and is influenced by frequency.

acoustic neuritis Inflammatory or degenerative lesions of the auditory nerve.

acoustic neuroma A tumor involving the nerve sheath of the auditory nerve.

acoustic reflex Contraction of one or both of the middle-ear muscles in response to an intense sound.

acoustic reflex arc The path of an acoustic stimulus that ascends from the outer ear to the brain stem and then descends via the facial nerves on both sides of the head to innervate the stapedial muscles in both middle ears.

acoustic reflex decay A decrease in the magnitude of the middle-ear reflex that occurs with constant acoustic stimulation.

acoustic reflex threshold (ART) The lowest intensity at which a stimulus can produce the acoustic reflex.

acoustic trauma notch A precipitous increase in hearing loss in the 3000 to 6000 Hz range, with recovery of hearing function at higher frequencies. It is usually, but not exclusively, associated with patients with noise-induced hearing loss.

acquired immune deficiency syndrome (AIDS) *See* human immunodeficiency virus.

action potential (AP) Change in voltage measured on the surface of a neuron when it fires.

acute Characterized by rapid onset, frequently of short duration.

aditus ad antrum A space in the middle ear containing the head of the malleus and the greater part of the incus. It communicates upward and backward with the mastoid antrum.

afferent Carrying impulses from the periphery toward the brain.

air-bone gap (ABG) The amount by which the air-conduction threshold of a patient exceeds the bone-conduction threshold at any frequency in the same ear.

air conduction The course of sounds that are conducted to the inner ear by way of the outer ear and middle ear.

allele One of two or more forms of a gene occupying corresponding locations on corresponding chromosomes.

alternate binaural loudness balance (ABLB) test Procedure that tests for recruitment in unilateral hearing losses. The growth of loudness of pure tones in the impaired ear is compared with that of the opposite (normal) ear as a function of increasing intensity.

Alzheimer's disease Condition associated with aging that accounts for about 60 to 70 percent of senile dementias and is associated with a variety of symptoms, most notably memory loss.

American National Standards Institute (ANSI) An organization established to oversee the creation and use of guidelines that affect all centers of U.S. business. These include acoustical devices like audiometers, construction equipment, and much more. It is also involved in accreditation of a variety of programs.

Americans with Disabilities Act A public law (P.L. 101-336) passed in 1990 to provide equal opportunity for individuals with disabilities.

amplitude The extent of the vibratory movement of a mass from its position of rest to that point farthest from the position of rest.

amplitude distortion The presence of frequencies in the output of an electroacoustic system that were not present at the input, resulting in a disproportional difference between the input and output waves.

ampulla The widened end of each of the three semicircular canals where they return to the utricle. Each ampulla contains an end organ for the sense of equilibrium.

analog hearing aid An amplification system in which the electrical signal is analogous to the input acoustical signal in frequency, intensity, and temporal patterns.

anechoic chamber A specially built room with large wedges of sound-absorbing material on all walls, the floor, and the ceiling, whose purpose is to provide maximum sound absorption and to keep reverberation to an absolute minimum.

annulus The ring of tissue around the periphery of the tympanic membrane that holds it in position at the end of the external auditory canal.

anotia Absence of the pinna.

anoxia Deprivation of oxygen to specific cells of the body, which affects their normal metabolism.

aperiodic sound Complex sound that varies randomly over time and does not have a fundamental frequency.

aperiodic wave A waveform that does not repeat over time.

Apgar test Method for evaluating the status of infants immediately and shortly after birth. Observations are made of the child's respiration, heart rate, muscle tone, color, and reflex irritability.

artificial ear Device for calibrating air-conduction earphones. It consists of a 6 cm^3 coupler to connect an earphone to a condenser microphone with cathode follower and a meter that reads in dB SPL. When calibrating insert earphones, a 2 cm^3 coupler must be used.

artificial mastoid Device for calibrating bone-conduction vibrators consisting of a resilient surface that simulates the vibrating properties of the mastoid process of the skull and an accelerometer. It is connected to a meter that reads in either decibels or units of force.

assistive listening devices (ALDs) Adjunct hearing instruments to improve signal-to-noise ratio. They may include personal amplifiers, FM systems, TV sets, or telephone amplifiers.

athetosis One of the three major categories of cerebral palsy, characterized by squirming or writhing movements.

atresia Congenital closure of a normally open body orifice, such as the external auditory canal.

attenuation The reduction of energy (e.g., sound).

audiocoil Recommended name to reflect this circuit's increasingly wider use beyond the telephone. Also known as *telecoil*.

audiogram Graphic representation of audiometric findings showing hearing thresholds as a function of frequency.

audiological rehabilitation Treatment of those with adventitious hearing loss to improve communication through hearing aids, hearing therapy, speechreading, and counseling. Audiological *habilitation* of children may also include speech and language therapy, auditory training, and manual communication. Also known as *aural rehabilitation*.

audiometer Device for determining the thresholds of hearing. Pure tones at various frequencies are generated, and their levels are increased and decreased until thresholds are found. Outputs may include earphones for air-conduction testing, a bone-conduction vibrator for bone-conduction testing, and one or more loudspeakers for sound-field testing.

audiometric Weber test An extension of the tuning-fork Weber test. The bone-conduction vibrator of the audiometer is applied to the forehead of a patient, and tones are presented above threshold. The patient is directed to respond by stating whether the tone was heard in the right ear, the left ear, or the midline.

auditory Referring to the sense of hearing.

auditory brain stem response (ABR) The seven wavelets that appear within 10 milliseconds after signal presentation.

auditory event-related potentials (ERPs) Auditory-evoked potentials (AEPs) that occur after latencies of about 60 milliseconds, with the largest positive wave at about 300 milliseconds.

The earliest AEP requiring active participation by subjects to generate the response.

auditory-evoked potentials (AEPs) The use of summing or averaging computers to observe the very small electrical responses to sound from the cochlea, brain stem, and cortex.

auditory late responses (ALRs) Those auditory-evoked potentials evident after about 60 milliseconds, usually of larger amplitude than the earlier responses. Pure tones may be used as stimuli, and frequency-specific information may be available.

auditory middle-latency responses (AMLRs) Responses that occur 10 to 50 milliseconds after signal onset and are thought to arise from the upper brain stem.

auditory nerve The VIIIth cranial nerve, which comprises auditory and vestibular branches, passing from the inner ear to the brain stem.

auditory neuropathy spectrum disorder (ANSD) Formerly referred to as auditory neuropathy/auditory dys-synchrony (AN/ADys), this disorder presents as a mild to moderate sensory/neural hearing loss with speech-recognition difficulties disproportionate to the degree of loss. In contrast to acoustic neuroma, there is an unexpected absence of ABR waveforms and a normal MRI.

auditory placode Thickened plate near the hindbrain in the human embryo that develops into the inner ear.

auditory processing disorder (APD) Difficulty in the development of language and other communication skills associated with disorders of the auditory centers in the brain.

auditory radiations Bundle of nerve fibers passing from the medial geniculate body to the temporal gyri of the cerebral cortex.

auditory steady-state response (ASSR) An auditory evoked potential for providing reliable frequency-specific threshold predictions in a clinically efficient time frame when behavioral thresholds cannot be obtained.

auditory training The training of the patient with a hearing loss in the optimum use of residual hearing.

auditory tube *See* eustachian tube.

aural rehabilitation Treatment to improve communication ability of those with hearing loss acquired after the development of spoken language.

auricle The cartilaginous appendage of the external ear.

auropalpebral reflex (APR) Contraction of the ring muscles of the eyes in response to a sudden, unexpected sound.

autism A condition of withdrawal and introspection manifested by asocial behavior.

autoimmune inner-ear disease (AIED) An inflammatory condition that arises when the body's immune system attacks the cells of the inner ear. The result may be a bilateral fluctuating and progressive sensory/neural hearing loss. Associated with tinnitus, aural fullness, and vertigo.

automatic gain control Special circuit within a hearing aid that prevents sounds from being overamplified for the impaired ear.

autophony A condition produced by some middle-ear or eustachian tube abnormalities, in which individuals' voices seem louder than normal to themselves.

autosomal dominant The capacity of a gene to express itself when carried by only one of a pair of homologous chromosomes.

autosomal recessive The inability of a gene to express a trait unless it is carried by both members of a pair of homologous chromosomes.

autosome Any chromosome other than a sex chromosome. There are 22 pairs in humans.

axon The efferent portion of a neuron.

barotrauma Damage to the ear by sudden changes in pressure, as in flying or diving.

basilar membrane A membrane extending the entire length of the cochlea, separating the scala tympani from the scala media and supporting the organ of Corti.

beats Periodic variations of the amplitude of a tone when a second tone of slightly different frequency is produced simultaneously.

behavioral observation audiometry (BOA) Observation of changes in the activity state of an infant in response to sound.

Békésy audiometry Automatic audiometry wherein patients track their own auditory thresholds for both pulsed and continuous pure tones by depressing a switch when the tone becomes audible and releasing it when the tone is inaudible. Results are traced on a special audiogram blank. This test is no longer popular.

Bel Unit for expressing ratios of sound pressures in base 10 logarithms.

Bell's palsy Paralysis of the peripheral branch of the facial (VIIth cranial) nerve.

BiCROS hearing aid A modification of the CROS hearing aid (*see* CROS) in which there is one microphone on each side of the head, delivering signals to the better-hearing ear when one ear is unaidable.

binaural Listening with both ears to either the same or different stimuli.

Bing test A tuning-fork test that utilizes the occlusion effect to test for the presence or absence of conductive hearing loss.

bone conduction The course of sounds that are conducted to the inner ear by way of the bones of the skull.

Brownian motion The constant random colliding movement of molecules in a medium.

calibration The electroacoustic or psychoacoustic determination that an audiometer is performing properly in terms of its acoustic output, attenuator linearity, frequency accuracy, harmonic distortion, and so on.

California Consonant Test A closed-message word-recognition test, with the emphasis on unvoiced consonants to tax the abilities of patients with high-frequency hearing losses.

caloric test Irrigation of the external auditory canal with warm or cold water to stimulate the vestibular labyrinth. In normal patients, the result is nystagmus with some sensation of vertigo.

cancellation The reduction of the amplitude of a sound wave to zero. This results when two tones of the same frequency and amplitude are introduced 180 degrees out of phase.

Carhart notch Artifact in the bone-conduction audiograms of patients with otosclerosis that makes it appear as though their sensorineural sensitivity is slightly poorer than it truly is. It is most evident at 2,000 Hz and often disappears following corrective surgery.

carotid artery The main large artery on either side of the neck. It passes beneath the anterior wall of the middle ear.

carrier A phenotypically normal individual, whose body contains a recessive gene for an abnormal trait, along with its normal allele.

carrier phrase A phrase, such as "Say the word . . ." or "You will say . . .," that precedes the stimulus word during speech audiometry. It is designed to prepare the patient for the test word and to assist the clinician (if monitored live voice is used) in controlling the input loudness of the test word.

cell body The central portion of a nerve cell.

central auditory processing disorder (CAPD) Impairment of the central auditory nervous system interfering with decoding of acoustic signals, including difficulties in sound localization and speech discrimination in noise. This term is often replaced by the less anatomically, more operationally defined term *auditory processing disorder.*

central masking The shift in the auditory threshold of a tone produced by a noise in the opposite ear when the level of the noise is not sufficient to cause peripheral masking by cross-conduction.

cerebellopontine angle (CPA) That area at the base of the brain at the junction of the cerebellum, medulla, and pons.

cerebellum The lower part of the brain above the medulla and the pons and behind the brain stem. It is the seat of posture and integrated movements.

cerebral palsy Motor disorder produced by damage to the brain; it usually occurs prenatally, perinatally, or in early infant life.

cerebrovascular accident (CVA) Clot or hemorrhage of one of the arteries within the cerebrum; stroke.

cerumen Earwax.

cerumenolytic Chemical substance (such as carbamide peroxide and glycerin) that is used to soften cerumen prior to removal.

CHARGE syndrome Congenital condition involving a number of body organs and almost every part of the auditory system.

cholesteatoma Tumor, usually occurring in the middle ear and mastoid, that combines fats and epithelium from outside the middle-ear space.

chorda tympani nerve Branch of the facial (VIIth cranial) nerve that passes through the middle ear. It conveys information about taste from the anterior two-thirds of one side of the tongue.

chromosome Structure in every animal cell nucleus that bears the genetic information.

chronic Characterized by long duration.

cilia Eyelash-like projections of some cells that beat rhythmically to move certain substances over their surfaces.

clinical decision analysis (CDA) Procedures by which tests can be assessed in terms of their sensitivity, specificity, efficiency, and predictive value.

cochlea Cavity in the inner ear resembling a snail shell and responsible for converting sound waves into an electrochemical signal that can be sent to the brain for interpretation.

cochlear duct *See* scala media.

cochlear implant Coil and series of electrodes surgically placed in the mastoid and inner ear. It is designed to provide sound to a patient with a profound hearing loss through a processor and external coil.

cochlear microphonic (CM) The measurable electrical response of the hair cells of the cochlea.

cold running speech Rapidly delivered speech, either prerecorded or by monitored live voice, in which the output is monotonous and the peaks of the words strike zero on the VU (volume units) meter.

commissures Nerve fibers connecting similar structures on both sides of the brain.

complex wave Sound wave made up of a number of different sinusoids, each with a different frequency.

compliance The inverse of stiffness.

component Pure-tone constituent of a complex wave.

compression (1) That portion of a sound wave where the molecules of the medium are compressed together; also known as *condensation*. (2) Decrease in pressure. In a hearing aid, a method of limiting the amplification of louder sounds relative to weaker sounds.

computed tomography (CT) Procedure for imaging the inside of the body by representing portions of it as a series of sections. The many pictures taken are resolved by computer into one image.

computerized audiometry The process of testing human hearing sensitivity by having computers programmed to present the stimuli and interpret the threshold results.

computerized dynamic posturography (CDP) Quantitative assessment of balance function for postural stability, performed by a computer-based moving platform and motion transducers.

conditioned orientation reflex (COR) Technique for testing young children in the sound field by having them look in the direction of a sound source in search of a flashing light.

conductive hearing loss Loss of sound sensitivity produced by abnormalities of the outer ear and/or middle ear.

condyle Rounded projection, or process, of a bone. The condyle of the mandible comes to rest in a fossa (a hollowed or depressed area) just below the osseocartilaginous junction of the external auditory canal.

Connected Speech Test (CST) A procedure by which the intelligibility of speech passages is measured on a sentence-by-sentence basis in the presence of a related background babble.

consonant-nucleus-consonant (CNC) words Monosyllabic words used in testing word recognition. Each word has three phonemes; the initial and final phonemes are consonants, and the middle phoneme is a vowel or diphthong.

CON-SOT-LOT Stands for "continuous tone, pulsed tone with a standard off-time (50 percent), and a lengthened off-time (80 percent)." A test for nonorganic hearing loss using a standard audiometer both ascending and descending from below and above the patient's threshold. The tones may be continuously on, pulsed on and off at the same rate, or on for only 20 percent of the time per pulse.

conversion disorder *See* psychogenic hearing loss.

conversion neurosis Freudian concept by which emotional disorders become transferred into physical manifestations (e.g., hearing loss or blindness).

Corti's arch Series of arches made up of the rods of Corti in the cochlear duct.

cosine wave Sound wave representing simple harmonic motion that begins at 90 degrees.

critical band Portion of a continuous band of noise surrounding a pure tone. When the sound-pressure level of this narrow band is the same as the sound-pressure level of the tone, the tone is barely perceptible.

CROS Stands for "contralateral routing of offside signals." A hearing aid originally developed for patients with unilateral hearing losses. The microphone is mounted on the side of the poorer ear, and the signal is routed to the better ear and presented by an "open" earmold.

cross hearing The reception of a sound signal during a hearing test (either by air conduction or bone conduction) at the ear opposite the ear under test.

crura Legs, as of the stapes.

crus Singular of crura.

cued speech System of handshapes or "cues" positioned near the mouth devised to augment speechreading by differentiating similar visual patterns of speech.

cyberknife Noninvasive alternative to surgery for the treatment of tumors anywhere in the body, including the VIIIth nerve. The system delivers beams of high-dose radiation with extreme accuracy.

cycle The complete sequence of events of a single sine wave through 360 degrees.

cytomegalovirus (CMV) Common virus that is a member of the herpes family of viruses and can cause congenital hearing loss when contracted by a pregnant woman.

damage-risk criteria The maximum safe allowable noise levels for different bandwidths.

damping Progressive diminution in the amplitude of a vibrating body. Systems are said to be heavily damped when the amplitude decays rapidly, lightly damped when the amplitude decays slowly, and critically damped if all vibration ceases before the completion of one cycle.

decibel (dB) Unit for expressing the ratio between two sound pressures or two sound powers; it is equal to one-tenth of a Bel.

decruitment The less-than-normal growth in loudness of a signal as the intensity is increased. It is suggestive of a loss of nerve units. Also known as *subtractive hearing loss*.

decussation Crossing over, as of nerve fibers connecting both sides of the brain.

delayed auditory feedback (DAF) The delay in time between a subject's creation of a sound (e.g., speech) and his or her hearing of that sound.

dementia The impairment of cognitive and intellectual functions. It is usually progressive and age-related, and is usually characterized by disorientation and impaired memory, judgment, and intellect.

dendrite The branched portion of a neuron that carries the nerve impulse to the cell body.

dichotic Stimulation of both ears by different stimuli. This is usually accomplished with earphones and two channels of an audio player.

dichotic digits test Test for central auditory disorders performed by presenting two pairs of digits simultaneously to both ears.

difference tone The perceived pitch of a tone resulting from the simultaneous presentation of two tones of different frequencies. The tone perceived has a frequency equal to the difference in hertz between the other two tones.

digital hearing aid Amplification system in which the input signal is stored, as by a computer, as sets of binary digits that represent the frequency, intensity, and temporal patterns of the input acoustical signal.

diotic Stimulation of both ears with stimuli that are approximately identical, as through a stethoscope.

diplacusis binauralis Hearing a tone of a single frequency as different pitches in the two ears.

diplacusis monauralis Hearing a single frequency in one ear as a chord or noise.

distortion In a hearing aid, the result of an inexact copy of the input signal by the output signal. Distortion is usually caused by the microphone, speaker, and/or amplifier.

distortional bone conduction The response to a sound stimulus evoked when the skull is deformed by a bone-conduction vibrator, distorting the cochlea and giving rise to electrochemical activity within the cochlea.

distortion-product otoacoustic emission (DPOAE) The emission of a sound from the cochlea, measured in the external auditory canal, which is the result of inner-ear distortion generated when two tones of different frequencies are introduced to the ear.

DNA Deoxyribonucleic acid, the fundamental molecular material that carries the genetic code.

Doerfler-Stewart test Binaural test for nonorganic hearing loss using spondaic words and a masking noise.

dorsal cochlear nucleus The smaller of two cochlear nuclei on each side of the brain, it receives fibers from the cochlea on the ipsilateral side.

Down syndrome Syndrome characterized by mental retardation; a small, slightly flattened skull; low-set ears; abnormal digits; and other unusual facial and body characteristics. Also known as *trisomy 21 syndrome.*

ductus reuniens Tube connecting the saccule with the scala media that carries endolymph to the cochlea.

dynamic range (DR) *See* range of comfortable loudness.

dyne (d) Unit of force just sufficient to accelerate a mass of 1 gram by 1 cm/sec^2.

dysacusis Distortion of an auditory signal that is associated with loss of auditory sensitivity. Evidenced by poor word recognition.

dysinhibition Bizarre behavior patterns often associated with brain-damaged individuals.

eardrum membrane The vibrating membrane that separates the outer ear from the middle ear; more correctly called the *tympanic membrane.*

ectoderm The outermost of the three primary embryonic germ layers.

effective masking (EM) The minimum amount of noise required just to mask out a signal (under the same earphone) at a given hearing level. For example, 40 dB EM will just mask out a 40 dB HL signal.

efferent Carrying impulses from the brain toward the periphery.

efficiency The percentage of time that a test correctly identifies a site of lesion and correctly eliminates an anatomical area as the site of lesion.

elasticity The ability of a mass to return to its natural shape.

electrocochleography (ECoG) Response to sound in the form of electrical potentials that occur within the first few milliseconds after signal presentation. The responses that arise from the cochlea are small in amplitude and must be summed on a computer after a number of presentations of clicks or tone pips.

electroencephalograph (EEG) Tracing showing changes in the electrical potentials in the brain.

electronystagmograph (ENG) Device used to monitor electrically the amount of nystagmus occurring spontaneously or from vestibular stimulation.

endogenous Produced or originating within the organism.

endolymph The fluid contained within the membranous labyrinth of the inner ear in both the auditory and vestibular portions.

entoderm The innermost of the three primary embryonic germ layers.

epitympanic recess That part of the middle ear above the upper level of the tympanic membrane. Also known as *attic of the middle ear.*

equivalent input noise level The inherent noise level within a hearing aid with the input signal turned off and the hearing aid set at the reference-test-gain level.

equivalent volume Method of approximating the compliance component of impedance; the volume (in cm^3) with a physical property equivalent to a similar property of the middle ear.

erg (e) Unit of work. One erg results when 1 dyne force displaces an object by 1 centimeter.

eustachian tube The channel connecting the middle ear with the nasopharynx on each side. It is lined with mucous membrane. Also known as *auditory tube* and *pharyngotympanic tube.*

evidence-based practice The conscious and clear use of the current best evidence, practitioner experience, and patient concerns and expectations in making decisions toward individualized patient care.

evoked otoacoustic emission (EOAE) Measurable echo produced by the cochlea in response to signals presented to the ear.

exogenous Produced or originating outside the organism.

exostoses Projections from the surfaces of bone, as the external auditory canal, that are usually covered with cartilage.

exponent Logarithm, or power, to which a number may be raised.

external auditory canal (EAC) The channel in the external ear from the concha of the auricle to the tympanic membrane.

external otitis Infection of the outer ear. Also known as *otitis externa.*

extra-axial Outside the brain stem.

false or exaggerated hearing loss *See* nonorganic hearing loss.

facial nerve The VIIth cranial nerve, which innervates the muscles of the face and the stapedius muscle.

factitious disorder *See* nonorganic hearing loss.

fallopian canal Bony channel, on the medial wall of the middle ear, through which the facial nerve passes. It is covered with a mucous membrane.

false negative response The failure of patients to respond during a hearing test when they have, in fact, heard the stimulus.

false positive response Response from a subject when no stimulus has been presented, or the stimulus is below threshold.

fascia Layers of tissue that form the sheaths of muscles.

fenestration Early operation designed to correct hearing loss from otosclerosis. A new window was created in the lateral balance canal of the inner ear, and the ossicular chain was bypassed.

fistula Abnormal opening, as by incomplete closure of a wound, that allows fluid to leak out.

footplate The base of the stapes, which occupies the oval window.

force The impetus required to institute or alter the velocity of a body.

forced vibration The vibration of a mass controlled and maintained by an external impetus.

formant Peak of energy in the spectrum of a vowel sound.

Fourier analysis The mathematical breakdown of any complex wave into its component parts, consisting of simple sinusoids of different frequencies.

free vibration The vibration of a mass independent of any external force.

frequency The number of complete oscillations of a vibrating body per unit of time. In acoustics, the unit of measurements is cycles per second (cps) or hertz (Hz).

frequency distortion Inexact reproduction of the frequencies in a sound wave.

frequency response The frequency range of amplification (as in a hearing aid), expressed in hertz, from the lowest to the highest frequency amplified.

functional gain The difference in decibels between unaided and aided thresholds of hearing.

functional hearing loss *See* nonorganic hearing loss.

fundamental frequency The lowest frequency of vibration in a complex wave.

furunculosis Infection of hair follicles, as in the external auditory canal.

gamma knife Removal of harmful tissue, such as tumors, by using gamma rays. These consist of penetrating electromagnetic radiation, which has shorter wavelengths than X-rays. The gamma rays arrest the growth of tumors without necessarily destroying them.

gene The unit of heredity, composed of a sequence of DNA, that is located in a specific position on a chromosome.

genotype The genetic constitution of an individual.

ground electrode The third electrode used in testing auditory evoked potentials to ground subjects so that their bodies cannot serve as an antenna.

harmonic Any whole-number multiple of the fundamental frequency of a complex wave. The fundamental frequency equals the first harmonic.

harmonic distortion The distortion created when harmonic frequencies are generated in an amplification system. Usually expressed in percentage of distortion.

Hearing Aid Industry Conference (HAIC) Organization of hearing aid manufacturers that provides standardization of measurement and reporting on hearing aid performance data.

hearing disability Difficulty in performing socially useful functions due to hearing loss. A given disability may or may not present a handicap.

hearing handicap The ways in which a hearing loss has a frustrating effect on individual roles or goals.

hearing impairment Abnormality of structure or function that is physiological, psychological, or anatomical.

hearing level (HL) The number of decibels above an average normal threshold for a given signal. The hearing-level dial of an audiometer is calibrated in dB HL.

hearing loss Any loss of sound sensitivity, partial or complete, produced by an abnormality anywhere in the auditory system.

hearing therapy Instruction, usually offered in groups, to enhance recognition of and intervention for those variables within the environment, or for poor speaker or listener habits, that impede successful communication.

helicotrema Passage at the apical end of the cochlea connecting the scala vestibuli with the scala tympani.

hemotympanum Bleeding in the middle ear.

hereditodegenerative hearing loss Hearing loss that has its onset after birth but is nonetheless hereditary.

hertz (Hz) Cycles per second (cps).

Heschl's gyrus *See* superior temporal gyrus.

heterozygous Possessing different genes at a specific site between paired chromosomes.

high-frequency average (HFA) American National Standards Institute (ANSI) hearing aid specification expressed as the average SPL at 1000, 1600, and 2500 Hz.

high-risk registry Set of criteria designed to help identify neonates whose probability of hearing loss is greater than normal.

homozygous Possessing identical genes at a specific site between paired chromosomes.

human immunodeficiency virus (HIV) Virus transmitted through body fluids that first appeared in the United States in the early 1980s. The virus affects the immune system and creates the possibilities of conductive, sensory, and neural hearing loss.

hypacusis Loss of hearing sensitivity.

hyperacusis Collapse of loudness tolerance with or without accompanying hearing loss.

hysterical deafness Older term for *psychogenic hearing loss.*

immittance Measurements made in the plane of the tympanic membrane.

impedance The opposition to sound-wave transmission. It comprises frictional resistance, mass, and stiffness, and is influenced by frequency.

incus The second bone in the ossicular chain, connecting the malleus to the stapes. It is named for its resemblance to an anvil.

individual education plan (IEP) Annually updated, federally mandated plan for the education of children with disabilities.

individual family service plan (IFSP) Annually updated, federally mandated plan for early intervention services for infants and toddlers with special needs and their families.

induction loop Continuous wire surrounding a room or listening area that radiates a magnetic field as electrical energy that is conducted through the wire from a microphone. The electromagnetic current flow from the wire is induced in the induction coil of a hearing aid (i.e., telecoil or audiocoil).

inertial bone conduction Stimulation of the cochlea caused by lag of the chain of middle-ear bones, or inner-ear fluids, when the skull is deformed, resulting in movement of the stapes in and out of the oval window.

inferior colliculus One of the central auditory pathways, found in the posterior portion of the midbrain.

initial masking (IM) The lowest level of effective masking presented to the nontest ear. For air-conduction tests, this level is equal to the threshold of the masked ear; for bone-conduction tests, the IM is equal to the air-conduction threshold of the masked ear plus the occlusion effect at each frequency.

inner ear That portion of the hearing mechanism, buried in the bones of the skull, that converts mechanical energy into electrochemical energy for transmission to the brain.

insertion gain The decibel difference between unaided and aided conditions as measured through a probe-tube microphone system. Also known as *real ear insertion gain (REIG).*

insertion loss The additional loss of hearing created by placing a hearing aid, turned off, within the ear.

insular Related to the insula, the central lobe of a cerebral hemisphere.

integrated circuit Inseparable unification of several transistors and resistors on a small piece of silicon maintaining an electrical isolation of the circuit components.

intensity The amount of sound energy per unit of area.

intensity level (IL) Expression of the power of a sound per unit of area. The reference level in decibels is 10^{-12} watt/m^2, or 10^{-16} watt/cm^2.

interaural attenuation (IA) The loss of energy of a sound presented by either air conduction or bone conduction as it travels from the test ear to the nontest ear; the number of decibels lost in cross hearing.

internal auditory canal Channel from the inner ear to the brain stem allowing passage of the auditory and vestibular branches of the VIIIth nerve, the VIIth nerve, and the internal auditory artery.

International Organization for Standardization (ISO) Worldwide consortium of 148 nations, based in Geneva, Switzerland, whose mandate is to oversee and set guidelines for literally thousands of devices, including audiometers. *See also* ISO.

intra-aural muscle reflex The contraction of the stapedius muscles produced by introduction of an intense sound to one ear. The reflex is a bilateral phenomenon.

intra-axial Inside the brain stem.

intraoperative monitoring The use of auditory evoked potentials, such as electrocochleography (ECoG) and auditory brain-stem response (ABR), for monitoring some of the electrophysiological states of the patient during neurosurgery.

inverse square law The intensity of a sound decreases as a function of the square of the distance from the source.

ISO Internationally accepted abbreviation derived from the Greek *isos,* meaning "equal." This single abbreviation is used in all languages to represent similar organizations that set standards for industry. *See also* International Organization for Standardization.

joule (J) The work obtained when a force of one Newton displaces an object one meter (one J is equal to 10 million ergs).

jugular bulb The bulbous protrusion of the jugular vein in the floor of the middle ear.

kernicterus Deposits of bile pigment in the central nervous system, especially the basal ganglia. It is associated with erythroblastosis and the Rh factor.

kinetic energy The energy of a mass that results from its motion.

labyrinth The system of interconnecting canals of the inner ear, composed of the bony labyrinth (filled with perilymph), that contains the membranous labyrinth (filled with endolymph).

labyrinthitis Inflammation of the labyrinth, resulting in hearing loss and vertigo.

latency The time delay between the presentation of a stimulus and the measured physiological response to that stimulus.

lateralization The impression that a sound introduced directly to the ears is heard in the right ear, the left ear, or the midline.

lateral lemniscus That portion of the auditory pathway running from the cochlear nuclei to the inferior colliculus and medial geniculate body.

lipreading *See* speechreading.

localization The ability of an animal to determine the specific location of a sound source.

logarithm The exponent that tells the power to which a number is raised; the number of times that a number (the base) is multiplied by itself.

Lombard test Test for nonorganic hearing loss based on the fact that speakers increase the loudness of their speech when a loud noise interferes with their normal auditory monitoring.

Lombard voice reflex The normal elevation of vocal intensity when the speaker listens to a loud noise.

longitudinal wave Wave in which the particles of the medium move along the same axis as the wave.

loudness The subjective impression of the power of a sound. The unit of measurement is the sone.

loudness discomfort level *See* uncomfortable loudness level.

loudness level The intensity above the reference level for a 1,000 Hz tone that is subjectively equal in loudness. The unit of measurement is the phon.

magnetic resonance imaging (MRI) System of visualizing the inside of the body without the use of X-rays. The body is placed in a magnetic field and bombarded with radio waves, some of which are reemitted and resolved by computer, which allows for viewing soft tissues and various abnormalities.

mainstreaming Integrating children with hearing impairments (or other disabilities) into the least restrictive educational setting. This often implies placement in a regular school classroom with special educational assistance, where necessary.

malingering The conscious, willful, and deliberate act of feigning or exaggerating a disability (such as hearing loss) for personal gain or exemption.

malleus The first and largest bone in the ossicular chain of the middle ear, connected to the tympanic membrane and the incus; so named because of its resemblance to a hammer (mallet).

Manually-Coded English Any communication system that expresses spoken English through a variety of hand signs and/or fingerspelling.

manubrium Process of the malleus embedded in the fibrous layer of the tympanic membrane.

masking Process by which the threshold of a sound is elevated by the simultaneous introduction of another sound.

masking-level difference (MLD) The binaural threshold for a pure tone is lower when a binaural noise is 180 degrees out of phase than when the noise is in phase between the two ears.

mass The quantity of a body as measured in terms of its relationship to inertia. The weight of a body divided by its acceleration due to gravity.

mass reactance The quantity that results from the formula $2\pi fM$ (two times pi times frequency times mass).

mastoidectomy Operation to remove infected cells of the mastoid. Mastoidectomies are termed as simple, radical, and modified radical, depending on the extent of surgery.

mastoiditis Infection of the mastoid.

mastoid process Protrusion of the temporal bone, behind the outer ear, one portion of which is pneumatized (filled with air cells).

maximum masking The highest level of noise that can be presented to one ear through an earphone before the noise crosses the skull and shifts the threshold of the opposite ear.

meatus Any passage, such as the external auditory canal.

medial geniculate body The final subcortical auditory relay station, found in the thalamus on each side of the brain.

medulla oblongata The lowest portion of the brain, connecting the pons with the spinal cord.

mel A unit of pitch measurement. One thousand mels is the pitch of a 1000 Hz tone at 40 dB SL, 2000 mels is the subjective pitch exactly double 1000 mels, and so on.

Ménière's disease Disease of the inner ear whose symptoms include tinnitus, vertigo, and hearing loss (usually fluctuating and unilateral).

meningitis Inflammation of the meninges, the three protective coverings of the brain and spinal cord.

meniscus The curved surface of a column of fluid. A meniscus is sometimes seen through the tympanic membrane when fluids are present in the middle ear.

mesenchyme Network of embryonic connective tissue in the mesoderm that forms the connective tissue, blood vessels, and lymph vessels of the body.

mesoderm The middlemost of the three primary embryonic germ layers, lying between the ectoderm and the entoderm.

metacognitive training Development of strategies to help a person to think about the process of thought in order to strengthen self-regulation of spoken language processing.

metalinguistic training Learning to think and communicate about language to aid in processing. Skill development may include use of mnemonics, rehearsal, paraphrasing, summarizing, and segmentation.

microbar (μbar) Pressure equal to one-millionth of standard atmospheric pressure (1 bar equals 1 dyne/cm^2).

microtia Congenitally abnormally small external ear.

middle ear Air-filled cavity containing a chain of three tiny bones whose function is to carry energy from the outer ear to the inner ear.

middle-ear cleft The space made up of the middle ear and the eustachian tube.

minimal auditory deficiency syndrome (MADS) Changes in the size of neurons in the central auditory nervous system caused by conductive hearing loss in early life. The result is difficulty in language learning.

minimum contralateral interference level On the Stenger test, the lowest intensity of a signal presented to the poorer ear that causes the patient to stop responding to the signal that is above threshold in the better ear.

minimum response level (MRL) The lowest level of response offered by a child to an acoustic stimulus. Depending on a variety of circumstances, the signal responded to may be either barely audible or well above threshold.

mismatch negativity (MMN) Small negative response evoked when subjects are instructed to attend to a set of stimuli in one ear while different signals are presented to the other ear.

mixed hearing loss Sensory/neural hearing loss with superimposed conductive hearing loss. The air-conduction level shows the entire loss; the bone-conduction level, the sensory/neural portion; and the air-bone gap, the conductive portion.

modiolus The central pillar of the cochlea.

monaural Listening with one ear.

monitored live voice (MLV) Introduction of a speech signal (as in speech audiometry) through a microphone. The loudness of the voice is monitored visually by means of a VU (volume units) meter (sometimes displayed as a series of light-emitting diodes).

Moro reflex Sudden embracing movement of the arms and drawing up of the legs of infants and small children in response to sudden loud sounds.

most comfortable loudness (MCL) The hearing level designated by a listener as the most comfortable listening level for speech.

mucous membrane Form of epithelium found in many parts of the body, including the mouth, nose, paranasal sinuses, eustachian tube, and middle ear. Its cells contain fluid-producing glands.

multifactorial genetic considerations Arising from the interaction of several genes and environmental factors.

multiple sclerosis (MS) A chronic disease showing hardening or demyelinization in different parts of the nervous system.

myringitis Any inflammation of the tympanic membrane.

myringoplasty Surgery for restoration or repair of the tympanic membrane.

myringotomy Incision of the tympanic membrane.

narrowband noise Restricted band of frequencies surrounding a particular frequency to be masked; usually obtained by band-pass filtering a broadband noise.

nasopharynx The area where the back of the nose and the throat communicate.

necrosis The death of living cells.

neoplasm Any new or aberrant growth, such as a tumor.

neuritis Inflammation of a nerve with accompanying sensory or motor dysfunction.

neurofibromatosis (NF) The presence of tumors on the skin or along peripheral nerves. Also known as *von Recklinghausen disease.*

neurofibromatosis type 2 Hereditary disorder characterized by bilateral tumors along the cochleovestibular nerve; associated with hearing loss and other intracranial tumors.

neuron Cell specializing as a conductor of nerve impulses.

neurotransmission The manner in which neurons communicate with one another neurochemically.

neurotransmitter Chemical substance that is released to bridge the gap between neurons so that neurotransmission can be facilitated.

Newton (N) The force required to give a 1 kg mass an acceleration of 1 m/sec^2 (one N equals 100,000 d).

nonorganic hearing loss The falsification or exaggeration of hearing ability for some conscious or unconscious reason.

Northwestern University Children's Perception of Speech (NUCHIPS) test A picture-identification test for measuring the word-recognition abilities of small children.

nystagmus Oscillatory motion of the eyes.

objective audiometry Procedures for testing the hearing function that do not require behavioral responses.

obscure auditory dysfunctions (OADs) Often difficult-to-diagnose auditory processing disorders.

occlusion effect (OE) The impression of increased loudness of a bone-conducted tone when the outer ear is tightly covered or occluded.

octave The difference between two tones separated by a frequency ratio of 2:1.

ohm (Ω) Unit of impedance.

operant conditioning audiometry (OCA) The use of tangible reinforcement, such as edible items, to condition difficult-to-test patients for pure-tone audiometry.

organ of Corti The end organ of hearing found within the scala media of the cochlea.

oscillation The back-and-forth movement of a vibrating body.

osseocartilaginous junction The union between the bony and cartilaginous portions of the external auditory canal.

osseotympanic bone conduction The contribution to hearing by bone conduction created when the vibrating skull sets the air in the external ear canal into vibration, causing sound waves to pass down the canal, impinge on the eardrum membrane, and be conducted through the middle ear to the cochlea.

ossicles The chain of three tiny bones (malleus, incus, and stapes) found in each middle ear.

osteitis Inflammation of bone marked by tenderness, enlargement, and pain.

osteomyelitis Inflammation of bone caused by a purulent infection.

otalgia Pain in the ear.

otitis media Any infection of the middle ear.

otoacoustic emissions (OAEs) Sounds emanating from the cochlea that can be detected in the external auditory canal with probe-tube microphones.

otocyst The auditory vesicle (sac) of the human embryo.

otology Subspecialty of medicine devoted to the diagnosis and treatment of diseases of the ear.

otomycosis Fungal infection of the external ear.

otoplasty Any plastic surgery of the outer ear.

otorrhea Any discharge from the external auditory canal or from the middle ear.

otosclerosis The laying down of new bone in the middle ear, usually around the footplate of the stapes. When it interferes with stapedial vibration, it produces a progressive conductive hearing loss.

otoscope Special flashlight device with a funnel-like speculum on the end, designed to observe the tympanic membrane.

otospongiosis *See* otosclerosis.

ototoxic Poisonous to the ear.

outer ear The outermost portion of the hearing mechanism, filled with air, whose primary function is to carry sounds to the middle ear.

output sound-pressure level (OSPL) The newer term for maximum power output of a hearing aid; the highest sound-pressure level to leave the receiver of a hearing aid, regardless of the input level.

oval window A tiny, oval-shaped aperture beneath the footplate of the stapes. The oval window separates the middle ear from the inner ear.

overmasking (OM) When a masking noise presented to the non-test ear is of sufficient intensity to shift the threshold in the test ear beyond its true value. In overmasking, the masking noise crosses from the masked ear to the test ear by bone conduction.

overtone Any whole-number multiple of the fundamental frequency of a complex wave. It differs from the harmonic only in the numbering used (e.g., the first overtone is equal to the second harmonic).

paracusis willisii Condition found among patients with conductive hearing loss in which they understand speech better in noisy than in quiet surroundings.

parietal lobe The division of each side of the cerebral cortex between the frontal and occipital lobes.

pars flaccida The loose folds of epithelium of the tympanic membrane above the malleus. Also known as *Shrapnell's membrane.*

pars tensa All of the remaining (taut) portion of the tympanic membrane besides the pars flaccida.

Pascal (Pa) Unit of pressure equal to 1 N/m^2.

PB Max The highest word-recognition score obtained with phonetically balanced (PB) word lists on a performance-intensity function, regardless of level.

performance-intensity function for PB word lists (PI-PB) Graph showing the percentage of correctly identified word-recognition materials as a function of intensity. The graph usually shows the word-recognition score on the ordinate and the sensation level on the abscissa.

perilymph The fluid contained in both the auditory and vestibular portions of the bony labyrinth of the inner ear.

period The duration (in seconds) of one cycle of vibration. The period is the reciprocal of frequency (e.g., the period of a 1,000 Hz tone is 1/1,000 second).

periodic sound Complex sound that repeats over time.

permanent threshold shift (PTS) Permanent sensory/neural loss of hearing, usually associated with exposure to intense noise.

perseveration Persistent repetition of an activity.

pharyngeal arches Paired embryonic arches that modify, in humans, into structures of the ear and neck. In fish, they modify into gills.

pharyngotympanic tube *See* eustachian tube.

phase The relationship in time between two or more waves.

phenotype The observable makeup of an individual that is determined by genetic or a combination of genetic and environmental factors.

phon The unit of loudness level. It corresponds to the loudness of a signal at other frequencies equal to the intensity of a 1,000 Hz tone.

phonemic regression Slowness in auditory comprehension associated with advanced age.

phonetically balanced (PB) word lists Lists of monosyllabic words used for determining word-recognition scores. Theoretically, each list contains the same distribution of phonemes that occurs in connected English discourse.

physical-volume test (PVT) High sound intensity, suggesting a large volume of air (greater than 5 cm^3) may be observed on c_1 during immittance measures. This indicates that a patent PE tube or tympanic membrane perforation is present.

Picture Identification Task (PIT) Word-recognition test using pictures of rhyming CNC (consonant-nucleus-consonant) words.

pinna The auricle of the external ear.

pinnaplasty Cosmetic operation designed to improve the appearance of the pinna.

pitch The subjective impression of the highness or lowness of a sound; the psychological correlate of frequency.

place theory of hearing The explanation for pitch perception based on a precise place on the organ of Corti, which, when stimulated, results in the perception of a specific pitch.

plasticity The ability of cells, such as those in the auditory centers of the brain, to become altered in order to conform to their immediate environment.

plateau (1) The theoretical point in clinical masking at which the level of noise in the nontest ear may be raised or lowered about 15 dB without affecting the threshold of the signal in the test ear. (2) The levels between undermasking and overmasking at which the true threshold of the test ear may be seen.

pneumatic mastoid The formation of air cavities in tissues, as in the temporal bones of the skull.

politzerization Inflation of the middle ear via the eustachian tube by forcing air through the nose.

pons Bridge of fibers and neurons that connect the two sides of the brain at its base.

positron emission tomography (PET) Medical imaging procedure that can indicate changes in the brain with a minimum of patient exposure to radioactivity. It is useful in identifying biochemical changes in the brain.

postlinguistic hearing loss Hearing loss acquired by children after they have developed some language skills.

posttraumatic stress disorder (PTSD) Development of dramatic symptoms, including cognitive dysfunction, following a psychologically traumatic event.

potential energy Energy resulting from a fixed and relative position, as in a coiled spring.

power The rate at which work is done. Units of measurement are watts or ergs/second.

predictive value The percentage of all positive test results that are truly positive and the percentage of all negative test results that are truly negative.

prelinguistic hearing loss Hearing loss that is either congenital or acquired before language skills have been developed.

presbycusis Hearing loss associated with old age.

pressure Force over an area of surface.

pressure-equalizing (PE) tube Short tube or grommet placed through a myringotomy incision in a tympanic membrane to allow for middle-ear ventilation.

prevalence The number of existing cases of a disease or condition within a population at any given time.

probe-tube microphone Microphone used to provide electroacoustic measures of hearing aid performance as the instrument is worn. The test is performed by placing a thin silicone tube, which is connected to a microphone that is inserted into the external auditory canal.

promontory Obtrusion into the middle ear, at its labyrinthine wall, produced by the basal turn of the cochlea.

pseudohypacusis *See* nonorganic hearing loss.

psychogenic hearing loss Nonorganic hearing loss, possibly produced at the unconscious level, for example, by an anxiety state.

psychophysical tuning curve (PTC) The measurable response in the cochlea to specific frequencies introduced into the ear.

pure tone Tone of only one frequency (i.e., no harmonics).

pure-tone average (PTA) The average of the hearing levels at frequencies 500, 1000, and 2000 Hz for each ear, as obtained on a pure-tone hearing test. Sometimes the pure-tone average is computed by averaging the two lowest thresholds obtained at 500, 1000, and 2000 Hz.

purulent Related to the formation of pus.

quality The sharpness of resonance of a sound system; the vividness or identifying characteristics of a sound; the subjective counterpart of spectrum; timbre.

range of comfortable loudness (RCL) The difference, in decibels, between the threshold for speech and the point at which speech becomes uncomfortably loud. It is determined by subtracting the SRT from the UCL. Also called the dynamic range (DR) for speech.

Rapidly Alternating Speech Perception (RASP) test Test for central auditory disorders in which sentences are rapidly switched from the left ear to the right ear. Normal brain-stem function is required for discrimination.

rarefaction That portion of a sound wave where the molecules become less densely packed per unit of space.

ratio The mathematical result of a quantity divided by another quantity of the same kind, often expressed as a fraction.

reactance The contribution to total acoustic impedance provided by mass, stiffness, and frequency.

recruitment Large increase in the perceived loudness of a signal produced by relatively small increases in intensity above threshold; it is symptomatic of some hearing losses produced by damage to the cochlea.

reference test gain The acoustic gain of a hearing aid as measured in a hearing aid test box. The gain control of the aid is set to amplify an input signal of 60 dB SPL to a level 17 dB below the OSPL90 value. The average values at 1000, 1600, and 2500 Hz determine the reference test gain.

reflex-activating stimulus (RAS) Pure tone or other acoustic signal of high intensity designed to cause the stapedial muscle to contract. The RAS can be presented through the probe assembly of an immittance meter to observe an acoustic reflex in the ear that houses the probe tip (the ipsilateral reflex), or it can be presented via an earphone in the ear opposite the probe (the contralateral acoustic reflex).

Reissner's membrane Membrane extending the entire length of the cochlea, separating the scala media from the scala vestibuli.

resistance The opposition to a force.

resonance The ability of a mass to vibrate at a particular frequency with a minimum application of external force.

resonance theory of hearing Nineteenth-century theory of pitch perception that suggested that the cochlea consisted of a series of resonating tubes, each tuned to a specific frequency.

resonance-volley theory of hearing Combination of the place and frequency theories of hearing; it suggests that nerve units in the auditory nerve fire in volleys, allowing pitch perception up to about 4000 Hz. Perception of pitch above 4000 Hz is determined by the point of greatest excitation on the basilar membrane.

resonant frequency The frequency at which a mass vibrates with the least amount of external force; the natural frequency of vibration of a mass.

retrocochlear Located behind the cochlea.

reverberation Short-term echo, or the continuation of a sound in a closed area after the source has stopped vibrating, resulting from reflection and refraction of sound waves.

Rh factor Pertaining to the protein factor found on the surface of the red blood cells in most humans. Named for the Rhesus monkey, in which it was first observed.

Rinne test Tuning-fork test that compares hearing by air conduction with hearing by bone conduction.

rotary chair testing Test of vestibular function using a chair that rotates with varying velocity in both clockwise and counterclockwise directions. During rotation, electronystagmographic findings are recorded.

round window Small, round aperture containing a thin but tough membrane. The round window separates the middle ear from the inner ear.

saccule The smaller of the two sacs found in the membranous vestibular labyrinth; it contains an end organ of equilibrium.

scala media The duct in the cochlea separating the scala vestibuli from the scala tympani. It is filled with endolymph and contains the organ of Corti.

scala tympani The duct in the cochlea below the scala media; it is filled with perilymph.

scala vestibuli The duct in the cochlea above the scala media; it is filled with perilymph.

Schwabach test Tuning-fork test that compares an individual's hearing by bone conduction with the hearing of an examiner (who is presumed to have normal hearing).

Schwartze sign Red glow seen through the tympanic membrane and produced by increased vascularity of the promontory in some cases of otosclerosis.

Screening Test for Auditory Processing Disorders (SCAN) Rapid test for central auditory processing disorders comprising three subtests: filtered words, auditory figure ground, and dichotic listening.

semicircular canals Three loops in the vestibular portion of the inner ear responsible for the sensation of turning.

sensation level (SL) The number of decibels above the hearing threshold of a given subject for a given signal.

sensitivity The percentage of time a test correctly identifies a site of lesion.

sensitivity prediction from the acoustic reflex (SPAR) Test designed to identify the presence and approximate degree of sensory/neural hearing loss through comparison of acoustic reflex thresholds elicited with pure tones and with broadband noise.

sensory/neural hearing loss Formerly called perceptive loss or nerve loss; the loss of hearing sensitivity produced by damage or alteration of the sensory mechanism of the cochlea or the neural structures that lie beyond.

serous effusion The collection of fluid in the middle-ear space, with possible drainage into the external ear canal. Also known as *serous otitis media.*

short increment sensitivity index (SISI) Test designed to determine a patient's ability to detect small changes (1 dB) in intensity of a pure tone presented at 20 dB SL.

Shrapnell's membrane The pars flaccida of the tympanic membrane.

signal-to-noise ratio (SNR) The difference, in decibels, between a signal (such as speech) and a noise presented to the same ear(s). When the speech has greater intensity than the noise, a positive sign is used; when the noise has greater intensity than the signal, a negative sign is used.

sine wave *See* sinusoidal wave.

sinusoidal wave The waveform of a pure tone showing simple harmonic motion. Also known as *sine wave.*

site of lesion The precise area in the auditory system producing symptoms of abnormal auditory function.

somatosensory Spatial orientation provided by proprioceptive input, as by the support the body receives on a surface.

sone The unit of loudness measurement. One sone equals the loudness of a 1,000 Hz tone at 40 dB SPL.

sound-evoked muscle reflex Reflex believed to be generated from acoustical stimulation of the saccule. It is used in the diagnosis of vestibular disorders.

sound-level meter Device designed for measurement of the intensity of sound waves in air. It consists of a microphone, an amplifier, a frequency-weighting circuit, and a meter calibrated in decibels with a reference of 20 µPa.

sound-pressure level (SPL) An expression of the pressure of a sound. The reference level in decibels is 20 µPa.

specificity The percentage of time a test correctly rejects an incorrect diagnosis.

spectrum The sum of the components of a complex wave.

speech conservation Therapy to maintain clear articulation when the auditory feedback for speech production has been hindered by postlinguistic hearing loss.

speech-detection threshold (SDT) The hearing level at which a listener can just detect the presence of an ongoing speech signal and identify it as speech. Also known as *speech awareness threshold (SAT).*

speech-language pathology The study of speech, language, and voice disorders in children and adults for the purposes of diagnosis and treatment.

Speech Perception in Noise (SPIN) test Prerecorded sentence test with a voice babble recorded on the second channel of the same recording.

speechreading The use of visual (primarily facial) cues to determine the words of a speaker.

speech-recognition score (SRS) The percentage of correctly identified items on a speech-recognition test.

speech-recognition threshold (SRT) The threshold of intelligibility of speech; the lowest intensity at which at least 50 percent of a list of spondees can be identified correctly.

speech spectrum The overall level and frequency composition of the energy of everyday conversational speech.

spiral ligament The thickened outer portion of the periosteum of the cochlear duct that forms a spiral band and attaches to the basilar membrane.

spondaic word Two-syllable word pronounced with equal stress on both syllables. Also known as *spondee.*

spontaneous otoacoustic emission (SOAE) Weak sound, emanating from the cochlea with no external stimulation, that travels through the middle ear and can be measured by a sensitive microphone placed in the external auditory canal.

stacked ABR Composite auditory brain-stem response reflecting activity from all frequency regions of the cochlea attained by aligning (in time) and adding the amplitudes of derived narrowband ABRs obtained using a high-pass noise/subtraction technique. The result yields a measure more sensitive to identification of small acoustic neuromas.

Staggered Spondaic Word (SSW) test A test for central auditory disorders utilizing the dichotic listening task of two spondaic words so that the second syllable presented to one ear is heard simultaneously with the first syllable presented to the other ear.

stapedectomy Operation designed to improve hearing in cases of otosclerosis by removing the affected stapes and replacing it with a prosthesis.

stapedius muscle Tiny muscle that is innervated by the facial nerve and connected to the stapes in the middle ear by the stapedius tendon. Both stapedius muscles normally contract, causing a change in the resting position of the tympanic membrane when either ear is stimulated by an intense sound.

stapedotomy Small fenestra stapedectomy.

stapes The third and smallest bone in the ossicular chain of the middle ear, connected to the incus and standing in the oval window; so named because of its resemblance to a stirrup.

stapes mobilization Operation to improve hearing in cases of otosclerosis by breaking the stapes free of its fixation in the oval window and allowing normal vibration. It is no longer commonly performed.

static acoustic compliance Measurement of the mobility of the tympanic membrane.

Stenger principle When two tones of the same frequency are presented to both ears simultaneously, only the louder one is perceived.

Stenger test Test for unilateral nonorganic hearing loss based on the Stenger principle.

stenosis Abnormal narrowing, as of the external auditory canal.

stereocilia Protoplasmic filament on the surface of a cell (e.g., a hair cell).

sternocleidomastoid muscle Large muscle that runs from the mastoid process to the joint between the collarbones and the sternum at the base of the throat. Also known as *trapezius muscle.*

stiffness The flexibility or pliancy of a mass. The inverse of compliance.

stiffness reactance The quantity that results when the stiffness of a body is divided by $2\pi f$ (two times pi times frequency).

stria vascularis Vascular strip that lies along the outer wall of the scala media. It is responsible for the secretion and absorption of endolymph, it supplies oxygen and nutrients to the organ of Corti, and it affects the positive DC potential of the endolymph.

subluxation Incomplete dislocation or sprain.

sudden idiopathic sensory/neural hearing loss (SISNHL) This condition refers to a hearing loss, usually unilateral, that may develop over the course of a few days or occur seemingly instantaneously with no known etiology.

superior olivary complex (SOC) One of the auditory relay stations in the midbrain, largely comprising units from the cochlear nuclei.

superior temporal gyrus The convolution of the temporal lobe believed to be the seat of language comprehension of the auditory system.

suppurative Producing pus.

synapse The area of communication between neurons where a nerve impulse passes from an axon of one neuron to the cell body or dendrite of another.

syndrome Set of symptoms that appear together to indicate a specific pathological condition.

synthetic sentence identification (SSI) Method for determining word-recognition scores by means of 10 seven-word sentences that are grammatically correct but meaningless.

tactile response The response obtained during bone-conduction (and occasionally air-conduction) audiometry to signals that have been felt, rather than heard, by the patient.

tangible reinforcement operant conditioning audiometry (TROCA) Form of operant audiometry using tangible reinforcers, such as food or tokens.

tectorial membrane Gossamer membrane above the organ of Corti in the scala media in which the tips of the cilia of the hair cells are embedded.

tele-audiology Delivery of audiological services through phone calls, within synchronous sessions through the phone or using real-time, encrypted videoconferencing, or Internet chats, or within an asynchronous format through the forwarding of documents, electronic records, video clips, and so on, for review and online comment for subsequent discussion.

telecoil Induction coil frequently built into hearing aids that picks up electromagnetic signals from a telephone or loop induction system. Also known as *audiocoil* and *t-coil*.

temporal lobe The part of the cerebral hemispheres usually associated with perception of sound. The auditory language areas are located in the temporal lobes.

temporary threshold shift (TTS) Temporary sensory/neural hearing loss, usually associated with exposure to intense noise.

temporomandibular joint (TMJ) syndrome Pain often felt in the ear but referred from a neuralgia of the temporomandibular joint.

tensor tympani muscle Small muscle that is innervated by the trigeminal nerve and inserted into the malleus in the middle ear. It is one of two small muscles in the middle ear that contract in response to intense acoustic stimulation.

tetrachoric table Table containing four cells designed to test the efficiency and accuracy of hearing screening measures.

thalamus Located in the brain base, it sends projecting fibers to, and receives fibers from, all parts of the cortex.

threshold In audiometry, the level at which a stimulus, such as a pure tone, is barely perceptible. Usual clinical criteria demand that the level be just high enough for the subject to be aware of the sound at least 50 percent of the times it is presented.

threshold of discomfort (TD) *See* uncomfortable loudness level.

time-compressed speech System of recording speech so that it is accelerated, and therefore distorted, but the words remain discriminable.

tinnitus Ear or head noises, usually described as ringing, roaring, or hissing.

tolerance level *See* uncomfortable loudness level.

tone decay The loss of audibility of a sound produced when the ear is constantly stimulated by a pure tone.

tonotopic Arranged anatomically according to best frequency of stimulation.

Toynbee maneuver Method for forcing the eustachian tube open by swallowing with the nostrils and jaw closed.

tragus Small cartilaginous flap forming the anterior portion of the pinna.

transduce To convert one form of power to another (e.g., pressure waves to electricity, as in a microphone).

transient-evoked otoacoustic emission (TEOAE) Otoacoustic emission evoked in the cochlea by very brief acoustic stimuli like clicks or tone pips.

transistor Electronic device, with low power consumption and small space requirements, that amplifies electric current through the use of the semiconducting properties of an element such as silicon.

transverse wave Wave in which the motion of the molecules of the medium is perpendicular to the direction of the wave.

trapezius muscle Large, superficial muscle at the back of the neck and upper part of the thorax, or chest. It originates in the occipital bone at the base of the skull. Also known as *sternocleidomastoid muscle*.

trapezoid body Nerve fibers in the pons that connect the ventral cochlear nucleus on one side of the brain with the lateral lemniscus on the other side.

traveling wave theory Theory that sound waves move in the cochlea from its base to its apex along the basilar membrane. The crest of the wave resonates at a particular point on the basilar membrane, resulting in the perception of a specific pitch.

trigeminal nerve The Vth cranial nerve; it innervates the tensor tympani and also some of the palatal muscles.

trisomy The presence of an additional (third) chromosome.

tuning fork Metal instrument with a stem and two tines. When struck, it vibrates, producing an audible, near-perfect tone.

tympanic membrane Thin vibrating membrane between the outer and middle ears, located at the end of the external auditory canal. It comprises an outer layer of skin, a middle layer of connective tissue, and an inner layer of mucous membrane.

tympanogram Graphic representation of a pressure-compliance function.

tympanometry Measurement of the pressure-compliance function of the tympanic membrane.

tympanoplasty Surgical procedure designed to restore the hearing function to a middle ear that has been partially destroyed (for example, by otitis media).

tympanosclerosis Formation of whitish plaques in the tympanic membrane and masses of hard connective tissue around the bones of the middle ear. It occurs secondary to otitis media and may result in fixation of the ossicular chain.

umbo Slight indentation at the approximate center of the tympanic membrane at the tip of the malleus; the point at which the tympanic membrane is most retracted.

uncomfortable loudness level (UCL) That intensity at which speech becomes uncomfortably loud.

undermasking Presenting a masking noise of insufficient intensity to the nontest ear to prevent the test signal from being heard in that ear.

utricle The larger of the two sacs found in the membranous vestibular labyrinth; it contains an end organ of equilibrium.

vacuum tube Glass enclosure designed to regulate the flow of electric current.

valsalva Autoinflation of the middle ear by closing off the mouth and nose and forcing air up the eustachian tube.

variable expressivity The extent to which an inheritable trait is manifested.

variable pure-tone average (VPTA) The average pure-tone threshold of the poorest three frequencies of 500, 1,000, 2,000, and 4,000 Hz, used for the assignment of hearing-loss-impairment labels. Allows for a representation of hearing loss of either flat configuration or isolated primarily within either the lower or higher frequency range.

Varying Intensity Story Test (VIST) Portions of a story are presented above the admitted "threshold" and portions below. If the patient remembers information presented below the admitted threshold, then the examiner has prima facie evidence that the hearing loss in that ear is exaggerated.

vasospasm The violent constriction of a blood vessel, usually an artery.

velocity The speed of a sound wave in a given direction.

ventral cochlear nucleus The larger of the two cochlear nuclei on each side of the brain; it receives the fibers of the cochlea on the ipsilateral side.

vertigo The sensation that a person (or his or her surroundings) is whirling or spinning.

vestibular-evoked myogenic potential (VEMP) A sound-evoked muscle reflex believed to be generated from acoustical stimulation of the saccule. It is used in the diagnosis of vestibular disorders.

vestibule The cavity of the inner ear containing the organs of equilibrium and giving access to the cochlea.

vibration The to-and-fro movements of a mass. In a free vibration, the mass is displaced from its position of rest and allowed to oscillate without outside influence. In a forced vibration, the mass is moved back and forth by applying an external force.

vibrotactile aid Device that delivers amplified vibratory energy to the surface of the skin by special transducers; it is designed for patients whose hearing losses are so severe that assistance in speechreading cannot be obtained from traditional hearing aids.

visual reinforcement audiometry (VRA) The use of a light or picture to reinforce a child's response to a sound.

volley theory of hearing Variation of the frequency theory in which some neurons fire during the refractory periods of other neurons.

warble tone Pure tone that is frequency modulated. The modulation is usually expressed as a percentage; for example, a 1,000 Hz tone warbled at 5 percent would vary from 950 to 1,050 Hz).

watt Unit of power.

wave Series of moving impulses set up by a vibration.

wavelength The distance between the same point (in degrees) on two successive cycles of a tone.

Weber test Tuning-fork test performed in cases of hearing loss in one ear to determine if the impairment in the poorer ear is conductive or sensory/neural.

white noise Broadband noise with approximately equal energy per cycle.

Word Intelligibility by Picture Identification (WIPI) test Test that uses pictures to determine word-recognition ability in young children.

word-recognition score (WRS) The percentage of correctly identified items on a word-recognition test.

work Energy expended by displacement of a mass. The unit of measurement is the erg or joule.

X-linked Characteristics transmitted by genes on the X chromosome (sex-linked).

References

Abouchacra, K. S., & Letowski, T. (1999). Comparison of air-conduction and bone-conduction hearing thresholds for pure tones and octave-band filtered sound effects. *Journal of the American Academy of Audiology, 10,* 422–428.

Abujamra, A. L., Escosteguy, J. B., Dall'lgna, C, Manica, D., Cigana, L. F., Coradini, P., Brunetto, A., & Gregianin, L. J. (2013). The use of high-frequency audiometry increases the diagnosis of asymptomatic hearing loss in pediatric patients treated with cisplatin-based chemotherapy. *Pediatric Blood & Cancer, 60,* 474–478.

Academy of Dispensing Audiologists. (1988). *Proceedings, ADA Conference on Professional Education.* October 7–8, Chicago.

Alford, B. (1968). Rubella: A challenge for modern medical science. *Archives of Otolaryngology, 88,* 27–28.

Allen, J. B., & Lonsbury-Martin, B. L. (1993). Otoacoustic emissions. *Journal of the Acoustical Society of America, 93,* 568–569.

Alpiner, J. G., & McCarthy, P. A. (2000). *Rehabilitative audiology: Children and adults.* Baltimore, MD: Lippincott Williams & Wilkins.

Altman, E. (1996). Meeting the needs of adolescents with impaired hearing. In F. N. Martin & J. G. Clark (Eds.), *Hearing care for children* (pp. 197–210). Boston: Allyn & Bacon.

American Academy of Audiology. (1997). Position statement and guidelines of the consensus panel on support personnel in audiology. *Audiology Today, 9*(3), 27–28.

American Academy of Audiology. (2000). *Audiologic guidelines for the diagnosis and management of tinnitus patients.* Retrieved July 4, 2004, from www.audiology.org/professional/position/tinnitus/php

American Academy of Audiology. (2000). Position statement: Audiologic guidelines for the diagnosis and treatment of otitis media in children. *Audiology Today, 12,* 3.

American Academy of Audiology. (2003, October). Pediatric amplification protocol. Retrieved, July 24, 2004, from www.audiology.org/professional/positions/pedamp.pdf

American Academy of Audiology. (2004). Considerations for the use of support personnel for newborn hearing screening. Retrieved August 6, 2004, from www.audiology.org/professional/positions/usp4nhs.pdf

American Academy of Audiology. (2004a). Audiology: Scope of practice. *Audiology Today, 16*(3), 44–45.

American Academy of Audiology. (2004b). *Position statement on the audiologist's role in the diagnosis and treatment of vestibular disorders.* Retrieved July 4, 2004, from www.audiology.org/professional/position/vestibular/php/

American Academy of Audiology. (2006). Audiologic management of adult hearing impairment: Summary guidelines. *Audiology Today, 18,* 32–36.

American Academy of Audiology. (2010). *Membership demographics.* Reston, VA.

American Academy of Audiology. (2011). Clinical practice guidelines: Childhood hearing screening. Retreived May 15, 2013, from www.audiology.org/resources/documentlibrary/Documents/ChildhoodScreeningGuidelines.pdf

American Academy of Ophthalmology and Otolaryngology. (1979). Committee on Hearing and Equilibrium and the American Council of Otolaryngology Committee on the Medical Aspects of Noise. Guide for the evaluation of hearing handicap. *Journal of the American Medical Association, 241,* 2055–2059.

American National Standards Institute. (1992). *Standard reference zero for the calibration of pure-tone bone-conduction audiometers.* S3.43-1992. New York: Author.

American National Standards Institute. (1999). *Maximum permissible ambient noise levels for audiometric test rooms.* ANSI S3.1-1999. New York: Author.

American National Standards Institute. (2003). *American National Standard for specification of hearing aid characteristics.* ANSI S3.22–2003. New York: Author.

American National Standards Institute. (2004). *American National Standard specification for audiometers.* ANSI S3.6-2004. New York: Author.

American National Standards Institute. (2007). *American National Standard specifications for instruments to measure aural acoustic impedance and admittance (aural acoustic immittance) (Revised).* ANSI S3.39-1987 [R2002]. New York: Author.

American Speech-Language-Hearing Association. (1978). Guidelines for manual pure-tone audiometry. *Asha, 20,* 297–301.

American Speech-Language-Hearing Association. (1984). Proposed guidelines for identification audiometry. *Asha, 26,* 47–50.

American Speech-Language-Hearing Association. (1988). Guidelines for determining the threshold for speech. *Asha, 30,* 85–89.

American Speech-Language-Hearing Association. (1990). Guidelines for audiometric symbols. *Asha, 32* (Suppl.), 25–30.

American Speech-Language-Hearing Association. (1992). Considerations in screening adults/older persons for handicapping hearing impairments. *Asha, 34,* 81–87.

American Speech-Language-Hearing Association. (1993). Guidelines for audiology services in the schools. *Asha, 35* (Suppl. 10), 24–32.

American Speech-Language-Hearing Association. (1994). Guidelines for the audiologic management of individuals receiving cochleotoxic drug therapy. *Asha, 36,* 11–19.

American Speech-Language-Hearing Association. (1997). *Guidelines for audiologic screening.* Rockville, MD: Author.

American Speech-Language-Hearing Association. (2001). *Scope of practice in speech-language pathology.* Rockville, MD: Author.

American Speech-Language-Hearing Association. (2002a). *Communication development and disorders in multicultural populations: Readings and related materials.* Retrieved August 10, 2004, from www.asha.org/about/leadership-projects/multicultural/readings/OMA_fact_sheets.htm

American Speech-Language-Hearing Association. (2002b). *Guidelines for audiology service provision in and for schools.* Rockville, MD: Author.

American Speech-Language-Hearing Association. (2004). Clinical practice by certificate holders in the profession in which they are not certified, *Asha, 24*(Suppl.), 39–40.

American Speech-Language-Hearing Association. (2004). *Guidelines for the audiological assessment of children from birth to 5 years of age* [Guidelines]. Retrieved from www.asha.org/policy

American Speech-Language-Hearing Association. (2004a). *Auditory processing disorders: Technical report and guidelines.* Retrieved August 10, 2004, from www.asha.org/cdonlyres/50287290-1945-4A4A-B5FF-104D61F1A271/0/APDTRDraft526.pdf-199.82KB

American Speech-Language-Hearing Association. (2004b). Scope of practice in audiology. *ASHA Supplement 24,* 27–35.

American Speech-Language-Hearing Association. (2004c). Knowledge and skills needed by speech-language pathologists and audiologists to provide culturally and linguistically appropriate services. *Asha, 24*(Suppl.), 152–158.

American Speech-Language-Hearing Association. (2004d). Scope of practice in audiology. *Asha, 24*(Suppl.), 27–35.

American Speech-Language-Hearing Association. (2004e). *Auditory integration training* [Position Statement]. Available from www.asha.org/policy.

American Speech-Language-Hearing Association. (2005). Guidelines for manual pure-tone threshold audiometry. Retrieved from www.asha.org/policy

Americans with Disabilities Act (ADA). (1991). Public Law 101-336. United States Architectural and Transportation Barriers Compliance Board accessibility guidelines for buildings and facilities. *Federal Register, 56*(144), 35455–35542.

Amlani, A. M. (2001). Efficacy of directional microphone hearing aids: A meta-analytic perspective. *Journal of the American Academy of Audiology, 12,* 202–214.

Andaz, C., Heyworth, T., & Rowe, S. (1995). Nonorganic hearing loss in children—A two-year study. *Journal of Oto-Rhino-Laryngology and Its Related Specialties, 57,* 33–55.

Anderson, E. E., & Barr, B. (1971). Conductive high-tone hearing loss. *Archives of Otolaryngology, 93,* 599–605.

Anderson, H., Barr, B., & Wedenberg, E. (1969). Intra-aural reflexes in retrocochlear lesions. In C. A. Hamberger & J. Wersall (Eds.), *Disorders of the skull base region* (pp. 49–55). New York: Wiley.

Anderson, H., Barr, B., & Wedenberg, E. (1970). Early diagnosis of VIIIth nerve tumors by acoustic reflex tests. *Acta Otolaryngologica, 264,* 232–237.

Anderson, K. L. (1989). *Screening instrument for targeting educational risk (SIFTER).* Tampa, FL: Educational Audiology Association.

Anderson, K. L. (2002). Early listening function (ELF). Retrieved October 7, 2010, from www.nlsec.k12.mn.us/downloads/ELF-Early_Listening_Function.pdf

Anderson, K. L., & Smaldino, J. (2000). Children's home inventory of listening difficulties (CHILD). *Educational Audiology Review, 17* (suppl.), 3.

Antonelli, A., & Calearo, C. (1968). Further investigations on cortical deafness. *Acta Otolaryngologica* (Stockholm), *66,* 97–100.

Apgar, V. (1953). A proposal for a new method of evaluation of the newborn infant. *Anesthesia Analgesia, 32,* 260–266.

Atkins, D. V. (1994). Counseling children with hearing loss and their families. In J. G. Clark & F. N. Martin (Eds.), *Effective counseling in audiology: Perspectives and practice* (pp. 116–146). Englewood Cliffs, NJ: Prentice Hall.

Auer, E. T., Bernstein, L. E., & Coulter, D. C. (1998). Temporal and spatio-temporal vibrotactile displays for voice fundamental frequency: An initial evaluation of a new vibrotactile speech perception aid with normal-hearing and hearing-impaired individuals. *Journal of the Acoustical Society of America, 24,* 77–89.

Austen, S., & Lynch, C. (2004). Non-organic hearing loss redefined: Understanding, categorizing and managing non-organic behavior. *International Journal of Audiology, 45,* 283–284.

Azah, H., & Moore, B. C. J. (2007). The value of routine real ear measurement of the gain of digital hearing aids. *Journal of the American Academy of Audiology, 18*(8), 653–664.

Bailey, H. A. T., & Graham, S. S. (1984). Reducing risk in stapedectomy: The small fenestra stapedectomy technique. *Audiology: A Journal for Continuing Education, 9,* 1–3.

Ballachanda, B. (2001). Audiological assessment of linguistically and culturally diverse populations. *Audiology Today, 13*(4), 34–35.

Barany, E. A. (1938). A contribution to the physiology of bone conduction. *Acta Otolaryngologica* (Stockholm), *26* (Suppl.).

Barry, S. J. (1994). Can bone conduction thresholds really be poorer than air? *American Journal of Audiology, 3,* 21–22.

Barry, S. J., & Gaddis, S. (1978). Physical and physiological constraints on the use of bone conduction speech audiometry. *Journal of Speech and Hearing Disorders, 43,* 220–226.

Bass, J. K., & White, S. T. (2008). Radiation-induced hearing loss. *Audiology Today, 20*(2), 22–24.

Bassim, M. K., & Fayad, J. N. (2010). Implantable middle ear hearing devices: A review. *Seminars in Hearing, 31*(1), 28–36.

Beasley, W. C. (1938). National Health Survey (1935–1936), preliminary reports. *Hearing Study Series Bulletin,* 1–7. Washington, DC: U.S. Public Health Service.

Békésy, G. V. (1947). A new audiometer. *Acta Otolaryngologica* (Stockholm), *35,* 411–422.

Békésy, G. von (1960). Wave motion in the cochlea. In E. G. Wever (Ed.), *Experiments in hearing* (pp. 485–534). New York: McGraw-Hill.

Berger, E. H., & Casali, J. G. (2000). Hearing protection devices. In M. Valente, H. Hosford-Dunn, & R. J. Roeser (Eds.), *Audiology treatment* (pp. 669–690). New York: Thieme.

Berger, K. W. (1988). History and development of hearing aids. In M. C. Pollack (Ed.), *Amplification for the hearing impaired* (3rd ed., pp. 1–20). Orlando, FL: Grune & Stratton.

Bergman, M., Hirsch, S., Solzi, P., & Mankowitz, Z. (1987). The threshold-of-interference test: A new test of interhemispheric suppression in brain injury. *Ear and Hearing, 8,* 147–150.

Berrick, J. M., Shubow, G. F., Schultz, M. C., Freed, H., Fournier, S. R., & Hughes, J. P. (1984). Auditory processing tests for children: Normative and clinical results on the SSW test. *Journal of Speech and Hearing Disorders, 49,* 318–325.

Bess, F. H., Lichtenstein, M. D., Logan, S. A., Burger, M. C., & Nelson, E. (1989). Hearing impairment as a determinant of function in the elderly. *Journal of the American Geriatrics Society, 37,* 123–128.

Bilger, R. C., Nuetzel, J. M., Rabinowitz, W. M., & Rzeczkowski, C. (1984). Standardization of a test of speech perception in noise. *Journal of Speech and Hearing Research, 27,* 32–48.

Blair, J. C. (1996). Educational audiology. In F. N. Martin & J. G. Clark (Eds.), *Hearing care for children* (pp. 316–334). Boston: Allyn & Bacon.

Bocca, E. (1955). Binaural hearing: Another approach. *Laryngoscope, 65,* 1164–1175.

Bocca, E. (1967). Distorted speech tests. In A. B. Graham (Ed.), *Sensorineural hearing processes and disorders* (Henry Ford Hospital International Symposium). Boston: Little, Brown.

Bocca, E., & Calearo, C. (1963). Central hearing process. In J. Jerger (Ed.), *Modern developments in audiology* (pp. 337–370). New York: Academic Press.

Bocca, E., Calearo, C., & Cassinari, V. (1954). A new method for testing hearing in temporal lobe tumors: Preliminary report. *Acta Otolaryngologica* (Stockholm), *44,* 219–221.

Boothroyd, A. (1968). Developments in speech audiometry. *British Journal of Audiology, 2,* 3–10.

Bratt, G. W., Rosenfeld, M. A. L., & Williams, D. W. (2007). NICD/VA hearing aid clinical trial and follow-up: Background. *Journal of the American Academy of Audiology, 18,* 274–281.

Brookhouser, P. E., Cyr, D. G., & Beauchaine, K. (1982). Vestibular findings in the deaf and hard of hearing. *Otolaryngology, Head and Neck Surgery, 90,* 773–777.

Brooks, A. C. (1994). Middle ear infections in children. *Science News, 146,* 332–333.

Brooks, D. N., & Goeghegan, P. M. (1992). Non-organic hearing loss in young persons: Transient episode or indicator of deep-seated difficulty? *British Journal of Audiology, 26,* 347–350.

Brunt, M. A. (2002). Cochlear and retrocochlear behavioral tests. In J. Katz (Ed.), *Handbook of clinical audiology* (4th ed., pp. 111–123). Baltimore, MD: Lippincott Williams & Wilkins.

Buchanan, M. A., Wilkinson, J. M., Fitzgerald, J. E., and Prinsley, P. R. (2008). Is golf bad for your hearing? *British Medical Journal.* Retrieved February 12, 2009, from bmj2008;337:a2835

Burgoon, J. D., Buller, D. B., & Woodall, W. G. (1989). *Nonverbal communication: The unspoken dialogue.* New York: Harper & Row.

Burk, M. H., & Wiley, T. L. (2004). Continuous versus pulsed tones in audiometry. *American Journal of Audiology, 13,* 54–61.

Burke, L. E., & Nerbonne, M. A. (1978). The influence of the guess factor on the speech reception threshold. *Journal of the American Auditory Society, 4,* 87–90.

Cacace, A. T. (2007). Aging, Alzheimer's disease, and hearing impairment: Highlighting relevant issues for additional research. Editorial. *American Journal of Audiology, 16,* 2–3.

Caissie, R., Campbell, M. M., Frenette, W. L., Scott, L., Howell, I., & Roy, A. (2005). Clear speech for adults with a hearing loss: Does intervention with communication partners make a difference? *Journal of the American Academy of Audiology, 16,* 157–171.

Calearo, C. (1957). Binaural summation in lesions of the temporal lobe. *Acta Otolaryngologica* (Stockholm), *47,* 392–395.

Cameron, S., Dillon, H., & Newall, P. (2006). The Listening in Spacialized Noise test: An auditory processing disorder study. *Journal of the American Academy of Audiology, 17,* 306–320.

Campanelli, P. (1963). Simulated hearing losses in school children following identification audiometry. *Journal of Auditory Research 3,* 91–108.

CareerCast. (2013). Jobs Rated 2013: Ranking 200 Jobs from Best to Worst. Retrieved June 4, 2013, from http://www.career-cast.com/jobs-rated/best-worst-jobs-2013

Carhart, R. (1946). Tests for selection of hearing aids. *Laryngoscope, 56,* 780–794.

Carhart, R. (1952). Bone conduction advances following fenestration surgery. *Transactions of the American Academy of Ophthalmology and Otolaryngology, 56,* 621–629.

Carhart, R. (1961). Tests for malingering. *Transactions of the American Academy of Ophthalmology and Otolaryngology, 65,* 437.

Carhart, R. (1964). Audiometric manifestations of preclinical stapes fixation. *Annals of Otology, Rhinology and Laryngology, 3,* 740–755.

Carhart, R. (1965). Problems in the measurement of speech discrimination. *Archives of Otolaryngology, 32,* 253–260.

Carhart, R. (1975). Introduction. In M. C. Pollack (Ed.), *Amplification for the hearing-impaired* (pp. xix–xxxvi). New York: Grune & Stratton.

Carhart, R., & Jerger, J. F. (1959). Preferred method for clinical determination of pure-tone thresholds. *Journal of Speech and Hearing Disorders, 24,* 330–345.

Carhart, R., & Porter, L. S. (1971). Audiometric configuration and prediction of threshold for spondees. *Journal of Speech and Hearing Research, 14,* 486–495.

Carter, A. S., Noe, C. M., & Wilson, R. H. (2001). Listeners who prefer monaural to binaural hearing aids. *Journal of the American Academy of Audiology, 12,* 261–272.

Cassell, E. J. (1989). Making the subjective objective. In M. Stewart & D. Roter (Eds.), *Communicating with medical patients* (pp. 13–23). Newbury Park, CA: Sage.

Cevette, M. J., Robinette, M. S., Carter, J., & Knops, J. L. (1995). Otoacoustic emissions in sudden unilateral hearing loss associated with multiple sclerosis. *Journal of the American Academy of Audiology, 6,* 197–202.

Chaiklin, J. B. (1967). Interaural attenuation and cross-hearing in air-conduction audiometry. *Journal of Auditory Research, 7,* 413–424.

Chaiklin, J. B. (1990). A descending LOT-Békésy screening test for functional hearing loss. *Journal of Speech and Hearing Disorders, 55,* 67–74.

Chermak, G. D., & Musiek, F. E. (1997). *Central auditory processing disorders: New perspectives.* San Diego, CA: Singular Publishing Group.

Cherry, R., & Ventry, I. (1976). The ascending-descending gap: A tool for identifying a suprathreshold response. *Journal of Auditory Research, 16,* 181–187.

Ching, T. Y. C., Hill, M., Dillon, H., & van Wanrooy, E. (2004). Fitting and evaluating a hearing aid for recipients of a unilateral cochlear implant: The NAL approach. *The Hearing Review, 14*(7), 14–22.

Chisolm, T. H., Johnson, C. E., Danhauer, J. L., Portz, L. J. P., Abrams, H. B., Lesner, S., McCarthy, P. A., & Newman, C. W. (2007). American Academy of Audiology task force of the health-related quality of life benefits of amplification in adults. *Journal of the American Academy of Audiology, 18,* 151–183.

Christensen, L., Smith-Olinde, L., Kimberlain, J., Richter, G. T., & Dornhoffer, J. L. (2010). Comparison of traditional bone-conduction hearing aids with the Baha® system. *Journal of the American Academy of Audiology, 21,* 267–273.

Chute, P. M., & Nevins, M. E. (2000). Cochlear implants in children. In M. Valente, H. Hosford-Dunn, & R. J. Roeser (Eds.), *Audiology treatment* (pp. 511–535). New York: Thieme.

Ciletti, L., & Flamme, G. A. (2009). Prevalence of hearing impairment by gender and audiometric configuration: Results from the National Health and Nutrition Examination Survey (1999–2004) and the Keokuk County Rural Health Study (1994–1998). *Journal of the American Academy of Audiology, 19,* 672–685.

Cinotti, T. M. (1998). The Fast ForWord program: A clinician's perspective. In M. G. Masters, N. A. Stecker, & J. Katz (Eds.), *Central auditory processing disorders.* Boston: Allyn & Bacon.

Clark, J. G. (1980). Central auditory dysfunction in school children: A compilation of management suggestions. *Speech, Language, and Hearing Services in Schools, 11*(4), 208–213.

Clark, J. G. (1981). Uses and abuses of hearing loss classification. *Asha, 23,* 493–500.

Clark, J. G. (1982). Percent hearing handicap: Clinical utility or sophistry? *Hearing Instruments, 33*(3), 37.

Clark, J. G. (1983). Beyond diagnosis: The professional's role in education consultation. *Hearing Journal, 36,* 20–25.

Clark, J. G. (1984). Tinnitus: An overview. In J. G. Clark & P. Yanick (Eds.), *Tinnitus and its management: A clinical text for audiologists* (pp. 3–14). Springfield, IL: Thomas.

Clark, J. G. (1992). *The ABC's to better hearing.* Cincinnati: HearCare.

Clark, J. G. (1994). Audiologist's counseling purview. In J. G. Clark & F. N. Martin (Eds.), *Effective counseling in audiology: Perspectives and practice* (pp. 1–17). Englewood Cliffs, NJ: Prentice Hall.

Clark, J. G. (1996). Pediatric amplification: Selection and verification. In F. N. Martin & J. G. Clark (Eds.), *Hearing care for children* (pp. 213–232). Boston: Allyn & Bacon.

Clark, J. G. (1999). Working with challenging patients: An opportunity to improve our counseling skills. *Audiology Today, 11*(5), 13–15.

Clark, J. G. (2000). Profiles in aural rehabilitation: An interview with Richard Carmen. *The Hearing Journal, 53*(7), 28, 30–33.

Clark, J. G. (2001). Hearing aid dispensing: Have we missed the point? *The Hearing Journal, 54,* 10ff.

Clark, J. G. (2002). Adding closure to the dispensing process. *The Hearing Review, 9*(3), 48–51.

Clark, J. G. (2002). If it's not hearing loss, then what: Confronting nonorganic hearing loss in children. *Audiologyonline.com/Article/October,14*

Clark, J. G. (2007). Patient-centered practice: Aligning professional ethics with patient goals. *Seminars in Hearing, 28*(3), 163–170.

Clark, J. G. (2009, January 21). Adult hearing loss management: Evening the legs of a three-legged stool. Audiology-Online Audio presentation.

Clark, J. G. (2010). Sisyphus personified: Audiology's attempts to rehabilitate adult hearing loss. *Hearing Journal, 63* (4), 26–28.

Clark, J. G., & English, K. E. (2004). *Audiologic counseling: Helping patients and families adjust to hearing loss.* Boston: Allyn & Bacon.

Clark, J. G., & English, K. E. (2014). *Counseling-infused audiologic care.* Boston: Allyn & Bacon.

Clark, J. G., & Jaindl, M. (1996). Conductive hearing loss in children: Etiology and pathology. In F. N. Martin & J. G. Clark (Eds.), *Hearing care for children* (pp. 45–72). Boston: Allyn & Bacon.

Clark, J. G., Kricos, P., & Sweetow, R. W. (2010). The circle of life: A possible rehabilitative journey leading to improved patient outcomes. *Audiology Today, 22*(1), 36–39.

Coles, R. R. A., & Priede, V. M. (1968). Clinical and subjective acoustics. *Institution of Sound and Vibration Research, 26,* Chapter 3A.

Comprehensive Telehealth Act of 1997. www.gpo.gov/fdsys/pkg/BILLS-105s385is/pdf/BILLS-105s385is.pdf. Retrieved 11/1/2013.

Cone-Wesson, B., Dowell, R., Tolin, D., Rance, G., & Min, W. J. (2002). The auditory steady-state response: Comparisons with the auditory brainstem response. *Journal of the American Academy of Audiology, 13,* 173–187.

Connor, C. M., Craig, H. K., Raudenbush, S. W., Heavner, K., & Zwolan, T. A. (2006). The age at which young deaf children receive cochlear implants and their vocabulary and speech-production growth: Is there an added value to early implantation? *Ear & Hearing, 27,* 628–644.

Cornett, R. O. (1967). Cued speech. *American Annals of the Deaf, 112,* 3–13.

Cosby, J., Culbertson, D., Hudson, S., Bengala, D., & Joyner, R. (2009). Pediatric cochlear implants: Knowledge and skills of speech-language pathologists. *ASHA Leader, 2*(6), 7, 18.

Cox, R. M. (2005). Evidence-based practice in provision of amplification. *Journal of the American Academy of Audiology, 16,* 419–438.

Cox, R. M., Alexander, G. C., & Gilmore, C. (1987). Development of the Connected Speech Test (CST). *Ear and Hearing, 8,* 119–126 (Suppl.).

Cox, R. M., Alexander, G. C., Gilmore, C., & Pusakulich, K. M. (1988). Use of the Connected Speech Test with hearing-impaired listeners. *Ear and Hearing, 9,* 198–207.

Crandell, C. C. (1998). Hearing aids: Their effects on functional health status. *The Hearing Journal, 51,* 22–32.

Cullen, J. K., Ellis, M. S., Berlin, C. I., & Lousteau, R. J. (1972). Human acoustic nerve action potential recordings from the tympanic membrane without anesthesia. *Acta Otolaryngologica, 74,* 15–22.

Cureoglu, S., Schchern, P., Paparella, M., & Lindgren, R. (2004). Cochlear changes in chronic otitis media. *Laryngoscope, 114*(4), 622–626.

Cyr, D. G., & Møller, C. G. (1988). Rationale for the assessment of vestibular function in children. *The Hearing Journal, 41,* 38–39, 45–46, 48–49.

Davis, A., & Refaie, A. E. (2000). Epidemiology of tinnitus. In R. Tyler (Ed.), *Tinnitus handbook* (pp. 1–23). San Diego, CA: Singular Publishing Group.

Davis, B. M., Richards, D. L., & Martin, D. R. (2007). Hearing protection as a factor of personal training. Poster session, Ohio Academy of Audiology Conference, Columbus, OH.

Davis, H., & Silverman, S. R. (1978). *Hearing and deafness* (4th ed.). New York: Holt, Rinehart and Winston.

Davis, J. (1986). Remediation of hearing, speech and language deficits resulting from otitis media. In J. F. Kavanagh (Ed.), *Otitis media and child development* (pp. 182–191). Parkton, MD: York Press.

Davis, P. B. (2006). Music and the acoustic desensitization protocol for tinnitus. In R. Tyler (Ed,) *Tinnitus treatment* (pp. 146–160). New York: Thieme.

Davis, P. B., Paki, B., & Hanley, P. J. (2007). Neuromonics tinnitus treatment: Third clinical trial. *Ear and Hearing, 28,* 242–259.

De Jonge, R. R., & Valente, M. (1979). Interpreting ear differences in static compliance measurements. *Journal of Speech and Hearing Disorders, 44,* 209–213.

Dean, M. S., & Martin, F. N. (1997). Auditory and tactile bone-conduction thresholds. *Journal of the American Academy of Audiology, 8,* 227–232.

Dean, M. S., & Martin, F. N. (2000). Insert earphone depth and the occlusion effect. *American Journal of Audiology, 9,* 131–134.

Derebery, M. J., Vermiglio, A., Berliner, K. I., Potthoff, M., & Holguin, K. (2012). Facing the music: Pre- and postconcert assessment of hearing in teenagers. *Otology & Neurotology, 33*(7), 1136–1141.

Desmon, A. L. (2000). Vestibular rehabilitation. In M. Valente, H. Hosford-Dunn, & R. J. Roeser (Eds.), *Audiology treatment* (pp. 639–667). New York: Thieme.

DeVries, S. M., & Decker, T. N. (1992). Otoacoustic emissions: Overview of measurement methodologies. *Seminars in Hearing, 13,* 15–22.

DeWeese, D., & Vernon, J. (1975). The American Tinnitus Association. *Hearing Instruments, 18,* 19–25.

Dhar, S., & Hall, J. W. (2011). *Otoacoustic emissions: Principles, procedures, and protocols.* San Diego, CA: Plural Publishing.

DiCarlo, L. M., Kendall, D. C., & Goldstein, R. (1962). Diagnostic procedures for auditory disorders in children. *Folia Phoniatrica, 14,* 206–264.

Diefendorf, A. O. (1996). Hearing loss and its effects. In F. N. Martin & J. G. Clark (Eds.), *Hearing care for children* (pp. 3–19). Boston: Allyn & Bacon.

DiGiovani, J. J., & Repka, J. N. (2007). Response method in audiometry. *American Journal of Audiology, 16,* 145–148.

Dillon, H. (2012). *Hearing aids* (2nd ed.) Turramurra, Austrailia: Boomerang Press.

Dix, M. R., & Hallpike, C. S. (1947). The peep show: A new technique for pure tone audiometry in young children. *British Medical Journal, 2,* 719–723.

Doerfler, L. G., & Stewart, K. (1946). Malingering and psychogenic deafness. *Journal of Speech Disorders, 11,* 181–186.

Don, M., & Kwong, B. (2009). Auditory brainstem response: Differential diagnosis. In J. Katz, L. Medwedwetsky, R. Burkard, & L. Hood (Eds.), *Handbook of clinical audiology* (6th ed., pp. 375–381). Baltimore, MD: Lippincott Williams & Wilkins.

Don, M., Masuda, A., Nelson, R. A., & Brackmann, D. E. (1997). Successful detection of small acoustic tumors using the stacked derived band ABR method. *American Journal of Otology, 18,* 608–621.

Downs, M. P., & Sterritt, G. M. (1967). A guide to newborn and infant screening programs. *Archives of Otolaryngology, 85,* 15–22.

Dufresne, R. M., Alleyne, B. C., & Reesal, M. R. (1988). Asymmetric hearing loss in truck drivers. *Ear and Hearing, 9,* 41–42.

Durrant, J. D., & Collet, L. (2002). Integrating otoacoustic emission and electrophysiological measures. In M. S. Robinette & Glattke, T. J. (Eds.), *Otoacoustic emissions* (2nd ed., pp. 273–296). New York: Thieme.

Edgerton, B. J., & Danhauer, J. L. (1979). *Clinical implications of speech discrimination testing using nonsense stimuli.* Baltimore: University Park Press.

Education for All Handicapped Children Act of 1975. Public Law 94–142. U.S. Congress, 94th Congress, 1st Session. U.S. Code, Section 1041–1456. Washington, DC: U.S. Government Printing Office.

Education of the Handicapped Amendments. (1986). Public Law 99–457. U.S. Statutes at Large, 100, 1145–1176. Washington, DC: U.S. Government Printing Office.

Egan, J. P. (1948). Articulation testing methods. *Laryngoscope, 58,* 955–991.

Eggermont, J. J. (2012). Current issues in tinnitus. In K. E. Tremblay & R. F. (Eds.), *Translational perspectives in auditory neuroscience.* San Diego, CA: Plural Publishing.

Eldert, M. A., & Davis, H. (1951). The articulation function of patients with conductive deafness. *Laryngoscope, 61,* 891–909.

Elliott, L. L., & Katz, D. (1980). *Development of a new children's test of speech discrimination.* St. Louis, MO: Auditec.

Elpern, B. S., & Naunton, R. F. (1963). The stability of the occlusion effect. *Archives of Otolaryngology, 77,* 376–382.

Engelberg, M. (1968). Test-retest variability in speech discrimination testing. *Laryngoscope, 78,* 1582–1589.

Etymōtic Research. (2001). Quick SIN: Speech-in-noise test, version 1.30. Elk Grove, IL: Author.

Everberg, G. (1957). Deafness following mumps. *Acta Otolaryngologica, 48,* 397–403.

Ewertson, H. W. (1973). Epidemiology of professional noise-induced hearing loss. *Audiology, 12,* 453–458.

Ewing, I., & Ewing, A. (1944). The ascertainment of deafness in infancy and early childhood. *Journal of Laryngology, 59,* 309–333.

Fagelson, M. A. (2007). The association between tinnitus and posttraumatic stress disorders. *American Journal of Audiology, 16,* 107–117.

Fagelson, M., & Martin, F. N. (1994). Sound pressure in the external auditory canal during bone conduction testing. *Journal of the American Academy of Audiology, 5,* 379–383.

Fairbanks, G. (1958). Test of phonemic differentiation: The rhyme test. *Journal of the Acoustical Society of America, 30,* 596–601.

Ferraro, J. A. (1992). Electrocochleography: What and why. *Audiology Today, 4,* 25–27.

Fisch U. (1982) Stapedotomy versus stapedectomy. *Otology & Neurotology, 4,* 112–117.

Fisch, U. (2009). Commentary: Stapedotomy versus stapedectomy. *Otology & Neurotology, 30*(8), 1166–1167.

Fletcher, H. (1950). Method of calculating hearing loss for speech from an audiogram. *Journal of the Acoustical Society of America, 22,* 1–5.

Fletcher, H., & Munson, W. A. (1933). Loudness, its definition, measurement, and calculation. *Journal of the Acoustical Society of America, 5,* 82–107.

Flexer, C. (1999). *Facilitating hearing and listening in young children* (2nd ed.). San Diego, CA: Singular Publishing Group.

Flexer, C., & Gans, D. (1985). Comparative evaluation of the auditory responsiveness of normal infants and profoundly multihandicapped children. *Journal of Speech and Hearing Research, 28,* 163–168.

Flexer, C., Wray, D., & Ireland, J. A. (1989). Preferential seating is *not* enough: Issues in classroom management of hearing-impaired students. *Language, Speech and Hearing Services in Schools, 20,* 11–21.

Flores, P., Martin, F. N., & Champlin, C. A. (1996). Providing audiological services to Spanish speakers. *American Journal of Audiology, 5,* 69–73.

Food and Drug Administration. (2000). Center for devices and radiologic health. Vibrant soundbridge P990052. Retrieved September 20, 2007, from www.fda.gov/cdrh/pdf/p990052.html

Fowler, C. G., & King, J. L. (2008). Sudden bilateral sensorineural hearing loss following speedballing. *Journal of the American Academy of Audiology, 19,* 461–464.

Frank, T. (1976). Yes-no test for nonorganic hearing loss. *Archives of Otolaryngology, 102,* 162–165.

Franklin, B. (1966). The effect on consonant discrimination of combining a low-frequency passband in one ear and a high-frequency passband in the other ear. *Journal of Auditory Research, 9,* 365–378.

Franklin, C., Johnson, K., Smith-Olinde, L., & Nicholson, N. (2009). The relationship of audiometric thresholds elicited with pulsed, warbled, and pulsed warbled tones in adults with normal hearing. *Ear and Hearing, 30,* 485–487.

Franks, J. R., Engel, D. P., & Themann, C. L. (1992). Real ear attenuation at threshold for three audiometric headphone devices: Implications for maximum permissible ambient noise level standards. *Ear and Hearing, 13,* 2–10.

Freeman, B. A., & Doyle, L. (2001). Falling in line with professionalism. *Advance for Audiologists, 3*(3), 18–19.

French, M. R., & Steinberg, J. C. (1947). Factors governing the intelligibility of speech sounds. *Journal of the Acoustical Society of America, 19,* 90–119.

Fulcher, A., Purcell, A. A., Baker, E., & Munro, N. (2012). Listen up: Children with early identified hearing loss achieve age-appropriate speech/language outcomes by 3 years-of-age. *International Journal of Pediatric Otolaryngology, 76,* 1785–1794.

Gaeth, J. H. (1948). *A study of phonemic regression in relation to hearing loss.* Doctoral dissertation, Northwestern University, Evanston, IL.

Galvin, K. L., Cowan, R. S. C., Sarant, J. Z., Alcantara, J. I., Blamey, P. J., & Clark, G. M. (1991). Use of a multichannel electrotactile speech processor by profoundly hearing-impaired children in a total communication environment. *Journal of the American Academy of Audiology, 2,* 214–225.

Gang, R. P. (1976). The effects of age on the diagnostic utility of the rollover phenomenon. *Journal of Speech and Hearing Disorders, 41,* 63–69.

Gardner, H. J. (1971). Application of a high frequency consonant discrimination word list in hearing-aid evaluation. *Journal of Speech and Hearing Disorders, 36,* 354–355.

Gates, G. A., Mills, D., Nam, B. H., D'Agostino, R., & Rubel, E. W. (2002). Effects of age on the distortion product otoacoustic emission growth functions. *Hearing Research, 163,* 53–60.

Geier, K. (1997). *Handbook of self-assessments and verification measures of communication performance.* Available from the Academy of Dispensing Audiologists, 3008 Millwood Avenue, Columbia SC 29205, 800/445-8629. Retrieved from www.audiologist.com

Gelfand, S. A., & Silman, S. (1993). Apparent auditory deprivation in children: Implications of monaural versus binaural amplification. *Journal of the American Academy of Audiology, 4,* 313–318.

Gelfand, S. T. (2002). The acoustic reflex. In J. Katz (Ed.), *Handbook of clinical audiology* (4th ed., pp. 205–232). Baltimore, MD: Lippincott Williams & Wilkins.

Ghossaini, S. N., Spitzer, J. B., & Borik, J. (2010). Use of the bone-anchored cochlear stimulator (Baha) and satisfaction among long-term users. *Seminars in Hearing, 31*(1), 3–14.

Giebink, G. S. (1984). Epidemiology and natural history of otitis media. In D. Lim, C. Bluestone, J. Klein, & J. Nelson (Eds.), *Recent advances in otitis media.* Philadelphia: B. C. Decker.

Gladstone, V. S. (1984). Advanced acoustic immittance considerations. In H. Kaplan, V. S. Gladstone, & J. Katz (Eds.), *Site of lesion testing: Audiometric interpretation* (Vol. 2, pp. 59–79). Baltimore: University Park Press.

Glass, L. (1990). Hearing impairment in geriatrics. In B. Kemp, K. Brummel-Smith, & J. W. Ramsdell (Eds.), *Geriatric rehabilitation.* Boston: College-Hill Press.

Glass, L. E., & Elliot, H. H. (1992 January/February). The professionals told me what it was, but that's not enough. *SHHH Journal,* 26–28.

Goetzinger, C. P. (1978). Word discrimination testing. In J. Katz (Ed.), *Handbook of clinical audiology* (2nd ed., pp. 149–158). Baltimore: Williams & Wilkins.

Goetzinger, C. P., & Angell, S. (1965). Audiological assessment in acoustic tumors and cortical lesions. *Eye, Ear, Nose and Throat Monthly, 44,* 39–49.

Goetzinger, C. P., & Proud, G. O. (1955). Speech audiometry by bone conduction. *Archives of Otolaryngology, 62,* 632–635.

Gollegly, K. M. (1994). *Otoacoustic emissions and pseudohypacusis.* Poster session presented at the Annual Convention of the American Speech-Language-Hearing Association, New Orleans, LA.

Gollegly, K. M., Bornstein, S. P., & Musiek, F. E. (1992). *Otoacoustic emissions and pseudohypacusis.* Poster session presented at the Annual Convention of the American Speech-Language-Hearing Association, San Antonio, TX.

Goodhill, V. (1950). Nuclear deafness and the nerve-deaf child: The importance of the Rh factor. *Transactions of the American Academy of Ophthalmology and Otolaryngology, 54,* 671–687.

Goodman, A. (1965). Reference zero levels for pure-tone audiometer. *Asha, 7,* 262–263.

Goodwin, P. E. (1984). The tinnitus evaluation. In J. G. Clark & P. Yanick (Eds.), *Tinnitus and its management: A clinical text for audiologists* (pp. 72–94). Springfield, IL: Thomas.

Gorga, M. P., Neely, S. T., Ohlrich, B., Hoover, B., Redner, J., & Peters, J. (1997). From laboratory to clinic: A large-scale study of distortion product otoacoustic emissions in ears with normal hearing and ears with hearing loss. *Ear and Hearing, 18,* 440–455.

Gorga, M. P., Preissler, K., Simmons, J., Walker, L., & Hoover, B. (2001). Some issues relevant to establishing a universal newborn screening program. *Journal of the American Academy of Audiology, 12,* 101–112.

Graham, J. (1987). Tinnitus in hearing-impaired children. In J. W. P. Hazel (Ed.), *Tinnitus* (pp. 131–143). Edinburgh: Churchill Livingston.

Graham, J., & Newby, H. (1962). Acoustical characteristics of tinnitus. *Archives of Otolaryngology, 75,* 162–167.

Guilford, F. R., & Haug, C. O. (1952). Diagnosis of deafness in the very young child. *Archives of Otolaryngology, 55,* 101–106.

Guinness World Records (2013). Loudest crowd roar at a sports stadium. http://www.guinnessworldrecords.com/records-1/loudest-crowd-roar-at-a-sports-stadium/ Retreived October 24, 2013.

Gunnarson, A., & Finitzo, T. (1991). Conductive hearing loss during infancy: Effects on later auditory brain stem electrophysiology. *Journal of Speech and Hearing Research, 34,* 1207–1215.

Gustafson, G. (1989, October/November). Early identification of hearing-impaired infants: A review of Israeli and American progress. *Volta Review, 91,* 291–294.

Hahlbrock, K. H. (1962). Bone conduction speech audiometry. *International Audiology, 1,* 186–188.

Hall, J. W. (2007). *New handbook of auditory evoked responses.* Boston: Pearson/Allyn & Bacon.

Hall, J. W., & Mueller, H. G. (1997). *Audiologists' desk reference,* Vol. I. San Diego, CA: Singular Publishing Group.

Hall, J. W., Smith, S. D., & Popelka, G. R. (2004). Newborn hearing screening with combined otoacoustic emissions and auditory brainstem response. *Journal of the American Academy of Audiology, 15,* 414–425.

Halpern, M. T., Palmer, C. S., & Seidlin, M. (1999). Treatment patterns for otitis externa. *Journal of the American Board of Family Practicet, 12*(1), 1–7.

Halpin, C. (2007). Incidence of responses at the lower audiometric limits. *American Journal of Audiology, 16,* 96–99.

Harford, E., & Barry, L. (1965). A rehabilitative approach to the problem of unilateral hearing impairment: The contralateral routing of signals (CROS). *Journal of Speech and Hearing Disorders, 30,* 121–138.

Harkrider, A. W., & Martin, F. N. (1998). Quantifying air-conducted acoustic radiation from the bone-conduction vibrator. *Journal of the American Academy of Audiology, 9,* 410–416.

Harris, D. A. (1958). A rapid and simple technique for the detection of nonorganic hearing loss. *Archives of Otolaryngology* (Chicago), *6X,* 758–760.

Harris, J. D. (1986). Anatomy and physiology of the peripheral auditory mechanism. In *The Pro-Ed studies in communication disorders.* Austin, TX: Pro-Ed.

Harrison, M., Roush, J., & Wallace, J. (2003). Trends in age of identification and intervention in infants with hearing loss. *Ear & Hearing, 24,* 89–95.

Haskins, H. (1949). *A phonetically balanced test of speech discrimination for children.* Master's thesis, Northwestern University.

Hattler, K. W. (1970). Lengthened off time: A self-recording screening device for nonorganicity. *Journal of Speech and Hearing Disorders, 35,* 113–122.

Haug, M., & Lavin, B. (1983). *Consumerism in medicine: Challenging physician authority.* Beverly Hills, CA: Sage.

Haug, O., Baccaro, P., & Guilford, F. (1967). A pure-tone audiogram on the infant: The PIWI technique. *Archives of Otolaryngology, 86,* 435–440.

Hawkins, D. B. (1990). Technology and hearing aids: How does the audiologist fit in? *Asha, 32,* 42–43.

Hayashi, R., Ohta, F., & Morimoto, M. (1966). Binaural fusion test: A diagnostic approach to the central auditory disorders. *International Audiology, 5,* 133–135.

Hayes, D., & Northern, J. L. (1996). *Infants and hearing.* San Diego, CA: Singular Publishing Group.

Health Insurance Portability and Accountability Act of 1996. (1996). Public Law 104-191, 104th Congress.

Hearing Aid Industry Conference. (1961). *Standard method of expressing hearing aid performance.* New York: Author.

Hearing Aid Industry Conference. (1975). *Standards for hearing aids.* New York: Author.

Hempton, G., & Grossman, J. (2009). *One square inch of silence.* New York: Free Press.

Henoch, M. A. (1979). *Aural rehabilitation for the elderly.* New York: Grune & Stratton.

Henry, D. F., & DiBartolomeo, J. R. (1993). Patulous eustachian tube identification using tympanometry. *Journal of the American Academy of Audiology, 4,* 53–57.

Henry, J. A., Schechter, M. A., Zaugg, T. L., Griest, S., Jastreboff, P. J., Vernon, J. A., Kaelin, C., Meikle, M. B., Lyons, K. S., & Stewart, B. J. (2006). Outcomes of clinical trial: Tinnitus masking versus tinnitus retraining therapy. *Ear and Hearing, 17,* 104–132.

Hirsh, I. (1948). The influence of interaural phase on interaural summation and inhibition. *Journal of the Acoustical Society of America, 23,* 384–386.

Hirsh, I., Davis, H., Silverman, S. R., Reynolds, E., Eldert, E., & Benson, R. W. (1952). Development of materials for speech audiometry. *Journal of Speech and Hearing Disorders, 17,* 321–337.

Hitselberger, W. E., & Telischi, F. F. (1994). Auditory brainstem implant. In D. E. Brackmann (Ed.), *Otologic surgery* (pp. 699–708). Philadelphia, PA: W. B. Saunders.

Hodgetts, W. E., Rieger, J. M., & Szarko, R. A. (2007). The effects of listening environment and earphone style on preferred listening levels of normal hearing adults using an MP3 player. *Ear and Hearing, 28,* 290–297.

Hodgson, W. (1967). Audiological report of a patient with left hemispherectomy. *Journal of Speech and Hearing Disorders, 32,* 39–45.

Hodgson, W. R. & Tillman, T. (1966). Reliability of bone conduction occlusion effects in normals. *Journal of Auditory Research, 6,* 141–153.

Holcomb, L. M., Nerbonne, M. A., & Konkle, D. F. (2000). Articulation index and hearing handicap. *Journal of the American Academy of Audiology, 11,* 224–229.

Hood, J. D. (1960). The principles and practice of bone-conduction audiometry: A review of the present position. *Laryngoscope, 70,* 1211–1228.

Hood, L. J. (2007). Auditory neuropathy and dys-synchrony. In R. F. Burkhard & D. M. Eggermont (Eds.), *Auditory evoked potentials: Basic principles and clinical applications.* Baltimore, MD: Lippincott Williams & Wilkins.

Hood, W. H., Campbell, R. A., & Hutton, C. L. (1964). An evaluation of the Békésy ascending descending gap. *Journal of Speech and Hearing Research, 7,* 123–132.

House, A. S., Williams, C. E., Hecker, M. H. L., & Kryter, K. D. (1965). Articulation testing methods: Consonantal differentiation with a closed-response set. *Journal of the Acoustical Society of America, 37,* 158–166.

House, W. F. (1982). Surgical considerations in cochlear implants. *Annals of Otology, Rhinology, and Laryngology, 91,* 15–20.

Individuals with Disabilities Education Act of 1990. (1990). Public Law 101-476. U.S.C. 1400et seq.: *U.S. Statutes at Large, 104,* 1103–1151.

Individuals with Disabilities Education Amendments of 1997. (1997). Public Law 105-17. *U.S. Statutes at Large, 111,* 37–157.

Jacobson, E., Downs, M., & Fletcher, J. (1969). Clinical findings in high-frequency thresholds during known ototoxic drug usage. *Journal of Auditory Research, 81,* 379–385.

Jahn, A. F. (1993). Middle ear ventilation with HydroxyVent tube: Review of the initial series. *Otolaryngology—Head and Neck Surgery, 108,* 701–705.

Jastreboff, P. J., & Hazell, J. W. P. (1998). Treatment of tinnitus based on a neurophysiological model. In J. A. Vernon (Ed.), *Tinnitus: Treatment and relief* (pp. 201–217). Boston: Allyn & Bacon.

Jereczek-Fossa, B. A., Zarowski, A., Milini, F., & Orecchia, R. (2003). Radiotherapy-induced ear toxicity. *Cancer Treatment Review, 29,* 417–430.

Jerger, J. (1960). Observations on auditory behavior in lesions of the central auditory pathways. *Archives of Otolaryngology* (Chicago), *71,* 797–806.

Jerger, J. (1970). Clinical experience with impedance audiometry. *Archives of Otolaryngology, 92,* 311–324.

Jerger, J. (1973). Diagnostic audiometry. In J. Jerger (Ed.), *Modern developments in audiology* (2nd ed., pp. 75–115). New York: Academic Press.

Jerger, J. F. (1960). Békésy audiometry in analysis of auditory disorders. *Journal of Speech and Hearing Research, 3,* 275–287.

Jerger, J. F., Shedd, J., & Harford, E. R. (1959). On the detection of extremely small changes in sound intensity. *Archives of Otolaryngology, 69,* 200–211.

Jerger, J., & Hayes, D. (1976). The cross-check principle in pediatric audiometry. *Archives of Otolaryngology, 102,* 614–620.

Jerger, J., & Herer, G. (1961). An unexpected dividend in Békésy audiometry. *Journal of Speech and Hearing Disorders, 26,* 390–391.

Jerger, J., & Jerger, S. (1971). Diagnostic significance of PB word functions. *Archives of Otolaryngology, 93,* 573–580.

Jerger, J., & Musiek, F. (2000). Report of the consensus conference on the diagnosis of auditory processing disorders in school children. *Journal of the American Academy of Audiology, ii,* 467–474.

Jerger, J., Ali, A., Fong, K., & Tseng, E. (1992). Otoacoustic emissions, audiometric sensitivity loss, and speech understanding: A case study. *Journal of the American Academy of Audiology, 3,* 283–286.

Jerger, J., Burney, P., Maudlin, L., & Crump, B. (1974). Predicting hearing loss from the acoustic reflex. *Journal of Speech and Hearing Disorders, 39,* 11–22.

Jerger, J., Chmiel, R., Stach, B., & Spretnjak, M. (1993). Gender affects audiometric shape in presbyacusis. *Journal of the American Academy of Audiology, 4,* 42–49.

Jerger, J., Johnson, K., & Jerger, S. (1988). Effect of response criterion on measures of speech understanding in the elderly. *Ear and Hearing, 9,* 49–56.

Jerger, J., Oliver, T. A., & Jenkins, H. (1987). Suprathreshold abnormalities of the stapedius reflex in acoustic tumors. *Ear and Hearing, 8,* 131–139.

Jerger, J., Speaks, C., & Trammell, J. L. (1968). A new approach to speech audiometry. *Journal of Speech and Hearing Disorders, 33,* 318–328.

Jerger, S., & Jerger, J. (1975). Extra- and intraaxial brain stem auditory disorders. *Audiology, 14,* 93–117.

Jewett, D. L. (1970). Volume-conducted potentials in response to auditory stimuli as detected by averaging in the cat. *Electro-encephalography and Clinical Neurophysiology, 28,* 609–618.

Johns Hopkins Medical Center. One in five Americans has hearing loss. Retrieved May 2, 2013, from http://www.hopkinsmedicine.org/news/media/releases/one_in_five_americans_has_hearing_loss

Johnson, C. D. (1994). Educational consultation: Talking with parents and school personnel. In J. G. Clark & F. N. Martin (Eds.), *Effective counseling in audiology: Principles and practice* (pp. 184–209). Englewood Cliffs, NJ: Prentice Hall.

Johnson, C. D., & Benson, P. V. (2000). *Educational audiology handbook* [CD ROM]. San Diego, CA: Singular Publishing.

Johnson, C. D., & Seaton, J. B. (2011). *Educational audiology handbook* (2nd ed.). Independence, KY: Cengage Learning.

Johnson, E. W. (1977). Auditory test results in 500 cases of acoustic neuroma. *Archives of Otolaryngology, 103,* 152–158.

Johnson, J., Weissman, M. M., & Klerman, G. L. (1992). Service utilization and social morbidity associated with depressive symptoms in the community. *Journal of the American Medical Association, 267,* 1478–1483.

Johnson, L. G., & Hawkins, J. E. (1976). Degeneration patterns in human ears exposed to noise. *Annals of Otology, 85,* 725–739.

Johnson, R., Meikle, M., Vernon, J., & Schleuning, A. (1988). An implantable bone conduction hearing device. *American Journal of Otology, 9,* 93–100.

Johnson, S. J., Hosford-Dunn, H., Paryani, S., Yeager, A. S., & Malachowski, N. (1986). Prevalence of sensorineural hearing loss in premature and sick term infants with perinatally acquired cytomegalovirus infection. *Ear and Hearing, 7,* 325–327.

Joint Committee on Infant Hearing. (1994). Joint Committee on Infant Hearing 1994 position statement. *Asha, 38,* 38–41.

Joint Committee on Infant Hearing. (2000, August). Joint Committee on Infant Hearing 2000 position statement: Principles and guidelines for early hearing detection and intervention programs [Special Issue]. *Audiology Today.*

Joint Committee on Infant Hearing. (2007). Year 2007 Position statement: Principles and guidelines for early hearing detection and intervention programs. *Pediatrics, 120,* 898–921.

Joint Committee on Infant Hearing. (2013). Supplement to the JCIH 2007 position statement: Principles and guidelines for early intervention after confirmation that a child is deaf or hard of hearing. *Pediatrics, 131*(4), e1324–e1349.

Josey, A. F. (1987). Audiologic manifestations of tumors of the VIIIth nerve. *Ear and Hearing, 8,* 198–218.

Josey, A. F., Glasscock, M. E., & Musiek, F. E. (1988). Correlation of ABR and medical imaging in patients with cerebello pontine angle tumors. *The American Journal of Otology, 9*(Suppl.), 12–16.

Kalikow, D. M., Stevens, K. N., & Elliott, L. L. (1977). Development of a test of speech intelligibility in noise using sentence materials with controlled predictability. *Journal of the Acoustical Society of America, 61,* 1337–1351.

Karmody, C. (1969). Asymptomatic maternal rubella and congenital deafness. *Archives of Otolaryngology, 89,* 720–726.

Katz, J. (1962). The use of staggered spondaic words for assessing the integrity of the central auditory nervous system. *Journal of Auditory Research, 2,* 327–337.

Katz, J. (1968). The SSW test: An interim report. *Journal of Speech and Hearing Disorders, 33,* 132–146.

Katz, J. (1978). The effects of conductive hearing loss on auditory function. *Asha 20,* 879–886.

Keith, R. W. (1981). Tests of central auditory function. In R. J. Roeser & M. P. Downs (Eds.), *Auditory disorders in school children* (pp. 159–173). New York: Thieme-Stratton.

Keith, R. W. (1986). *SCAN: A screening test for auditory processing disorders.* San Antonio, TX: The Psychological Corporation, Harcourt Brace Jovanovich.

Keith, R. W. (1994). SCAN-A: Test for auditory processing disorders in adolescents and adults. San Antonio, TX: The Psychological Corporation, Harcourt Brace Jovanovich.

Keith, R. W. (1995). Development and standardization of SCAN-A: Test of auditory processing disorders in adolescents and adults. *Journal of the American Academy of Audiology, 7,* 286–292.

Keith, R. W. (2000). *Random Gap Detection Test.* St. Louis, MO: Auditec.

Keith, R. W., Rudy, J., Donahue, P. A., & Katfamma, B. (1989). Comparison of SCAN results with other auditory and language measures in a clinical population. *Ear and Hearing, 10,* 382–386.

Kemp, D. T. (1978). Stimulated acoustic emissions from within the human auditory system. *Journal of the Acoustical Society of America, 65,* 1386–1391.

Kemp, D. T. (1979). Evidence of mechanical nonlinearity and frequency selective wave amplification in the cochlea. *Archives of Oto-Rhino-Laryngology, 221,* 37–45.

Kemp, D. T. (1981). Physiologically active cochlear micromechanics—one source of tinnitus. In D. Evered & G. Lawrenson (Eds.), *Tinnitus, Ciba Foundation Symposium* (Vol. 85, pp. 54–81). Bath, England: Pittman Books.

Kemp, D. T. (2002). Exploring cochlear status with otoacoustic emissions. In M. S. Robinette & T. J. Glattke (Eds.), *Otoacoustic emissions* (2nd ed., pp. 1–47). New York: Thieme.

Kemp, R. J., Roeser, R. J., Pearson, D., & Ballachanda, B. B. (1995). *Infection control for the professions of audiology and speech-language pathology.* San Diego, CA: Singular Publishing Group.

Kenworthy, O. T., Klee, T., & Tharpe, A. M. (1990). Speech recognition of children with unilateral sensorineural hearing loss as a function of speech stimuli and listening conditions. *Ear and Hearing, 11,* 4.

Keogh, T., Kei, J., Driscoll, C., Cahill, L., Hoffman, A., Wilce, E., Kondamuri, P., & Marinac, J. (2005). Measuring the ability of school children with a history of otitis media to understand everyday speech. *Journal of the American Academy of Audiology, 16,* 301–311.

Kibbe-Michal, K., Verkest, S. B., Gollegly, K. M., & Musiek, F. E. (1986). Late auditory potentials and the P300. *Hearing Instruments, 37,* 22–24.

Killion, M. C., Mueller, H. G., Pavlovic, C. V., & Humes, L. E. (1993). A is for audibility. *The Hearing Journal, 46*(4), 29.

Killion, M. C., Wilber, L. A., & Gudmundsen, G. I. (1985). Insert earphones for more interaural attenuation. *Hearing Instruments, 36,* 34–36.

Kim, L. J., Klopfenstein, J. D., Porter, R. W., & Syms, M. S. (2004). Acoustic neuromas, symptoms and diagnosis. *BNI Quarterly, 20,* 4–16.

Kirkwood, D. (2004). Survey finds most dispensers bullish, but not on over-the-counter devices. *The Hearing Journal 57,* 19–30.

Kochkin, S., & Rogin, C. M. (2000). Quantifying the obvious: The impact of hearing instruments on quality of life. *The Hearing Review, 7*(1), 6–34.

Kochkin, S., Tyler, R., & Born, J. (2011). MarkeTrak VIII: The prevalence of tinnitus in the United States and the self-reported efficacy of various treatments. *Hearing Review, 18*(12), 10–26.

Konkle, D. F., & Berry, G. A. (1983). Masking in speech audiometry. In D. F. Konkle & W. F. Rintelmann (Eds.), *Principles of speech audiometry* (pp. 285–319). Baltimore: University Park Press.

Konkle, D. F., & Rintelmann, W. F. (1983). Introduction to speech audiometry. In D. F. Konkle & W. F. Rintelmann (Eds.), *Principles of speech audiometry* (pp. 1–10). Baltimore: University Park Press.

Kraemer, M. J., Richardson, M. A., Weiss, N. S., Furukawa, C. T., Shapiro, G. G., Pierson, W. E., & Bierman, C. W. (1983). Risk factors for persistent middle-ear effusions. *Journal of the American Medical Association, 249,* 1022–1025.

Kricos, P., & McCarthy, P. (2007). From ear to there: A historical perspective on auditory training. *Seminars in Hearing, 28*(2), 89–98.

Kumazawa, T. (1985). Three acoustic impedance recording methods. *Annals of Otology, Rhinology and Laryngology, 94,* 25–26.

Kurdziel, S., Noffsinger, D., & Olsen, W. (1976). Performance by cortical lesion patients on 40 and 60% time compressed materials. *Journal of the American Audiology Society, 2,* 3–7.

Lamb, L. E., & Peterson, J. L. (1967). Middle ear reflex measurements in pseudohypacusis. *Journal of Speech and Hearing Disorders, 32,* 46–51.

Lane, H. (1987). Mainstreaming of deaf children—From bad to worse. *The Deaf American, 38,* 15.

Lane, H. (1992). *The mask of benevolence: Disabling the deaf community.* New York: Alfred A. Knopf.

Lane, H., & Bahan, B. (1998). Ethics of cochlear implantation in young children: A review and reply from a Deaf-World perspective. *Otolaryngology—Head and Neck Surgery, 119,* 297–314.

Larson, V. D., Williams, D. W., Henderson, W. G., Luethke, L. E., Beck, L. B., Noffsinger, D., Wilson, R. H., Dobie, R. A., Haskell, G. B., Bratt, G. W., Shanks, J. E., Stelmachowicz, P., Boyson, A. E., Donahue, A., Canalis, R., Fausti, S. A., & Rappaport, B. Z. (2000). Efficacy of 3 commonly used hearing aid circuits: A crossover trial. *Journal of the American Medical Association, 284*(14), 1806–1813.

Lawrence, J. (1987). HIV infections in infants and children. *Infections in Surgery, 8,* 249–255.

Lawrence, M. (1969). Labyrinthine fluids. *Archives of Otolaryngology, 89,* 85–89.

Legatt, A. D., Arezzo, J. C., & Vaughan, H. G. (1988). The anatomical and physiologic bases of brain stem auditory evoked potentials. *Neurologic Clinics, 6,* 681–704.

Lehiste, I., & Peterson, G. E. (1959). Linguistic considerations in the study of speech intelligibility. *Journal of the Acoustical Society of America, 31,* 280–286.

Lehiste, I., & Peterson, G. E. (1962). Revised CNC lists for auditory tests. *Journal of Speech and Hearing Disorders, 27,* 62–70.

Lempert, J. (1938). Improvement of hearing in cases of otosclerosis: A new one-stage surgical technique. *Archives of Otolaryngology, 28,* 42–97.

Liden, G., & Kankkonen, A. (1961). Visual reinforcement audiometry. *Acta Otolaryngologica* (Stockholm), *67,* 281–292.

Lieberthal, A. S., Carroll, A. E., Chonmaitree, T., Ganiats, T. G., Hoberman, A., Jackson, M. A., Joffee, M. D., Miller, D. T., Rosenfeld, R. M., Sevilla, X. D., Schwartz, R. H., Thomas, P. A., & Tunkel, D. E. (2013). *Pediatrics, 31,* 964–999.

Ling, D. (1989). *Foundations of spoken language for hearing impaired children.* Washington, DC: Alexander Graham Bell Association for the Deaf.

Ling, D., & Berlin, C. (1997). The six sound test. In D. Ling (Ed.), *Acoustics, audition and speech reception.* Alexandria, VA: Auditory-Verbal International.

Lipscomb, D. M. (1992). Fallacies and foibles in hearing conservation. *Audiology Today, 4,* 29–33.

Lloyd, L. L., Spradlin, J. E., & Reid, M. J. (1968). An operant audiometric procedure for difficult-to-test patients. *Journal of Speech and Hearing Disorders, 33,* 236–245.

Lockwood, A. H., Salvi, R. J., Coad, M. L., Tosley, M. S., Wack, D. S., & Murphy, B. W. (1998). The functional neuroanatomy of tinnitus: Evidence for limbic system links and neural plasticity. *Neurology, 50*(1), 114–122.

Lonsbury-Martin, B. L., & Martin, G. K. (2003). Otoacoustic emissions. *Current Opinion in Otolaryngology and Head & Neck Surgery, 11*(5), 361–366.

Lynn, G. E., & Gilroy, J. (1977). Evaluation of central auditory dysfunction in patients with neurological disorders. In R. W. Keith (Ed.), *Central auditory dysfunction* (pp. 177–222). New York: Grune & Stratton.

Mann, T., Cuttler, K., & Campbell, C. (2001). Newborn hearing screens may give a false sense of security. *Journal of the American Academy of Audiology, 12,* 215–219.

Maran, A. (1966). The causes of deafness in children. *Journal of Laryngology and Otology, 80,* 495–505.

Margolis, R. H. (1993). Detection of hearing impairment with the acoustic stapedius reflex. *Ear and Hearing, 14,* 3–10.

Margolis, R. H., & Goycoolea, H. G. (1993). Multifrequency tympanometry in normal adults. *Ear and Hearing, 14,* 408–413.

Margolis, R. H., & Hunter, L. L. (2000). Acoustic immittance measurements. In R. J. Roeser, M. Valente, & H. Hosford-Dunn (Eds.), *Audiology diagnosis* (pp. 381–423). New York: Thieme.

Martin, F. N. (1966). Speech audiometry and clinical masking. *Journal of Auditory Research, 6,* 199–203.

Martin, F. N. (1972). *Clinical audiometry and masking.* Indianapolis, IN: Bobbs-Merrill.

Martin, F. N. (1974). Minimum effective masking levels in threshold audiometry. *Journal of Speech and Hearing Disorders, 39,* 280–285.

Martin, F. N. (1994). Conveying diagnostic information. In J. G. Clark & F. N. Martin (Eds.), *Effective counseling in audiology: Principles and practice* (pp. 38–69). Englewood Cliffs, NJ: Prentice Hall.

Martin, F. N. (2009). Nonorganic hearing loss. In J. Katz, L. Medwetsky, R. Burkhard, & L. Hood (Eds.), *Handbook of clinical audiology* (6th ed., pp. 699–711). Baltimore, MD: Lippincott Williams and Wilkins.

Martin, F. N., & Blosser, D. (1970). Cross hearing—air conduction or bone conduction. *Psychonomic Science, 20,* 231.

Martin, F. N., & Blythe, M. (1977). On the cross-hearing of spondaic words. *Journal of Auditory Research, 17,* 221–224.

Martin, F. N., & Clark, J. G. (1977). Audiologic detection of auditory processing disorders in children. *Journal of the American Audiology Society, 3,* 140–146.

Martin, F. N., & Clark, J. G. (1996). Behavioral hearing tests with children. In F. N. Martin & J. G. Clark (Eds.), *Hearing care for children* (pp. 115–134). Boston, MA: Allyn & Bacon.

Martin, F. N., & Clark, J.G. (2012). *Introduction to audiology* (11th ed.). Boston: Allyn & Bacon.

Martin, F. N., & Coombes, S. (1976). A tangibly reinforced speech reception threshold procedure for use with small children. *Journal of Speech and Hearing Disorders, 41,* 333–338.

Martin, F. N., & DiGiovanni, D. (1979). Central masking effects on spondee thresholds as a function of masker sensation level and masker sound pressure level. *Journal of the American Audiology Society, 4,* 141–146.

Martin, F. N., & Dowdy, L. K. (1986). A modified spondee threshold procedure. *Journal of Auditory Research, 26,* 115–119.

Martin, F. N., & Fagelson, M. (1995). Bone conduction reconsidered. *Tejas, 20,* 26–27.

Martin, F. N., & Monro, D. A. (1975). The effects of sophistication on Type V Békésy patterns in simulated hearing loss. *Journal of Speech and Hearing Disorders, 40,* 508–513.

Martin, F. N., & Shipp, D. B. (1982). The effects of sophistication on three threshold tests for subjects with simulated hearing loss. *Ear and Hearing, 3,* 34–36.

Martin, F. N., & Stauffer, M. L. (1975). A modification of the Tillman-Olsen method for obtaining the speech reception threshold. *Journal of Speech and Hearing Disorders, 40,* 25–28.

Martin, F. N., & Wittich, W. W. (1966). A comparison of forehead and mastoid tactile bone conduction thresholds. *The Eye, Ear, Nose and Throat Monthly, 45,* 72–74.

Martin, F. N., Bailey, H. A. T., & Pappas, J. J. (1965). The effect of central masking on threshold for speech. *Journal of Auditory Research, 5,* 293–296.

Martin, F. N., Barr, M., & Bernstein, M. (1992). Professional attitudes regarding counseling of hearing-impaired adults. *American Journal of Otology, 13,* 279–287.

Martin, F. N., Bernstein, M. E., Daly, J. A., & Cody, J. P. (1988). Classroom teachers' knowledge of hearing disorders and attitudes about mainstreaming hard-of-hearing children. *Language, Speech and Hearing Services in Schools, 19,* 83–95.

Martin, F. N., Butler, E. C., & Burns, P. (1974), Audiometric Bing test for determination of minimum masking levels for bone conduction tests. *Journal of Speech and Hearing Disorders, 39,* 148–152.

Martin, F. N., Butler, E. C., & Burns, P. (1974). Audiometric Bing test for determination of minimum masking levels for bone-conduction tests. *Journal of Speech and Hearing Disorders, 39,* 148–152.

Martin, F. N., Champlin, C. A., & Chambers, J. (1998). Seventh survey of audiometric practices in the United States. *Journal of the American Academy of Audiology, 9,* 95–104.

Martin, F. N., Champlin, C. A., & Marchbanks, T. P. (1998). A varying intensity story test for simulated hearing loss. *American Journal of Audiology, 7,* 39–44.

Martin, F. N., Champlin, C. A., & McCreery, T. M. (2001). Strategies used in feigning hearing loss. *Journal of the American Academy of Audiology, 12,* 59–63.

Martin, F. N., Champlin, C. A., & Perez, D. D. (2000). The question of phonetic balance in word recognition testing. *Journal of the American Academy of Audiology, 11,* 489–493.

Martin, F. N., Champlin, C. A., & Streetman, P. S. (1997). Audiologists' professional satisfaction. *Journal of the American Academy of Audiology, 8,* 11–17.

Martin, F. N., George, K., O'Neal, J., & Daly, J. (1987). Audiologists' and parents' attitudes regarding counseling of families of hearing impaired children. *Asha, 29,* 27–33.

Martin, F. N., Krall, L., & O'Neal, J. (1989). The diagnosis of acquired hearing loss: Patient reactions. *Asha, 31,* 47–50.

Martin, F. N., Krueger, J. S., & Bernstein, M. (1990). Diagnostic information transfer to hearing-impaired adults. *Tejas, 16,* 29–32.

Martin, F. N., Severance, G. K., & Thibodeau, L. (1991). Insert earphones for speech recognition testing. *Journal of the American Academy of Audiology, 2,* 55–58.

Martin, J. S., Martin, F. N., & Champlin, C. A. (2000). The CON-SOT-LOT test for nonorganic hearing loss. *Journal of the American Academy of Audiology, 11,* 46–51.

Matzker, J. (1959). Two new methods for the assessment of central auditory functions in cases of brain disease. *Annals of Otology, Rhinology and Laryngology, 63,* 1185–1197.

McFadden, D., & Plattsmier, H. S. (1983). Aspirin can potentiate the temporary hearing loss induced by noise. *Hearing Research, 9,* 295–316.

Mehl, A. L., & Thomson, V. (1998). Newborn hearing screening: The great omission. *Pediatrics, 101,* 4e Retrieved from www .pediatrics.org

Mehra, S., Eavey, R. D. & Keamy, D. G. (2009). The epidemiology of hearing impairment in the United States: Newborns, children and adlolescents. *Otolaryngology–Head and Neck Surgery, 140,* 461–472.

Mehrpavar, A. H., Mirmohammadi, S. J., Ghoreyshi, A., Mollasadeghi, A., & Loukzadeh, Z. (2011). High-frequency adiometry: A means for early diagnosis of noise-induced hearing loss. *Noise Health, 13,* 402–406.

Melnick, W. (1984). Auditory effects of noise exposure. In M. Miller & C. Silverman (Eds.), *Occupational hearing conservation* (pp. 100–132). Englewood Cliffs, NJ: Prentice-Hall.

Mendel, L. L., Danhauer, J. L., & Singh, S. (1999). *Singular's illustrated dictionary of audiology.* San Diego, CA: Singular Publishing Group.

Meyerhoff, W. L. (1986). *Disorders of hearing.* Austin, TX: Pro-Ed.

Meyers, D. G. (2002). The coming audiocoil revolution. *Hearing Review, 9,* 28–31.

Meyers, D. G. (2010). Progress toward the looping of America—and doubled hearing aid functionality. *Hearing Review, 17*(2), 10–17.

Miller, D. A. & Sammeth, C.A. (2008). Middle ear implantable hearing devices. In M. Valente, H. Hosford Dunn, & R. J. Roeser (eds.), *Audiology treatment* (2nd ed. pp 324–343). New York: Thieme.

Møller, A. R. (2000). Intraoperative neurophysiological monitoring. In R. J. Roeser, M. Valente, & H. Hosford-Dunn (Eds.), *Audiology diagnosis* (pp. 545–570). New York: Thieme.

Monro, D. A., & Martin, F. N. (1977). The effects of sophistication on four tests for nonorganic hearing loss. *Journal of Speech and Hearing Disorders, 42,* 528–534.

Moore, J. M., Thompson, G., & Folsom, R. C. (1992). Auditory responsiveness of premature infants utilizing visual reinforcement audiometry. *Ear and Hearing, 13,* 187–194.

Moorehouse, A., Waddington, D., & Adams, M. (2005). Procedure for the assessment of low frequency noise complaints. University of Salford, Manchester, UK Contract No. NANR45.

Morrison, A. W., & Bundey, S. E. (1970). The inheritance of otosclerosis. *Journal of Laryngology and Otology, 84,* 921–932.

Moses, K. (1979). Parenting a hearing-impaired child. *Volta Review, 81,* 73–80.

Mueller, H. G. (1987a). An auditory test protocol for evaluation of neural trauma. *Seminars in Hearing, 8,* 223–238.

Mueller, H. G. (1987b). The Staggered Spondaic Word test: Practical use. *Seminars in Hearing, 8,* 267–277.

Mueller, H. G., Hawkins, D. B., & Northern, J. L. (1992). *Probe microphone measurements: Hearing aid selection and assessment.* San Diego, CA: Singular Publishing Group.

Musiek, F. E. (1983). The evaluation of brainstem disorders using ABR and central auditory tests. *Monographs in Contemporary Audiology, 4,* 1–24.

Musiek, F. E., & Baran, J. A. (2007). *The auditory system: Anatomy, physiology, and clinical correlates.* Boston: Allyn & Bacon.

Musiek, F. E. & Chermak, G. D. (2007). *Handbook of (central) auditory processing disorders.* Vol II. San Diego, CA: Singular Publishing.

Musiek, F. E., Bornstein, S. P., & Rintelmann, W. F. (1995). Transient evoked otoacoustic emissions and pseudohypacusis. *Journal of the American Academy of Audiology, 6,* 293–301.

Musiek, F. E., Shinn, J., Jirsa, R., Bamiou, D., Baran, J. A., & Zaidan, E. (2005). The GIN (Gaps-in-Noise) test performance in subjects with confirmed central auditory nervous system involvement. *Ear and Hearing, 6,* 608–618.

Näätänen, R. (1995). The mismatch negativity: A powerful tool for cognitive neuroscience. *Ear and Hearing, 16,* 6–18.

Nabelek, A. K., Freyaldenhoven, M. C., Tampas, J. W., Burchfield, S. B., & Muenchen, R. A. (2006). Acceptable noise level as a predictor of hearing aid use. *Journal of the American Academy of Audiology, 17,* 626–639.

Nadler, N. (1997, November/December). Noisy toys: Hidden hazards. *Hearing Health,* 18–21.

Nagel, R. F. (1964). RRLJ: A new technique for the noncooperative patient. *Journal of Speech and Hearing Disorders, 29,* 492–493.

Naseri, I., Jerris, R. C., & Sobol, S. E. (2009). Nationwide trends in pediatric *Staphylococcus aureus* head and neck infections. *Archives of Otolaryngology Head Neck Surgery, 135,* 14–16.

Nashner, L. M. (1993). Computerized dynamic posturography. In G. P. Jacobson, C. W. Newman, & J. M. Kartush, *Handbook of balance function testing* (pp. 280–307). St. Louis, MO: Mosby.

National American Precis Syndicated. (2007). Money matters: Hearing loss may mean income loss. Retrieved July 10, 2007, from www.napsnet.com/health/70980.html

National Institute for Occupational Safety and Health. (1998). *Criteria for a recommended standard: Occupational noise exposure* (Report No. 98–126). Cincinnati, OH: Author.

National Institute for Occupational Safety and Health. (2001). Work related hearing loss. (DHHS/NIOSH Pub. No. 2001-103). Cincinnati, OH: Author.

National Institute on Deafness and Other Communication Disorders. (2010a). Retrieved June 1, 2013, from http://www.nidcd.nih.gov/health/statistics/Pages/quick.aspx

National Institute on Deafness and Other Communication Disorders (2010b). Healthy People 2010 Hearing Health Progress Review. Retrieved June 3, 2013, from http://www.nidcd.nih.gov/health/healthyhearing/what_hh/pages/progress_review_04.aspx

National Institutes of Health (NIH) Consensus Statement. (1991). *Acoustic neuroma.* U.S. Department of Health and Human Services, NIH Consensus Development Conference, Bethesda, MD.

National Institutes of Health. (1993). *Early identification of hearing impairment in infants and young children.* NIH Consensus Statement, *11,* 1–24.

Negley, C., Katbamna, B., Crumpton, C., & Lawson, G. D. (2007). Effects of cigarette smoking on distortion product otoacoustic emissions. *Journal of the American Academy of Audiology, 18,* 665–674.

Nelson, J. A., Henion, K. M., & Martin, F. N. (2000). Scoring Spanish word-recognition tests by nonnative Spanish speakers. *Tejas, 24,* 10–13.

Nemes, J., (2010), Tele-audiology, a once-futuristic concept is growing into a worldwide reality. *The Hearing Journal, 63,* 19–20, 22–24.

Newby, H. A. (1948). Evaluating the efficiency of group screening tests of hearing. *Journal of Speech and Hearing Disorders, 13,* 236–240.

Nicholas, J. G., & Geers, A. E. (2003). Personal, social, and family adjustment in school-aged children with a cochlear implant. *Ear and Hearing, 24,* 69S–81S.

Nilsson, M., Soli, S., & Sullivan, J. (1994). Development of the hearing in noise test for the measurement of speech reception thresholds in quiet and in noise. *Journal of the Acoustical Society of America, 95,* 1085–1099.

Niquette, P., & Eply, J. (2010). *Hearing protection for musicians: Know you've done it right.* San Diego, CA: American Academy of Audiology Convention, April 15.

Niskar, A. S., Kieszak, S. M., Holmes, A. E., Estaban, E., Rubin, C., & Brody, D. J. (2001). Estimated prevalence of noise-induced hearing threshold shifts among children 6 to 19 years of age: The Third National Health and Nutrition Examination Survey, 1988–1994, United States. *Pediatrics, 108,* 40–43.

No Child Left Behind Act of 2001 (NCLB). (2001). Public Law 107–110. 107th Congress.

Nober, E. H. (1970). Cutile air and bone conduction thresholds of the deaf. *Exceptional Children, 36,* 571–579.

Noffsinger, D., Martinez, C., & Schaefer, A. (1985). Puretone techniques in evaluation of central auditory function. In J. Katz (Ed.), *Handbook of clinical audiology* (3rd ed., pp. 337–354). Baltimore, MD: Williams & Wilkins.

Northern, J. L., & Downs, M. P. (1991). *Hearing in children* (4th ed.). Baltimore: Williams and Wilkins.

O'Conner, A. F., & Shea, J. J. (1981). Autophony and the patulous eustachian tube. *Laryngoscope, 91,* 1427–1435.

Occupational Safety and Health Administration. (1983, March 8). Occupational noise exposure: Hearing conservation amendment; final rule. *Federal Register, 46,* 9738–9785.

Occupational Safety and Health Administration. (2010). Occupational noise exposure—1910–95. Retrieved January 25, 2010, from www.osha.gov/pls/oshaweb/owadisp.show_document?p_table=STANDARDS&p_id=9735

Olsen, W. O., & Noffsinger, D. (1976). Masking level differences for cochlear and brainstem lesions. *Annals of Otology, Rhinology and Laryngology, 85,* 820–825.

Orchik, D. J., Schumaier, D. R., Shea, J. J., & Xianxi, G. (1995). Middle ear and inner ear effects on clinical bone-conduction threshold. *Journal of the American Academy of Audiology, 6,* 256–260.

Oviatt, D. L., & Kileny, P. (1984). Normative characteristics of ipsilateral acoustic reflex adaptations. *Ear and Hearing, 5,* 145–152.

Owens, E., & Schubert, E. D. (1977). Development of the California Consonant Test. *Journal of Speech and Hearing Research, 20,* 463–474.

Palmer, C. V. (2009). Best practices: It's a matter of ethics. *Audiology Today, 28*(5), 30–35.

Palva, A., & Jokinen, K. (1975). The role of the binaural test in filtered speech audiometry. *Acta Otolaryngologica, 79,* 310–314.

Pascoe, D. P. (1991). *Hearing aids: Who needs them?* St. Louis, MO: Big Bend Books.

Pascoe, D. R. (1975). Frequency responses of hearing aids and their effects on the speech perception of hearing impaired subjects. *Annals of Otology, Rhinology and Laryngology, 23*(Suppl.), 1–40.

Patrick, P. E. (1987). Identification audiometry. In F. N. Martin (Ed.), *Hearing disorders in children* (pp. 399–425). Austin, TX: Pro-Ed.

Peck, J. E. (2011). *Pseudohypacusis: False and exagerated hearing loss.* San Diego, CA: Plural Publishing.

Peck, J. E. (2011). Pseudohypacusis: False and exaggerated hearing loss. In R. Seewald & A. M. Tharpe (Eds.), *Comprehensive handbook of pediatric audiology* (pp. 269–280). San Diego, CA: Plural Publishing.

Pedersen, E., van den Berg, F., Bakker, R., & Bouma, J. (2009). Response to noise from modern wind farms in the Netherlands. *Journal of the Acoustical Society of America, 126,* 634–643.

Pick, G. F. (1980). Level dependence of psychological frequency resolution and auditory filter shape. *Journal of the Acoustical Society of America, 68,* 1085–1095.

Picton, T. W. (1995). The neurophysiological evaluation of auditory discrimination. *Ear and Hearing, 16,* 1–5.

Picton, T. W., Durieux-Smith, A., Champagne, S. C., Whittingham, J., Moran, L. M., Giguere, C., & Beauregard, Y. (1998). Objective evaluation of aided thresholds using auditory steady-state responses. *Journal of the American Academy of Audiology, 9,* 315–331.

Pirvola, U., Xing-Qun, L., Virkkala, J., Saarma, M., Murakata, C., Camoratto, A., Walton, K., & Ylikoski, J. (2000). Rescue of hearing, auditory hair cells, and neurons by CEP-1347/KT7515, an inhibitor of c-Jun N-terminal kinase activation. *Journal of Neuroscience, 20*(1), 43–50.

Plant, G. (1998). Training in the use of a tactile supplement to lipreading: A long-term case study. *Ear and Hearing, 19,* 394–406.

Plate, S., Johnsen, M. N. J., Pederson, N., & Thompsen, K. A. (1979). The frequency of patulous eustachian tubes in pregnancy. *Clinical Otolaryngology, 4,* 393–400.

Pool, J. I., Pava, A. A., & Greenfield, E. C. (1970). *Acoustic nerve tumors: Early diagnosis and treatment* (2nd ed.). Springfield, IL: Thomas.

Popelka, G. R. (1983). Basic acoustic immittance measures. *Audiology: A Journal for Continuing Education, 8,* 1–16.

Press, L., & Vernon, J. (1997). Tinnitus in the elderly. *Hearing Health, 13,* 6ff.

Price, G. R., & Kalb, J. T. (1999). Auditory hazard from airbag noise exposure. *Journal of the Acoustical Society of America, 106*(4), 2629–2637.

Prieve, B. A., Gorga, M. P., Schmidt, A., Neely, S., Peters, J., Schulte, L., & Jesteadt, W. (1993). Analysis of transient-evoked otoacoustic emissions in normal-hearing and hearing-impaired ears. *Journal of the Acoustical Society of America, 93,* 3308–3319.

Prieve, B., & Fitzgerald, T. (2009). Otoacoustic emissions. In J. Katz, L. Medwedwetsky, R. Burkard, & L. Hood (Eds.), *Handbook of clinical audiology* (6th ed., pp. 497–528). Baltimore, MD: Lippincott Williams & Wilkins.

Probst, R., Lonsbury-Martin, B. L., & Martin, G. K. (1991). A review of otoacoustic emissions. *Journal of the Acoustical Society of America, 89,* 2027–2067.

Pulec, J. (1996). Ménière's disease. In J. L. Northern (Ed.), *Hearing disorders* (3rd ed., pp. 165–176). Boston: Allyn & Bacon.

Rapin, I., & Gravel, J. S. (2006). Auditory neuropathy: A biologically inappropriate label unless acoustic nerve involvement is documented. *Journal of the American Academy of Audiology, 17,* 147–150.

Reich, G., & Griest, S. (1991). *American Tinnitus Association hyperacousis survey.* Fourth International Tinnitus Seminar, Bordeaux, France.

Rentschler, G. J., & Rupp, R. R. (1984). Conductive hearing loss: Cause for concern. *Hearing Instruments, 35,* 12–14.

Riedner, E. D., & Efros, P. L. (1995). Nonorganic hearing loss and child abuse: Beyond the sound booth. *British Journal of Audiology, 29,* 195–197.

Roberts, J. E., Burchinal, M. R., & Zeisel, S. A. (2002). Otitis media in early childhood in relation to children's school-age language and academic skills. *Pediatrics, 110,* 696–706.

Robeznieks, A. (2003, September). First embryos screened for deafness gene. *American Medical News.* Retrieved September 20, 2007, from Amednews.com

Rock, E. H. (1974). Practical otologic applications and considerations in impedance audiometry. *Impedance Newsletter, 3*(Suppl.). New York: American Electromedics Corporation.

Roeser, R. J., Buckley, K. A., & Stickney, G. S. (2000). Pure tone tests. In R. J. Roeser, M. Valente, & H. Hosford-Dunn (Eds.), *Audiology diagnosis* (pp. 227–251). New York: Thieme.

Rose, D. S. (1983). The fundamental role of hearing in psychological development. *Hearing Instruments, 34,* 22–26.

Roseberry-McKibbin, C. (1997). Working with linguistically and culturally diverse clients. In K. G. Shipley (Ed.), *Interviewing and counseling in communicative disorders* (pp. 151–173). Boston: Allyn & Bacon.

Rosen, S. (1953). Mobilization of the stapes to restore hearing in otosclerosis. *New York Journal of Medicine, 53,* 2650–2653.

Rosen, S., Bergman, M., Plester, D., El-Mofty, A., & Hammed, H. (1962). Presbycusis study of a relatively noise-free population in the Sudan. *Annals of Otology, Rhinology and Laryngology, 71,* 727–743.

Rosenfeld, R. M., Schwartz, S. R., Pynnonen, M. A., Tunkel, D. E., Hussey, H. M., Fichera, J. S.… Schellhase, K. G. (2013). Clinical practice guideline: Tympanosotm tubes in children—executive summary. *Otoloaryngol Head Necu Surg, 149 (1) 8-16*

Ross, M. (1964). The variable intensity pulse count method (VIPCM) for the detection and measurement of the pure-tone threshold of children with functional hearing losses. *Journal of Speech and Hearing Disorders, 29,* 477–482.

Ross, M. (2002). Telecoils: The powerful assistive listening device. *Hearing Review, 9,* 22–26.

Ross, M., & Calvert, D. R. (1967). The semantics of deafness. *Volta Review, 69,* 644–649.

Ross, M., & Huntington, D. A. (1962). Concerning the reliability and equivalency of the CID W-22 auditory tests. *Journal of Auditory Research, 2,* 220–228.

Ross, M., & Lerman, J. (1970). A picture identification test for hearing impaired children. *Journal of Speech and Hearing Research, 13,* 44–53.

Ross, M., & Matkin, N. (1967). The rising audiometric configuration. *Journal of Speech and Hearing Disorders, 32,* 377–382.

Ross, M., Brackett, D., & Maxon, A. (1991). *Assessment and management of mainstreamed hearing-impaired children.* Austin: Pro-Ed.

Rowsowski, J. J., Nakajima, H. H., & Merchant, S. N. (2008). Clinical utility of Laser-Doppler Vibrometer measurements in live normal and pathologic human ears. *Ear and Hearing, 29,* 3–19.

Ruhm, H. B., & Cooper, W. A., Jr. (1962). Low sensation level effects of pure-tone delayed auditory feedback. *Journal of Speech and Hearing Research, 5,* 185–193.

Ryals, B. M. (2000). Regeneration of the auditory pathway. In M. Valente, H. Hosford-Dunn, & R. J. Roeser (Eds.), *Audiology treatment* (pp. 755–771). New York: Thieme.

Sackett, D. L., Rosenberg, W. M., Gray, J. A., Haynes, R. B., & Richardson, W. S. (1996). Evidence-based medicine: What it is and what it isn't. *British Medical Journal, 312,* 71–72.

Sanderson-Leepa, M. E., & Rintelmann, W. F. (1976). Articulation function and test-retest performance of normal-hearing children on three speech discrimination tests: WIPI, PBK 50 and NU Auditory Test No. 6. *Journal of Speech and Hearing Disorders, 41,* 503–519.

Sandlin, R. E., & Olsson, R. T. (2000). Subjective tinnitus: Its mechanisms and treatment. In M. Valente, H. Hosford-Dunn, & R. J. Roeser (Eds.), *Audiology treatment* (pp. 691–714). New York: Thieme.

Sataloff, J., Sataloff, R. T., & Vassallo, L. A. (1980). *Hearing loss* (2nd ed.). Philadelphia: Lippincott.

Saunders, G. H., & Haggard, M. P. (1989). The clinical assessment of obscure auditory dysfunction, 1: Auditory and psychological factors. *Ear and Hearing, 10,* 200–208.

Saunders, G. H., & Haggard, M. P. (1993). The influence of personality-related factors upon consultation for two different "marginal" organic pathologies with and without reports of auditory symptomatology. *Ear and Hearing, 14,* 242–248.

Schechter, M. A., McDermott, J. C., & Fausti, S. A. (1992). The incidence of psychological dysfunction in a group of patients fitted with tinnitus maskers. *Audiology Today, 4,* 34–35.

Scheifele, L, Clark, J. G. & Scheifele, P. M. (2012). Canine hearing loss management. In B. L. Njaa & L. K. Cole (Eds.). Otology and otic disease. *Veterinary Clinics of North America: Small Animal Practice.* 1225–1239.

Scheifele, P. M., Clark, J. G., Miller, J. H., Gaglione, E., & Starke, K. (2009). Ballroom music spillover into a beluga whale aquarium exhibit. *Advances in Acoustics and Vibration,* vol. 2012, Article ID 402130, 7 pages doi:10.1155/2012/ 402130.

Schlauch, R. S., Arnce, K. D., Lindsay, M. O., Sanchez, S., & Doyle, T. N. (1998), Identification of pseudohypacusis using speech recognition thresholds. *Ear and Hearing, 17,* 229–236.

Schmida, M. J., Peterson, H. J., & Tharpe, A. M. (2003). Visual reinforcement audiometry using digital video disc and conventional reinforcers. *American Journal of Audiology, 12,* 35–40.

Schuknecht, H. F. (1993). *Pathology of the ear* (2nd ed.). Philadelphia, PA: Lea & Febiger.

Schum, D. J., & Matthews, L. J. (1992). SPIN test performance of elderly hearing-impaired listeners. *Journal of the American Academy of Audiology, 3,* 303–307.

Schwaber, M. (1992). Neuroplasticity of the adult primate auditory cortex. *Audiology Today, 4,* 19–20.

Self Help for Hard of Hearing People, Inc. (1996). Position statement on group hearing aid orientation programs. *SHHH, 3,* 29.

Sells, J. P., Hurley, R. M., Morehouse, C. R., & Douglas, J. E. (1997). Validity of the ipsilateral acoustic reflex as a screening parameter. *Journal of the American Academy of Audiology, 8,* 132–136.

Shahrokh, N. C., & Hales, R. E. (Eds.). (2003). *American psychiatric glossary* (8th ed.). Washington, DC: American Psychiatric Publishing.

Shanks, J. E., Lilly, D. J., Margolis, R. H., Wiley, T. L., & Wilson, R. H. (1988). Tympanometry. *Journal of Speech and Hearing Disorders, 53,* 354–377.

Shargorodsky, J., Curhan, G. C., & Farwell, W. R. (2010). Prevalence and characteristics of tinnitus among US adults. *American Journal of Medicine, 123*(8), 711–718.

Shea, J. J. (1958). Fenestration of the oval window. *Annals of Otology, Rhinology and Laryngology, 67,* 932–951.

Shenk, H., & Dancer, J. (2004). *The dangers of ear candling.* Retrieved August 10, 2004, from www.advanceforaud.com/ common/Editorial/Editorial.aspx?CC=36427

Shepherd, D. C. (1978). Pediatric audiology. In D. E. Rose (Ed.), *Audiological assessment* (2nd ed., pp. 261–300). Englewood Cliffs, NJ: Prentice-Hall.

Silver, F. W. (1996). Management of conversion disorder. *American Journal of Physical Medical Rehabilitation, 75,* 134–140.

Silverman, C. A., Silman, S., Emmer, M. B., Schoepflin, J. R., & Lutolf, J. J. (2006). Auditory deprivation in adults with asymmetric, sensorineural hearing impairment. *Journal of the American Academy of Audiology, 17,* 747–762.

Silverstein, H., Thompson, J., Rosenberg, S. I., Brown, N., & Light, J. (2004). Silverstein microwick. *Otolaryngologic Clinics of North America, 37*(5), 1019–1034.

Simons-McCandless, M., & Parkin, J. (1997). Patient reported benefit and objective outcome data in adult cochlear implant patients. *Audiology Today, 9*(6), 27, 29, 31.

Sivian, L. J., & White, S. D. (1933). On minimum audible sound fields. *Journal of the Acoustical Society of America, 4,* 288–321.

Skafte, M. D. (1990). Fifty years of hearing health care. *Hearing Instruments,* Commemorative Issue, *41*(9), 38, 52–54.

Skafte, M. D. (2000). The 1999 hearing instrument market: The dispenser's perspective. *Hearing Review, 7*(6), 8–40.

Sklare, D. A., & Denenberg, L. J. (1987). Interaural attenuation for Tubephone insert earphones. *Ear and Hearing, 8,* 298–300.

Smith, B., & Resnick, D. (1972). An auditory test for assessing brain stem integrity: Preliminary report. *Laryngoscope, 82,* 414–424.

Smith, S. D. (1994). Genetic counseling. In J. G. Clark & F. N. Martin (Eds.), *Effective counseling in audiology: Perspectives and practice* (pp. 70–91). Englewood Cliffs, NJ: Prentice Hall.

Snyder, J. M. (2001). Audiological evaluation for exaggerated hearing loss. In R. A. Dobie (Ed.), *Medical-legal evaluation of hearing loss* (2nd ed., pp. 49–88). San Diego: Singular Thomsen Learning.

Spitzer, J. B., Ghossaini, S. N., & Wazen, J. J. (2002). Evolving applications in the use of bone-anchored hearing aids. *American Journal of Audiology, 11,* 96–103.

Spradlin, J. E., & Lloyd, L. L. (1965). Operant conditioning audiometry with low level retardates: A preliminary report. In L. L. Lloyd & D. R. Frisina (Eds.), *The audiological assessment of the mentally retarded: Proceedings of a national conference* (pp. 45–58). Parsons, KS: Parsons State Hospital and Training Center.

Stach, B. A. (2003). *Comprehensive dictionary of audiology: Illustrated* (2nd ed.). Clifton Park, NY: Delmar Learning.

Starr, A., Picton, T. W., Sininger, Y., Hood, L., & Berlin, C. I. (1996). Auditory neuropathy. *Brain, 119,* 741–753.

Stewart, J. M., & Downs, M. P. (1984). Medical management of the hearing-handicapped child. In J. L. Northern (Ed.), *Hearing disorders* (2nd ed., pp. 267–278). Boston: Little, Brown.

Stika, C. J., Ross, M., & Cuevas, C. (2002 May/June). Hearing aid services and satisfaction: The consumer viewpoint. *Hearing Loss (SHHH),* 25–31.

Strasnick, B., Glasscock, M. E., Haynes, D., McMenomey, S. O., & Minor, L. B. (1994). The natural history of untreated acoustic neuromas. *Laryngoscope, 104,* 1115–1119.

Strom, K. (2004). The HR 2004 dispenser survey. *Hearing Review, 11*(6), 14–32.

Studebaker, G. A. (1962). Placement of vibrator in bone conduction testing. *Journal of Speech and Hearing Research, 5,* 321–331.

Studebaker, G. A. (1967). Intertest variability and the air-bone gap. *Journal of Speech and Hearing Disorders, 32,* 82–86.

Suzuki, T., & Ogiba, Y. (1961). Conditioned orientation reflex audiometry. *Archives of Otolaryngology, 74,* 84–90.

Svirsky, M. A., Robbins, A. M., Kirk, K. I., Pisoni, D. B., & Miyamoto, R. T. (2000). Language development in profoundly deaf children with cochlear implants. *Psychological Science, 11*(2), 153–158.

Sweetow, R. W., & Sabes, J. H. (2006). The need for and development of an adaptive listening and communication enhancement (LACE™) program. *Journal of the American Academy of Audiology, 17,* 538–558.

Telian, S. A., & Kileny, P. R. (1988). Pitfalls in neurotologic diagnosis. *Ear and Hearing, 9,* 86–91.

Telian, S. A., Kileny, P. R., Niparko, J. K., Kemink, J. L., & Graham, M. D. (1989). Normal auditory brainstem response in patients with acoustic neuroma. *Laryngoscope, 99,* 10–14.

Telischi, F. F., Widick, M. P., Lonsbury-Martin, B. L., & McCoy, M. J. (1995). Monitoring cochlear function intraoperatively using distortion product otoacoustic emissions. *American Journal of Otology, 16,* 597–608.

Tharpe, A. M., & Bess, F. H. (1991). Identification and management of children with minimal hearing loss. *International Journal of Otorhinolaryngology, 21,* 41–50.

Thelin, J. W. (1997). *Ascending-descending test for functional hearing loss.* Poster presented at the 1997 convention of the American Academy of Audiology, Fort Lauderdale, FL.

Thelin, J. W., & Swanson, L. A. (2006). CHARGE syndrome, *The ASHA Leader,* 6–7.

Thornton, A. R., & Raffin, M. J. M. (1978). Speech discrimination scores modified as a binomial variable. *Journal of Speech and Hearing Research, 21,* 507–518.

Tillman, T. W., & Carhart, R. (1966). An expanded test for speech discrimination utilizing CNC monosyllabic words. Northwestern University Auditory Test No. 6, *Technical Report, SAM-TR-66-55.* Brooks Air Force Base, TX: USAF School of Aerospace Medicine, Aerospace Medical Division (AFSC).

Tillman, T. W., Carhart, R., & Wilber, L. (1963). A test for speech discrimination composed of CNC monosyllabic words. Northwestern University Auditory Test No. 4, *Technical Report, SAM-TDR-62-135.* Brooks Air Force Base, TX: USAF School of Aerospace Medicine, Aerospace Medical Division (AFSC).

Tillman, T. W., & Olsen, W. O. (1973). Speech audiometry. In J. Jerger (Ed.), *Modern developments in audiology* (2nd ed., pp. 37–74). New York: Academic Press.

Tobey, E. A., Devous, M. D., Buckley, K., Overson, G., Harris, T., Ringe, W., & Martinez-Verhoff, J. (2005). Pharmacological enhancement of aural habilitation in adult cochlear implant users. *Ear and Hearing, 26,* 45S–56S.

Tobias, J. V. (1964). On phonemic analysis of speech discrimination tests. *Journal of Speech and Hearing Research, 7,* 98–100.

Tonry, K. L. (1988). A comparison of discrimination scores using the short isophonemic and CID W-22 word lists. Unpublished master's thesis, University of Cincinnati.

Torres-Russotto, D., Landau, W. M., Harding, G. W., Bohne, B. A., Sun, K., & Sinatra, P. M. (2009). Calibrated finger rub auditory screening test (CALFRAST). *Neurology, 72,* 1595–1600.

Tremblay, K. L., & Kraus, N. (2002). Auditory training induces asymmetrical changes in cortical neural activity. *Journal of Speech, Language and Hearing Research, 45,* 564–572.

Tremblay, K. L., Kraus, N., Carrell, T. D., & McGee, T. (1997). Central auditory system plasticity: Generalization to novel stimuli following listening training. *Journal of the Acoustical Society of America, 102,* 3762–3773.

Trychin, S. (1994). Helping people cope with hearing loss. In J. G. Clark & F. N. Martin (Eds.), *Effective counseling in audiology: Perspectives and practice* (pp. 247–277). Englewood Cliffs, NJ: Prentice Hall.

Turner, R. G., Robinette, M. S., & Bauch, C. D. (1999). Clinical decisions. In F. E. Musiek & W. F. Rintelmann (Eds.), *Contemporary perspectives in hearing assessment* (pp. 437–463). Boston: Allyn and Bacon.

21st Century Communications and Video Accessability Act. (2010). Public Law 111-260. http://www.gpo.gov/fdsys/pkg/PLAW-111publ260/pdf/PLAW-111publ260.pdf. Retrieved 11/1/2013.

Tyler, R. S., & Schum, D. J. (1995). *Assistive devices for persons with hearing impairment.* Boston: Allyn & Bacon.

U.S. Bureau of the Census. (1990). *Statistical abstract of the United States: 1990* (110th ed.). Washington, DC: Government Printing Office.

U.S. Bureau of the Census. (2000). *Statistical abstract of the United States: 2000* (119th ed.). Washington, DC: U.S. Department of Commerce.

U.S. Department of Health and Human Resources. (1993). *Prevalence of selected chronic conditions: United States, 1986–88.* Washington, DC: Centers for Disease Control and Prevention, National Center for Health Statistics.

U.S. Department of Veterans Affairs (2008). Annual Benefits Report FY 2008. Veterans Benefits Administration. Retrieved September 22, 2009, from www.vba.va.gov/REPORTS/abr/208_abr.pdf

Utley, J. (1946). A test of lipreading ability. *Journal of Speech and Hearing Disorders, 11,* 109–116.

Valente, M., Peterein, J., Goebel, J., & Neely, J. G. (1995). Four cases of acoustic neuromas with normal hearing. *Journal of the American Academy of Audiology, 6,* 203–210.

Valente, M., Valente, M., & Goebel, J. (1992). High-frequency thresholds: Circumaural earphone versus insert earphone. *Journal of the American Academy of Audiology, 3,* 410–418.

Van Bergeijk, W. A., Pierce, J. R., & David, E. E. (1960). *Waves and the ear.* New York: Doubleday.

Vaugn, G. R., Lightfoot, R. K., & Teter, D. L. (1988). Assistive listening devices and systems (ALDS) enhance the lifestyles of hearing impaired persons. *American Journal of Otology, 9,* 101–106.

Veniar, F. A., & Salston, R. S. (1983). An approach to the treatment of pseudohypacusis in children. *American Journal of Disorders of Childhood, 137,* 34–36.

Ventry, I. M., & Chaiklin, J. B. (1962). Functional hearing loss: A problem in terminology. *Asha, 4,* 251–254.

Vernon, J., & Press, L. (1998). Treatment for hyperacusis. In J. Vernon (Ed.), *Tinnitus: Treatment and relief* (pp. 223–227). Boston: Allyn & Bacon.

Vernon, M., & Mindel, E. (1978). Psychological and psychiatric aspects of profound hearing loss. In D. Rose (Ed.), *Audiological assessment* (pp. 99–145). Englewood Cliffs, NJ: Prentice-Hall.

Vittitow, M., Windmill, I. M., Yates, J. W., & Cunningham, D. R. (1994). Effect of simultaneous exercise and noise exposure (music) on hearing. *Journal of the American Academy of Audiology, 5,* 343–348.

Walker, J. D. (2003). *Universal Newborn Screening: Saving Monday, saving lives.* Invited Scientific, 2003 Annual Meeting of the Texas Chapter of the American Academy of Pediatrics, Galveston, TX.

Watermeyer, J., Kanji, A. & Cohen, A. (2012). Caregiver recall and understanding of paediatric diagnostic information and assessment feedback. *International Journal of Audiology, 51,* 864–869.

Wayner, D. S., & Abrahamson, J. E. (1996). *Learning to hear again: An audiological curriculum guide.* Austin, TX: Hear Again Publishing. Retrieved from www.hearagainpublishing.com

Wazen, J. J., Spitzer, J. B., Ghossaini, S. N., Fayad, J. N., Niparko, J. K., Cox, K., Brackmann, D. E., & Soli, S. D. (2003). Transcranial contralateral cochlear stimulation in unilateral deafness. *Otolaryngology—Head and Neck Surgery, 129,* 248–254.

Weaver, N. J., Wardell, F. N., & Martin, F. N. (1979). Comparison of tangibly reinforced speech-reception and pure-tone thresholds of mentally retarded children. *American Journal of Mental Deficiency, 33,* 512–517.

Weber, P. C. (2002). Medical and surgical considerations for implantable hearing prosthetic devices. *American Journal of Audiology, 11,* 134–138.

Webster, D. B., & Webster, M. (1977). Neonatal sound deprivation affects brain stem auditory nuclei. *Archives of Otolaryngology, 103,* 392–396.

Wedenberg, E. (1956). Auditory test in newborn infants. *Acta Otolaryngologica, 46,* 446–461.

Wegel, R. L., & Lane, G. I. (1924). The auditory masking of one pure tone by another and its probable relation to the dynamics of the inner ear. *Physiological Review, 23,* 266–285.

Whitehead, M. L., Lonsbury-Martin, B. L., & Martin, G. K. (1992). Relevance of animal models to the clinical application of otoacoustic emissions. *Seminars in Hearing, 13,* 81–101.

Wild, D. C., Brewster, M. J., & Banerjee, A. R. (2005). Noise-induced hearing loss is exacerbated by long term smoking. *Clinical Otolaryngology, 30,* 517–520.

Wilder, R. T., Flick, R. P., Sprung, J., Katusic, S. K., Barbaresi, W. J., Mickelson, C., Gleich, S. J., Schroeder, D. R., Weaver, A. L., & Warner, D. O. (2009). Early exposure to anesthesia and learning disabilities in a population-based birth cohort. *Anesthesiology, 110*(4), 796–804.

Wiley, T. L., Stoppenbach, D. T., Feldhake, L. J., Moses, K. A., & Thordardottir, E. T. (1994). Audiologic practices: What is popular versus what is supported by evidence. *American Journal of Audiology, 4,* 26–34.

Williams, C. J., & Jacobs, A. M. (2009). The impact of otitis media on cognitive and educational outcomes. *Medical Journal of Australia,* Supplement 9, S69–S72.

Williams, P. S. (1975). A tympanometry pressure swallow test for assessment of eustachian tube function. *Annals of Otology, Rhinology and Laryngology, 84,* 339–343.

Williford, J. A. (1977). Differential diagnosis of central auditory dysfunction. *Audiology: An Audio Journal for Continuing Education, 2.*

Wilson, R. H., & Antablin, J. K. (1980). A picture identification task as an estimate of the word-recognition performance of nonverbal adults. *Journal of Speech and Hearing Disorders, 45,* 223–238.

Wilson, R. H., & Margolis, R. H. (1983). Measurements of auditory thresholds for speech stimuli. In D. F. Konkle & W. F. Rintelmann (Eds.), *Principles of speech audiometry* (pp. 79–126). Baltimore: University Park Press.

Wilson, R. H., Moncrieff, D. W., Townsend, E. A., & Pillion, A. L. (2003). Development of a 500-Hz masking-level difference protocol for clinical use. *Journal of the American Academy of Audiology, 14,* 1–8.

Wittich, W. W., Wood, T. J., & Mahaffey, R. B. (1971). Computerized speech audiometric procedures. *Journal of Auditory Research, 11,* 335–344.

Woodford, C. M., Harris, G., Marquette, M. L., Perry, L., & Barnhart, A. (1997). A screening test for pseudohypacusis. *The Hearing Journal, 4,* 23–26.

Woods, A. G., Pena, L. D., & Martin, F. N. (2004). Exploring possible sociocultural bias on the SCAN-C. *Journal of the American Academy of Audiology, 13,* 173–184.

Woodward, J. (1972). Implications of sociolinguistics research among the deaf. *Sign Language Studies, 1,* 1–7.

World Health Organization. (1980). *International classification of impairments, disabilities, and handicaps: A manual of classification relating to the consequences of disease* (pp. 25–43). Geneva, Switzerland: Author.

World Health Organization. (2001). *International classification of functioning, disability and health*. Geneva, Switzerland: Author. Retrieved from www.who.int/icidh

Yoshinaga-Itano, C., Sedley, A., Coulter, D., & Mehl, A. (1998). Language of early- and later-identified children with hearing loss. *Pediatrics, 102*, 1161–1171.

Yost, W. A., & Nielson, D. W. (2000). *Fundamentals of hearing: An introduction* (4th ed.). New York: Holt, Rinehart and Winston.

Zadeh, M. H., Storper, I. S., & Spitzer, J. B. (2003). Diagnosis and treatment of sudden-onset sensorineural hearing loss: A study of 51 patients. *Archives of Otolaryngology, Head and Neck Surgery, 128*, 92–98.

Zhou, G., Gopen, Q., & Poe, D. S. (2007). Clinical and diagnostic characterization of canal dehiscence syndrome: A great otologic mimicker. *Otology & Neurotology, 28*(7), 920–926.

Zumach, A., Gerrits, E., Chenault, M., & Anteunis, L. (2010). Long-term effects of early-life otitis media on language development. *Journal of Speech-Language-Hearing Research, 53*, 34–43.

Zwislocki, J. (1950). Acoustic attenuation between ears. *Journal of the Acoustical Society of America, 25*, 752–759.

Zwolan, T. A., Kileny, P. R., & Telian, S. A. (1997). Self-report of cochlear implant use and satisfaction by prelingually deafened adults. *Ear and Hearing, 17*, 198–210.

Author Index

Abouchacra, K. S., 199
Abrahamson, J. E., 415
Academy of Dispensing
    Audiologists, 6
Adams, M., 429
Alexander, G. C., 112
Alford, B., 190
Ali, A., 339
Allen, J. B., 283
Alleyne, B. C., 297
Alpiner, J. G., 402
Altman, E., 8
American Academy of
    Audiology, 5, 13, 192, 208,
    414, 428, 429
American National Standards
    Institute, 48, 59, 71, 368
American Speech-Language-
    Hearing Association, 5, 103,
    160, 195, 208, 418, 420, 424,
    425, 429, 431
Amlani, A. M., 367
Andaz, C., 357
Anderson, E. E., 260
Anderson, H., 165, 321
Anderson, K. L., 386
Angell, S., 334
Antablin, J. K., 110
Anteunis, L., 7
Antonelli, A., 334
Apgar, V., 189
Arezzo, J. C., 171
Arnce, K. D., 354
Atkins, D. V., 412, 431
Auer, E. T., 379
Austen, S., 345
Azah, H., 384

Baccaro, P., 198
Bahan, B., 381
Bailey, H. A. T., 144, 267
Baker, E., 188, 193
Bakker, R., 302
Ballachanda, B., 229, 431
Banerjee, A. R., 303
Baran, J. A., 316
Barany, E. A., 86
Barnhart, A., 354
Barr, B., 165, 260, 321
Barr, M., 409
Barry, L., 376

Barry, S. J., 92, 104
Bass, J. K., 303
Bassim, M. K., 378
Bauch, C. D., 327
Beasley, W. C., 48
Beauchaine, K., 276
Békésy, G. v., 93, 283, 284
Bell, A. G., 44
Bengala, D., 381
Benson, P. V., 406
Berger, E. H., 298
Berger, K. W., 365
Bergman, M., 297, 336
Berlin, C. I., 171, 200, 326
Berliner, K. I., 300
Bernstein, L. E., 379
Bernstein, M., 407, 409
Bernstein, M. E., 420
Berrick, J. M., 337
Berry, G. A., 144
Bess, F. H., 188, 415
Bilger, R. C., 112
Blair, J. C., 406
Blosser, D., 127
Blythe, M., 143
Bocca, E., 334
Boothroyd, A., 110
Borik, J., 377
Born, J., 426
Bornstein, S. P., 351
Bouma, J., 302
Brackett, D., 419
Brackmann, D. E., 172
Bratt, G. W., 415
Brewster, M. J., 303
Brookhouser, P. E., 276
Brooks, D. N., 346
Brown, N., 304
Brunt, M. A., 184
Buchanan, M. A., 300
Buckley, K. A., 344
Buller, D. B., 346
Bundey, S. E., 262
Burchfield, S. B., 383
Burchinal, M. R., 7
Bureau of the Census, U.S., 431
Burger, M. C., 415
Burgoon, J. D., 346
Burk, M. H., 79
Burke, L. E., 103
Burney, P., 164, 350

Burns, P., 139
Butler, E. C., 139

Cacace, A. T., 414
Caissie, R., 418
Calearo, C., 334, 335
Calvert, D. R., 421
Cameron, S., 334
Campanelli, P., 211
Campbell, C., 191
Campbell, R. A., 354
Canfield, N., 5
CareerCast, 9
Carhart, R., 5, 6, 79, 104, 109, 262,
    344, 383
Carrell, T. D., 179
Carter, A. S., 371
Carter, J., 339
Casali, J. G., 298
Cassell, E. J., 406
Cassinari, V., 334
Cevette, M. J., 339
Chaiklin, J. B., 127, 344, 353
Chambers, J. A., 86, 103, 128,
    180, 353
Champlin, C. A., 9, 86, 103,
    108, 128, 180, 333, 346, 353,
    354
Chenault, M., 7
Chermak, G. D., 206, 338, 339
Cherry, R., 354
Ching, T. Y. C., 381
Chisolm, T. H., 415
Chmiel, R., 310
Christensen, L., 377
Chute, P. M., 381
Ciletti, L., 88, 286, 310
Cinotti, T. M., 425
Clark, J. G., 7, 8, 9, 13, 82, 116,
    187, 205, 206, 207, 212, 300,
    335, 344, 357, 385, 406, 409,
    410, 411, 412, 414, 415, 416,
    417, 424, 426, 431, 435
Cody, J. P., 420
Cohen, A., 408
Coles, R. R. A., 127
Collet, L., 180
Cone-Wesson, B., 176
Connor, C. M., 381
Coombes, S., 202
Cooper, W. A., Jr., 353

Cornett, R. O., 423
Cosby, J., 381
Coulter, D. C., 193, 379
Cox, R. M., 112, 434
Craig, H. K., 381
Crandell, C. C., 415
Crump, B., 164, 350
Cuevas, C., 409
Culbertson, D., 381
Cullen, J. K., 171
Cunningham, D. R, 300
Cureoglu, S., 254
Curhan, G. C., 301
Cuttler, K., 191
Cyr, D. G., 276

D'Agostino, R., 310
Daly, J. A., 408, 420
Dancer, J., 232
Danhauer, J. L., 109, 344
David, E. E., 50
Davis, A., 426
Davis, B. M., 298, 428
Davis, H., 111, 115
Davis, J., 8
Dean, M. S., 87, 92, 130
Decker, T. N., 284
De Jonge, R. R., 260
Denenberg, L. J., 127
Department of Health and Human
    Resources, U.S., 189
Department of Veterans
    Affairs, U.S., 300
Derebery, M. J., 300
Desmon, A. L., 430
DeVries, S. M., 284
DeWeese, D., 427
Dhar, S., 192
DiBartolomeo, J. R., 262
DiCarlo, L. M., 202
Diefendorf, A. O., 8
DiGiovanni, D., 144
Dillon, H., 334, 376, 381
Dix, M. R., 202
Doerfler, L. G., 352
Don, M., 172
Donahue, P. A., 338
Douglas, J., 208
Dowdy, L. K., 102
Dowell, R., 176
Downs, M. P., 8, 82, 190, 293

Doyle, L., 13, 354
Dufresne, R. M., 297
Durrant, J. D., 180

Eavey, R. D., 187
Edgerton, B. J., 109
Efros, P. L., 346
Egan, J. P., 108
Eggermont, J. J., 426
Eldert, M. A., 115
Elliot, H. H., 409
Elliott, L. L., 111, 112
Ellis, M. S., 171
El-Mofty, A., 297
Elpern, B. S., 87
Emmer, M. B., 371
Engel, D. P., 72
Engelberg, M., 115
English, K. E., 8, 9, 357, 406, 409,
    410, 412, 414, 415, 416, 417,
    426, 431, 435
Eply, J., 298
Etymotic Research, 112
Everberg, G., 292
Ewertson, H. W., 295
Ewing, A., 196
Ewing, I., 196

Fagelson, M. A., 86, 87, 427
Fairbanks, G., 110
Farwell, W. R., 301
Fausti, S. A., 428
Fayad, J. N., 378
Feldhake, L. J., 114
Ferraro, J. A., 171, 306
Finitzo, T., 330
Fisch, U., 268
Fitzgerald, J. E., 300
Fitzgerald, T., 168
Flamme, G. A., 88, 286, 310
Fletcher, H., 60, 104
Fletcher, J., 293
Flexer, C., 207, 391, 420
Flores, P., 431
Folsom, R. C., 199
Fong, K., 339
Food and Drug Administration, 378
Fowler, C. G., 294
Frank, T., 355
Franklin, B., 335
Franklin, C., 79
Franks, J. R., 72
Freeman, B. A., 13
French, M. R., 108
Freyaldenhoven, M. C., 383
Fulcher, A., 188, 193

Gaddis, S., 104
Gaeth, J. H., 310
Gaglione, E., 300
Galvin, K. L., 379
Gang, R. P., 333
Gans, D., 207
Gardner, H. J., 109
Gates, G. A., 310
Geers, A. E., 381
Geier, K., 402
Gelfand, S. A., 371
Gelfand, S. T., 159
George, K., 408

Gerrits, E., 7
Ghoreyshi, A., 297
Ghossaini, S. N., 377
Giebink, G. S., 248
Gilmore, C., 112
Gilroy, J., 334
Gladstone, V. S., 258
Glass, L. E., 310, 409
Glasscock, M. E., 320, 327
Goebel, J., 294, 323
Goeghegan, P. M., 346
Goetzinger, C. P., 106, 116, 334
Goldstein, R., 202
Gollegly, K. M., 178, 351
Goodhill, V., 328
Goodman, A., 385
Goodwin, P. E., 426
Gopen, Q., 308
Gorga, M. P., 192, 351
Goycoolea, H. G., 263
Graham, J., 426
Graham, M. D., 319
Graham, S. S., 267
Gravel, J. S., 326
Gray, J. A., 432
Greenfield, E. C., 320
Griest, S., 428
Grossman, J., 302
Gudmundsen, G. L., 130
Guilford, F., 198
Guilford, F. R., 202
Guinness World Records, 300
Gunnarson, A., 330
Gustafson, G., 188

Haggard, M. P., 329
Hahlbrock, K. H., 106
Hales, R. E., 345
Hall, J. W., 176, 192, 206, 424
Hallpike, C. S., 202
Halpin, C., 83
Hammed, H., 297
Hanley, P. J., 428
Harford, E. R., 181, 376
Harkrider, A. W., 89
Harris, D. A., 354
Harris, G., 354
Harris, J. D., 221
Harrison, M., 188
Haskins, H., 109
Hattler, K. W., 353
Haug, C. O., 202, 407
Haug, O., 198
Hawkins, D. B., 8, 384
Hawkins, J. E., 295
Hayashi, R., 335
Hayes, D., 199
Haynes, D., 432
Hazell, J. W. P., 428
Heavner, K., 381
Hecker, M. H. L., 110
Hempton, G., 302
Henion, K. M., 99
Henoch, M. A., 5
Henry, D. F., 262
Henry, J. A., 428
Herer, G., 353
Heyworth, T., 357
Hill, M., 381
Hirsch, S., 336

Hirsh, I., 108, 332
Hitselberger, W. E., 382
Hodgetts, W. E., 301, 302
Hodgson, W., 334
Holcomb, L. M., 116
Holguin, K., 300
Hood, J. D., 135
Hood, L., 326
Hood, L. J., 326
Hood, W. H., 354
Hoover, B., 192
Hosford-Dunn, H., 290
House, A. S., 110
House, W. F., 379
Hudson, S., 381
Humes, L. E., 116
Hunter, L. L., 156
Huntington, D. A., 108
Hurley, R. M., 208
Hutton, C. L., 354

Ireland, J. A., 420

Jacobs, A. M., 8
Jacobson, E., 293
Jahn, A. F., 257
Jaindl, M., 7
Jastreboff, M. M., 428
Jenkins, H., 322
Jereczek-Fossa, B. A., 303
Jerger, J., 111, 114, 157, 164, 182,
    199, 206, 264, 310, 322, 329,
    334, 335, 336, 339, 350, 353
Jerger, J. F., 79, 100, 181, 333
Jerger, S., 100, 329, 333
Jerris, R. C., 246
Jewett, D. L., 172
Johnsen, M. N. J., 261
Johnson, C. D., 10, 406
Johnson, E. W., 319
Johnson, J., 346
Johnson, K., 79, 100, 377
Johnson, L. G., 295
Johnson, L. G., 295
Johnson, S. J., 290
Joint Committee on Infant
    Hearing, 190
Jokinen, K., 335
Josey, A. F., 323, 324, 327
Joyner, R., 381

Kalb, J. T., 299
Kalikow, D. M., 112
Kanji, A., 408
Kankkonen, A., 198
Karmody, C., 290
Katfamma, B., 338
Katz, D., 111
Katz, J., 330, 337
Keamy, D. G., 187
Keith, R. W., 331, 337, 338
Kemp, D. T., 165, 166, 283
Kemp, R. J., 229
Kendall, D. C., 202
Kenworthy, O. T., 376
Keogh, T., 7
Kibbe-Michal, K., 178
Kileny, P. R., 165, 319, 327, 381
Killion, M. C., 116, 130
Kim, L. J., 320
Kimberlain, J., 377

King, J. L., 294
Kirk, K. I., 381
Kirkwood, D., 366
Klee, T., 376
Klerman, G. L., 346
Klopfenstein, J. D., 320
Knops, J. L., 339
Kochkin, S., 415, 426
Konkle, D. F., 101, 107,
    116, 144
Kraemer, M. J., 249
Krall, L., 8, 409
Kraus, N., 179
Kricos, P., 415
Krueger, J. S., 407
Kryter, K. D., 110
Kumazawa, T., 261
Kurdziel, S., 337
Kwong, B., 172

Lamb, L. E., 348
Lane, G. I., 133
Lane, H., 381, 419, 423
Larson, V. D., 415
Lavin, B., 407
Lawrence, J., 290
Legatt, A. D., 171
Lehiste, I., 109
Lempert, J., 266
Lerman, J., 110
Letowski, T., 199
Lichtenstein, M. D., 415
Liden, G., 198
Lieberthal, A. S., 254
Lightfoot, R. K., 392
Lilly, D. J., 156
Lindsay, M. O., 354
Ling, D., 200
Lipscomb, D. M., 298
Lloyd, L. L., 201
Lockwood, A. H., 427
Logan, S. A., 415
Lonsbury-Martin, B. L., 166, 283,
    284, 339
Loukzadeh, Z., 297
Lousteau, R. J., 171
Lutolf, J. J., 371
Lynch, C., 345
Lynn, G. E., 334

Mahaffey, R. B., 118
Malachowski, N., 290
Mankowitz, Z., 336
Maran, A., 211
Marchbanks, T. P., 354
Margolis, R. H., 104, 156, 263, 350
Marquette, M. L., 354
Martin, D. R., 298
Martin, F. N., 8, 9, 86, 87, 89, 92,
    99, 102, 103, 106, 108, 109,
    110, 114, 127, 128, 130, 133,
    134, 139, 143, 144, 145, 146,
    181, 187, 198, 202, 205, 207,
    283, 333, 335, 338, 344, 345,
    346, 353, 354, 406, 407, 408,
    409, 420
Martin, G. K., 166
Martin, J. S., 354
Martinez, C., 332
Masuda, A., 172

Matkin, N., 196
Matthews, L. J., 112
Matzker, J., 335
Mauldin, L., 164, 350
Maxon, A. B., 419
McCarthy, P. A., 402, 415
McCoy, M. J., 339
McCreery, T. M., 346
McDermott, J. C., 428
McFadden, D., 295
McGee, T., 179
McMenomey, S. O., 320
Mehl, A. L., 190, 193
Mehra, S., 187
Mehrpavar, A. H., 297
Meikle, M., 377
Melnick, W., 298
Mendel, L. L., 344
Merchant, S. N., 168
Meyerhoff, W. L., 258, 269
Meyers, D. G., 391
Milini, F., 303
Miller, D. A., 377
Miller, J. H., 300
Mills, D., 310
Min, W. J., 176
Mindel, E., 423
Minor, L. B., 320
Mirmohammadi, S. J., 297
Miyamoto, R. T., 381
Mollasadeghi, A., 297
Møller, A. R., 179
Møller, C. G., 276
Moncrieff, D. W., 332
Monro, D. A., 354
Moore, J. M., 199, 384
Moorehouse, A., 429
Morehouse, C. R., 208
Morimoto, M., 335
Morrison, A. W., 262
Moses, K., 114, 408
Mueller, H. G., 116, 206, 332, 337, 384, 424
Muenchen, R. A., 383
Munro, N., 188, 193
Munson, W. A., 60
Musiek, F. E., 178, 206, 316, 327, 329, 332, 338, 339, 351

Näätänen, R., 179
Nabelek, A. K., 383
Nadler, N., 295
Nagel, R. F., 354
Nakajima, H. H., 168
Nam, B. H., 310
Naseri, I., 246
Nashner, L. M., 277
National American Precis Syndicated, 8
National Institute for Occupational Safety and Health, 297
National Institute on Deafness and Other Communication Disorders, 7
National Institutes of Health, 188, 320
Naunton, R. F., 87
Neely, S. T., 323
Negley, C., 303

Nelson, E., 415
Nelson, J. A., 99
Nelson, R. A., 172
Nemes, J., 12, 432
Nerbonne, M. A., 103, 116
Nevins, M. E., 381
Newall, P., 334
Newby, H. A., 209, 426
Nicholas, J. G., 381
Nicholson, N., 79
Nielson, D. W., 316
Nilsson, M., 112
Niparko, J. K., 319
Niquette, P., 298
Niskar, A. S., 295
Nober, E. H., 92
Noe, C. M., 371
Noffsinger, D., 332, 337
Northern, J. L., 8, 384
Nuetzel, J. M., 112

O'Conner, A. F., 261
Ogiba, Y., 198
Ohta, F., 335
Oliver, T. A., 322
Olsen, W. O., 102, 332, 337
Olsson, R. T., 427
O'Neal, J., 8, 408, 409
Orchik, D. J., 245
Orecchia, R., 303
Oviatt, D. L., 165
Owens, E., 110

Paki, B., 428
Palmer, C. S., 228
Palmer, C. V., 384
Palva, A., 335
Pappas, J. J., 144
Parkin, J., 381
Paryani, S., 290
Pascoe, D. P., 366
Patrick, P. E., 208
Pava, A. A., 320
Pavlovic, C. V., 116
Pearson, D., 229
Peck, J. E., 212, 345, 357
Pedersen, E., 302
Pederson, N., 261
Pena, L. D., 338
Perez, D. D., 108, 333
Perry, L., 354
Peterein, J., 323
Peterson, G. E., 109
Peterson, H. J., 198
Peterson, J. L., 348
Pick, G. F., 285
Picton, T. W., 176, 178, 326
Pierce, J. R., 50
Pirvola, U., 286
Plant, G., 379
Plate, S., 261
Plattsmier, H. S., 295
Plester, D., 297
Poe, D. S., 308
Pool, J. I., 320
Popelka, G. R., 192
Porter, L. S., 104
Porter, R. W., 320
Potthoff, M., 300
Preissler, K., 192

Press, L., 427, 429
Price, G. R., 299
Priede, V. M., 127
Prieve, B. A., 168, 351
Prinsley, P. R., 300
Probst, R., 284
Proud, G. O., 104
Pulec, J., 305
Purcell, A. A., 188, 193
Pusakulich, K. M., 112

Rabinowitz, W. M., 112
Raffin, M. J. M., 110, 115
Rance, G., 176
Rapin, I., 326
Raudenbush, S. W., 381
Reesal, M. R., 297
Refaie, A. E., 426
Reich, G., 428
Reid, M. J., 201
Rentschler, G. J., 330
Repka, J. N., 75
Resnick, D., 335
Richards, D. L., 298
Richardson, M. A., 432
Richter, G. T., 377
Riedner, E. D., 346
Rieger, J. M., 301
Rintelmann, W. F., 101, 107, 109, 351
Robbins, A. M., 381
Roberts, J. E., 7
Robeznieks, A., 404
Robinette, M. S., 327, 339
Rock, E. H., 258
Roeser, R. J., 229, 344
Rogin, C. M., 415
Rose, D. S., 207
Roseberry-McKibbin, C., 431
Rosen, S., 266, 297
Rosenberg, S. I., 304
Rosenberg, W. M., 432
Rosenfeld, M. A. L., 258, 415
Ross, M., 108, 110, 196, 212, 346, 354, 367, 391, 409, 419, 421
Roush, J., 188
Rowe, S., 357
Rowsowski, J. J., 168
Rubel, E. W., 310
Rudy, J., 338
Ruhm, H. B., 353
Rupp, R. R., 330
Ryals, B. M., 286
Rzeczkowski, C., 112

Sabes, J. H., 415
Sackett, D. L., 432
Salston, R. S., 356
Sammeth, C. A., 377
Sanchez, S., 354
Sanderson-Leepa, M. E., 109
Sandlin, R. E., 427
Sataloff, J., 82
Sataloff, R. T., 82
Saunders, G. H., 329
Schaefer, A., 332
Schechter, M. A., 428
Scheifele, P. M., 13, 300
Schlauch, R. S., 354
Schleuning, A., 377

Schmida, M. J., 198
Schoepflin, J. R., 371
Schubert, E. D., 110
Schuknecht, H. F., 308, 310
Schum, D. J., 112, 391
Schumaier, D. R., 245
Schwaber, M., 330
Seaton, J. B., 10
Sedley, A., 193
Self Help for Hard of Hearing People, Inc., 416
Sells, J. P., 208
Severance, G. K., 146
Shahrokh, N. C., 345
Shanks, J. E., 156
Shargorodsky, J., 301
Shea, J. J., 245, 261, 266
Shedd, J., 181
Shenk, H., 232
Shepherd, D. C., 188
Shier, M., 5
Shipp, D. B., 354
Silman, S., 371
Silver, F. W., 356
Silverman, C. A., 371
Silverman, S. R., 111
Silverstein, H., 304
Simmons, J., 192
Simons-McCandless, M., 381
Singh, S., 344
Sininger, Y., 326
Sivian, L. J., 60
Skafte, M. D., 416
Sklare, D. A., 127
Smaldino, J., 386
Smith, B., 335
Smith, S. D., 192, 404
Smith-Olinde, L., 79, 377
Snyder, J. M., 345
Sobol, S. E., 246
Soli, S., 112
Solzi, P., 336
Speaks, C., 111
Spitzer, J. B., 304, 377
Spradlin, J. E., 201
Spretnjak, M., 310
Stach, B. A., 310, 344
Starke, K., 300
Starr, A., 326
Stauffer, M. L., 102
Steinberg, J. C., 108
Sterritt, G. M., 190
Stevens, K. N., 112
Stewart, J. M., 82
Stewart, K., 352
Stickney, G. S., 344
Stika, C. J., 409
Stoppenbach, D. T., 114
Storper, I. S., 304
Strasnick, B., 320
Streetman, P. S., 9
Strom, K., 371
Studebaker, G. A., 86, 92
Sullivan, J., 112
Suzuki, T., 198
Svirsky, M. A., 381
Swanson, L. A., 226
Sweetow, R. W., 415
Syms, M. J., 320
Szarko, R. A., 301

Tampas, J. W., 383
Telian, S. A., 319, 327, 381
Telischi, F. F., 339, 382
Teter, D. L., 392
Tharpe, A. M., 188, 198, 376
Thelin, J. W., 226, 354
Themann, C. L., 72
Thibodeau, L., 146
Thompsen, K. A., 261
Thompson, G., 199
Thompson, J., 304
Thomson, V., 190
Thordardottir, E. T., 114
Thornton, A. R., 110, 115
Tillman, T. W., 102, 109
Tobey, E. A., 415
Tobias, J. V., 110
Tolin, D., 176
Tonry, K. L., 110
Torres-Russotto, D., 211
Townsend, E. A., 332
Trammell, J. L., 111
Tremblay, K. L., 179
Trychin, S., 426
Tseng, E., 339

Turner, R. G., 327
Tyler, R. S., 391, 426

Utley, J., 355

Valente, M., 260, 294, 323
van Bergeijk, W. A., 50
van den Berg, F., 302
van Wanrooy, E., 381
Vassallo, L. A., 82
Vaughan, H. G., 171
Vaugn, G. R., 392
Veniar, F. A., 356
Ventry, I. M., 344, 354
Verkest, S. B., 178
Vermiglio, A., 300
Vernon, J., 377, 427, 429
Vernon, M., 423
Vittitow, M., 300

Waddington, D., 429
Walker, J. D., 189, 192
Wallace, J., 188
Wardell, F. N., 202
Watermeyer, J., 408

Wayner, D. S., 415
Wazen, J. J., 377
Weaver, N. J., 202
Weber, P. C., 382
Webster, D. B., 330
Webster, M., 330
Wedenberg, E., 165, 189, 190, 321
Wegel, R. L., 133
Weissman, M. M., 346
White, S. D., 60
White, S. T., 303
Whitehead, M. L., 284
Widick, M. P., 339
Wilber, L. A., 109, 130
Wild, D. C., 303
Wilder, R. T., 257
Wiley, T. L., 79, 114, 157
Wilkinson, J. M., 300
Williams, C. E., 110
Williams, C. J., 8
Williams, D. W., 415
Williams, P. S., 246
Williford, J. A., 336
Wilson, R. H., 104, 110, 157, 332, 371

Windmill, I. M., 300
Wittich, W. W., 92, 118
Wood, T. J., 118
Woodall, W. G., 346
Woodford, C. M., 354
Woods, A. G., 338
Woodward, J., 423
World Health Organization, 413
Wray, D., 420

Xianxi, G., 245

Yates, J. W., 300
Yeager, A. S., 290
Yoshinaga-Itano, C., 193
Yost, W. A., 316

Zadeh, M. H., 304
Zarowski, A., 303
Zeisel, S. A., 7
Zhou, G., 308
Zumach, A., 7
Zwislocki, J., 127
Zwolan, T. A., 381

Subject Index

AAA. *See* American Academy of Audiology
AAOO. *See* American Academy of Ophthalmology and Otolaryngology
ABG. *See* Air-bone gap
ABIs. *See* Auditory brain-stem implants
ABLB. *See* Alternate binaural loudness balance test
ABRs. *See* Auditory brain-stem responses
AC. *See* Air conduction
Academic preparation, in audiology, 5–6
Academy of Dispensing Audiologists, 6
Academy of Doctors of Audiology, 14
Academy of Rehabilitative Audiology, 14
Acceleration
  angular, 275
  linear, 275
Acceptable noise levels, 58–59, 383
Acoupedics, 422
Acoustic admittance, 159
Acoustic feedback, 372, 374
Acoustic gain, 367, 368–369
Acoustic immittance, 151
  for eustachian tube function, 258
  factors governing, 153
  measurements on, 152
  middle-ear measurement equipment, 153–154
  static acoustic compliance, 155–156
  for tube patency, 258
  tympanometry, 156–159
Acoustic impedance, 151
Acoustic neuritis, 324
Acoustic neuroma, 320–324
Acoustic reflex, 152, 159–165, 265
  contralateral, 160, 161, 164
  decay test, 164–165
  defined, 159
  implications of, 160–162
  interpreting, 162–164
  ipsilateral, 160, 161, 164
  measuring, 160
  SPAR, 164, 350
Acoustic reflex arc, 160

Acoustic reflex test, 338, 350–351
Acoustic reflex threshold (ART), 160, 164, 348
Acoustic trauma, 296
Acoustic trauma notch, 296–297, 301
Acquired immune deficiency syndrome (AIDS), 247, 290
Action potential (AP), 282
Activity limitations, 413
Acute suppurative otitis media, 249, 254
A/D. *See* Analog-to-digital converter
ADHD. *See* Attention deficit hyperactivity disorder
Aditus ad antrum, 240
Adults
  ADP management in, 425–426
  hearing aids and, 381, 382–385, 387
  hearing impairment management, 413–418
  nonorganic hearing loss in, 212
  speechreading training with, 417–418
AEPs. *See* Auditory-evoked potentials
Aerobic instructors, 300
Afferent system, 282, 318
Aging process, 426
AI. *See* Audibility index
Aided threshold goals, 385
AIDS. *See* Acquired immune deficiency syndrome
AIED. *See* Autoimmune inner-ear disease
Airbag deployment, 299
Air-bone gap (ABG), 88, 90
  low-frequency, 262
Air-bone relationships, 91–92
Air conduction (AC), 16, 17
  audiometry, 77–84, 127–128
  masking methods for, 133–134
  pure-tone audiometer and, 55–56
  speech audiometer and, 57
  thresholds, 90
Air-pressure differentials, 240
AIT. *See* Auditory integration training
ALDs. *See* Assistive listening devices

Alerting units, 392
Alexander Graham Bell Association for the Deaf and Hard of Hearing, 14, 413
Alleles, 287
ALRs. *See* Auditory late responses
Alternate binaural loudness balance test (ABLB), 180–181
Alzheimer's disease, 414
American Academy of Audiology (AAA), 6, 14, 330
American Academy of Ophthalmology and Otolaryngology (AAOO), 82–83
American Auditory Society, 14
American Board of Audiology, 381
American National Standards Institute (ANSI), 48, 71, 92
American Sign Language (ASL), 422, 423–424
American Speech-Language-Hearing Association (ASHA), 9, 11, 14, 128, 208, 399
  air-conduction audiometry and, 78–79, 84
  licensing and certification, 6
  SRT testing and, 102–103
American Standards Association (ASA), 48
Americans with Disabilities Act (1991), 413
American Tinnitus Association, 427
AMLR. *See* Auditory middle latency response
Amplification/sensory systems, 364–396
  bilateral/binaural amplification, 371
  case studies on, 392–396
  dispensing hearing aids, 388–389
  electroacoustic characteristics of hearing aids, 367–371
  hearing aid acceptance and orientation, 387
  hearing aid circuit overview, 366–367
  hearing aid development, 365–366
  hearing aid selection for adults, 381, 382–385, 387

  hearing aid selection for children, 386
  hearing aid types, 371–382
  hearing assistance technologies, 389–392
Amplitude, 36, 169
Amplitude distortion, 369
Ampullae, 274
AN/AD. *See* Auditory neuropathy/dys-synchrony
Analog hearing aids, 366
Analog-to-digital converter (A/D), 366
Anatomy
  of central auditory pathways, 316–318
  of ear, 17
  of inner ear, 274–285
  of middle ear, 239–244
  of outer ear, 219–223
Anechoic chambers, 52, 53, 73
Anger, 409–410
Angular acceleration, 275
Animal audiology, 12–13
Annulus, 223
Anomalies, of ear, 226
Anotia, 224
Anoxia, 290–291, 328
ANSD. *See* Auditory neuropathy spectrum disorder
ANSI. *See* American National Standards Institute
Antibiotics, 252–254
Antioxidants, 302
AP. *See* Action potential
APDs. *See* Auditory processing disorders
Aperiodic sounds, 39
Apgar test, 189
APR. *See* Auropalpebral reflex
ART. *See* Acoustic reflex threshold
Art, audiology as, 8–9
Articulation, 114
Articulation index, 116
Artificial ear, 60
Artificial mastoid, 60, 63
ASA. *See* American Standards Association
Ascending auditory pathways, 316
ASHA. *See* American Speech-Language-Hearing Association
ASL. *See* American Sign Language

Aspirin, 295
Assessment of hearing
  masking, 126–148
  physiological tests, 150–182
  pure-tone audiometry, 70–95
  speech audiometry, 98–120
Assistants, 6
Assistive listening devices (ALDs),
  389
ASSR. *See* Auditory steady-state
  response
Athetosis, 289
Atresia, of EAC, 225–226
Atresia choanae, 226
Attention deficit hyperactivity
  disorder (ADHD), 205
Attenuation, 18
AuD. *See* Doctor of audiology
Audibility index (AI), 116–118
Audiocoils, 367
Audiograms, 70, 78, 84
  interpretation of, 88–92
  plotting masked results on,
    140–142
  pure-tone, 104
  split, 129
Audiological counseling, 406–413
  adult hearing impairment
    management, 413–418
  diagnostic counseling, 407–408
  emotional response to hearing
    loss, 408–410
  personal adjustment counseling,
    410–412
  support groups, 412–413
"Audiological Problems in
  Education" (Auricular
  Foundation Institute of
  Audiology), 5
Audiological rehabilitation, 413
Audiological treatment, 398–436.
  See also Surgical treatments
  adult hearing impairment
    management, 413–418
  APD management, 424–426
  audiological counseling, 406–413
  case studies on, 433–436
  childhood hearing impairment
    management, 418–423
  Deaf community, 423–424
  evidence-based practice,
    432–433
  hyperacusis, 428–429
  multicultural considerations,
    431–432
  outcome measures, 433
  patient histories, 399–402
  referral to other specialists,
    402–406
  speechreading training with
    adults, 417–418
  tinnitus management, 426–428
  vestibular rehabilitation,
    429–430
Audiology, 4–14. *See also* Pediatric
  audiology
  academic preparation in, 5–6
  for animals, 12–13
  as art and science, 8–9
  case studies on, 24–27

clinical, 52
dispensing, 11
educational, 10, 406
employment settings, 13
evolution of, 5–6
industrial, 11
licensing and certification for, 6
medical, 9–10
prevalence and impact of hearing
  loss, 7–8
professional societies, 14
recreational, 12–13, 300
rehabilitative, 11
specialists of, 9–13
tele-audiology, 11–12, 432
Audiometers, 47–48, 70
  acceptable noise levels for, 58–59
  calibration of, 59–65
  diagnostic, 99
  pure-tone, 54–56, 64, 71
  speech, 57–58
Audiometric Bing test, 139–140
Audiometric earphones, 55, 77
Audiometric suites, 73
Audiometric Weber test, 88
Audiometric zero, 48, 56
Audiometry. *See also* Pure-
  tone audiometry; Speech
  audiometry
  air-conduction, 77–84, 127–128
  automatic, 93
  behavioral observation, 196
  Békésy, 93, 182, 353–354
  bone-conduction, 85–87,
    127–128
  computerized, 93
  data form, 81
  impedance, 152
  objective, 351
  operant conditioning, 201–202
  play, 202–203
  sound-field, 197–199
  suppurative otitis media and,
    250–252
  TROCA, 201
  visual reinforcement, 198
Auditory brain-stem implants
  (ABIs), 382
Auditory brain-stem responses
  (ABRs), 169, 171–174, 204,
    315, 322–323
  neonatal screening with, 191
  stacked, 172
  suppurative otitis media and,
    251–252
Auditory event-related potentials
  (ERPs), 169
Auditory-evoked potentials
  (AEPs), 169–180, 338–339, 351
  auditory brain-stem responses,
    171–174
  auditory late responses, 177–179
  auditory middle latency
    response, 176–177
  auditory steady-state response,
    174–176
  cortical, 177
  electrocochleography, 170–171
  intraoperative monitoring,
    179–180

Auditory-global approach, 422
Auditory integration training
  (AIT), 425
Auditory late responses (ALRs),
  169, 177–179
Auditory mechanism, 278–279
Auditory middle latency response
  (AMLR), 169, 176–177
Auditory nerve, 17, 315, 317
  case study on, 340
  development of, 318
  disorders of, 319–327
  hearing loss and, 319
Auditory neuron, 281
Auditory neuropathy, 207
Auditory neuropathy/dys-
  synchrony (AN/AD), 192
Auditory neuropathy spectrum
  disorder (ANSD), 326–327
Auditory placode, 285
Auditory processing disorders
  (APDs), 206, 329–330
  management of, 424–426
  tests for, 331–339
Auditory radiations, 317
Auditory responses, 187–188
Auditory retraining, 415–416
Auditory steady-state response
  (ASSR), 174–176, 204
Auditory tract, 16
Auditory training, 415
  with children, 418–419
Auditory tube, 239–240
Auditory-verbal approach, 422
Aural/oral method, 422
Aural rehabilitation, 5, 413
Auricle, 219
  disorders of, 224–225
Auropalpebral reflex (APR), 189
Autism, 205
Autoimmune inner-ear disease
  (AIED), 308
Automatic audiometry, 93
Automatic gain control, 369
Autophony, 260, 308
Autosomal dominant hearing
  losses, 287
Autosomal recessive inheritance,
  287
Autosomes, 286
Axon, 281

Babbling, 188
Bacterial infections, 252
Bacterial meningitis, 291
BADGE. *See* Békésy ascending
  descending gap evaluation
Balance retraining, 429–430
Band-pass binaural speech
  audiometry, 335
Barotrauma, 246, 294
Basal cell carcinoma, 225
Basilar membrane, 278, 279, 280, 305
Beats, 39
Behavioral measures, 340, 386
Behavioral observation
  audiometry (BOA), 196
Behavioral testing, 196–204, 351
  electrophysiological hearing
    tests, 204

operant conditioning
  audiometry, 201–202
  play audiometry, 202–203
  pure-tone audiometry, 201
  sound-field audiometry, 197–199
  sound-field test stimuli, 199
  speech audiometry, 200–201
Behind-the-ear hearing aids
  (BTE), 372
Békésy ascending descending gap
  evaluation (BADGE), 354
Békésy audiometry, 93, 182,
  353–354
Bel, 44
Bell's palsy, 260
Bell Telephone Laboratories, 365
BiCROS hearing aid, 376
Bilateral amplification, 371
Binary digits, 366
Binaural, 99
Binaural amplification, 371
Bing test, 22–23
  audiometric, 139–140
Biofeedback, 428
Biological determinism, 287
Bits, 366
Blue babies, 205
BOA. *See* Behavioral observation
  audiometry
Body-type hearing aids, 372
Boilermaker's disease, 297
Bone conduction (BC), 16, 17, 71
  audiometry, 85–87, 127–128
  distortional, 85
  inertial, 85
  masking methods for, 138–140
  osseotympanic, 85
  pure-tone audiometer and, 56
  speech-recognition testing, 116
  SRT, 104–106
  thresholds, 87, 90
Bone-conduction hearing aids,
  376–377
  implantable, 377–378
Bones, in middle ear, 241–242
Brownian motion, 31
Bruton Conference, 339
BTE. *See* Behind-the-ear
  hearing aids
Bureau of Education of the
  Handicapped, 419

CAEP. *See* Cortical auditory-
  evoked potential
CALFRAST. *See* Calibrated finger
  rub auditory screening test
Calibrated finger rub auditory
  screening test (CALFRAST), 211
Calibration, 72
  of audiometers, 59–65
  psychoacoustic, 143
  of pure-tone masking noises,
    130–133
  of speech-masking noises,
    143–144
California consonant test, 110
Caloric test, 275
Canalith repositioning, 429
Cancellation, 39
Canine hearing loss, 12–13

CAPD. *See* Central auditory processing disorder
Captioned telephones, 392
Carhart notch, 262–263
Carotid artery, 239
Carrier phrase, 102
Carriers, 287
CAT. *See* Computerized axial tomography
CCM. *See* Contralateral competing message
CDA. *See* Clinical decision analysis
CDP. *See* Computerized dynamic posturography
Cell body, 281
Central auditory nervous system, 318
Central auditory pathways anatomy of, 316–318
hearing loss and, 319
physiology of, 316–318
Central auditory processing disorder (CAPD), 329
Central deafness, 331
Central Institute for the Deaf (CID), 111
Central masking, 130
compensation for, 146
for speech, 144
Cerebellopontine angle (CPA), 317
Cerebellum, 274, 317
Cerebral palsy, 289
Cerebrovascular accidents (CVAs), 328
Certificate of Clinical Competence in Audiology, 6
Certification, 6
Cerumen, 220
in EAC, 229–232
Cerumenolytic, 232
CF. *See* Correction factor
CGS. *See* Metric centimeter-gramsecond system
CHARGE syndrome, 225
Chemical hypothesis, 283
Chemotherapy, 303
Child Find, 420
Childhood communication development checklist, 193–194
Childhood motor developmental checklist, 194
Children, 10. *See also* Pediatric audiology
APD management of, 424–425
auditory processing disorders, 206
auditory training with, 418–419
hearing aids and, 370, 374, 377, 379–381, 386, 387
hearing impairment management, 418–423
hearing loss in, 7–8, 176
myringotomy and, 257
nonorganic hearing loss and, 211–212, 346, 357
otitis media and, 246–248, 330
parents' emotional responses and, 408–410

speechreading training with, 419
teachers of, 405
Cholesteatoma, 258–259, 260
Chorda tympani nerve, 243
Chromosomes, 286
Chronic suppurative otitis media, 249, 254
CIC. *See* Completely-in-the-canal hearing aids
CID. *See* Central Institute for the Deaf; Cytomegalic inclusion disease
CID Auditory Test W-22, 108
Cigarette smoke, 247, 303
Cilia, 239
Circumaural audiometric earphones, 55
Classroom management, 424
Clinical audiology, 52
Clinical decision analysis (CDA), 69
Clinical psychologists, 404
Clinicians
in pure-tone audiometry, 76–77
in speech audiometry, 100
CM. *See* Cochlear microphonic
CMV. *See* Cytomegalovirus
CNC. *See* Consonant-nucleus-consonant words
Cochlea, 17, 278–279
central auditory pathways and, 316
efferent system of, 282
fluids of, 281–282
frequency analysis in, 284–285
hearing loss from surgical complications, 303–304
osseointegrated cochlear stimulator, 377
physiology of, 280
toxic causes of hearing loss, 293–294
Cochlear BAHA, 378
Cochlear conductive presbycusis, 310
Cochlear dust, 278, 280
Cochlear implants, 378–382
Cochlear microphonic (CM), 282
Cochlear nuclei
disorders of, 327–328
dorsal, 317
ventral, 317
Cochleotoxic drugs, 293–294
Cold running speech, 101
SRT testing with, 102
Coloboma, 225
Commercial earmuffs, 299
Commercial earplugs, 299
Commissures, 317
Communication impact, 424
Communication methodologies, 421
ASL, 422
auditory-verbal approach, 422
aural/oral method, 422
cued speech, 423
manually coded English, 423
Competing sentence test (CST), 336
Completely-in-the-canal hearing aids (CIC), 375

Complex sounds
fundamental frequency, 39
harmonics, 39
spectrum of, 39, 40–41
Compliance, 151
pressure-compliance function, 264
static acoustic, 152, 155–156
Components, 39
Comprehensive Telehealth Act (1997), 432
Compressions, 31, 367
Computed tomography (CT), 326
Computerized audiometry, 93
Computerized axial tomography (CAT), 327
Computerized dynamic posturography (CDP), 276–277
Computerized speech audiometry, 118
Conditioned orientation reflex (COR), 198
Conductive hearing loss, 18–19
amplification/sensory systems and, 393–394
audiological treatment and, 433–434
hearing tests and, 24, 25–26
masking and, 147
middle ear and, 245, 269–270
outer ear disorders and, 234
pure-tone audiometry and, 88–89, 94
speech audiometry and, 118–119
Condyle, 220
Congenital malformations, 269
Congenital rubella syndrome (CRS), 289
Connected speech test (CST), 112
Consonant-nucleus-consonant words (CNC), 109, 335
CON-SOT-LOT, 354
Contralateral acoustic reflex, 160, 161, 164
Contralateral competing message (CCM), 336
Contralateral response pathway, 161
Contralateral routing of offside signal. *See* CROS hearing aids
Conversion disorder, 345
Conversion neurosis, 347
COR. *See* Conditioned orientation reflex
Correction factor (CF), 139, 145
Cortical auditory-evoked potential (CAEP), 177
Corti's arch, 279
Cosine waves, 33
Counseling, 406–413
adult hearing impairment management, 413–418
diagnostic counseling, 407–408
emotional response to hearing loss, 408–410
personal adjustment counseling, 410–412
support groups, 412–413
Counting with a loudness reference, 346

COWS (cold—opposite, warm—same), 275
CPA. *See* Cerebellopontine angle
Crista, 274
Critical band, 130
CROS hearing aids (contralateral routing of offside signals), 376
Cross hearing, 92, 348
masking and, 127–128
in SRT tests, 142–143, 145–146
CRS. *See* Congenital rubella syndrome
Crura, 241
Crus, 241
CST. *See* Competing sentence test; Connected speech test
CT. *See* Computed tomography
Cued speech, 326, 423
CVAs. *See* Cerebrovascular accidents
Cyanotic babies, 205
Cyberknife, 321
Cycle, 33
Cytomegalic inclusion disease (CID), 290
Cytomegalovirus (CMV), 290

D/A. *See* Digital-to-analog converter
DAF. *See* Delayed auditory feedback
Damage-risk criteria, 297
Damping, 34
DC. *See* Direct current
Deaf community, 423–424
Deafness
central, 331
hysterical, 345
nuclear, 328
semantics of, 421
Deception, 346
Decibels (dB), 43
hearing level, 47
intensity level, 44–46
logarithms of, 44
sensation level, 48
sound-pressure level, 46–47
Decongestants, 256
Decruitment, 180
Decussations, 317
Delayed auditory feedback (DAF), 353
Dementia, 414
Dendrites, 281
Denial, 409
Deoxyribonucleic acid. *See* DNA
Department of Defense, U.S., 302
Department of Health, U.S., 11
Department of Veteran Affairs, 356
Developmental disabilities, 207
Diagnostic audiometer, 99
Diagnostic counseling, 407–408
Diagnostic imperative, 189
Dichotic, 335
Dichotic digits test, 332
Difference tone, 39
Digital hearing aids, 366
Digital-to-analog converter (D/A), 366

Dihydrostreptomycin, 293
Diminished Schwabach, 21
Diotic, 335
Diplacusis binauralis, 286
Diplacusis monauralis, 286
Direct current (DC), 281
Disorders
  of auditory nerve, 319–327
  auditory processing, 206,
    329–339, 424–426
  of auricle, 224–225
  of cochlear nuclei, 327–328
  conversion, 345
  factitious, 345
  of heart, 226
  hereditary, 286–287
  of higher auditory pathways,
    329–331
  of inner ear, 286–311
  language, 205–206
  of middle ear, 245–268
  of outer ear, 224–234
  psychological, 207
  PTSD, 427
  SCAN, 337–338
  symbolic, 205
Dispensing audiology, 11
Disposable hearing aids, 375–376
Distortion, 367, 369
Distortional bone conduction, 85
Distortion-product otoacoustic
  emissions (DPOAEs), 166, 195
DNA (deoxyribonucleic acid), 286
Doctor of audiology (AuD), 6
Doerfler-Stewart test, 352
Dogs, 12–13
Dormant otitis media, 254
Dorsal cochlear nucleus, 317
Down syndrome, 224, 287
DPOAEs. See Distortion-product
  otoacoustic emissions
DR. See Dynamic range
Drugs
  cochleotoxic, 293–294
  ototoxic, 293
  recreational, 294
Ductus reuniens, 278
Dynamic range (DR), 107
Dyne (d), 42
Dysacusis, 286
Dysinhibition, 205

EAC. See External auditory canal
Ear. See also Inner ear; Middle ear;
  Outer ear
  anatomy of, 17
  anomalies of, 226
  artificial, 60
  pathways of sound, 17–18
  physiology of, 17
Earbuds, 301
Ear candling, 232
Eardrum, 220
Eardrum membrane. See
  Tympanic membrane
Ear infections
  in children, 7–8
  external otitis, 228–229
  MRSA and, 246
  suppurative otitis media, 246–254

Early cortical auditory-evoked
  potential, 176
Early hearing detection and
  intervention (EHDI), 189
Earmuffs, 299
Earobics, 425
Earphones
  attenuation devices, 72
  audiometric, 55, 77
  earbuds, 301
  insert, 72, 77
Earplugs, 299
Earwax. See Cerumen
ECoG. See Electrocochleography
Ectoderm, 223
Education, 419–421. See also
  Schools
  for audiology, 5–6
Educational audiology, 10, 406
Educational Audiology
  Association, 14
Education for All Handicapped
  Children Act (1975), 10, 405
Education for the Handicapped
  Amendments (1986), 10
EEG. See Electroencephalograph
Effective masking (EM), 130–132
Efferent system, 318
  of cochlea, 282
Efficiency, 69, 211
EHDI. See Early hearing detection
  and intervention
Elasticity, 31
Elderly citizens, 310–311
Electrical hypothesis, 283
Electroacoustic immittance meter,
  152, 154
Electrocochleography (ECoG),
  169, 170–171
Electroencephalograph (EEG),
  169–170
Electronic hearing tests, 24
Electronystagmograph (ENG),
  267, 275–276
Electrophysiological hearing
  tests, 204
EM. See Effective masking
Embolisms, 328
Embryonic genetic screenings, 404
Emotional disturbance, 205
Emotional response, to hearing
  loss, 408–410
Employment settings, 13
Endogenous causes, 286
Endolymph, 274, 281, 304–305
Energy, 34
ENG. See Electronystagmograph
English, 423
Entoderm, 223, 244
Environmental adaptations, 392
Environmental sounds, 49, 50
EOAEs. See Evoked otoacoustic
  emissions
Epitympanic recess, 239
Equivalent input noise level, 369
Equivalent volume, 155
Erg (e), 43
ERPs. See Auditory event-related
  potentials
Erroneous hearing loss, 344

ETD. See Eustachian-tube
  dysfunction
Eustachian tube, 239–240
  immittance testing for, 258
  patulous, 260–262
Eustachian-tube dysfunction
  (ETD), 245
Event related, 179
Everyday sentence test (CID), 111
Evidence-based practice, 432–433
Evoked otoacoustic emissions
  (EOAEs), 166
Exaggerated hearing loss, 345
Exogenous causes, 286
Exostoses, 229
Exponent, 44
External auditory canal (EAC),
  219–223
  atresia of, 225–226
  collapsing, 226–227
  earwax in, 229–232
  foreign bodies in, 227–228
  growths in, 229
External otitis, 228–229
Extra-axial lesions, 329
Extrinsic redundancy, 319
Eyeglass hearing aids, 372

Facial nerve, 162, 243
Facial palsy, 260
Factitious disorder, 345
Fallopian canal, 243
False hearing loss, 345
False negative responses, 75
False negative Rinne, 22
False normal Schwabach, 21
False positive responses, 75
False responses, 75, 100
Fascia, 267
Fast ForWord, 425
FDA. See Food and Drug
  Administration
Feedback
  acoustic, 372, 374
  biofeedback, 428
  delayed auditory, 353
Fenestration, 266
Filtered speech tests, 334–335
Fistula, 267
FM. See Frequency modulated
  system
Food and Drug Administration
  (FDA), 377, 378, 382
Footplate, 241
Force, 41, 42
Forced vibrations, 34–35
Formant, 41
Fourier analysis, 40
Fragile ears, 303
Free field, 52
Free vibrations, 34–35
Frequency, 33
  distortion, 369
  fundamental, 39
  high-frequency emphasis
    lists, 109
  length and, 35
  low-frequency ABGs, 262
  mass and, 35
  pitch and, 49–50

radio, 390
  resonant, 36
  response, 367, 369
  stiffness and, 36
Frequency analysis, in cochlea,
  284–285
Frequency modulated system
  (FM), 390
Friction, 34
Functional gain, 385
Functional hearing loss, 344
Fundamental frequency, 39
Furunculosis, 228

Gamma knife, 321
Gaps-in-noise test (GIN), 332
Gaussian noise, 130
Gender, presbycusis and, 310
Genes, 286
Genetic counselors, 404
Genitourinary abnormalities, 226
Genotype, 286
Georgia Aquarium, 300
Gerald R. Ford International
  Airport, 391
German measles, 289
GIN. See Gaps-in-noise test
Ground electrode, 171
Group communication training,
  416–417
"Guidelines for Determining
  Threshold Level for Speech"
  (ASHA), 101
Guilt, 410

Haemophilus influenza, 247
HAIC. See Hearing Aid Industry
  Conference
Hair cell transduction, hypotheses
  for, 283
Half lists, 110
Hand-held otoscope, 223
Harmonic distortion, 369
Harmonics, 39
Harvard University, 108
HCP. See Hearing-conservation
  program
Head trauma, 308–310, 329
Health Insurance Portability and
  Accountability Act (HIPAA),
  402
Hearing
  cross hearing, 92, 127–128,
    142–143, 145–146, 348
  disability, 413
  handicap, 413
  impairment, 413
  residual, 414
  therapy, 416
  UNHS, 190, 381
  zero hearing level, 48
Hearing Aid Industry Conference
  (HAIC), 367
Hearing aids, 11
  acceptance and orientation of,
    387
  for adults, 381, 382–385, 387
  auditory brain-stem implants,
    382
  behind-the-ear, 372

body-type, 372
bone-conduction, 376–377
for children, 370, 374, 377,
379–381, 386, 387
circuit overview, 366–367
cochlear implants, 378–382
completely-in-the-canal, 375
CROS, 376
development of, 365–366
dispensing of, 388–389
electroacoustic characteristics of,
367–371
eyeglass, 372
implantable bone-conduction,
377–378
in-the-canal, 375
in-the-ear, 372, 375
invisible-in-the-canal, 375
middle-ear implants, 378
open-fit, 372–374
receiver in canal, 374
single-day-fit, 375–376
types of, 371–382
vacuum for, 388
verification and validation of
performance, 384–385, 386
vibrotactile, 379, 382
Hearing assessment
masking, 126–148
physiological tests, 150–182
pure-tone audiometry, 70–95
speech audiometry, 98–120
Hearing assistance technologies,
389–392
Hearing-conservation program
(HCP), 298
Hearing in noise test (HINT),
112
Hearing level (HL), 47, 145
Hearing loss. *See also* Conductive
hearing loss; Nonorganic
hearing loss; Sensory/neural
hearing loss
auditory nerve and, 319
central auditory pathways and,
319
in children, 7–8, 176
emotional response to,
408–410
erroneous, 344
functional, 344
hereditodegenerative, 191, 286
impact of, 7–8
in infants, 188–193
inner ear disorders and, 286
middle ear and, 245
mixed, 19, 88, 91, 291
noise-induced, 294–302
outer ear and, 224
postlinguistic, 418
prelinguistic, 418
prevalence of, 7–8
pseudohypacusis, 344
psychogenic, 20, 344–345
radiation-induced, 303
in schools, 207–211
from surgical complications,
303–304
Hearing Loss Association of
America, 14, 413

Hearing loss management
amplification/sensory systems,
364–396
audiological treatment, 398–436
Hearing pill, 302
Hearing screening
in infants, 189–191
measures, 208
reliability of measures, 208–211
UNHS, 190, 381
Hearing sensitivity, loss of, 319
Hearing tests, 70. *See also*
Physiological tests; Testing;
Tuning-fork tests
for APDs, 331–339
electronic, 24
electrophysiological, 204
for nonorganic hearing loss, 25,
26–27, 350–355
performance on, 347–349
Hearing theories
place theory, 282–283
resonance, 282
resonance-volley, 283
traveling wave theory, 283
volley theory, 283
Heart disorders, 226
Helicotrema, 278
Hematomas, 226
Hemotympanum, 249
Hereditary disorders, 286–287
Hereditodegenerative hearing loss,
191, 286
Hertz (Hz), 35
Heschl's gyrus, 318
Heterozygous, 287
HFA. *See* High-frequency average
Higher auditory pathways,
disorders of, 329–331
High-frequency average (HFA), 368
High-frequency emphasis lists, 109
High-risk registry, 190
HINT. *See* Hearing in noise test
HIPAA. *See* Health Insurance
Portability and Accountability
Act
HIV. *See* Human
immunodeficiency virus
HL. *See* Hearing level
Homozygous, 287
Human Genome Project, 287
Human immunodeficiency virus
(HIV), 290
Hybrid hearing instruments, 367
Hypacusis, 286
Hyperacusis, 428–429
Hypertension, 301
Hypotheses, for hair cell
transduction, 283
Hysterical deafness, 345
Hz. *See* Hertz

IA. *See* Interaural attenuation
ICM. *See* Ipsilateral competing
message
IEP. *See* Individual education plan
IFSP. *See* Individual family service
plan
IIC. *See* Invisible-in-the-canal
hearing aids

IL. *See* Intensity level
IM. *See* Initial masking
Imaging, medical, 326–327
Immittance, 151. *See also* Acoustic
immittance
Impedance, 53–54
acoustic, 151
audiometry, 152
matcher, 242–243
Implantable bone-conduction
hearing aids, 377–378
Incus, 241
Individual education plan (IEP),
420
Individual family service plan
(IFSP), 420
Individuals with Disabilities
Education Act (1990), 420
Individuals with Disabilities
Education Act Amendments
(1997), 420
Induction loop, 390–391
Industrial audiology, 11
Industrial noise, 297
Industrial revolution, 294
Inertial bone conduction, 85
Infants. *See also* Neonatal
screening
eustachian tube in, 240
hearing loss in, 188–193
hearing screening in, 189–191
Infection-control procedures, 72
Infections. *See also* Ear infections
bacterial, 252
postoperative, 265
staph, 246
viral, 289
Inferior colliculus, 317
Infrared systems (IR), 390
Initial masking (IM), 134
Inner ear, 17, 273–311
anatomy of, 274–285
case study of, 311
development of, 285
disorders of, 286–311
physiology of, 274–285
Insert earphones, 72, 77
Insertion gain, 384
Insertion loss, 384
In situ measurements, 374
Instantaneous velocity, 37
Insular area, 318
Integrated circuits, 365
Intensity
force, 41, 42
latency-intensity functions, 309
performance intensity, 103,
114–115, 333–334
power, 43
pressure, 42–43
VIST, 354–355
work, 43
Intensity level (IL), 44–46
Interaural attenuation (IA), 127,
138, 146
Interference, 38–39
Internal auditory canal, 316
International Organization for
Standardization (ISO), 48
International System of Units (SI), 43

In-the-canal hearing aids (ITC),
375
In-the-ear hearing aids (ITE),
372, 375
Intra-aural muscle reflex, 159
Intra-axial lesions, 329
Intraoperative monitoring,
179–180
Intrinsic redundancy, 319
Inverse square law, 43
Invisible-in-the-canal hearing aids
(IIC), 375
iPods, 301
Ipsilateral acoustic reflex, 160,
161, 164
Ipsilateral competing message
(ICM), 335–336
Ipsilateral response pathway, 161
IR. *See* Infrared systems
ISO. *See* International
Organization for
Standardization
ITC. *See* In-the-canal hearing aids
ITE. *See* In-the-ear hearing aids

Joint Committee on Infant
Hearing (JCIH), 190
Joules (J), 43
Jugular bulb, 239

Kanamycin, 293
KEMAR. *See* Knowles Electronic
Manikin for Acoustic Research
Kemp echoes, 284
Kernicterus, 328
Kidney disease, 293
Kinetic energy, 34
Knowles Electronic Manikin for
Acoustic Research (KEMAR), 53

Labyrinth, 273
Labyrinthitis, 293
LACE. *See* Listening and
communication enhancement
Language disorders, 205–206
Laser-Doppler Vibrometer (LDV),
168
Latency, 169
Latency-intensity functions, 309
Lateralization, 23
Lateral lemniscus, 317
Lateral line, 242
LDL. *See* Loudness discomfort
level
LDV. *See* Laser-Doppler
Vibrometer
Licensure, 6
Linear acceleration, 275
Ling Six sound test, 200
Linguistics of Visual English
(LOVE), 423
Lipreading, 355, 417. *See also*
Speechreading training
Listening and communication
enhancement (LACE), 415, 417
Listening in spacialized noise
test, 334
Localization, 52
Logarithms, 44
Lombard test, 353

Lombard voice reflex, 262
Longitudinal waves, 32
Loudness, 50–52
  alternate binaural loudness balance test, 180–181
  balancing, 180–181
  counting with a loudness reference, 346
  decreased tolerance of, 428–429
  judgment, 346
  level, 50
  most comfortable loudness, 106
  range of comfortable loudness, 107
  reference, 346
  uncomfortable loudness, 106–107
Loudness discomfort level (LDL), 106–107
LOVE. See Linguistics of Visual English
Low-frequency ABG, 262

Macula acoustica sacculi, 274
Macula acoustica utriculi, 274
MADS. See Minimal auditory deficiency syndrome
MAF. See Minimum audible field
Magnetic resonance imaging (MRI), 326, 414
Mainstreaming, 419
Malaria, 293
Malingering, 20, 345, 357
Malleus, 221, 241
Manual alphabet, 422
Manualists, 421
Manually-coded English, 423
Manubrium, 241
MAP. See Minimum audible pressure
Mapping, 381
Masked thresholds, 83
Masking, 52, 71, 126–148
  for air conduction, 133–134
  for bone conduction, 138–140
  calibration of noises, 130–133
  case studies on, 147–148
  central, 130, 144, 146
  cross hearing, 127–128
  effective masking, 130–132
  initial masking, 134
  maximum, 130, 134–135
  noises used in, 130
  overmasking, 133, 135, 136, 144
  plateau method, 135–138
  plotting results on audiogram, 140–142
  pure-tone, 130–133
  speech-masking noises, 143–144
  for SRT, 142–146
  undermasking, 135, 136
Masking-level difference (MLD), 332
Mass, 153
  frequency and, 35
  reactance, 54
Mastoid, 240
  artificial, 60, 63
  process, 21, 85–86, 239
Mastoidectomy, 259

Mastoiditis, 249
Maximum masking, 130, 134–135
May Better Hearing and Speech Month, 295
MCL. See Most comfortable loudness
MCRs. See Message-to-competition ratios
Measles, 291
Measurement of sound
  acceptable noise levels, 58–59
  calibration of audiometers, 59–65
  pure-tone audiometer, 54–56
  sound-level meters, 58
  speech audiometer, 57–58
Meatus, 219
Mechanical hypothesis, 283
Medial geniculate body, 317
Medical audiology, 9–10
Medical imaging, 326–327
Medicare, 377
Medulla oblongata, 317
Mel scale, 51
Ménière's disease, 171, 304–307
Meningitis, 291
Meniscus, 254
Mental retardation, 205
Mesenchyme, 224, 244
Mesoderm, 223
Message-to-competition ratios (MCRs), 336
Metacognitive training, 206
Metalinguistic training, 206
Meter-kilogram-second system (MKS), 43
Methicillin-resistant staphylococcus aureus (MRSA), 246
Metric centimeter-gramsecond system (CGS), 43
Microbar (μbar), 47
Microcircuitry, 167
Micropascals, 43
Microtia, 224
Middle ear, 17, 238
  anatomy of, 239–244
  bones in, 241–242
  case study on, 269–270
  development of, 244
  disorders of, 245–268
  hearing loss and, 245
  measurements, 152, 153–154
  nonauditory structures of, 243–244
  physiology of, 239–244
  serous effusion of, 254–258
  windows of, 241
Middle-ear cleft, 239
Middle-ear implants, 378
Military veterans, 297, 300–301
Minimal auditory deficiency syndrome (MADS), 330–331
Minimum audible field (MAF), 60
Minimum audible pressure (MAP), 60
Minimum contralateral interference level, 352
Minimum-noise method, 133–134

Minimum response levels (MRLs), 187
Mismatch negativity (MMN), 178–179
Mixed hearing loss, 19, 88, 91, 291
MKS. See Meter-kilogram-second system
MLD. See Masking-level difference
MLV. See Monitored live-voice
MMN. See Mismatch negativity
Mobilization, of stapes, 266
Modified rhyme test, 110
Modified Stenger test, 352
Modiolus, 278
Monaural, 99
Monitored live-voice (MLV), 99, 114
Moro reflex, 198
Most comfortable loudness (MCL), 106
MP3 players, 301
MPD. See Myofacial pain dysfunction syndrome
MRI. See Magnetic resonance imaging
MRLs. See Minimum response levels
MRSA. See Methicillin-resistant staphylococcus aureus
MS. See Multiple sclerosis
Mucous membrane, 239
Mucous otitis media, 258
Multicultural considerations, 431–432
Multifactorial genetic considerations, 287
Multiple sclerosis (MS), 324
Multisensory approach, 422
Mumps, 291–292
Muscles
  intra-aural reflex, 159
  sound-evoked reflex, 277
  stapedius, 159, 244
  sternocleidomastoid, 277
  tensor tympani, 159, 244
  trapezius, 277
Music, 301
Musicians, 300
Myofacial pain dysfunction syndrome (MPD), 220
Myringitis, 229
Myringocentesis, 257
Myringoplasty, 233
Myringostomy, 256, 304
Myringotomy, 256–257

Narrowband noise, 130
Nasopharynx, 239, 248
National Council on Aging (NCOA), 415
National Institute for Occupational Safety and Health (NIOSH), 297
NCLB. See No Child Left Behind Act
NCOA. See National Council on Aging
Neck loop, 391
Necrosis, 249
Negative Bing, 23

Negative charge, 275
Negative middle-ear pressure, 245–246
Negative Rinne, 22
Neomycin, 293
Neonatal hypothyroidism, 189
Neonatal screening
  with ABRs, 191
  with OAEs, 192
Neoplasm, 320
Nerves. See also Auditory nerve
  chorda tympani, 243
  facial, 162, 243
  loss of, 19
  trigeminal, 244
Neural presbycusis, 310
Neuritis, 305
Neurofibromatosis (NF), 320
Neurofibromatosis type 2, 382
Neuromonics, 428
Neurons, 281
Neuropathy, auditory, 207
Neurosurgery, 321
Neurotransmission, 281
Neurotransmitters, 281
Newtons, 42
NF. See Neurofibromatosis
NIOSH. See National Institute for Occupational Safety and Health
No Child Left Behind Act (NCLB), 420
Noise, 302
  acceptable levels of, 58–59, 383
  calibration of, 130–133
  dosimeters, 298
  equivalent input noise level, 369
  exposure to, 11
  gaps-in-noise test, 332
  Gaussian, 130
  hearing in noise test, 112
  industrial, 297
  for masking, 130
  minimum-noise method, 133–134
  narrowband, 130
  pure-tone masking, 130–133
  quick SIN test, 112
  signal-to-noise ratio, 111, 166, 391, 424
  speech-masking, 143–144
  speech perception in noise test, 112
  thermal, 130
  white, 130
Noise-induced hearing loss, 294–302
Nonauditory structures, of middle ear, 243–244
Nonorganic hearing loss, 20, 343–358
  in adults, 212
  amplification/sensory systems and, 395
  audiological treatment and, 435–436
  case study on, 358
  in children, 211–212, 346, 357
  hearing tests for, 25, 26–27, 350–355

indications of, 347
management of patients with, 356–358
masking and, 147–148
objective testing for, 350–355
patients with, 345–347, 356–358
performance on routine hearing tests, 347–349
pure-tone audiometry and, 95
speech audiometry and, 119–120
terminology for, 344–345
tests for, 350–355
tinnitus and, 356
Nonprofessional counselors, 411
Nonsense-syllable lists, 109–110
Normal Schwabach, 21
Northwestern University Children's Perception of Speech test (NUCHIPS), 111
Nuclear deafness, 328
Nystagmus, 267, 275

OAD. *See* Obscure auditory dysfunction
OAEs. *See* Otoacoustic emissions
Objective audiometry, 351
Objective testing
for nonorganic hearing loss, 350–355
in pediatric hearing evaluation, 193–195
Obscure auditory dysfunction (OAD), 329
OCA. *See* Operant conditioning audiometry
Occlusion effect (OE), 22, 87, 139
Occupational Safety and Health Administration (OSHA), 297, 298
Octave, 50
October Audiology Awareness Month, 295
OE. *See* Occlusion effect
Ohm, 54
OM. *See* Overmasking
Open-fit hearing aids, 372–374
Operant conditioning audiometry (OCA), 201–202
Oralists, 421
Organ of Corti, 278, 280
Oscillation, 33, 85
OSHA. *See* Occupational Safety and Health Administration
OSPL. *See* Output sound-pressure level
Osseocartilaginous junction, 220
Osseointegrated auditory prosthesis, 377–378
Osseointegrated cochlear stimulator, 377
Osseotympanic bone conduction, 85
Ossicles, 241
Ossicular chain, 242
Osteitis, 229
Osteomyelitis, 229
Otalgia, 220
Otitis media, 291, 303, 330
dormant, 254
mucous, 258

suppurative, 246–254
Otoacoustic emissions (OAEs), 165, 283–284, 315, 324, 339
distortion-product, 166, 195
evoked, 166
interpreting, 168
measuring, 167–168
neonatal screening with, 192
spontaneous, 165, 284
transient-evoked, 166, 168, 284, 351
Otocyst, 285
Otolaryngologists, 403–404
Otology, 5
Otomycosis, 228
Otoplasty, 224
Otorrhea, 259
Otosclerosis, 262–268, 294
Otoscope, 221–223
Otospongiosis, 262
Ototoxic drugs, 293
Outcome measures, 433
Outer ear, 17, 218–235
anatomy of, 219–223
case study on, 234
development of, 223–224
disorders of, 224–234
hearing loss and, 224
physiology of, 219–223
Output sound-pressure level (OSPL), 367, 368
Oval window, 241
Overmasking (OM), 133, 135, 136, 144
Overtones, 39

Paracentesis of the tympanic membrane, 257
Paracusis willisii, 262
Parents, emotional responses to hearing loss by, 408–410
Parietal lobe, 318
Parotitis, 291
Pars flaccida, 223
Pars tensa, 223
Participation restriction, 413
Pascals (Pa), 42–43
Pathways of sound, 17–18
Patients
histories of, 399–402
with nonorganic hearing loss, 345–347, 356–358
position of, 76–77
in pure-tone audiology, 74–75
response of, 74–75
speech audiometry and, 99–100
well-patient model, 406
Patulous eustachian tube (PET), 260–262
PB. *See* Phonetically balanced word lists
PB Max, 115
PE. *See* Pressure-equalizing tubes
Pediatric audiology, 11, 25, 27, 95, 120, 148, 186–213
amplification/sensory systems and, 395–396
audiological treatment and, 436
auditory neuropathy, 207

auditory processing disorders, 206
auditory responses, 187–188
behavioral testing, 196–204
case studies on, 212–213
developmental disabilities, 207
hearing loss in infants, 188–193
hearing loss in schools, 207–211
language disorders, 205–206
nonorganic hearing loss, 211–212
objective testing in, 193–195
psychological disorders, 207
Perceptive loss, 19
Perforations, 256
of tympanic membrane, 232–234
Performance intensity (PI), 103, 114–115
Performance-intensity function for PB words (PI-PB), 115, 333–334
Perilymph, 274, 281–282
Perinatal causes, of inner ear disorders, 290
Period, 35
Periodic sounds, 39
Permanent threshold shift (PTS), 295
Perseveration, 205
Personal adjustment counseling, 410–412
Personal listening system, 391
PET. *See* Positron emission tomography
Pharyngeal arches, 223
Pharyngotympanic tube, 239–240
Phase
beats, 39
interference, 38–39
Phenotype, 286
Phenylketonuria (PKU), 189
Phon, 50
Phonemic regression, 310
Phonetically balanced word lists (PB), 108–109
performance-intensity function for, 115
Physical-volume test (PVT), 258
Physiological tests, 150
acoustic immittance, 151–159
acoustic reflex, 159–165
auditory-evoked potentials, 169–180
case studies on, 182
combined speech and pure-tone audiometry, 151
historical, 180–182
Laser-Doppler Vibrometer measurement, 168
otoacoustic emissions, 165–168
Physiology
of central auditory pathways, 316–318
of cochlea, 280
of ear, 17
of inner ear, 274–285
of middle ear, 239–244
of outer ear, 219–223
PI. *See* Performance intensity
Picture identification task (PIT), 110

Pidgin Sign English (PSE), 423
Pinna, 78, 219
Pinnaplasty, 224
PI-PB. *See* Performance-intensity function for PB words
PIT. *See* Picture identification task
Pitch, 49–50
PIWI. *See* Puppet in the window illuminated
PKU. *See* Phenylketonuria
Place theory of hearing, 282–283
Plasticity, 330
Plateau method, 135–138, 144
Play audiometry, 202–203
Pneumatic mastoid, 240
Pocketalker, 392
Politzerization, 246
Pons, 317
Position, of patients during testing, 76–77
Positive Bing, 23
Positive charge, 275
Positive Rinne, 22
Positron emission tomography (PET), 327, 414
Postlinguistic hearing loss, 418
Postmortem electron microscope studies, 295
Postnatal causes, of inner ear disorders, 291–293
Postoperative infection, 265
Posttraumatic stress disorder (PTSD), 427
Potential energy, 34
Power, 43
Predictive value, 69
Pregnancy, 261–262
smoking and, 303
Prelinguistic hearing loss, 418
Prematurity, 291
Prenatal causes, of inner ear disorders, 286–290
Presbycusis, 310–311
Pressure, 42–43
Pressure-compliance function, 264
Pressure-equalizing tubes (PE), 232, 256
Prevalence, of hearing loss, 7–8
Primary tones, 166
Private practice, 13
Probe-tube microphone, 369
Professional societies, 14
Programmable hearing aids, 367
Prolonged Schwabach, 21
Promontory, 241, 278
Prosthesis, 267–268
PSE. *See* Pidgin Sign English
Pseudohypacusis, 344
Psychoacoustic calibration, 143
Psychoacoustic Laboratories, Harvard University, 108
Psychoacoustic method, 59
Psychoacoustics
localization, 52
loudness, 50–52
masking, 52
pitch, 49–50
Psychogenic hearing loss, 20, 344–345
Psychological disorders, 207

Psychophysical tuning curve (PTC), 285
Psychotherapy, 411
PTA. *See* Pure-tone average
PTC. *See* Psychophysical tuning curve
PTS. *See* Permanent threshold shift
PTSD. *See* Posttraumatic stress disorder
Puppet in the window illuminated (PIWI), 198
Pure tone, 33
  complex sounds and, 39–40
  stimuli, 92
Pure-tone audiograms, 104
Pure-tone audiometer, 54, 64, 71
  air conduction, 55–56
  bone conduction, 56
Pure-tone audiometry, 70–95, 298
  air-conduction audiometry, 77–84
  audiogram interpretation, 88–92
  audiometers, 71
  audiometric Weber test, 88
  automatic audiometry, 93
  behavioral testing and, 201
  bone-conduction audiometry, 85–87
  case studies on, 94–95
  clinician's role in, 76–77
  computerized audiometry, 93
  with immittance measures, 151
  patient's role in, 74–75
  test environment for, 72–74
Pure-tone average (PTA), 82, 106, 336, 347–348, 413–414
Pure-tone DAF test, 353
Pure-tone masking
  calibration of noises, 130–133
  noises used in, 130
Purulent organisms, 249
PVT. *See* Physical-volume test

Quality, of sound, 31
Quick speech in noise test (quick SIN test), 112
Quinine, 293

Radiation-induced hearing loss, 303
Radio frequency (RF), 390
Radiosurgery, 321
Random gap detection test (RGDT), 332
Range of comfortable loudness (RCL), 107
Rapidly alternating speech perception test (RASP), 336–337
Rarefactions, 31
RAS. *See* Reflex-activating stimulus
RASP. *See* Rapidly alternating speech perception test
Ratios, 44
  rollover, 333
  signal-to-noise, 111, 166, 391, 424
RCL. *See* Range of comfortable loudness

Reactance, 53–54, 153
Receiver in canal hearing aids (RIC), 374
Receiver-in-the-ear hearing aids (RITE), 374
Receptive language skills, 386
Recreational audiology, 12–13, 300
Recreational drugs, 294
Recruitment, 180
Reference Equivalent Threshold Force Levels (RETFLs), 63
Reference Equivalent Threshold Sound Pressure Levels (RETSPLs), 62, 64
Reference test gain, 369
Referral to other specialists, 402
  clinical psychologists, 404
  genetic counselors, 404
  otolaryngologists, 403–404
  regular school classroom teachers, 405–406
  speech-language pathologists, 404–405
  teachers of children with hearing impairment, 405
Reflex-activating stimulus (RAS), 160
Rehabilitation
  audiological, 413
  aural, 5, 413
  vestibular, 429–430
Rehabilitative audiology, 11
Reissner's membrane, 278, 280
Reliability, 69
  of hearing screening measures, 208–211
  test-retest, 107, 115
Residual hearing, 414
Resistance, 53, 153
Resonance, 36, 53
Resonance theory of hearing, 282
Resonance-volley theory, 283
Resonant frequency, 36
Retarded growth and development, 226
RETFLs. *See* Reference Equivalent Threshold Force Levels
Retrocochlear, 283
RETSPLs. *See* Reference Equivalent Threshold Sound Pressure Levels
Reverberation, 52
RF. *See* Radio frequency
RGDT. *See* Random gap detection test
Rh factor (rhesus factor), 289
Rh incompatibility, 328
RIC. *See* Receiver in canal hearing aids
Rinne test, 22, 70
RITE. *See* Receiver-in-the-ear hearing aids
Rochester Method, 423
Rollover ratios, 333
Rotary chair testing, 275
Round window, 241
Rubella, 289–290
Rubeola, 291

Saccule, 274
SAT. *See* Speech-awareness threshold
Saturation sound-pressure level (SSPL), 368
Scala media, 278
Scala tympani, 278
Scala vestibuli, 278
SCAN. *See* Screening test for auditory processing disorders
SCDS. *See* Semicircular canal dehiscence syndrome
Schools
  hearing screening measures in, 208
  identifying hearing loss in, 207–211
  regular classroom teachers, 405–406
  reliability of screening measures in, 208–211
Schwabach test, 21, 70
Schwartze sign, 262
Science, audiology as, 8–9
Screening test for auditory processing disorders (SCAN), 337–338
SDS. *See* Speech-discrimination score
SDT. *See* Speech-detection threshold
SE. *See* Signed English
Sedatives, 305
SEE 1. *See* Signing Essential English
SEE 2. *See* Signing Exact English
Semantics of deafness, 421
Semicircular canal dehiscence syndrome (SCDS), 307–308
Semicircular canals, 274
Sensation level (SL), 48, 163
Sensitivity, 69
Sensitivity prediction from the acoustic reflex test (SPAR), 164, 350
Sensory/neural hearing loss, 19, 285
  amplification/sensory systems and, 394–395
  audiological treatment and, 434–435
  auditory nerve disorders and, 319, 340
  hearing tests and, 24–25, 26
  inner ear disorders and, 311
  masking and, 147
  pure-tone audiometry and, 88, 90, 94–95
  speech audiometry and, 119
  tobacco smoke and, 303
Sensory presbycusis, 310
Serous effusion, 261, 263
  of middle ear, 254–258
Sexton Conversation Tube, 365
Short increment sensitivity index (SISI), 181
Short isophonemic word lists, 110
Shotgun approach, 133
Shrapnell's membrane, 223

SI. *See* International System of Units
SIDS. *See* Sudden Infant Death Syndrome
Signaling units, 392
Signal-to-noise ratio (SNR), 111, 166, 391, 424
Signed English (SE), 423
Signing Essential English (SEE 1), 423
Signing Exact English (SEE 2), 423
Sine waves, 32–33
Single-day-fit hearing aids, 375–376
Sinusoidal waves, 33
SISI. *See* Short increment sensitivity index
SISNHL. *See* Sudden idiopathic sensory/neural hearing loss
Site of lesion, 182
Skull fractures, 269
SL. *See* Sensation level
Smoking, 247, 303
SNR. *See* Signal-to-noise ratio
SOAEs. *See* Spontaneous otoacoustic emissions
SOC. *See* Superior olivary complex
Somatosensory stimuli, 274
Sone, 51
Sound, 30
  aperiodic, 39
  complex sounds, 39–41
  decibel, 43, 44–48
  defined, 31
  environmental, 49, 50
  frequency, 35–36
  impedance, 53–54
  intensity, 41–43
  pathways of, 17–18
  periodic, 39
  phase, 38–39
  psychoacoustics, 49–52
  quality of, 31
  resonance, 36
  velocity, 36–37
  vibrations, 34–35
  wavelength, 37–38
  waves, 31–33
Sound-evoked muscle reflex, 277
Sound field, 58
  audiometry, 197–199
  test stimuli, 199
Sound-isolated chambers, 73–74
Sound-level meters, 47, 58, 297
Sound measurement
  acceptable noise levels, 58–59
  calibration of audiometers, 59–65
  pure-tone audiometer, 54–56
  sound-level meters, 58
  speech audiometer, 57–58
Sound-pressure level (SPL), 46–47
Sound velocity, 36–37
Sound waves
  cosine, 33
  longitudinal, 32
  sine, 32–33
  sinusoidal, 33
  transverse, 31–32
  traveling wave theory, 283

Spanish word-recognition tests, 99
SPAR. *See* Sensitivity prediction from the acoustic reflex test
Specialists
  animal audiology, 12–13
  dispensing audiology, 11
  educational audiology, 10
  industrial audiology, 11
  medical audiology, 9–10
  pediatric audiology, 11
  recreational audiology, 12–13
  referral to, 402–406
  rehabilitative audiology, 11
  tele-audiology, 11–12
Specialized goggles, 276
Specificity, 69
Spectrum
  auditory neuropathy spectrum disorder, 326–327
  of complex sound, 39, 40–41
  speech, 385
Speech
  central masking for, 144
  cued, 326, 423
  filtered tests, 334–335
  quick SIN test, 112
  time-compressed, 337
Speech audiometer
  air conduction, 57
  sound field, 58
Speech audiometry, 98–120
  band-pass binaural, 335
  behavioral testing and, 200–201
  bone-conduction SRT, 104–106
  clinician's role in, 100
  computerized, 118
  diagnostic audiometer, 99
  with immittance measures, 151
  most comfortable loudness level, 106
  patient's role in, 99–100
  range of comfortable loudness, 107
  speech-recognition testing, 107–118
  speech-threshold testing, 100–101
  test environment, 99
  uncomfortable loudness level, 106–107
  worksheet for, 105
Speech-awareness threshold (SAT), 101
Speech conservation, 420
Speech-detection threshold (SDT), 100, 104, 200
Speech-discrimination score (SDS), 107
Speech-language pathologists, 404–405
Speech-language pathology, 5, 9, 160, 371
Speech-masking noises, 143–144
Speech perception in noise test (SPIN), 112
Speechreading training
  with adults, 417–418
  with children, 419
Speech-reception threshold, 101
Speech-recognition score (SRS), 107

Speech-recognition testing, 107, 333
  administration of, 113
  audibility index and, 116–118
  bone-conduction, 116
  with competition, 111–113
  consonant-nucleus-consonant words, 109
  high-frequency emphasis lists, 109
  nonsense-syllable lists, 109–110
  performance-intensity functions in, 114–115
  phonetically balanced word lists, 108–109
  problems in, 115–116
  recording test results for, 113
  with sentences, 111
  short isophonemic word lists, 110
  stimuli, materials, and response method for, 114
  testing word recognition with half lists, 110
  test presentation level, 115
Speech-recognition threshold (SRT), 100–101, 200, 347–348
  bone-conduction, 104–106
  with cold running speech, 102
  cross hearing in, 142–143, 145–146
  masking for, 142–146
  recording results for, 104
  with spondaic words, 102–104
Speech spectrum, 385
Speech Stenger test, 352
Speech-threshold testing, 100–101
  recording SRT results, 104
  speech-detection threshold, 101
  speech-recognition threshold, 101–102
  SRT testing with cold running speech, 102
  SRT testing with spondaic words, 102–104
SPIN. *See* Speech perception in noise test
Spiral ligament, 278
SPL. *See* Sound-pressure level
Split audiograms, 129
Spondaic words (spondees), 101
  SRT testing with, 102–104
  SSW test, 337
Spontaneous otoacoustic emissions (SOAEs), 165, 284
Sports, 300
SRS. *See* Speech-recognition score
SRT. *See* Speech-recognition threshold
SSEP. *See* Steady-state evoked potential
SSI. *See* Synthetic sentence identification test
SSPL. *See* Saturation sound-pressure level
SSW. *See* Staggered spondaic word test
Stacked ABR, 172
Staggered spondaic word test (SSW), 337

Stapedectomy, 266, 303
Stapedius muscle, 159, 244
Stapedotomies, 267
Stapes, 241, 264–265
  mobilization of, 266
Staph infection, 246
Static acoustic compliance, 152
  measurements of, 155–156
  normal values for, 155–156
  recording and interpreting, 156
Steady-state evoked potential (SSEP), 174–176
Stenger principle, 23, 351
Stenger test, 351–352, 358
Stenosis, 226
Stenotic EACs, 226
Stereocilia, 279
Sternocleidomastoid muscles, 277
Stiffness, 153
  frequency and, 36
  reactance, 54
Strial presbycusis, 310
Stria vascularis, 278, 304
Strokes, 328
Subluxations, 260
Sudden idiopathic sensory/neural hearing loss (SISNHL), 304
Sudden Infant Death Syndrome (SIDS), 189
Superior olivary complex (SOC), 317
Superior temporal gyrus, 318
Support groups, 412–413
Suppurative otitis media, 246–254
  antibiotics for, 252–254
  audiometric findings in, 250–252
Supra-aural audiometric earphones, 55, 77
Surgical complications, cochlear hearing loss following, 303–304
Surgical treatments
  for fenestration, 266
  for Ménière's disease, 305–306
  for middle-ear fluid, 256
  neurosurgery, 321
Symbolic disorders, 205
Synapses, 281
Syndromes, 287. *See also specific syndromes*
Synthetic sentence identification test (SSI), 111, 335–336
Syphilis, 292–293, 328

Tactile response, 92
Tangible reinforcement operant conditioning audiometry (TROCA), 201
TC. *See* Total communication
TD. *See* Threshold of discomfort
TDDs. *See* Telecommunication devices for the deaf
Teachers
  of children with hearing impairment, 405
  regular classroom, 405–406
Tectorial membrane, 280
Teen support groups, 412
Tele-audiology, 11–12, 432
Telecoils, 367

Telecommunication devices for the deaf (TDDs), 392
Temporal lobes, 318
Temporary threshold shift (TTS), 295
Temporomandibular joint syndrome (TMJ), 220
Tensor tympani muscle, 159, 244
TEOAEs. *See* Transient-evoked otoacoustic emissions
Test environment, 99
  earphone attenuation devices for, 72
  insert earphones for, 72
  sound-isolated chambers for, 73–74
Testing. *See also* Behavioral testing; Hearing tests; Physiological tests; Speech-recognition testing; Speech-threshold testing
  acoustic reflex, 338, 350–351
  Apgar, 189
  Bing, 22–23, 139–140
  California consonant, 110
  caloric, 275
  competing sentence, 336
  connected speech, 112
  dichotic digits, 332
  Doerfler-Stewart, 352
  everyday sentence, 111
  filtered speech, 334–335
  gaps-in-noise, 332
  immittance, 258
  Ling Six, 200
  listening in spacialized noise, 334
  Lombard, 353
  modified rhyme, 110
  objective, 193–195, 350–355
  patients' position during, 76–77
  quick SIN, 112
  RASP, 336–337
  reference test gain, 369
  RGDT, 112
  Rinne, 22, 70
  rotary chair, 275
  SCAN, 337–338
  Schwabach, 21, 70
  sensitivity prediction from the acoustic reflex, 164, 350
  SSI, 111, 335–336
  SSW, 337
  Stenger, 351–352, 358
  tuning fork, 16, 20–23, 88, 139–140
  VIST, 354–355
  Weber, 23, 88
  WIPI, 111, 335
  word-recognition, 116
Test presentation level, 115
Test-retest reliability, 107, 115
Tetrachoric table, 209, 210
Text telephones (TTs), 392
Thalamus, 317
Thalidomide, 289
Theories of hearing
  place theory, 282–283
  resonance, 282
  resonance-volley, 283
  traveling wave theory, 283
  volley theory, 283

Therapy, hearing, 416
Thermal noise, 130
Threshold of discomfort (TD), 106–107
Thresholds, 48, 71, 83. *See also* Speech-recognition threshold; Speech-threshold testing
  acoustic reflex, 160, 164, 348
  aided goals, 385
  air-conduction, 90
  bone-conduction, 87, 90
  masked, 83
  permanent shift, 295
  RETFLs, 63
  RETSPLs, 62, 64
  speech-awareness, 101
  speech-detection, 100, 104, 200
  speech-reception, 101
  temporary shift, 295
  unmasked, 83
Thromboses, 328
Time-compressed speech, 337
Tinnitus, 262, 301, 356
  management of, 426–428
Tinnitus retraining therapy (TRT), 428
TMJ. *See* Temporomandibular joint syndrome
Tobacco smoke, 247, 303
Tolerance level, 106–107
Tone. *See also* Pure tone
  decay, 181
  difference, 39
  overtones, 39
  primary, 166
  warble, 79
Tonotopicity, 317
Total communication (TC), 423
Total impedance, 53
Toxic causes, of cochlear hearing loss, 293–294
Toynbee maneuver, 246
TPP. *See* Tympanometric peak pressure
Tragus, 219
Tranquilizers, 305
Transcranial routing of signal (TROS), 377
Transduce, 273
Transient-evoked otoacoustic emissions (TEOAEs), 166, 168, 284, 351
Transistor, 365
Transverse waves, 31–32
Trapezius muscles, 277
Trapezoid body, 317
Traveling wave theory, 283
Treacher Collins syndrome, 225

Treatment, 398–436. *See also* Surgical treatments
  adult hearing impairment management, 413–418
  APD management, 424–426
  audiological counseling, 406–413
  case studies on, 433–436
  childhood hearing impairment management, 418–423
  Deaf community, 423–424
  evidence-based practice, 432–433
  hyperacusis, 428–429
  multicultural considerations, 431–432
  outcome measures, 433
  patient histories, 399–402
  referral to other specialists, 402–406
  speechreading training with adults, 417–418
  tinnitus management, 426–428
  vestibular rehabilitation, 429–430
Trigeminal nerve, 244
Trisomy, 287
TROCA. *See* Tangible reinforcement operant conditioning audiometry
TROS. *See* Transcranial routing of signal
TRT. *See* Tinnitus retraining therapy
TTs. *See* Text telephones
TTS. *See* Temporary threshold shift
Tuberculosis, 293
Tumors, 269
  of auditory nerve, 320–324
Tuning-fork tests, 16, 20, 70
  Bing test, 22–23, 139–140
  Rinne test, 22
  Schwabach test, 21
  Weber test, 23, 88
TW. *See* Tympanometric width
21st Century Communications and Video Accessibility Act (2010), 413
Tympanic membrane, 220–223, 242
  paracentesis of, 257
  perforations of, 232–234
Tympanograms, 157–159, 265
Tympanometric peak pressure (TPP), 159
Tympanometric width (TW), 159
Tympanometry, 152, 156–159, 195
Tympanoplasty, 259–260
Tympanosclerosis, 233–234, 258
Tympanostomy, 257
Tympanotomy, 257
Type V pattern, 353

UCL. *See* Uncomfortable loudness
Umbo, 221
Uncomfortable loudness (UCL), 106–107
Undermasking, 135, 136
UNHS. *See* Universal newborn hearing screening
Unisensory approach, 422
Universal newborn hearing screening (UNHS), 190, 381
Unmasked thresholds, 83
Utricle, 274

VA. *See* Veterans Administration
Vacuum tube, 365
Validation
  of hearing aid performance for adults, 384–385
  of hearing aid performance for children, 386
Validity, 69
Valsalva, 246
Variable expressivity, 287
Variable pure-tone average (VPTA), 82, 414
Varying intensity story test (VIST), 354–355
Vascular accidents, 328
Vasospasm, 304
Velocity, 36–37
VEMP. *See* Vestibular-evoked myogenic potential
Ventral cochlear nucleus, 317
Verification
  of hearing aid performance for adults, 384–385
  of hearing aid performance for children, 386
Vertigo, 275, 305
Vestibular-evoked myogenic potential (VEMP), 277, 308
Vestibular rehabilitation, 429–430
Vestibular schwannoma, 320
Vestibular suppressants, 305
Vestibule, 274–277
Veterans, 297, 300–301
Veterans Administration (VA), 356
Vibrations, 31
  energy and, 34
  forced, 34–35
  free, 34–35
Vibrotactile aids, 379, 382
Video otoscope, 223
Viomycin, 293
Viral infections, 289
VIST. *See* Varying intensity story test

Visual reinforcement audiometry (VRA), 198
Vocalizations, 196–197
Volley theory of hearing, 283
Volume units (VU), 57, 99, 114
von Recklinghausen disease, 320
VPTA. *See* Variable pure-tone average
VRA. *See* Visual reinforcement audiometry
VU. *See* Volume units

Warble tones, 79
Watts, 44
Wavelength, 37–38
Waves
  cosine, 33
  longitudinal, 32
  sine, 32–33
  sinusoidal, 33
  transverse, 31–32
  traveling wave theory, 283
Weber test, 23
  audiometric, 88
Weighting networks, 58–59
Well-patient model, 406
White noise, 130
WHO. *See* World Health Organization
Windows, of middle ear, 241
Wind turbines, 302
Word intelligibility by picture identification test (WIPI), 111, 335
Word lists
  consonant-nucleus-consonant, 109, 335
  half, 110
  nonsense-syllable, 109–110
  phonetically balanced, 108–109, 115
  short isophonemic, 110
Word-recognition scores (WRS), 105, 107
Word-recognition tests, 116
Work, 43
World Health Organization (WHO), 432
World War II, 4, 5, 114, 254, 300
WRS. *See* Word-recognition scores

X-linked, 287

Yes-no method, 355

Zero hearing level, 48